Case Studies in Hematologic Malignancies

Case Studies in Hematologic Malignancies

Editor: Ronan Allen

AMERICAN
MEDICAL PUBLISHERS
www.americanmedicalpublishers.com

AMERICAN
MEDICAL PUBLISHERS
www.americanmedicalpublishers.com

Cataloging-in-Publication Data

Case studies in hematologic malignancies / edited by Ronan Allen.
p. cm.
Includes bibliographical references and index.
ISBN 979-8-88740-601-5
1. Lymphoproliferative disorders. 2. Lymphomas. 3. Lymphatics--Diseases.
4. Immunological deficiency syndromes. 5. Cell proliferaltion. 6. Blood--Diseases.
I. Allen, Ronan.
RC646.2 .N49 2023
61642--dc23

American Medical Publishers,
41 Flatbush Avenue,
1st Floor, New York,
NY 11217, USA

ISBN 979-8-88740-601-5 (Hardback)

Contents

Preface

The purpose of the book is to provide a glimpse into the dynamics and to present opinions and studies of some of the scientists engaged in the development of new ideas in the field from very different standpoints. This book will prove useful to students and researchers owing to its high content quality.

Hematologic malignancies, also known as blood cancers, refer to a wide range of cancers that originate in the bone marrow or the lymphatic system. These cancers can affect the production and function of blood cells, including white blood cells, red blood cells and platelets. Hematologic malignancies include leukemia, lymphoma, and multiple myeloma. The treatment of hematologic malignancies depends on the specific type and stage of the cancer, as well as individual patient factors. These malignancies can be treated through radiation therapy, chemotherapy, immunotherapy, targeted therapy and stem cell transplantation. Radiation therapy uses high-energy radiation to target and kill cancer cells. Chemotherapy makes use of powerful medications to destroy cancer cells or prevent their growth. This book brings forth some of the most innovative concepts and elucidates the unexplored aspects of hematological malignancies. It will serve as a valuable source of reference for graduate and postgraduate students.

At the end, I would like to appreciate all the efforts made by the authors in completing their chapters professionally. I express my deepest gratitude to all of them for contributing to this book by sharing their valuable works. A special thanks to my family and friends for their constant support in this journey.

Editor

1

Complete Response to R-EPOCH in Primary Cardiac Lymphoma

Kartik Anand[1], **Sai Ravi Pingali**[1], **Barry Trachtenberg**[2] and **Swaminathan Padmanabhan Iyer**[1,3]

[1]*Houston Methodist Cancer Center, Weill Cornell Medicine, Houston, TX, USA*
[2]*Division of Cardiology, DeBakey Heart & Vascular Institute, Houston Methodist Hospital, Houston, TX, USA*
[3]*Department of Lymphoma/Myeloma, UT MD Anderson Cancer Center, Houston, TX, USA*

Correspondence should be addressed to Kartik Anand; kartikanand88@gmail.com

Academic Editor: Sylvain Choquet

Primary cardiac lymphoma (PCL) is a rare extranodal lymphoma involving only the heart and/or the pericardium. Most common presenting signs and symptoms are nonspecific including dyspnea, pericardial effusion, and arrhythmia. Prognosis of PCL patients remain poor compared to non-cardiac lymphoma patients. Since most of the information about PCL comes from case reports or case series, there is no treatment consensus. Anthracycline containing chemotherapy remains main treatment modality which is potentially cardiotoxic. We present a case of PCL that achieved complete remission using R-EPOCH (rituximab, etoposide, prednisone, vincristine, cyclophosphamide, and doxorubicin). We also used dexrazoxane in an effort to reduce cardiotoxicity of chemotherapy.

1. Introduction

Primary cardiac lymphoma (PCL) is a rare malignancy, accounting only for 1.3% of cardiac tumors and 0.5% of extranodal lymphoma [1]. PCL was first described in a German publication in 1939 [2]. PCL is defined by the WHO as an extranodal lymphoma, involving only the heart and/or the pericardium [3]. Most common presenting signs and symptoms of PCL are dyspnea, arrhythmia, congestive heart failure, and pericardial effusion, as these signs and symptoms are nonspecific, making prompt diagnosis of PCL challenging. Before the advent of cardiac imaging (e.g. echocardiography), most cases were diagnosed at autopsy. Likely due to the increased frequency of cardiac imaging, more cases are being diagnosed each year [4]. The most common histologic subtype for PCL is diffuse large B-cell lymphoma [5]. Currently, there is no treatment consensus for PCL due to its rare presentation, and most of the literature comes from case reports. Anthracycline containing chemotherapy remains the most frequently used treatment modality [4]. SEER database analysis shows that median overall survival for cardiac lymphoma patients remains poor compared to non-cardiac lymphoma patients [5]. Herein, we report a case of PCL with treatment using dose adjusted R-EPOCH (rituximab, etoposide, prednisone, vincristine, cyclophosphamide, and doxorubicin) which leads to complete remission (CR). We also explore other interesting clinical considerations in this case, including the use of dexrazoxane in the treatment of PCL.

2. Case Presentation

A 69-year-old Caucasian male presented to the hospital with new onset dyspnea on exertion on walking 50 feet for past 3 weeks. Past medical history included hypertension, hyperlipidemia, atrial fibrillation of 2-month duration, and complete atrioventricular block status after permanent pacemaker placement a year preceding to current presentation. His home medications included lisinopril, metoprolol, apixiban, and atorvastatin. His laboratory workup on presentation was unremarkable except mild elevation of uric acid at 8.5 mg/dl. HIV status was checked and was negative. Transthoracic echocardiography revealed pericardial effusion with evidence of pericardial tamponade and right ventricular wall hypertrophy. Pericardial window was performed, and pericardial fluid cytology was negative for

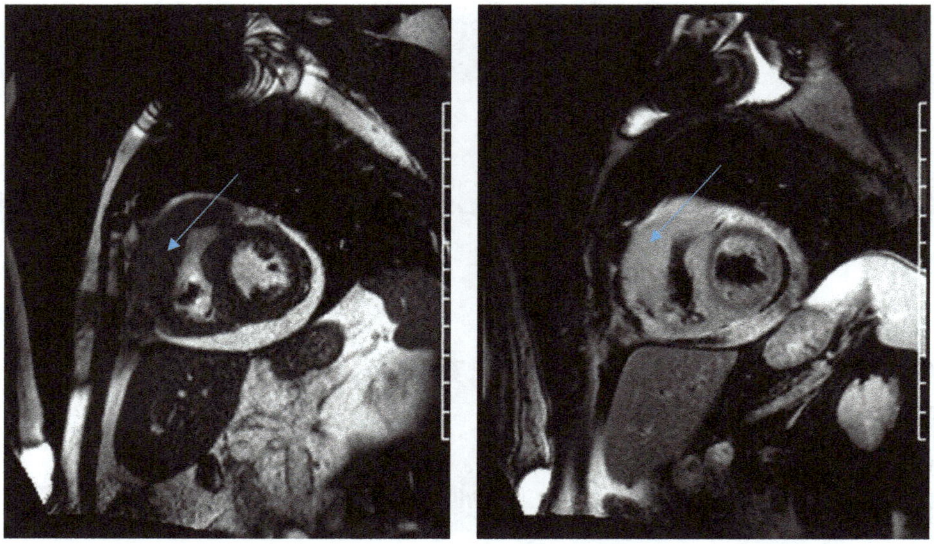

(a) (b)

Figure 1: Cardiac MRI showing mass in lateral wall of the left ventricle on T1 and T2 imaging.

any malignant cells. The patient was eventually discharged and referred to a heart failure specialist due to concerns for cardiac amyloidosis based on the right ventricular hypertrophy and conduction disease. A cardiac MRI was performed and showed a large mass, involving right ventricular (RV) lateral wall with a maximum thickness of 3 cm. Mass was hyperintense to myocardium on T2 and isointense on T1 (Figure 1). Left ventricular ejection fraction (EF) calculated using cardiac MRI was 41–43%. Cardiac biopsy of the RV mass was performed using an endovascular approach via the right internal jugular vein in the cardiac catheterization lab, assisted by intracardiac echocardiography. Additional work-up at that time included a coronary angiogram that showed absence of obstructive coronary disease. Immunohistochemistry (IHC) markers on the mass were positive for CD45, CD20, PAX-5, BCL2, BCL6, and MUM-1 and negative for CD5, CD10, and cyclin D1 (Figure 2). Ki-67 on the mass was 50–60%; EBER was negative along with FISH for MYC, BCL2, and BCL6. Findings from IHC were consistent with diffuse large B-cell lymphoma, nongerminal center subtype. Bone marrow biopsy performed as staging work-up was negative for any lymphoma involvement. The PET scan showed increased FDG (F-18 fluorodeoxyglucose) uptake in right atrium, right ventricle, and left ventricle with no abnormal uptake outside of the heart (Figure 3). The patient after getting a transthoracic echocardiography which confirmed EF at 45% was started on dose-adjusted R-EPOCH with 20% dose reduction in doxorubicin dose for the first cycle. In addition, he was noted to be chronically RV paced (99%) on pacemaker interrogation. It was decided that he may have had cardiomyopathy due to the RV pacing, and thus, he was upgraded to a biventricular pacemaker. After tolerating the first cycle, the patient was given full-dose doxorubicin starting the 2nd cycle. The interim PET scan after 2 cycles of R-EPOCH showed complete response (CR). The patient subsequently received 4 more cycles of R-EPOCH and continues to be in CR (confirmed by PET scan) 18 months after treatment. The patient also received dexrazoxane with 2nd, 3rd, and 4th cycles of chemotherapy to reduce cardiotoxicity of doxorubicin, given his existing cardiomyopathy. After chemotherapy, the patient's left ventricular EF is stable at 47% along with improvement in his atrial fibrillation. He remains on surveillance with 6 monthly echocardiography with a plan of getting cardiac MRI at 2 years after treatment completion.

3. Discussion

PCL is a rare disease and is less frequent than secondary cardiac involvement by lymphoma [6]. Most of the information comes from case reports and case series. Immune suppression by HIV is a major risk factor [7]. Petrich et al. [4] analyzed 197 cases of PCL described in the literature from 1949 to 2009. Immune status was only known for 64 cases, out of which 41% had HIV. The median age of PCL presentation is 63 years with male to female predominance by 2 : 1 [4]. Most common presenting signs/symptoms of PCL are nonspecific, including dyspnea, pericardial effusion, and arrhythmia [4, 8]. Echocardiography is important for diagnosis of PCL and has improved ability to detect cases antemortem, as before the first use of echocardiography in 1981 for PCL 64% of cases were at postmortem which has gone to 15% [4]. Cardiac MRI is an important diagnostic technique as it helps to differentiate PCL from other causes of primary cardiac masses such as sarcoma. Lymphoma appears hypo- or isointense on T1-weighted imaging or iso- or hyperintense on T2-weighted imaging [9]. PET scan is also important in diagnosis as well as following outcomes after treatment [10]. The right atrium is the most common site affected by PCL [4, 8]. The most common histological subtype for PCL is diffuse large-cell lymphoma, consisting of 72% of total PCL cases in SEER database analysis and 77% in analysis of 197 cases of PCL from 1949–2009 by Petrich et al. [4, 5]. Treatment mainly consists of anthracycline-based

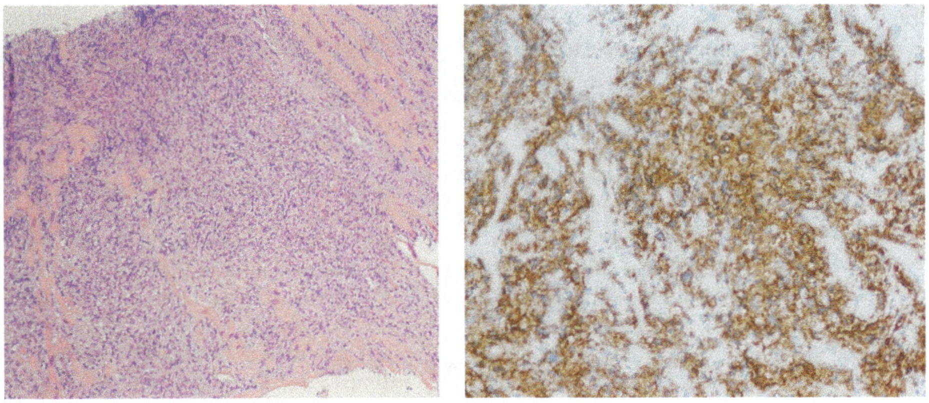

(a) (b)

Figure 2: (a) H&E section of cardiac biopsy showing diffuse infiltration of large cells. (b) Immunohistochemistry staining positive for CD20.

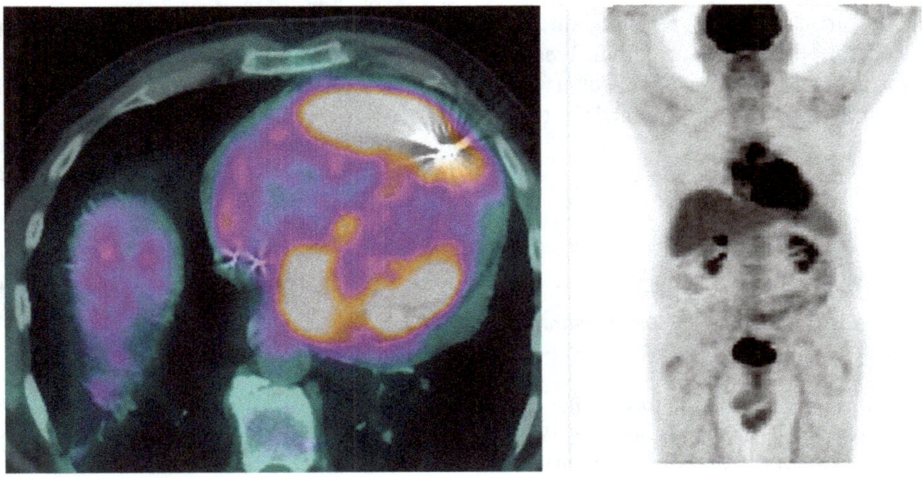

(a) (b)

Figure 3: PET scan showing (a) increased FDG uptake in the cardiac tissue and (b) no extra cardiac FDG uptake.

Table 1: Previous publications using R-EPOCH in PCL.

Publication	Patient age	Presenting signs/symptoms	Site of disease	Response to R-EPOCH	Follow-up
Rogers et al. [13]	72 years	Palpitations, dyspnea, dizziness	Right atrium, right ventricle	CR after 2 cycles	Chemotherapy discontinued after 3 cycles due to decline in performance status
Thiagraj et al. [14]	50 years	Abdominal pain, thromboembolism, pericardial tamponade	Left ventricle	CR after 2 cycles	Completed 6 cycles of chemotherapy, remains in CR at 1-year follow-up

chemotherapy CHOP (cyclophosphamide, doxorubicin, vincristine, and prednisone) plus rituximab (anti-CD20 monoclonal antibody) [4]. Overall response rate (ORR) to chemotherapy is high, in analysis by Petrich et al. ORR to chemotherapy was 79% with 59% achieving CR, and in a single-center retrospective study by Carras et al., the ORR to chemotherapy was 85% with 62% of the patients achieving CR. Heart failure and sepsis remain two major causes of mortality [4]. As there is a risk of cardiac wall rupture with chemotherapy [11], for our patient, we used dose-adjusted R-EPOCH with 20% dose reduction in the first cycle. In R-EPOCH, doxorubicin is given in as an infusion over 72 hours and is less cardiotoxic compared to bolus doxorubicin given in R-CHOP [12]. To our knowledge, there are only two other published cases of PCL treated using R-EPOCH; in both cases, patients were able to achieve CR after only 2 cycles of chemotherapy (Table 1) [13, 14]. Our patient also received IV dexrazoxane with 2nd, 3rd, and 4th cycle in an attempt to reduce cardiotoxicity. Dexrazoxane has been shown to be cardioprotective without compromising the efficacy of chemotherapy and increasing the rate of secondary malignancies [15, 16]. Till date, there has been no published report of dexrazoxane use in PCL. Although more studies are needed to quantify benefit of using

R-EPOCH plus dexrazoxane in PCL cases, these studies are difficult to complete due to low number of cases each year.

4. Conclusion

PCL is a rare malignancy with nonspecific presenting signs and symptoms. R-EPOCH should be used as front-line treatment for PCL due to less cardiotoxicity. Addition of dexrazoxane in the treatment strategy for PCL needs to be explored further.

Authors' Contributions

Kartik Anand was involved in conducting research, drafting the article, critical revision, and approval of the article to be published. Sai Ravi Pingali and Barry Trachtenberg were involved in drafting the article, critical revision, and approval of the article to be published. Swaminathan Iyer was involved in drafting the article, critical revision, supervision of research findings, and approval of the article to be published.

References

[1] J. Jeudy, J. Kirsch, F. Tavora et al., "From the radiologic pathology archives: cardiac lymphoma: radiologic-pathologic correlation," *Radiographics*, vol. 32, no. 5, pp. 1369–1380, 2012.

[2] C. M. Whorton, "Primary malignant tumors of the heart report of a case," *Cancer*, vol. 2, no. 2, pp. 245–260, 1949.

[3] J. J. Maleszweski and E. S. Jaffe, "Cardiac lymphomas," in *WHO Classification of Tumors of the Lung, Pleura, Thymus and Heart*, W. D. Travis, A. Marx, E. Barambilla, A. Nicholson, and A. Burke, Eds., pp. 340-341, IARC, Lyon, France, 2015.

[4] A. Petrich, S. I. Cho, and H. Billett, "Primary cardiac lymphoma," *Cancer*, vol. 117, no. 3, pp. 581–589, 2011.

[5] G. H. Oliveira, S. G. Al-Kindi, C. Hoimes, and S. J. Park, "Characteristics and survival of malignant cardiac tumors: a 40-year analysis of over 500 patients," *Circulation*, vol. 132, no. 25, pp. 2395–2402, 2015.

[6] M. L. Grebenc, M. L. Rosado de Christenson, A. P. Burke, C. E. Green, and J. R. Galvin, "Primary cardiac and pericardial neoplasms: radiologic-pathologic correlation," *Radiographics* vol. 20, no. 4, pp. 1073–1103, 2000.

[7] J. Guarner, R. K. Brynes, W. C. Chan, G. Birdsong, and G. Hertzler, "Primary non-Hodgkin's lymphoma of the heart in two patients with the acquired immunodeficiency syndrome," *Archives of Pathology & Laboratory Medicine* vol. 111, no. 3, pp. 254–256, 1987.

[8] S. Carras, F. Berger, L. Chalabreysse et al., "Primary cardiac lymphoma: diagnosis, treatment and outcome in a modern series," *Hematological Oncology*, vol. 35, no. 4, pp. 510–519, 2017.

[9] A. Luna, R. Ribes, P. Caro, J. Vida, and J. J. Erasmus, "Evaluation of cardiac tumors with magnetic resonance imaging," *European Radiology*, vol. 15, no. 7, pp. 1446–1455, 2005.

[10] J. B. Castelli, L. Alexandre, G. Futuro, M. Scanavacca, and J. Soares Júnior, "Primary cardiac lymphoma detected by 18F-FDG PET scan: a case report," *Journal of Nuclear Cardiology*, vol. 18, no. 5, pp. 974–977, 2011.

[11] D. O'mahony, R. L. Piekarz, W. P. Bandettini, A. E. Arai, W. H. Wilson, and S. E. Bates, "Cardiac involvement with lymphoma: a review of the literature," *Clinical Lymphoma and Myeloma*, vol. 8, no. 4, pp. 249–252, 2008.

[12] S. S. Legha, "Reduction of doxorubicin cardiotoxicity by prolonged continuous intravenous infusion," *Annals of Internal Medicine*, vol. 96, no. 2, pp. 133–139, 1982.

[13] S. C. Rogers, O. A. O'Connor, G. Granati, and K. Yaddanapudi, "The first case of primary cardiac lymphoma, diffuse large B-cell type, successfully treated with EPOCH-R," *Blood*, vol. 128, no. 22, p. 5418, 2016.

[14] A. Thiagaraj, P. Kalamkar, R. Rahman, V. Farah, and I. Poornima, "An unprecedented case report of primary cardiac lymphoma exclusive to left ventricle: a diagnostic and therapeutic challenge," *European Heart Journal-Case Reports*, vol. 2, no. 2, pp. 1–6, 2018.

[15] B. L. Asselin, M. Devidas, L. Chen et al., "Cardioprotection and safety of dexrazoxane in patients treated for newly diagnosed T-cell acute lymphoblastic leukemia or advanced-stage lymphoblastic non-hodgkin lymphoma: a report of the children's oncology group randomized trial pediatric oncology group 9404," *Journal of Clinical Oncology*, vol. 34, no. 8, pp. 854–862, 2016.

[16] S. M. Swain, F. S. Whaley, M. C. Gerber et al., "Cardioprotection with dexrazoxane for doxorubicin-containing therapy in advanced breast cancer," *Journal of Clinical Oncology*, vol. 15, no. 4, pp. 1318–1332, 1997.

2

Severe Aplastic Anemia Developed after Thymectomy: A Case Report and Literature Review

Bruna Cristine Duarte Rodrigues[1] **Pedro José Galvão Freire,**[1] **Beatriz Pinto e Siqueira Campos,**[1] **Juliana Oliveira Vieira,**[2] **and Pedro Alves da Cruz Gouveia**[1]

[1]*Internal Medicine Service, Federal University of Pernambuco, Recife, PE, Brazil*
[2]*Hematology Service, Federal University of Pernambuco, Recife, PE, Brazil*

Correspondence should be addressed to Bruna Cristine Duarte Rodrigues; brunacristinedr@hotmail.com

Academic Editor: Håkon Reikvam

Thymus neoplasms are frequently related to paraneoplastic autoimmune manifestations. Its most common associations are myasthenia gravis and pure red cell aplasia. Aplastic anemia has been increasingly documented as an initial presentation of thymoma. Nevertheless, its development after successful surgical resection of thymoma is a rare condition. We report a case of a 53-year-old man with severe aplastic anemia preceded by amegakaryocytic thrombocytopenia three years after thymectomy with no signs of disease recurrence. He underwent immunosuppressive therapy with cyclosporine 5 mg/kg/day and prednisone 2 mg/kg/day for six weeks. Considering the availability of a compatible donor, allogeneic stem cell transplantation was carried out. However, the patient died 11 days after transplant. A literature review was conducted, and another ten cases of aplastic anemia, diagnosed three months to four years after thymectomy, were identified. These cases suggest persistence of peripheral self-reactive T lymphocytes even years after tumor definitive treatment.

1. Introduction

Thymus neoplasms are known for their association with different paraneoplastic autoimmune manifestations. Its most common associations are myasthenia gravis and pure red cell aplasia [1, 2]. Other less frequently found hematologic complications are aplastic anemia, autoimmune hemolytic anemia, pernicious anemia, immune thrombocytopenic purpura, agranulocytosis, and hypogammaglobulinemia [3]. Although being an uncommon association, over the last years several case reports of aplastic anemia following thymecotymy have been published. However, development of such autoimmune manifestation after successful surgical resection of the tumor is rarely described in the literature [2–10]. We report a case of a 53-year-old man with severe aplastic anemia three years after thymectomy with no signs of disease recurrence.

2. Case Presentation

A 53-year-old man was admitted for investigation of dyspnea on moderate exertion, which started in the previous month. On admission, he presented with pancytopenia with a hemoglobin level of 3.4 g/dL, white blood count of 1960/mm^3 without dysplastic changes (1270 lymphocytes and 520 neutrophils), and platelet count of 3120/mm^3. Bone marrow biopsy showed 10% cellularity with hypoplasia of all hematopoietic series, predominantly myeloid series. There were no signs of anomalous cells, dysplastic changes, infiltration by malignant cells, or fibrosis. Histopathological findings were consistent with aplastic anemia (Figure 1).

The patient had previous history of asymptomatic mediastinal mass three years ago, diagnosed in preoperative exams for excision of gouty tophus on the elbow. The mediastinal tumor was resected, and pathological and

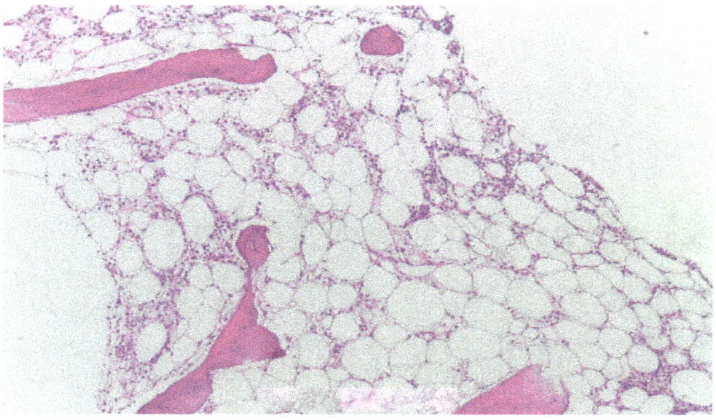

Figure 1: Fat-filled hypocellular bone marrow biopsy without fibrosis or anomalous cell infiltrate.

immunohistochemical studies were compatible with encapsulated type B1 thymoma with free surgical margins. In the same year, throughout postoperative follow-up, isolated thrombocytopenia was identified. Bone marrow showed hypocellular megakaryocytic clustering without dysplasia and other series without alterations. These findings were consistent with amegakaryocytic thrombocytopenia, which progressed about three years to current admission pancytopenia.

Search for secondary causes of aplastic anemia was performed, and there was no exposure to drugs, radiation, or chemicals. Normal levels of folic acid and vitamin B12 were found, besides negative serology for hepatitis B, C, human immunodeficiency virus (HIV), and Epstein-Barr virus (EBV). Flow cytometry did not identify paroxysmal nocturnal hemoglobinuria (PNH) clones. Serum protein electrophoresis showed no monoclonal protein or hypogammaglobulinemia. Abdominal ultrasound showed no signs of visceromegaly.

In order to investigate active thymoma, chest computed tomography (CT) was performed, but no alterations were found. To completely rule out recurrence of thymoma, an Fluorine(18)-fluorodeoxyglucose PET/CT scan was performed and showed a physiological distribution of the radiotracer. Thus, aplastic anemia therapy was initiated with cyclosporine 5 mg/kg/day and prednisone 2 mg/kg/day. Antithymocyte globulin was not available to complement the therapy. Treatment was maintained for six weeks, given the availability of a compatible HLA donor. The patient underwent allogeneic stem cell transplantation; however, on the 11th day after transplantation, he developed fusariosis and died of septic shock.

3. Discussion

Thymoma represents 20% of mediastinal neoplasms and highest prevalence in individuals between 40 and 60 years old, with similar incidence rates between both genders [11]. Its detection typically occurs when asymptomatic mediastinal masses, compressive symptoms, or paraneoplastic autoimmune manifestations are identified. In about 44% of cases, it is associated with myasthenia gravis, which leads to earlier diagnosis. On the other hand, when it presents with hematological paraneoplastic involvement, its identification tends to occur in later stages [12].

Pure red blood cell aplasia is the most common haematological abnormality, detected in about 15% of thymomas. Aplastic anemia is also an autoimmune disorder that is sometimes associated with thymoma [12]. In such cases, thymoma is usually diagnosed in etiological investigation of a previously diagnosed aplastic anemia [2, 13, 14]. However, the occurrence of this hematologic disease after thymectomy is uncommon as described in our case. Aplastic anemia may be preceded by isolated cytopenias such as amegakaryocytic thrombocytopenia reported here [1, 4, 6, 9].

A literature review was conducted in the PubMed database with English language case reports of patients who developed aplastic anemia after thymectomy. After reviewing publications from 1993 to 2018, we were able to identify a total of nine publications [2–10] with a total of ten cases that we summarize in Table 1. Six patients were male and four females. Pancytopenia was diagnosed between three months [5, 9] and four years [4] after thymectomy with an average of 19.6 months. In all cases, there were no signs of disease recurrence on CT scan; however, only the present case ruled out this possibility by also performing a PET/CT scan. Two patients were diagnosed with thymoma in the presence of signals and symptoms of myasthenia gravis [2, 6], while the other cases reported no systemic abnormalities other than hematologic ones. Regarding hematological progress, in one case aplastic anemia was preceded by immune thrombocytopenic purpura [4] and in three others by the association of pure red cell aplasia and amegakaryocytic thrombocytopenia [6, 9, 10]. The present case was only preceded by isolated amegakaryocytic thrombocytopenia. In all cases, except one whose treatment was not reported [6], the immunosuppressive regimen contained cyclosporin A and six demonstrated good response to immunosuppression [2–5, 7, 8]. Studies have demonstrated that increases in cell count may require different time intervals, besides exhibiting different follow-up times to evaluate disease recurrence. Most patients had an effective response to treatment; however, in two, the response was not described [6, 10]. In addition to our study, we were only able to identify one case where a patient underwent allogeneic stem cell transplantation and, in contrast to our case, long-term cure was documented [9].

Despite the association of thymoma with these autoimmune diseases, thymus resection may not completely reverse previously existing clinical manifestations. Specific treatment of these manifestations is often necessary even after thymectomy [7, 12]. This evolution corroborates the pathophysiology that was proposed by other studies suggesting the persistence of peripheral self-reactive T lymphocytes (originated from thymoma). These peripheral T lymphocytes could be responsible for promoting autoimmune phenomena, even at later times after curative thymectomy [2, 7, 8, 10]. We identified case reports of aplastic anemia developed three to 48 months after thymus resection [4, 5, 9].

Table 1: Review of published cases of aplastic anemia after thymectomy.

Authors	Ref.	Sex/ age	Treatment for thymoma	Interval between thymoma and AA	Progress of blood disorder	Associated diseases	Treatment for AA	Effect
Kobayashi et al.	[4]	F/63	TMT + RT	4 years	ITP ⟶ AA	ND	Splenectomy + CyA	E
Dinçol et al.	[5]	M/38	TMT	3 months	AA	ND	CyA + ATG + mPSL + G-CSF	E
Ritchie et al.	[2]	M/50	TMT + CT + RT	1 year	AA	Myasthenia gravis	mPSL + CyA + ATG	E
Park et al.	[3]	F/61	TMT	16 months	AA	ND	CyA	E
Maslovsky et al.	[6]	M/42	TMT + CT	12 months	PRCA + AT ⟶ AA	Myasthenia gravis	ND	ND
Bajel et al.	[7]	M/67	TMT	6 months	AA	ND	CyA + ATG	E
de Castro et al.	[8]	M/69	TMT	3 years	AA	ND	CyA	E
		F/59	TMT + RT	2 years	AA	ND	CyA + PDN	NE
Simkins et al.	[9]	F/61	CT + TMT	3 months	PRCA + AT ⟶ AA	ND	ATG + mPSL + CyA ⟶ SCT	NE/E
Dahal et al.	[10]	M/63	TMT + CT + RT	More than 3 years	PRCA + AT ⟶ AA	ND	CyA	ND
Present case	—	M/53	TMT	3 years	AT ⟶ AA	ND	CyA + PDN ⟶ SCT	NE

Ref.: reference; AA: aplastic anemia; age: age at diagnosis of AA; TMT: thymectomy; CT: chemotherapy; RT: radiotherapy; CyA: cyclosporin A; ITP: immune thrombocytopenia purpura; ATG: antithymocyte globulin; PDN: prednisone; mPSL: methylprednisolone; ND: not described; NE: not effective; E: effective; PRCA: pure red cell aplasia; AT: amegakaryocytic thrombocytopenia; AA: aplastic anemia; G-CSF: granulocyte-colony stimulating factor; SCT: stem cell transplantation.

Treatment of aplastic anemia after thymectomy usually requires prolonged immunosuppressive therapy and has a higher relapse rate after weaning off immunosuppressive therapy than other causes of aplastic anemia [2]. There are few reported cases of allogeneic stem cell transplantation in the treatment of autoimmune haematological diseases after thymectomy [9, 15]. This type of transplant should usually be the first line in the management of idiopathic aplastic anemia cases with good performance status and HLA-compatible donor, in patients aged under 50 years [16]. In the case reported here, antithymocyte globulin was not available and the patient had transplant conditions. However, the outcome was negative with the patient's death on the 11th postoperative day.

As for amegakaryocytic thrombocytopenia, management guidelines are even scarcer. Case reports suggest good response to immunosuppression also recommended for aplastic anemia treatment. This cytopenia may be, as observed in our case, an early presentation of aplastic anemia [6, 10].

Here we report a case of a late autoimmune manifestation suggesting persistence of peripheral self-reactive T lymphocytes even years after a curative thymectomy. This condition can lead to the development of hematological diseases such as severe aplastic anemia described here. We would emphasize that this hematological condition may be preceded by other blood abnormalities such as amegakaryocytic thrombocytopenia. This case suggests patients with thymoma should have periodic evaluations of their blood cell count, aiming at early identification of the most varied hematological alterations.

References

[1] A. Gaglia, A. Bobota, E. Pectasides, C. Kosmas, G. Papaxoinis, and D. Pectasides, "Successful treatment with cyclosporina of thymoma-related aplastic anemia," *Research Anticancer*, vol. 27, no. 4, pp. 3025–3028, 2007.

[2] D. S. Ritchie, C. Underhill, and A. P. Grigg, "Aplastic anemia as a late complication of thymoma in remission," *European Journal of Haematology*, vol. 68, no. 6, pp. 389–391, 2002.

[3] C. Y. Park, H. J. Kim, Y. J. Kim et al., "Very severe aplastic anemia appearing after thymectomy," *The Korean Journal of Internal Medicine*, vol. 18, no. 1, pp. 61–63, 2003.

[4] H. Kobayashi, K. Kitano, F. Ishida et al., "Aplastic anemia and idiopathic thrombocytopenic purpura with antibody to platelet glycoprotein llb/llla following resection of malignant thymoma," *Acta Haematologica*, vol. 90, no. 1, pp. 42–45, 1993.

[5] G. Dinçol, B. Saka, M. Aktan et al., "Very severe aplastic anemia following resection of lymphocytic thymoma: effectiveness of antilymphocyte globulin, cyclosporin A, and granulocyte-colony stimulating fator," *American Journal of Hematololy*, vol. 64, no. 1, pp. 78-79, 2000.

[6] I. Maslovsky, D. Gefel, L. Uriev, D. Ben Dor, and G. Lugassy, "Malignant thymoma complicated by amegakaryocytic thrombocytopenic purpura," *European Journal of Internal Medicine*, vol. 16, no. 7, pp. 523-524, 2005.

[7] A. Bajel, A. Ryan, S. Roy, and S. S. Opat, "Aplastic anemia: autoimmune sequel of thymoma," *British Journal of Haematology*, vol. 147, no. 5, p. 591, 2009.

[8] M. A. de Castro, M. A. de Castro, A. M. de Arantes, and M. R. Roberti, "Thymoma followed by aplastic anemia—two different responses to immunosuppressive therapy," *Revista Brasileira de Hematologia e Hemoterapia*, vol. 33, no. 6, pp. 476-477, 2011.

[9] A. Simkins, A. Maiti, N. J. Short et al., "Acquired amegakaryocytic thrombocytopenia and red cell aplasia in a patient with thymomaprogressing to aplastic anemia successfully

treated with allogenic stem cell transplantation," *Hematology Oncology Stem Cell Therapy*, vol. 12, no. 2, pp. 115–118, 2019.

[10] S. Dahal, E. Sharma, S. Dahal, B. Shrestha, and B. Bhattarai, "Acquired amegakaryocytic thrombocytopenia and pure red cell aplasia in thymoma," *Case Reports in Hematology*, vol. 2018, Article ID 5034741, 3 pages, 2018.

[11] N. Safieddine, G. Liu, K. Cuningham et al., "Prognostic factors for cure, recurrence and long-term survival after surgical resection of thymoma," *Journal of Thoracic Oncology*, vol. 9, no. 7, pp. 1018–1022, 2014.

[12] C. Bernard, H. Frih, F. Pasquet et al., "Thymoma associated with autoimmune diseases: 85 cases and literature review," *Autoimmunity Reviews*, vol. 15, no. 1, pp. 82–92, 2016.

[13] L. D. Grbelja, R. Vrhovac, and M. Ulamec, "Myasthenia gravis associated with thymoma and aplastic anemia: case report," *Acta Clinica Croatica*, vol. 56, no. 4, pp. 817–820, 2017.

[14] C. B. Falkson, A. Bezjak, G. Darling et al., "The management of thymoma: a systematic review and practice guideline," *Journal of Thoracic Oncology*, vol. 4, no. 7, pp. 911–919, 2009.

[15] V. Trisal, A. Nademanee, S. K. Lau, and F. W. Grannis Jr., "Thymoma-associated severe aplastic anemia treated with surgical resection followed by allogeneic stem-cell transplantation," *Journal of Clinical Oncology*, vol. 25, no. 22, pp. 3374-3375, 2007.

[16] J. C. W. Marsh, S. E. Ball, J. Cavenagh et al., "Guidelines for the diagnosis and management of aplastic anaemia," *British Journal of Haematology*, vol. 147, no. 1, pp. 43–70, 2009.

3

A Case of Histiocytic Sarcoma Arising from Mycosis Fungoides

Ethan A. Burns,[1] Cesar Gentille,[2] Saro Kasparian,[1] and Sai Ravi Pingali[2]

[1]Houston Methodist Hospital, Department of Medicine, 6550 Fannin St, Ste 1101, Houston, TX 77030, USA
[2]Houston Methodist Cancer Center, 6445 Main St Floor 24, Houston, TX 77030, USA

Correspondence should be addressed to Ethan A. Burns; eaburns312@gmail.com

Academic Editor: Masayuki Nagasawa

Histiocytic sarcoma (HS) is an uncommon malignant neoplasm arising from mature histiocytes and most commonly characterized by the immunophenotypic expression of CD68, CD163, or lysozyme. Although rare, HS arising as a second primary malignancy following hematolymphoid neoplasms has been reported. To our knowledge, this is the first reported case of HS occurring as a second primary malignancy in a patient with mycosis fungoides (MF), with the retained immunophenotype markers CD30 and CD4.

1. Introduction

The hematopoietic system is comprised of distinct cellular lineages uniquely delineated by morphologic, immunophenotypic, and functional characteristics [1, 2]. These cells are considered lineage committed once they are fully differentiated [2], which is defined by the expression of specific genes and phenotypic markers. However, under certain circumstances, fully differentiated cells may inherit mutations making it possible to undergo a transformation into a distinctly new cell line [2]. A rare, but well-documented example is HS arising as a secondary or concurrent malignancy in association with hematologic malignancies. This is the first known report of HS arising in a patient with previously diagnosed MF.

2. Case

The patient is a 61-year-old African American female with a long history of MF stage IB that first presented with symptoms of pruritic cutaneous lesions on her extremities at the age of 10 years, though the diagnosis of MF was not confirmed via skin biopsy until the age of 36 years. She had a long treatment course, but her disease was refractory to multiple modalities including psoralens and long-wave ultraviolet radiation, interferon, isotretinoin, nitrogen mustard, total body skin beam radiation, bexarotene, and acitretin. Two years prior to her admission, she developed a rapidly enlarging left hip tumor. Biopsies confirmed MF without large-cell transformation that was positive for CD4 and CD30. She received localized external beam radiation for 5 treatments (2,000 cGY). Following radiation therapy, she developed an ulcer in the tumor bed. A punch biopsy indicated chronic inflammation and scar but no evidence of tumor recurrence.

Several months after the biopsy, the patient developed weakness, fatigue, fever, and increasing serosanguinous discharge from her left hip wound and was admitted to the hospital for sepsis. Computed tomography (CT) scans were significant for diffuse diaphragmatic, abdominal, pelvic, and inguinal lymphadenopathy concerning for lymphoma, suspected to be metastatic visceral spread from her underlying MF. She had an excisional left inguinal lymph node biopsy which revealed an enlarged lymph node with effaced architecture due to diffuse proliferation of neoplastic spindle cells (Figures 1–6). Positive tumor markers included CD4, CD30, CD45, CD43, CD68, and CD163, with a 37% MIB-1 proliferative index, consistent with HS (Figures 1–6). Positron emission tomography (PET) imaging indicated widely metastatic disease, with increased uptake in numerous lymph nodes, pulmonary nodules, and the liver (Figure 7). She had a bone marrow biopsy without a clonal B-cell population, aberrant T-cell markers, or immunophenotypic myeloblasts. She was started on cyclophosphamide,

FIGURE 1: Low-power view of the left inguinal lymph node biopsy demonstrating complete effacement of normal lymph node architecture.

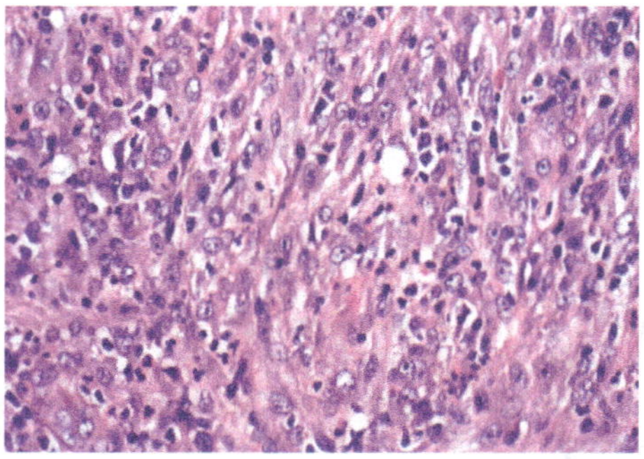

FIGURE 2: Effaced inguinal lymph node with spindled and epithelioid cells with eosinophilic cytoplasm. Large pleomorphic nuclei with abundant nucleoli.

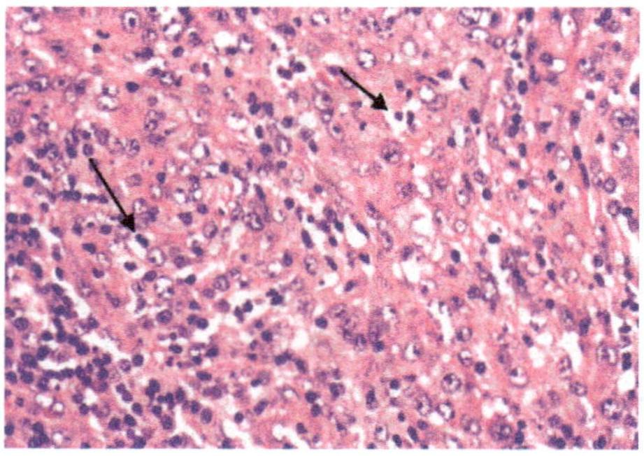

FIGURE 3: Effaced inguinal lymph node with frequent mitoses and apoptosis.

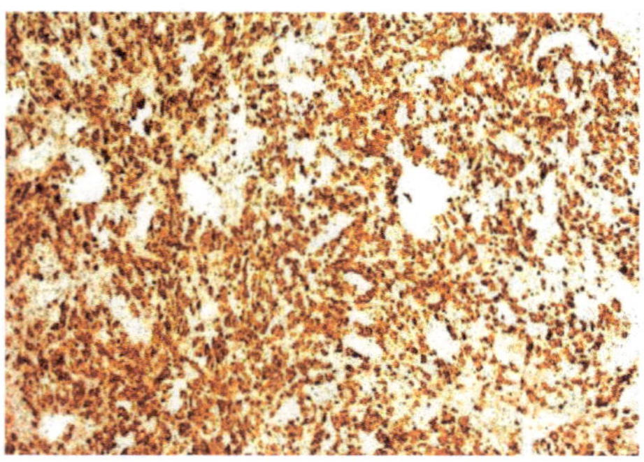

FIGURE 4: Inguinal lymph node CD30+ stain.

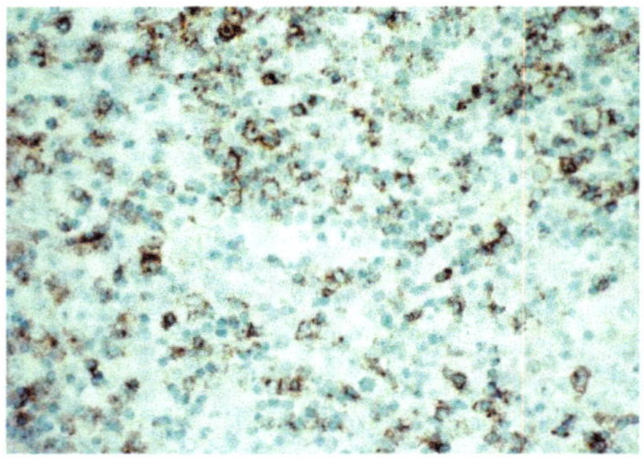

FIGURE 5: Inguinal lymph node CD4+ stain.

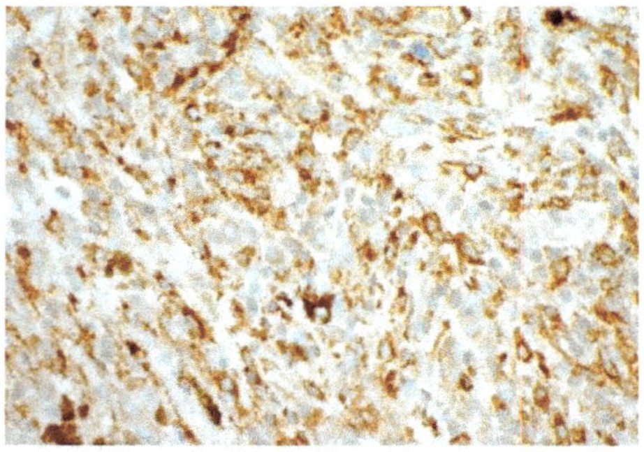

FIGURE 6: Inguinal lymph node CD163+ stain.

adriamycin, vincristine, prednisone, and etoposide (CHOEP) and was discharged with follow-up.

The patient had a repeat PET scan after completion of her third cycle of CHOEP that demonstrated a new lesion in the first lumbar vertebrae and increased uptake in her liver concerning for disease progression (Figure 8). She had a biopsy of the liver mass lesion which was identical to the HS noted on the previous excisional lymph node biopsy (Figures 2–9). Prior to resuming her chemotherapy, the patient developed nausea, vomiting, and abdominal pain and was admitted again. She had elevated alkaline phosphatase, bilirubin, and right upper quadrant pain concerning for acute cholangitis. Imaging revealed a large intrahepatic mass and extensive intra-abdominal and mediastinal lymphadenopathy. Due to her treatment-resistant disease, she was started on cladribine and cytarabine. Her hospital course was complicated by acute hypoxemic respiratory failure and ascending cholangitis requiring a delay in chemotherapy. She further progressed to multiorgan failure, so her family decided to proceed with comfort care measures.

3. Discussion

HS is an uncommon malignancy that arises from mature macrophages and diagnosed by the molecular expression of CD68, CD163, or lysozyme (Table 1) [3]. Clinically, it is associated with the typical "B" symptoms seen in non-Hodgkin lymphoma, including fevers, night sweats, and weight loss, and may also present with cytopenias, lymphadenopathy, or hepatosplenomegaly. The incidence is 0.17 per

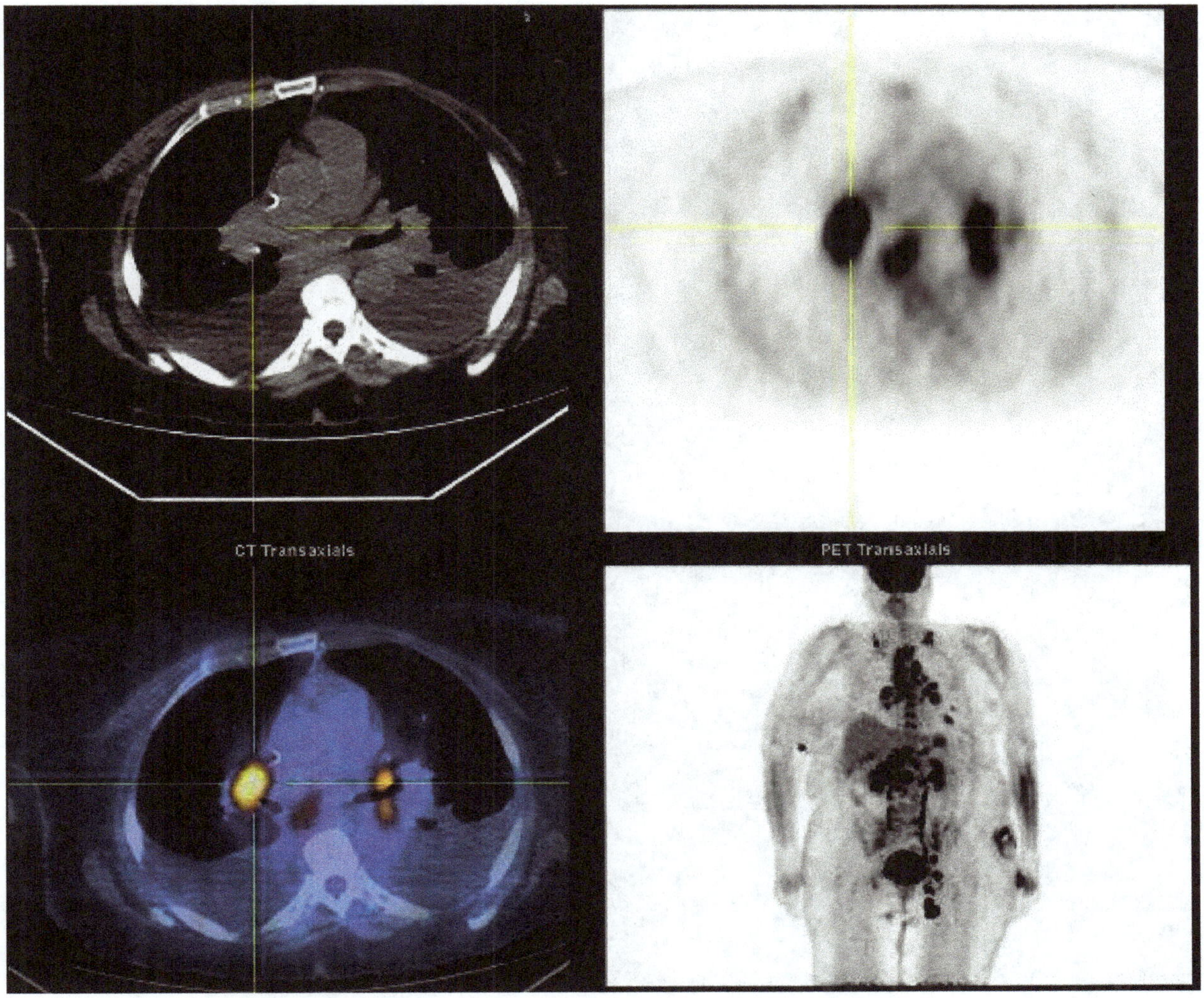

Figure 7: Positron emission tomography (PET) scan assessment of tumor burden before CHOEP chemotherapy initiation. Increased uptake in the bilateral supraclavicular (SUV 10.9), paratracheal (SUV 12.1), hilar (SUV 12.9), periportal (SUV 10.3), left inguinal (SUV 16.9) lymph nodes, pulmonary nodule (SUV 6.1), and right hepatic lobe (SUV 4.7). CHOEP: cyclophosphamide, Adriamycin, vincristine, etoposide, and prednisone.

1,000,000 individuals, occurs more frequently in Caucasian males, and has a median age of 63 years at diagnosis [4]. The most common initial sites of involvement include the skin and connective tissues (35.8%), lymph nodes (17%), respiratory tract (8.2%), and central nervous system (7.5%) [4]. Staging workup, including imaging studies such as CT or PET/CT, is helpful in determining the extent of disease spread, but excisional biopsy with tissue confirmation is necessary to confirm the diagnosis [5]. There is no standardized treatment algorithm for this aggressive malignancy. The overall median survival is 6 months, which appears to be independent of the primary site or ethnicity [4].

There is a clear, albeit rare association between HS and hematolymphoid malignancies via retained genetic and molecular abnormalities [5]. HS arising as a secondary malignancy occurs in approximately 21% of HS cases and is most often reported following hematologic malignancies arising from B-cell origin [4, 5]. The 2008 World Health Organization revised the diagnostic criteria for HS to include immunoglobulin heavy chain and T-cell receptor rearrangements that were classified as transdifferentiated forms of various other hematolymphoid malignancies [6].

The mechanism of HS transformation from hematolymphoid malignancies remains poorly understood and controversial. Transformation is believed to occur via three mechanisms. Transdifferentiation is a well-studied and reported process in malignancies arising from B cells, occurring when lineage-committed B cells convert into phenotypically distinct cells with similar genetic makeup [5]. The second theorized mechanism is a two-step process via dedifferentiation to a common precursor cell followed by transdifferentiation to a different cell line. Finally, transdetermination involves differentiation of a lineage committed but not fully differentiated cell into another [5, 7]. The latter has been reported in T-cell lymphoma but occurred concomitantly with two other malignancies [7]. This is the first reported case of HS arising in a patient with MF, interestingly, with retention of immunophenotypic markers of the initial malignancy. In this case, genetic tests were not conducted on the skin biopsies diagnostic of

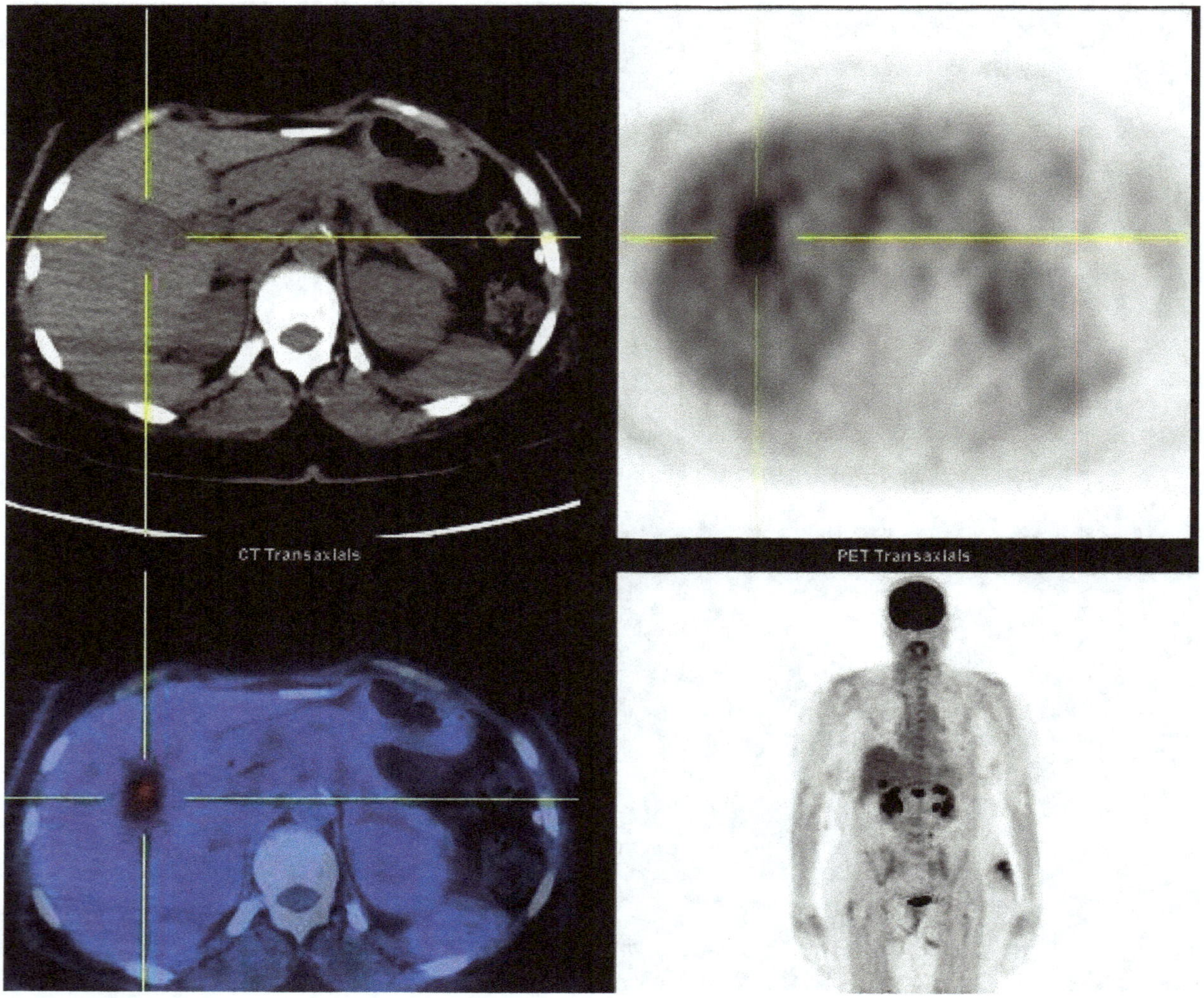

FIGURE 8: Follow-up PET after the 3rd cycle of CHOEP. Interval resolution of supraclavicular, hilar, and axillary uptake. Increased uptake in the right hepatic lobe (SUV 5.8). New uptake in L1 (SUV 8.8). PET: positron emission tomography; CHOEP: cyclophosphamide, Adriamycin, vincristine, etoposide, and prednisone.

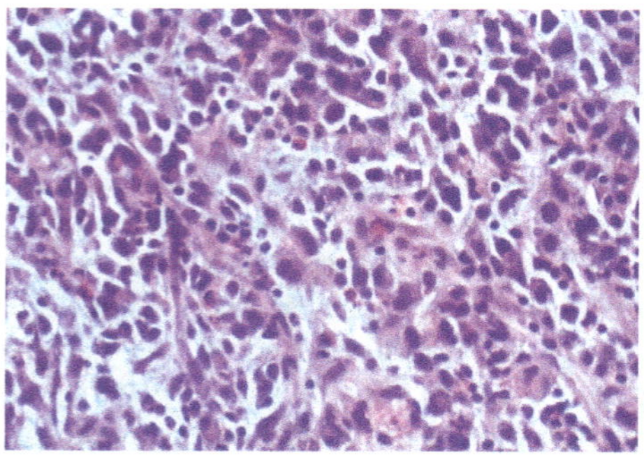

FIGURE 9: Liver parenchyma infiltrated with large spindle cells with abundant foamy clear to eosinophilic cytoplasm and large pleomorphic nuclei with abundant nucleoli. Mixed inflammatory infiltrates, consisting of neutrophils, eosinophils, lymphocytes, and plasma cells.

MF or on the lymph node biopsy diagnostic of HS, so a common genetic mutation definitively linking the two malignancies and thus transformation could not be established. Typically, when HS arises from a lymphoid neoplasm it has a distinctly unique immunophenotype with retained genetic mutations. However, in this case, there was evidence of retained immunophenotype markers CD30 and CD4, unique findings that introduces the possibility of a malignant transformation between the two malignancies. The mechanism by which the secondary HS arose following decades of treatment-resistant MF is not defined, but is likely to have occurred via a myriad of factors, including a combination of transcription factors and epigenetic modifications, a dynamic microenvironment resulting in severe immunosuppression [8], alteration in cytokine receptor signaling, and selection pressure (Figure 10).

In MF, disease pathogenesis is believed to stem from apoptotic resistance by the malignant monoclonal T-cell infiltrate, which has been linked to aberrant overexpression of the BCL11B transcription factor [9, 10]. Further augmenting this mechanism, cutaneous T-cell lymphoma (CTCL) cells have demonstrated resistance to FAS-mediated apoptosis and growth suppression by TGF-β [11]. With advancing tumor and disease stage in CTCL, BCL11B activity appears to increase, indicating a potential

Table 1: A comparison of the immunophenotypic, cytomorphologic, and clinical findings of HS and MF.

Malignancy	Histiocytic sarcoma	Mycosis fungoides
Immunophenotype	CD68 CD163 Lysozyme May be variable	CD4 CD8 CD56 CD4/8-CD30[¥]
Cytomorphology	Large and round oval nuclei with spindling; large, atypical pleomorphic lymphocytes with eosinophilic cytoplasm May be variable	T cells in epidermis and dermis with ceribriform nuclei; Pautrier micro abscesses in epidermis
Clinical findings	Unifocal to metastatic disease with systemic symptoms; preferentially involves skin, soft tissue, or the gastrointestinal tract	Cutaneous patches/plaques or tumors that may be localized or diffuse

[¥]CD30 (Ki-1) positivity may be seen in primary cutaneous anaplastic large-cell lymphoma, lymphomatoid papulosis, pagetoid reticulosis, and transformed MF.

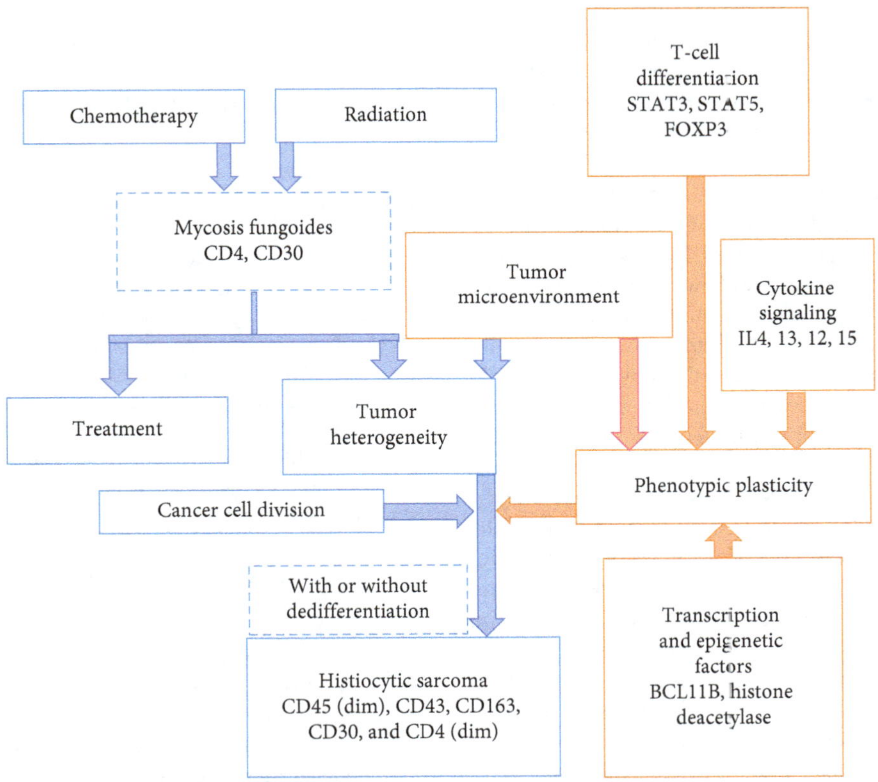

Figure 10: Theoretical malignant evolution and factors contributing to second primary HS in a patient with a protracted history of mycosis fungoides.

role in disease progression [9]. Moreover, BCL11B interacts with histone deacetylases, which are functional classes of epigenetic protein complexes involved in various arrays of cellular functions including regulation of gene expression and tumorigenesis [10, 12]. As MF advances, clonal dominance of the TH2 cytokines IL4 and IL13 predominate allowing for clonal proliferation [13], immune dysregulation, and subsequent disease progression [11, 14]. It is possible that over decades, alteration in this patient's aberrant transcription factors and epigenetic regulator modifications allowed for mutations that permitted cellular transformation.

T-cell lymphomas are a heterogenous group of lymphoproliferative malignancies, and the subgroup that comprises CTCL has a dynamic and alternating microenvironment with a high phenotypic plasticity. In general, phenotypic plasticity is due to a host of factors that work to evade antitumor immunity and ultimately results in severe immunosuppression [8]. In addition to genetic and epigenetic modifications, the tumor microenvironment plays a pivotal role in malignant heterogeneity [8]. STAT3 and STAT5 are important mediators of plasticity and important determinants of T-cell differentiation in CTCL. These serve to weaken antitumor immunity by promoting the differentiation to TH17 and Treg cells [15]. The cytokines IL-2 and IL-15 play a role in the stimulation of malignant T-cell phenotype through JAK3/JAK3 kinase phosphorylation cascades as well as IL-10 and FOXP3 expression [8]. Overtime, these factors culminate in severe immunosuppression, which appears to be due to disruption of the T-cell repertoire [16]. It is possible that hyperactivity of these factors impacting tumor heterogeneity and plasticity, coupled with tumor treatment resistance and selection pressure created an ideal environment that allowed for class switching to HS (Figure 10).

Cases of HS arising as a secondary malignancy directly attributed to selection pressure are lacking, so it is not known if this plays a direct or contributory role in malignant transformation. However, hematolymphoid malignancies and specifically CTCL are known to have tumor heterogeneity, so it is possible they are predisposed to treatment-driven selection pressure. Genetic heterogeneity may lead to subpopulations of treatment-sensitive and treatment-resistant clones, a phenomenon seen in various malignancies. Upon treatment initiation, the elimination of treatment-sensitive clones allows for "competitive release," or the minimalization of competitive forces of the treatment-sensitive dominant clone on the treatment-resistant subclone [17]. This allows for treatment-resistant subclones to repopulate and drive the tumor, which may be genetically distinct and carry more genetic abnormalities than the initial treatment-sensitive clone [18, 19]. For example, Tang et al. suggested that treatment with imatinib in chronic myeloid leukemia (CML) diminished CML clones with the most aggressive malignant potential [20]. However, CML clones have dichotomous kinetics that may allow more slowly dividing leukemic cell lines to relapse after discontinuation of imatinib [20]. In addition to "competitive release," chemotherapy-induced mutagenesis can further drive malignant evolution [17].

The carcinogenic potential of radiation therapy is well known and attributed to approximately 5% of second primary malignancies [21]. Ionizing radiation can precipitate breaks in double-stranded DNA and alteration in DNA repair, which may lead to malignant transformation of the irradiated cell and increase the risk of secondary malignancies [21, 22]. Radiation-induced sarcomas are the second most common malignancy that can arise following radiation therapy, and typically arise 10–12 years following radiation therapy, with an arbitrary cutoff period of 3–4 years to delineate sporadic sarcomas [23, 24]. There is an isolated case report of a central nervous system HS arising following radiation therapy (CD163, CD68, and CD4 positive) [25], and it is known that radiation therapy in patients with non-Hodgkin's lymphoma are at increased risk for second malignancies including sarcomas [26], so it is possible that radiation played a role in the formation of this second primary malignancy. The patient in this case had treatment-resistant and recurrent MF for five decades. Prior to radiation therapy, biopsy of her right hip tumor was positive for CD4 and CD30 without large-cell transformation. While selection pressure alone cannot be implicated as the primary cause of malignant transformation, it may have been one of a complex array of pathogenic mechanisms leading to this malignant transformation.

4. Conclusion

This is the first presentation of HS arising as a secondary malignancy from a patient with MF, supported by the retention of CD4 and CD30 immunophenotype from the primary cancer. Although uncommon, hematolymphoid malignancies of T-cell origin, including cutaneous T-cell lymphomas, may precipitate a secondary HS. This concerning and often fatal second malignancy should be considered in patients with ongoing or previous management of a hematolymphoid malignancy presenting with new or rapid disease progression.

Abbreviations

HS: Histiocytic sarcoma
MF: Mycosis fungoides
CT: Computed tomography
PET: Positron emission tomography
CHOEP: Cyclophosphamide, adriamycin, vincristine, etoposide, and prednisone
CTCL: Cutaneous T-cell lymphoma
CML: Chronic myeloid leukemia.

References

[1] K. Akashi, D. Traver, T. Miyamoto, and I. L. Weissman, "A clonogenic common myeloid progenitor that gives rise to all myeloid lineages," *Nature*, vol. 404, no. 6774, pp. 193–197, 2000.

[2] A. L. Feldman, D. A. Arber, S. Pittaluga et al., "Clonally related follicular lymphomas and histiocytic/dendritic cell sarcomas: evidence for transdifferentiation of the follicular lymphoma clone," *Blood*, vol. 111, no. 12, pp. 5433–5439, 2008.

[3] C. Yoshida and M. Takeuchi, "Histiocytic sarcoma: identification of its histiocytic origin using immunohistochemistry," *Internal Medicine*, vol. 47, no. 3, pp. 165–169, 2008.

[4] A. Kommalapati, S. H. Tella, M. Durkin, R. S. Go, and G. Goyal, "Histiocytic sarcoma: a population-based analysis of incidence, demographic disparities, and long-term outcomes," *Blood*, vol. 131, no. 2, pp. 265–268, 2017.

[5] J. Ansari, A. R. Naqash, R. Munker et al., "Histiocytic sarcoma as a secondary malignancy: pathobiology, diagnosis, and treatment," *European Journal of Haematology*, vol. 97, no. 1, pp. 9–16, 2016.

[6] E. Takahashi and S. Nakamura, "Histiocytic sarcoma: an updated literature review based on the 2008 WHO classification," *Journal of Clinical and Experimental Hematopathology*, vol. 53, no. 1, pp. 1–8, 2013.

[7] E. Waanders, K. M. Hebeda, E. J. Kamping et al., "Independent development of lymphoid and histiocytic malignancies from a shared early precursor," *Leukemia*, vol. 30, no. 4, pp. 955–958, 2015.

[8] R. M. Abraham, Q. Zhang, N. Odum, and M. A. Wasik, "The role of cytokine signaling in the pathogenesis of cutaneous T-cell lymphoma," *Cancer Biology & Therapy*, vol. 12, no. 12, pp. 1019–1022, 2011.

[9] X. Gu, Y. Wang, G. Zhang, W. Li, and P. Tu, "Aberrant expression of BCL11B in mycosis fungoides and its potential role in interferon-induced apoptosis," *The Journal of Dermatology*, vol. 40, no. 8, pp. 596–605, 2013.

[10] W. Fu, S. Yi, L. Qiu, J. Sun, P. Tu, and Y. Wang, "BCL11B-Mediated epigenetic repression is a crucial target for histone deacetylase inhibitors in cutaneous T-cell lymphoma," *Journal of Investigative Dermatology*, vol. 137, no. 7, pp. 1523–1532, 2017.

[11] E. J. Kim, S. Hess, S. K. Richardson et al., "Immunopathogenesis and therapy of cutaneous T cell lymphoma," *Journal of Clinical Investigation*, vol. 115, no. 4, pp. 798–812, 2005.
[12] E. Ceccacci and S. Minucci, "Inhibition of histone deacetylases in cancer therapy: lessons from leukaemia," *British Journal of Cancer*, vol. 114, no. 6, pp. 605–611, 2016.
[13] L. J. Geskin, S. Viragova, D. B. Stolz, and P. Fuschiotti, "Interleukin-13 is overexpressed in cutaneous T-cell lymphoma cells and regulates their proliferation," *Blood*, vol. 125, no. 18, pp. 2798–2805, 2015.
[14] E. Guenova, R. Watanabe, J. E. Teague et al., "TH2 cytokines from malignant cells suppress TH1 responses and enforce a global TH2 bias in leukemic cutaneous T-cell lymphoma," *Clinical Cancer Research*, vol. 19, no. 14, pp. 3755–3763, 2013.
[15] X. P. Yang, K. Ghoreschi, S. M. Steward-Tharp et al., "Opposing regulation of the locus encoding IL-17 through direct, reciprocal actions of STAT3 and STAT52011," *Nature Immunology*, vol. 12, no. 3, pp. 247–254, 2011.
[16] N. Yawalkar, K. Ferenczi, D. A. Jones et al., "Profound loss of T-cell receptor repertoire complexity in cutaneous T-cell lymphoma," *Blood*, vol. 102, no. 12, pp. 4059–4066, 2003.
[17] S. Venkatesan, C. Swanton, B. S. Taylor, and J. F. Costello, "Treatment-induced mutagenesis and selective pressure sculpt cancer evolution," *Cold Spring Harbor Perspectives in Medicine*, vol. 7, no. 8, article 026617, 2017.
[18] P. M. Enriquez-Navas, Y. Kam, T. Das et al., "Exploiting evolutionary principles to prolong tumor control in preclinical models of breast cancer," *Science Translational Medicine*, vol. 8, no. 327, article 327ra24, 2016.
[19] D. A. Landau, S. L. Carter, P. Stojanov et al., "Evolution and impact of subclonal mutations in chronic lymphocytic leukemia," *Cell*, vol. 152, no. 4, pp. 714–726, 2013.
[20] M. Tang, J. Foo, M. Gonen, J. Guilhot, F.-X. Mahon, and F. Michor, "Selection pressure exerted by imatinib therapy leads to disparate outcomes of imatinib discontinuation trials," *Haematologica*, vol. 97, no. 10, pp. 1553–1561, 2012.
[21] C. B. Dracham, A. Shankar, and R. Madan, "Radiation induced secondary malignancies: a review article," *Radiation Oncology Journal*, vol. 36, no. 2, pp. 85–94, 2018.
[22] L. Mullenders, M. Atkinson, H. Paretzke, L. Sabatier, and S. Bouffler, "Assessing cancer risks of low-dose radiation," *Nature Reviews Cancer*, vol. 9, no. 8, pp. 596–604, 2009.
[23] L. Giannini, F. Incandela, M. Fiore et al., "Radiation-induced sarcoma of the head and neck: a review of the literature," *Frontiers in Oncology*, vol. 8, p. 449, 2018.
[24] S. G. Patel, A. C. H. See, P. A. Williamson, D. J. Archer, and P. H. Rhys Evans, "Radiation induced sarcoma of the head and neck," *Head & Neck*, vol. 21, no. 4, pp. 346–354, 1999.
[25] W. Wu, A. Tanrivermis Sayit, H. V. Vinters, W. Pope, L. Mirsadraei, and J. Said, "Primary central nervous system histiocytic sarcoma presenting as a postradiation sarcoma: case report and literature review," *Human Pathology*, vol. 44, no. 6, pp. 1177–1183, 2013.
[26] J. D. Tward, M. M. M. Wendland, D. C. Shrieve, A. Szabo, and D. K. Gaffney, "The risk of secondary malignancies over 30 years after the treatment of non-Hodgkin lymphoma," *Cancer*, vol. 107, no. 1, pp. 108–115, 2006.

4

Chronic Eosinophilic Leukemia Presenting as Cardiac Failure

Nii Boi-Doku Pepra-Ameyaw[1] **William Kwasi Ghunney**[2] **Eugene Baafi Ampofo**[3] **and Edeghonghon Olayemi**[4]

[1]*Department of Haematology, Korle Bu Teaching Hospital, Accra, Ghana*
[2]*Ghana Institute of Clinical Genetics, Korle Bu, Accra, Ghana*
[3]*National Cardiothoracic Centre, Korle Bu Teaching Hospital, Accra, Ghana*
[4]*Department of Haematology, University of Ghana Medical School, Accra, Ghana*

Correspondence should be addressed to Edeghonghon Olayemi; eolayemi@ug.edu.gh

Academic Editor: Pier Paolo Piccaluga

Chronic eosinophilic leukemia (CEL) is a rare chronic myeloproliferative disorder characterized by sustained eosinophilia. Although the incidence of CEL is uncertain, it can be clinically devastating as it has a propensity to affect several important organ systems. This is of particular significance in Sub-Saharan Africa where helminthic infections are a more prevalent cause of eosinophilia. To the best of our knowledge, we present the first reported case of CEL complicated by cardiac disease in a Ghanaian. He presented with a history of orthopnoea and dyspnoea on exertion, and examination revealed a pansystolic murmur over the mitral region and moderate splenomegaly. Good symptomatic control was achieved using hydroxyurea after which haematologic and cytogenetic remission was achieved after 12 weeks on a tyrosine kinase inhibitor. Physicians working in low resource environments should exclude clonality in patients presenting with eosinophilia and end-organ damage.

1. Introduction

Chronic eosinophilic leukemia (CEL) is a rare chronic myeloproliferative disorder characterized by an absolute eosinophil count greater than 1.5×10^9 cells/L persisting for more than 6 months and the presence of myeloid cells that exhibit a clonal cytogenetic aberration [1]. It shares a clinicopathological overlap with idiopathic hypereosinophilic syndrome in which tissue damage is present without an associated identifiable cytogenetic aberration or blasts greater than 5% but less than 20% in the bone marrow [2]. In the United States, the age-adjusted incidence of hypereosinophilic syndrome is estimated to be approximately 0.036 per 100,000 person-years [3]. Eosinophilia with recurrent genetic abnormalities make up an even smaller subset of these cases.

The Revised 2016 World Health Organization Classification of Eosinophilic Disorders recognizes myeloid/lymphoid neoplasms with eosinophilia and rearrangement of PDGFRA, PDGFRB, or FGFR1, or with PCM-JAK2 as a distinct clinical entity [1]. The incidence of *FIP1L1-PDGFRA* in patients with idiopathic hypereosinophilia is approximately 10% [4]; this is of significant clinical consequence as this group of patients is uniquely sensitive to tyrosine kinase inhibitor therapy and is capable of achieving complete molecular remission [5]. *CHIC2* deletion is a surrogate for the *FIP1L1-PDGFRA* fusion.

2. Case Presentation

A 37-year-old man with no known history of hypertension, atherosclerosis, or heart disease presented with a year-long history of progressively worsening dyspnoea on exertion associated with orthopnoea and bipedal oedema. He had no known history of allergic disease or exposure to toxins. At presentation, his blood pressure was 90/67 mmHg. Further examination revealed a chronically ill looking adult male with raised jugular venous pressure and pitting bipedal oedema up to the level of the distal third of his tibia, a grossly enlarged spleen approximately 10 cm below the left costal

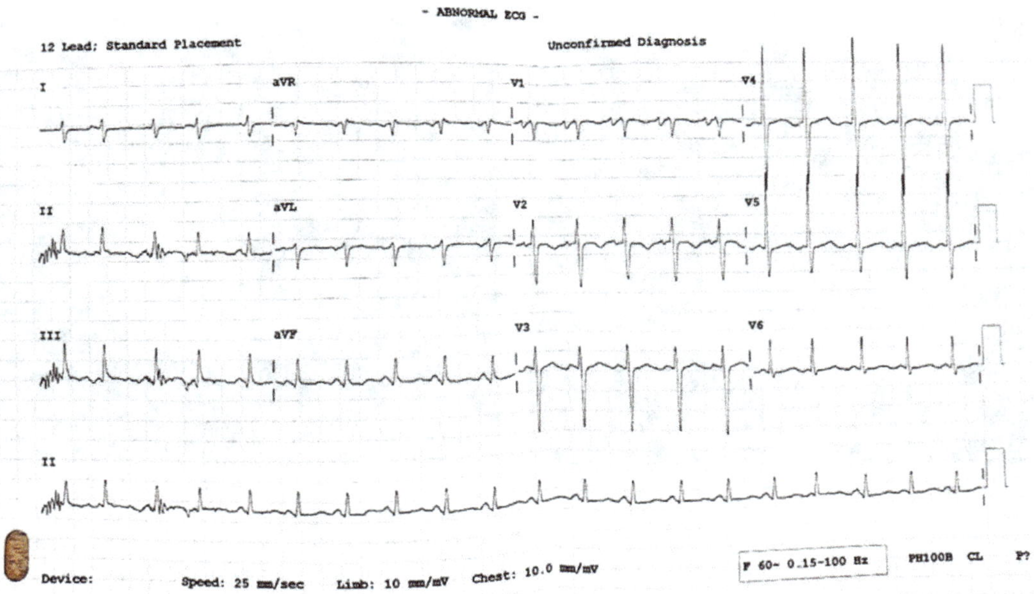

FIGURE 1: ECG at presentation showing sinus tachycardia and a right axis deviation. P wave duration of 120 ms with deep terminal portion > 1 mm (left atrial component) in V1 indicative of a dilated left atrium. The dilated left atrium is a result of an increased volume load from the severe mitral regurgitation.

margin, and ascites and bilateral inguinal lymphadenopathy. Auscultation revealed a pansystolic murmur over the mitral region.

Chest radiography displayed a cardiomegaly with cephalization of vessels. Sinus tachycardia and a right axis deviation were seen on the electrocardiogram (figure 1). An echocardiogram further revealed a thickened mitral valve with severe mitral regurgitation, mild tricuspid regurgitation, mild left atrial dilatation, mild pulmonary hypertension, and a pericardial effusion. Measured left ventricular ejection fraction was 63% (Figure 2). About 18 months prior, he had noticed insidious migratory pain that involved the shoulder, elbow, wrist, knee, and ankle joints, and this pain was severe enough to interfere with his activities of daily living with poor response to nonsteroidal anti-inflammatory drugs (NSAIDS).

A full blood count (FBC) showed a haemoglobin (Hb) concentration of 11.2 g/dl, total white blood cell (WBC) count of 153×10^9 cells/L (neutrophil count of 112×10^9 cells/L; eosinophil count of 30×10^9 cells/L), and a platelet count of 104×10^9 cells/L (Table 1). A leucoerythroblastic picture with a complete spectrum of myeloid cells was seen on the peripheral film. Bone marrow aspirate revealed a hypercellular marrow with increased granulocytes, 50% of which were comprised of eosinophils at different stages of development. No blasts were noted (Figure 3). RT-PCR for *BCR-ABL* transcripts was negative. FISH analysis was positive for deletion of *CHIC2* in 67% of interphase cells analysed (Figure 3). A diagnosis of chronic eosinophilic leukemia complicated by cardiac failure secondary to valvular heart disease was therefore made.

Before his arrival at our facility, he had received a course of ivermectin that proved ineffective. We initiated treatment with 1 g hydroxyurea twice daily to which the patient showed good haematologic response. After receipt of his FISH analysis, hydroxyurea was replaced with 400 mg daily of imatinib. Repeat FISH analysis 3 months after starting imatinib showed no evidence of *CHIC2* deletion in 100% of the interphase cells analysed (Figure 3). He has not required blood product transfusion since starting treatment and experienced no adverse drug effects of imatinib that required interruption or adjustment of therapeutic dosage. His cardiac failure is being managed with digoxin, diuretics (furosemide and spironolactone), and bisoprolol. Our patient has been unable to undergo a mitral valve replacement due to lack of funds. However, with the above mentioned treatment regimen, he has returned to his normal daily activities and is able to undertake tasks with no functional limitations.

3. Discussion

Hypereosinophilia may be reactive, clonal, or idiopathic. Helminthic infection is a well-recognized cause of reactive eosinophilia especially in developing countries. It is worthwhile to note that nonmyeloid malignancies such as T-cell lymphomas and Hodgkin disease can cause nonclonal eosinophilopoiesis due to the production of cytokines such as interleukin-5 which stimulate eosinophil precursor cell proliferation [6]. After exclusion of a reactive cause, investigation for a clonal cause should begin (Table 2).

A peripheral blood film and bone marrow aspirate examination may indicate well-defined WHO myeloid neoplasms such as chronic myeloid leukemia, acute myeloid leukemia, or systemic mastocytosis that may present with eosinophilia. These conditions usually have characteristic genetic markers such as the Philadelphia chromosome [7] or *KIT* gene mutations [8] that must be further investigated.

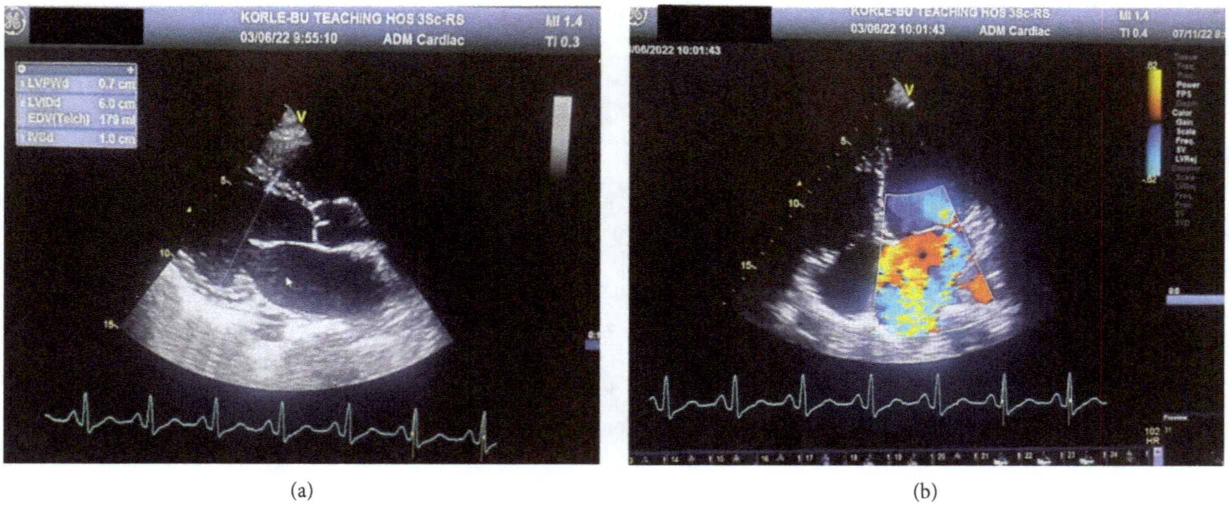

FIGURE 2: Echocardiogram 5 weeks post imatinib: (a) 2D parasternal long axis view showing dilated left ventricle, left atrium and thickened mitral valve leaflets. (b) 2D apical 4-chamber view showing severe mitral regurgitation on colour doppler.

TABLE 1: Series of full blood count results showing response to therapy.

	FBC at presentation	FBC after 2 weeks on hydroxyurea	FBC after 1 week on imatinib	FBC after 1 month on imatinib	Reference range
Hb concentration (g/dL)	11.2	7.9	10.3	10.2	11.0–18.0
WBC count (x 10^9/L)	153.17	7.05	5.84	6.80	2.5–8.5
Eosinophil count (x 10^9/L)	30.87	2.56	0.53	0.17	0.04–0.4
Neutrophil count (x 10^9/L)	112.43	2.43	1.82	3.13	2.0–7.0
Lymphocyte count (x 10^9/L)	4.60	1.66	3.15	3.00	1.0–3.0
Basophil count (x 10^9/L)	0.84	0.09	0.04	0.03	0.02–0.2
Monocyte count (x 10^9/L)	4.29	0.31	0.30	0.47	0.2–1.0
Platelet count (x 10^9/L)	104	149	271	359	150–450

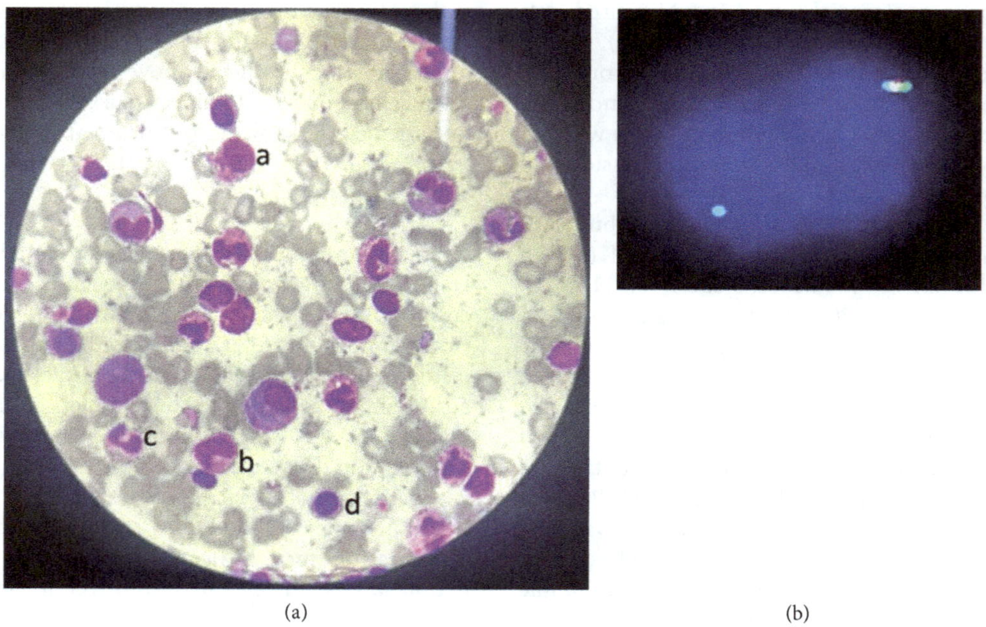

FIGURE 3: Continued.

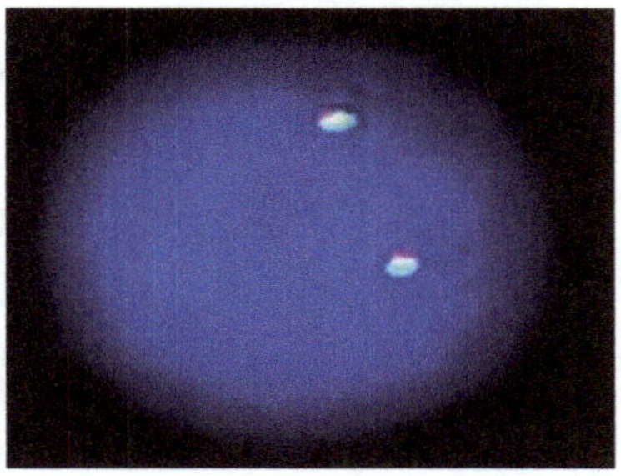

(c)

FIGURE 3: Bone marrow aspirate morphology and FISH result: (a) Bone marrow aspirate showing (i) eosinophilic myelocyte (ii) eosinophilic metamyelocyte (iii) eosinophilic band (iv) normoblast (b) FISH signal pattern at diagnosis indicative of deletion of CHIC2 gene. FISH signal patterns in nuclei having interstitial deletions of the orange probe target (CHIC2) should be observed as one tri-colour fusion and one green/ aqua fusion. (c) FISH signal pattern 3 months post imatinib showing no evidence of CHIC2 deletion.

TABLE 2: Differential diagnoses of hypereosinophilia.

Reactive	Helminthiasis T-cell lymphoma Lymphocyte-variant hypereosinophilic syndrome Hodgkin disease
Clonal	Chronic eosinophilic leukemia Chronic myeloid leukemia Acute myeloid leukemia Systemic mastocytosis
Idiopathic	Idiopathic hypereosinophilic syndrome Idiopathic hypereosinophilia

The Revised 2016 World Health Organization Classification of Eosinophilic Disorders recognizes myeloid/lymphoid neoplasms with eosinophilia and rearrangement of *PDGFRA*, *PDGFRB*, or *FGFR1*, or with *PCM-JAK2* as a distinct clinical entity. Chronic eosinophilic leukemia, not otherwise specified, and idiopathic hypereosinophilic syndrome are diagnoses of exclusion which require the elimination of a known reactive process, genetically defined myeloid malignancy, or a lymphocyte-variant hypereosinophilia (the clonal T-cell population produce a cytokine driven reactive eosinophilia) [9]. Chronic eosinophilic leukemia, not otherwise specified, and idiopathic hypereosinophilic syndrome are similar in that both conditions are associated with persistent hypereosinophilia (absolute eosinophil count $>1.5\times10^9$ cells/L) with evidence of tissue damage. The exact underlying mechanisms of injury have not been well elucidated. It is postulated to be related to direct eosinophil infiltration, fibrosis, or thrombosis ultimately affecting a diverse array of organs including the cranial nerves, oesophagus, lungs, kidneys, skin, and heart [10]. As seen in our patient, there have been infrequent reports of polyarthritis occurring with eosinophilia but without evidence of systemic involvement that is characteristically unresponsive to NSAIDS but ameliorated by corticosteroids [11, 12]. The distinction is made in favour of chronic eosinophilic leukemia, not otherwise specified, when a clonal cytogenetic or molecular genetic abnormality is established, or blast count is $\geq 2\%$ in the peripheral blood or $>5\%$ in the bone marrow [2]. In the absence of tissue damage, the term idiopathic hypereosinophilia is preferred.

The *FIP1L1-PDGFRA* fusion gene, a constitutively activated tyrosine kinase, arises as a result of a deletion on chromosome 4q12 [13]. The *CHIC2* gene is located in this region. As such, the *FIP1L1-PDGFRA* fusion gene is often referred to as "CHIC2 deletion" [14]. This is usually detected with FISH but can also be detected by RT-PCR. A significant majority of the patients with this fusion gene are sensitive to tyrosine kinase inhibitors [5] and primary or secondary resistance to imatinib is rare [15]. Discontinuation of therapy may, however, lead to relapse [16].

4. Conclusion

In conclusion, physicians should be on high alert when eosinophilia occurs with end-organ damage. The laboratory evaluation for such patients, after elimination of reactive causes, should include screening for the *FIP1L1-PDGFRA* fusion gene, and if found, treatment must be commenced with imatinib. In the absence of a tyrosine kinase inhibitor, hydroxyurea is a viable alternative.

Consent

The patient gave signed informed consent for the publication of this case report.

Acknowledgments

The authors wish to acknowledge the nurses of the haematology department, KBTH.

References

[1] D. A. Arber, A. Orazi, R. Hasserjian et al., "The 2016 revision to the World Health Organization classification of myeloid neoplasms and acute leukemia," *Blood*, vol. 127, no. 20, pp. 2391–2405, 2016.

[2] W. Shomali and J. Gotlib, "World Health Organization-defined eosinophilic disorders: 2022 update on diagnosis, risk stratification, and management," *American Journal of Hematology*, vol. 97, no. 1, pp. 129–148, 2022.

[3] M. M. Crane, C. M. Chang, M. G. Kobayashi, and P. F. Weller, "Incidence of myeloproliferative hypereosinophilic syndrome in the United States and an estimate of all hypereosinophilic syndrome incidence," *The Journal of Allergy and Clinical Immunology*, vol. 126, no. 1, pp. 179–181, 2010.

[4] A. Pardanani, S. R. Brockman, S. F. Paternoster et al., "FIP1L1-PDGFRA fusion: prevalence and clinicopathologic correlates in 89 consecutive patients with moderate to severe eosinophilia," *Blood*, vol. 104, no. 10, pp. 3038–3045, 2004.

[5] J. V. Jovanovic, J. Score, K. Waghorn et al., "Low-dose imatinib mesylate leads to rapid induction of major molecular responses and achievement of complete molecular remission in FIP1L1-PDGFRA-positive chronic eosinophilic leukemia," *Blood*, vol. 109, no. 11, pp. 4635–4640, 2007.

[6] P. Valent, A. D. Klion, H. P. Horny et al., "Contemporary consensus proposal on criteria and classification of eosinophilic disorders and related syndromes," *The Journal of Allergy and Clinical Immunology*, vol. 130, no. 3, pp. 607–612.e9, 2012.

[7] R. Kurzrock, H. M. Kantarjian, B. J. Druker, and M. Talpaz, "Philadelphia chromosome-positive leukemias: from basic mechanisms to molecular therapeutics," *Annals of Internal Medicine*, vol. 138, no. 10, pp. 819–830, 2003.

[8] I. Maric, J. Robyn, D. D. Metcalfe et al., "KIT D816V-associated systemic mastocytosis with eosinophilia and FIP1L1/PDGFRA-associated chronic eosinophilic leukemia are distinct entities," *The Journal of Allergy and Clinical Immunology*, vol. 120, no. 3, pp. 680–687, 2007.

[9] E. Cogan, L. Schandené, A. Crusiaux, P. Cochaux, T. Velu, and M. Goldman, "Brief report: clonal proliferation of type 2 helper T cells in a man with the hypereosinophilic syndrome," *New England Journal of Medicine*, vol. 330, no. 8, pp. 535–538, 1994.

[10] P. Akuthota and P. F. Weller, "Spectrum of eosinophilic end-organ manifestations," *Immunology and Allergy Clinics of North America*, vol. 35, no. 3, pp. 403–411, 2015.

[11] C. H. Tay, "Eosinophilic arthritis," *Rheumatology*, vol. 38, no. 12, pp. 1188–1194, 1999.

[12] H. Yamabe, F. Kudo, and M. Shimada, "Eosinophilic arthritis-a case report," *Clinical Case Reports*, vol. 9, no. 3, pp. 1220–1222, 2021.

[13] J. Cools, D. J. DeAngelo, J. Gotlib et al., "A tyrosine kinase created by fusion of the PDGFRA and FIP1L1 genes as a therapeutic target of imatinib in idiopathic hypereosinophilic syndrome," *New England Journal of Medicine*, vol. 348, no. 13, pp. 1201–1214, 2003.

[14] A. Pardanani, R. P. Ketterling, S. R. Brockman et al., "CHIC2 deletion, a surrogate for FIP1L1-PDGFRA fusion, occurs in systemic mastocytosis associated with eosinophilia and predicts response to imatinib mesylate therapy," *Blood*, vol. 102, no. 9, pp. 3093–3096, 2003.

[15] S. Q. Qu, T. J. Qin, Z. F. Xu et al., "Long-term outcomes of imatinib in patients with FIP1L1/PDGFRA associated chronic eosinophilic leukemia: experience of a single center in China," *Oncotarget*, vol. 7, no. 22, pp. 33229–33236, 2016.

[16] M. Baccarani, D. Cilloni, M. Rondoni et al., "The efficacy of imatinib mesylate in patients with FIP1L1-PDGFR-positive hypereosinophilic syndrome. Results of a multicenter prospective study," *Haematologica*, vol. 92, no. 9, pp. 1173–1179, 2007.

5

Epstein–Barr Virus Primary Infection Complicated by Hemophagocytic Lymphohistiocytosis and Plasmablastic Lymphoma in a HIV-Negative Patient

Nan Chen, Mike Perez, and Martha Mims

Baylor College of Medicine, 1 Baylor Plaza, Houston, TX 77030, USA

Correspondence should be addressed to Nan Chen; nanc@bcm.edu

Academic Editor: Kostas Konstantopoulos

EBV (Epstein–Barr virus) viremia causes immune dysregulation through various mechanisms, and we are understanding more that mutations in B, T, and NK (natural killer) cell signaling pathways allow EBV complications such as HLH (hemophagocytic lymphohistiocytosis) and lymphomas to arise. Here, we report a 20-year-old previously healthy, HIV- (human immunodeficiency virus-) negative male who presented with fevers, sore throat, and lymphadenopathy (LAD). He was found to have EBV viremia, pancytopenia, and elevated LFTs (liver function tests) suspicious for HLH. Bone marrow biopsy and elevated IL-2 (interleukin) receptor confirmed this diagnosis. Additionally, gastric biopsy confirmed diagnosis of plasmablastic lymphoma (PBL), a rare, aggressive HIV- and EBV-associated lymphoma. Both bone marrow and gastric biopsy showed evidence of EBV. Patients with EBV complications should have a rigorous workup to characterize the full extent of immune dysregulation including genetic testing at a high-volume center.

1. Case Presentation

The patient was a healthy 20-year-old M who presented with 3 weeks of intermittent fever, sore throat, and painful bilateral cervical lymph nodes. He went to an outside emergency room 5 days prior to presentation and was diagnosed with infectious mononucleosis via positive monospot and discharged with symptomatic treatment. He presented to our institution for 2 days of hematemesis, melena, jaundice, and continued fevers. On interview with his family, he had a healthy childhood without prior hospitalizations and one healthy younger male sibling.

On physical exam, he was febrile and tachycardic. He had bilateral cervical lymphadenopathy, decreased breath sounds in his bilateral lung bases, and hepatosplenomegaly. Initial laboratory testing showed the following: Hgb (hemoglobin) 12.3 g/dL, WBC (white blood cell) 5.2 k/uL, platelets 68 k/uL, aspartate aminotransferase 361 U/L, alanine aminotransferase 242 U/L, alkaline phosphatase 332 U/L, total bilirubin 10.7 mg/dL, prothrombin time 34.3 seconds, fibrinogen 95 mg/dL, and d-dimer 6.5 ug/mL. HIV (human immunodeficiency virus) and hepatitis panel were negative. CT (computed tomography) of chest, abdomen, and pelvis showed diffuse lymphadenopathy in axillary, mediastinal, hilar, retroperitoneal, and inguinal regions, numerous pulmonary nodules bilaterally, and hepatosplenomegaly. Over the following 24 hours, the patient's clinical condition deteriorated, and the following day, he was intubated for hypoxemic respiratory failure, started on broad-spectrum antibiotics, and given supportive transfusions. EBV viremia was confirmed with a viral load of 2 million copies/mL (Figure 1).

An EGD (esophagogastroduodenoscopy) was performed for bleeding, revealing multiple friable, superficial ulcers throughout the distal esophagus and stomach inconsistent with peptic ulcer disease, and biopsies were collected. With dropping blood counts, triglycerides of 289 mg/dL and ferritin of 13,000 ng/mL (Figure 2), there was concern for hemophagocytic lymphohistiocytosis (HLH), and a marrow exam was performed along with a left inguinal lymph node

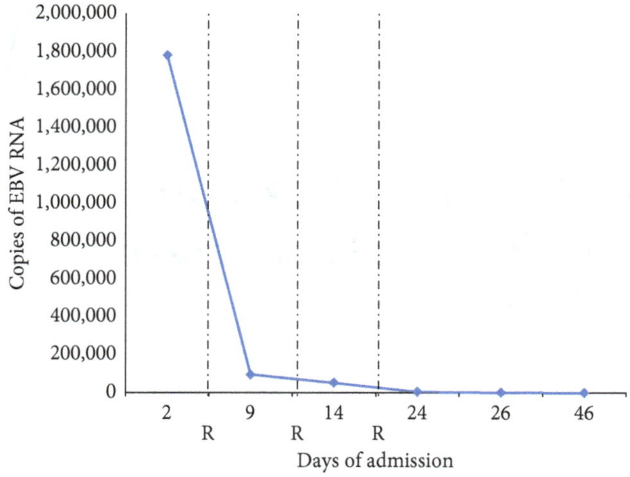

FIGURE 1: Epstein–Barr virus (EBV) viremia through days of admission. R = Rituximab administration at 375 mg/m^2.

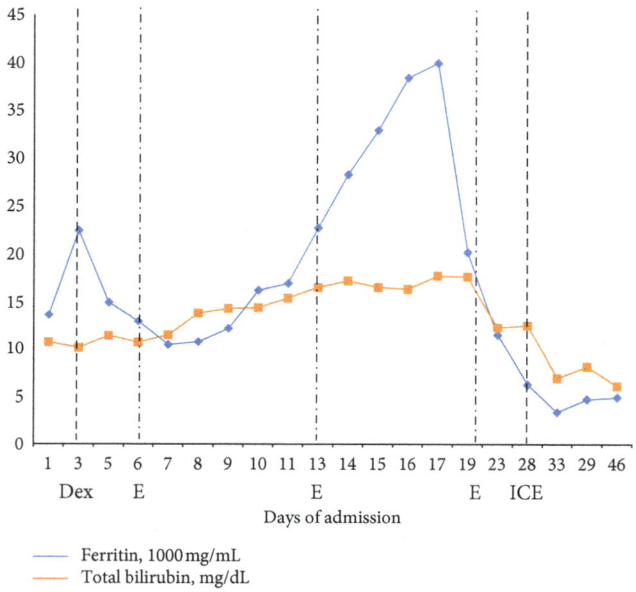

FIGURE 2: Ferritin and total bilirubin throughout hospital course. Dex = dexamethasone administration; E = etoposide administration; ICE = ifosfamide, carboplatin, and etoposide administration.

biopsy. Marrow demonstrated "areas with increased macrophages associated with hemophagocytosis and focal necrosis," consistent with HLH. Inguinal lymph node biopsy also showed hemophagocytosis but was uninvolved by lymphoma. The patient was started on dose-reduced dexamethasone and etoposide (for renal and hepatotoxicity) as per the HLH-94 protocol as well as IVIG (intravenous immunoglobulin) [1]. By day 8, despite numerous supportive transfusions and therapy, laboratory testing showed WBC 1.6 K/uL, Hgb 7.8 g/dL, platelets 13 K/uL, and fibrinogen 89 mg/dL. During this time, his ferritin rose to 28,000 ng/mL. Liver transaminases continued to rise and in conjunction with other laboratory values reflected acute liver failure. Serum immunoglobulins were low. His IL-2 (interleukin) soluble receptor sent earlier in admission returned at 36,000 U/mL (reference range 406–1100 U/mL).

Weekly rituximab was started for EBV viremia. On day 10 of hospital admission, gastric biopsies returned showing a neoplastic infiltrate positive for CD138, CD45, CD79a, CD43, BCL-2, and MUM-1 and negative for CD20 consistent with plasmablastic lymphoma (PBL). Both bone marrow and gastric biopsies were positive for EBER (Epstein–Barr virus-encoded small ribonucleic acids). Initiation of chemotherapy was held, while both HLH treatment and antibiotics for enterococcus bacteremia were ongoing. The patient remained with liver failure, disseminated intravascular coagulation (DIC) requiring daily supportive transfusions, and kidney failure requiring hemodialysis. The patient improved and by day 20 was extubated; EBV viral load decreased to 900 copies/mL, ferritin decreased to 7,000 ng/mL, and pancytopenia improved. Eventually, his blood cultures cleared, and on day 27 of his hospital admission, dose-reduced ifosfamide, carboplatin, and etoposide (ICE) was initiated. Adriamycin was omitted because of low ejection fraction in the setting of acute illness. He tolerated Cycle #1 without any immediate complications. However, 5 days after chemotherapy, despite improving coagulopathy, the patient reported abdominal pain and imaging revealed a nontraumatic, spontaneous retroperitoneal hematoma which was unable to be safely evacuated. Seven days after chemotherapy, he developed worsening pancytopenia and transaminitis, thought to be secondary to ICE as opposed to recurrent HLH. The patient developed neutropenic fever and septic shock, antibiotics were restarted, and CT chest showed right lower lobe pneumonia. Again, he went into respiratory failure, was reintubated, and on bronchoscopy, blood was seen in all lobes of the right lung, consistent with diffuse alveolar hemorrhage. The patient became comfort care and subsequently died.

2. Discussion

EBV is a common virus with pathogenic and oncogenic potential, a characteristic magnified in compromised immune systems [2]. Here, we describe a previously healthy patient presenting with EBV primary infection complicated by PBL and HLH resulting in multiorgan failure. The EBV virus was found in both bone marrow and gastric biopsy samples, implicating the important role it played in the pathogenesis of both processes (Figures 3 and 4). This report explores the relationship between EBV, immunity, and malignancy. In a healthy male, could his unique presentation be a manifestation of an underlying primary immunodeficient state?

In patients with normal immunity, EBV affects B cells but lies dormant until triggered by cellular stress. As the virus reproduces, it is recognized by cytotoxic immune cells and subsequently suppressed [2]. In patients with abnormalities in T and NK cell function, this can lead to inefficient immune cytotoxic activity, causing persistent immune activation and ultimately resulting in clinical HLH [2]. EBV is a well-recognized trigger for HLH, and a complicated clinical course of EBV primary infection should prompt an evaluation for immunodeficiencies. Studies conducted in

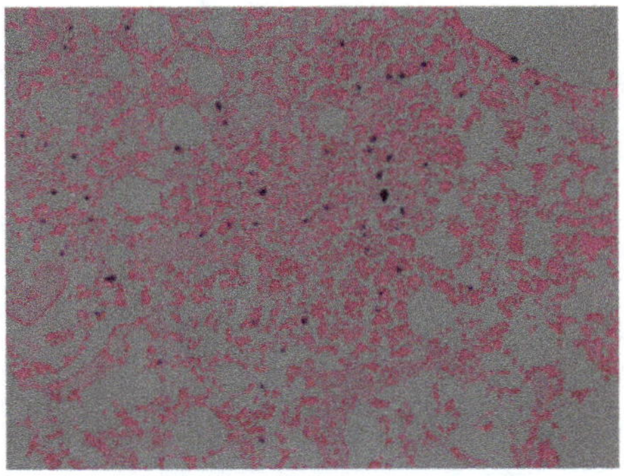

FIGURE 3: 40x of the EBER-ISH (EBV-encoded RNA-in situ hybridization) stain demonstrating EBV activity in the bone marrow.

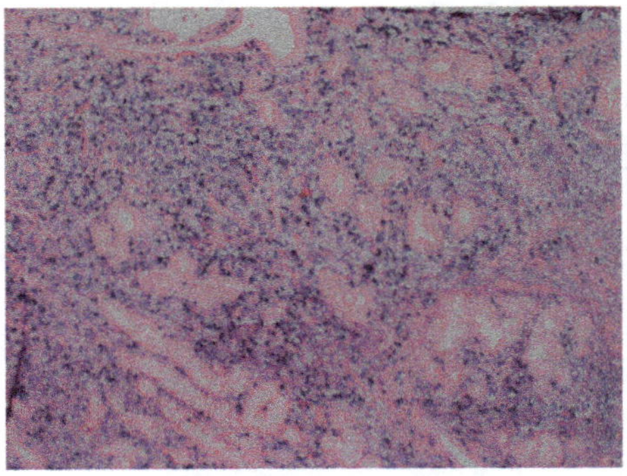

FIGURE 4: 40x of the EBER-ISH stain on gastric biopsy demonstrating PBL with extensive involvement by EBV.

post-stem cell transplant patients showed that chronically elevated EBV loads were associated with simultaneous T-cell activation and T-cell exhaustion suggesting that both an upregulated and a functional T-cell response are required to control EBV infection [3]. In both X-linked lymphoproliferative disorder (XLP) and X-linked inhibitor of apoptosis deficiency (XIAD), genetic mutations in T and NK cells impair cell-mediated immunity and lead to EBV proliferation [2, 4]. Even in chronic active EBV (CAEBV), an entity characterized by patients with persistent EBV infection and lack of known immunodeficiency, we are understanding more that it is likely due to lesser known B-cell mutations [5].

EBV is also recognized for its oncogenic potential. PBL is an aggressive B-cell malignancy of plasmablasts strongly associated with HIV. In affected patients, up to two thirds are HIV positive; however, among the HIV negative, fifty percent are positive for EBER [6, 7]. There have been no data to discuss the role of primary immunodeficiency or EBV in the pathogenesis of PBL, but EBV-associated lymphomas are well characterized. The myc rearrangement, the genetic hallmark of EBV-associated Burkitt's lymphoma, is also the most common cytogenetic finding in PBL [7]. Mutations in myc and its regulator, PRDM1/Blimp-1, can produce the PBL phenotype, and loss of function in this pathway was recently shown to produce more phenotypically aggressive diffuse large B-cell lymphomas [8, 9]. Nearly, all primary immunodeficiencies that are associated with EBV-driven malignancies are related to B, T, and NK cell function [10]. T and NK cells clear virally infected B cells but are also vitally important in clearing malignant cells [10]. EBV presence and viral load has even been studied as a potential prognostic marker of HIV-associated lymphomas [11]. Prognosis for PBL has been historically poor, with expected survival of less than 6 months in untreated patients [7]. Standard lymphoma regimens are most commonly followed such as CHOP (cyclophosphamide, doxorubicin, vincristine, and prednisone) or EPOCH (etoposide, cyclophosphamide, doxorubicin, vincristine, and prednisone); however, no standard of care exists [7]. Other immunomodulatory agents such as bortezomib and lenalidomide have had limited success and should be considered on an individual basis [12].

For our patient, initial workup for immunodeficiency was unrevealing. His HIV antibody and viral load were both negative repeatedly, and he had a normal karyotype. Further workup was not pursued as his acute illness worsened, but testing would have included B-cell phenotyping and genetic evaluation for common T, B, and NK cell mutations such as XLP (X-linked lymphoproliferative syndrome) and XIA (X-linked agammaglobulinemia), with a more targeted panel if those are negative. Patients with diagnosed genetic disorders should be considered for bone marrow transplant. This case illustrates the difficulties in diagnosing and managing the complications of EBV primary infection. It is imperative to consider an underlying primary immunodeficiency in patients with rare complications from EBV infection and to be aggressive about characterizing the full extent of immune dysregulation.

References

[1] J.-I. Henter, A. Samuelsson-Horne, M. Aricò et al., "Treatment of hemophagocytic lymphohistiocytosis with HLH-94 immunochemotherapy and bone marrow transplantation," *Blood*, vol. 100, no. 7, pp. 2367–2373, 2002.

[2] J. L. Kutok and F. Wang, "Spectrum of Epstein-Barr Virus-associated diseases," *Annual Review of Pathology: Mechanisms of Disease*, vol. 1, no. 1, pp. 375–404, 2006.

[3] C. Macedo, S. A. Webber, A. D. Donnenberg et al., "EBV-specific CD8+ T cells from asymptomatic pediatric thoracic transplant patients carrying chronic high EBV loads display contrasting features: activated phenotype and exhausted function," *The Journal of Immunology*, vol. 186, no. 10, pp. 5854–5862, 2011.

[4] N. Parvaneh, A. H. Filipovich, and A. Borkhardt, "Primary immunodeficiencies predisposed to Epstein-Barr virus-driven haematological diseases," *British Journal of Haematology*, vol. 162, no. 5, pp. 573–586, 2013.

[5] H. Kimura and J. I. Cohen, "Chronic active Epstein-Barr Virus disease," *Frontiers in Immunology*, vol. 8, p. 1867, 2017.

[6] M. Liu, B. Liu, B. Liu et al., "Human immunodeficiency virus-negative plasmablastic lymphoma: a comprehensive analysis of 114 cases," *Oncology Reports*, vol. 33, no. 4, pp. 1615–1620, 2015.

[7] J. J. Castillo, M. Bibas, and R. N. Miranda, "The biology and treatment of plasmablastic lymphoma," *Blood*, vol. 125, no. 15, pp. 2323–2330, 2015.

[8] S. Montes-Moreno, N. Martinez-Magunacelaya, T. Zecchini-Barrese et al., "Plasmablastic lymphoma phenotype is de-

termined by genetic alterations in MYC and PRDM1," *Modern Pathology*, vol. 30, no. 1, pp. 85–94, 2018.

[9] Y. Xia, Z. Y. Xu-Monette, A. Tzankov et al., "Loss of PRDM1/BLIMP-1 function contributes to poor prognosis of activated B-cell-like diffuse large B-cell lymphoma," *Leukemia*, vol. 31, no. 3, pp. 625–636, 2017.

[10] M. Shabani, K. E. Nichols, and N. Rezaei, "Primary immunodeficiencies associated with EBV-Induced lymphoproliferative disorders," *Critical Reviews in Oncology/Hematology*, vol. 108, pp. 109–127, 2016.

[11] J. Muncunill, M.-J. Baptista, Á. Hernandez-Rodríguez et al., "Plasma epstein-barr virus load as an early biomarker and prognostic factor of human immunodeficiency virus-related lymphomas," *Clinical Infectious Diseases*, vol. 68, no. 5, pp. 834–843, 2019.

[12] D. Pretscher, A. Kalisch, M. Wilhelm, and J. Birkmann, "Refractory plasmablastic lymphoma-a review of treatment options beyond standard therapy," *Annals of Hematology*, vol. 96, no. 6, pp. 967–970, 2017.

6

A Patient with Chronic Lymphocytic Leukemia with Pancreatic Involvement

Rajesh Essrani[1], **Matthew J. Sullivan**[2] **and Hiral Shah**[2]

[1]*General Internal Medicine, Lehigh Valley Health Network, Allentown, PA, USA*
[2]*Department of Gastroenterology, Lehigh Valley Health Network, Allentown, PA, USA*

Correspondence should be addressed to Rajesh Essrani; raj1_essrani@hotmail.com

Academic Editor: Marie-Christine Kyrtsonis

A 78-year-old female with a past medical history of hypertension, type 2 diabetes mellitus, and chronic lymphocytic leukemia was hospitalized for poor appetite, weight loss, and night sweats. On physical exam, there was no palpable lymphadenopathy, and her abdomen was soft and nondistended. Laboratory results showed a hemoglobin count of 13.3 g/dl, hematocrit 41.3%, white blood cell $68.4 \times 103\,\mu$L with lymphocytes 92.0%, total bilirubin 0.4 mg/dL, aspartate transaminase 14 U/L, and alanine transaminase 15 U/L. CT of the chest, abdomen, and pelvis showed hypodense lesions within the pancreatic body (1.4×1.4 cm) and medial aspect of the pancreatic head (1.2 cm) as well as mild splenomegaly (13 cm craniocaudally). She subsequently underwent endoscopic ultrasound (EUS) with fine needle aspiration (FNA) of the pancreatic mass. Flow cytometry revealed expression of CD5 and CD23, consistent with chronic lymphocytic leukemia.

1. Introduction

Chronic lymphocytic leukemia (CLL) is a malignancy of CD 5-positive B cells that is characterized by the accumulation of small, mature-appearing neoplastic lymphocytes in the blood, bone marrow, and secondary lymphoid tissues. This results in lymphocytosis, infiltration of the marrow, lymphadenopathy, and splenomegaly. CLL is the most common form of adult leukemia, accounting for 10% of hematologic malignancies. CLL is diagnosed by the detection of clonal B lymphocytes at a count of $\geq$5,000 μL in the peripheral blood, predominance of small, morphologically mature lymphocytes upon cytological examination of the blood smear, and coexpression of the B-cell antigens CD19, CD20, CD23, and T-cell antigen CD5 upon multiparametric immunophenotyping. Each clone of leukemia cells is restricted to expression of either kappa or lambda immunoglobulin light chains [1]. Due to its chronic course, patients with CLL usually do not require immediate treatment. A "watch-and-wait" strategy is the standard of care in patients with early-stage and asymptomatic CLL.

2. Case Report

A 78-year-old female with a past medical history of hypertension, type 2 diabetes mellitus, hypertension, and chronic lymphocytic leukemia was hospitalized for poor appetite, weight loss, and night sweats. On physical exam, her abdomen was soft and nondistended without palpable lymphadenopathy. Laboratory results showed a hemoglobin count of 13.3 g/dl, hematocrit 41.3%, white blood cell count $68.4 \times 103\,\mu$L with lymphocytes 92.0%, total bilirubin 0.4 mg/dL, aspartate transaminase 14 U/L, and alanine transaminase 15 U/L. CT of the chest, abdomen, and pelvis showed hypodense lesions within the pancreatic body (1.4×1.4 cm) and medial aspect of the pancreatic head (1.2 cm) as well as mild splenomegaly (13 cm craniocaudally) (Figure 1). She subsequently underwent EUS with FNA of the pancreatic mass (Figure 2). There was no blood contamination during the FNA procedure. Flow cytometry revealed coexpression of CD5 and CD23, consistent with CLL.

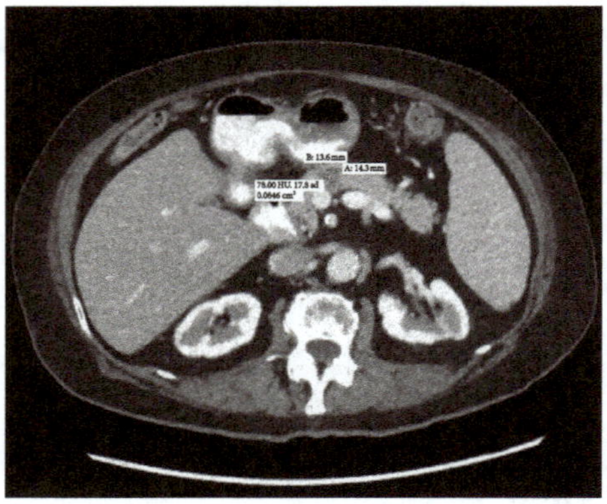

Figure 1: CT abdo/pelvis: hypodense lesions within the pancreatic body and medial aspect of the pancreatic head which are concerning for a neoplastic process.

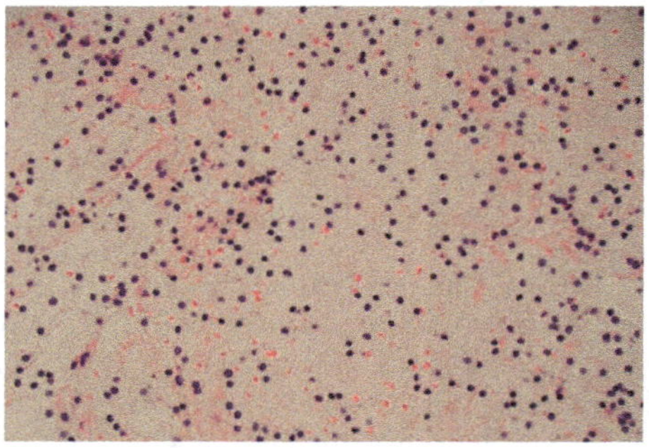

Figure 2: Histology slide for CLL.

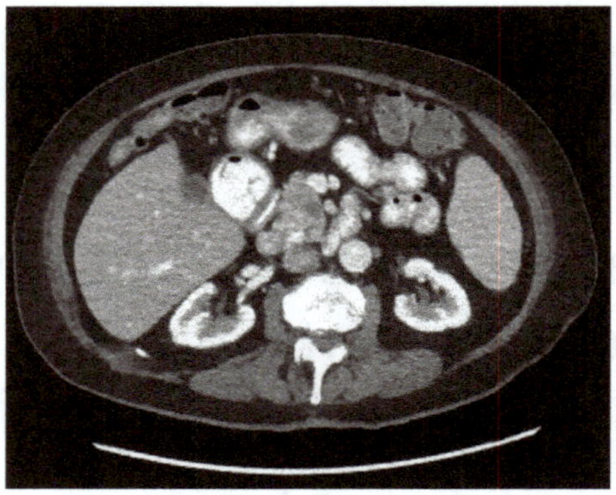

Figure 3: CT abdo/pelvis: normal-appearing pancreas.

She was initially diagnosed with CLL around 3 years prior to the pancreatic involvement. Initial flow cytometry demonstrated a CD5- and CD23-positive clonal B-cell population. Fluorescence in situ hybridization (FISH) showed 58% of nuclear positive for apparent trisomy 12 which has been shown to correlate with an intermediate prognosis. The results for CCND1/IGH, ATM, 13q, and TP53 were all normal. Bone marrow biopsy showed 47, XX + 12 with overall pathology consistent with CLL.

After the FNA results, she was re-evaluated by her oncologist who recommended close follow-up with interval imaging in 6 months. Repeat CT scan of the abdomen and pelvis was performed two months later due to an episode of an acute abdominal pain and demonstrated a normal-appearing pancreas (Figure 3). This unexpected finding represented a spontaneous resolution of CLL involvement of the pancreas. Her suspected B-cell symptoms also resolved other than occasional fatigue reported during subsequent office visits. She has remained asymptomatic and has not required treatment of her CLL.

3. Discussion

Chronic lymphocytic leukemia/small lymphocytic lymphoma (CLL/SLL) is a malignancy of CD 5-positive B cells that is characterized by the accumulation of small, mature-appearing lymphocytes in the blood, bone marrow, and lymphoid tissues. The term CLL is used when the disease manifests primarily in the blood, whereas the term SLL is used when lymph nodes are mainly involved. Patients are usually asymptomatic at presentation, with CLL identified by a relative lymphocytosis on a routine complete blood count. Some patients can present with painless swelling of lymph nodes, but uncommon presentations include constitutional "B-cell symptoms" of lymphoma (i.e., fevers, chills, and weight loss), symptoms related to an acquired immunodeficiency or autoimmune complications [2].

Patients with CLL are grouped prognostically according to the Rai and Binet staging systems which are based on the physical examination and CBC results [3, 4]. The Rai system is based on the concept that, in CLL, there is a gradual and progressive increase in the body burden of leukemic lymphocytes, starting in the blood and bone marrow (lymphocytosis), progressively involving lymph nodes (lymphadenopathy), and spleen and liver (organomegaly), with eventual compromise of bone marrow function (anemia and thrombocytopenia) [5]. The Binet staging system takes into consideration five potential sites of involvement: the cervical, axillary, and inguinal lymph nodes (whether unilateral or bilateral, each area is counted as one), the spleen, and the liver. Involvement is judged only by physical exam and does not take into consideration the results of imaging studies. Patients are classified according to the number of involved sites plus the presence of anemia (hemoglobin <10 g/dL) and/or thrombocytopenia (platelets <100,000 μL).

CT of the chest, abdomen, and pelvis is not routinely performed as part of the pretreatment evaluation. However, a CT scan should be done in any patient in whom enlarged abdominal or pelvic nodes are suspected based on evidence of complications such as obstructive jaundice or obstruction of the inferior vena cava or ureters [6].

Viadana et al. analyzed the involvement at every site of the human body in acute lymphoblastic, chronic lymphoblastic, acute myeloblastic, and chronic myelocytic leukemia during autopsy. CLL showed an excess of involvement in all lymph nodes (>80%), kidney (61–80%), adrenals, lungs (41–50% each), and heart (31%–40%) but rarely pancreas (11%) [7]. There was no organ involvement seen in 51–60% of autopsies. Outside of a few documented autopsy findings, there have been no case reports of CLL with pancreatic involvement reported in the literature [7, 8].

The differential diagnosis for a hypodense pancreatic lesion also includes granulomatous disease, infection, pseudocyst, cystic tumor, and solid tumors. Most pancreatic lesions are seen on CT, but MRI is more sensitive and specific.

Watchful waiting is an appropriate strategy for many asymptomatic patients with CLL. Therapy is indicated for patients with active disease as manifested by advanced stage, high tumor burden, severe disease-related "B-cell symptoms," or repeated infections [9–12]. Early stage I and II SLL are treated with radiation therapy, and more advanced SLL is treated with chemotherapy and anti-CD 20 antibodies. Symptomatic patients should undergo a pretreatment evaluation with a complete blood count with differential and chemistries including liver and renal function and electrolytes, alkaline phosphatase, lactate dehydrogenase (LDH), beta-2 microglobulin, direct antiglobulin test (DAT), HIV, hepatitis B and hepatitis C screening, CMV serology, and fluorescence in situ hybridization (FISH) for del17p, del11q, trisomy 12, and del13q. This workup can determine the extent of disease, patient performance status, and assessment of comorbidities [2, 13, 14]. CLL patients are at increased risk of secondary malignancies like large-cell lymphoma by Richter transformation and autoimmune diseases like immune thrombocytopenia and hemolytic anemia.

In summary, CLL is usually asymptomatic on presentation and can be observed without the need for therapy for decades. There have been a few reported cases of pancreas involvement discovered at autopsy, but no case reports of symptomatic CLL involving the pancreas have been reported in the literature.

Disclosure

This case was presented as an abstract in ACG 2018 Annual Scientific Meeting Abstracts, Philadelphia, Pennsylvania.

References

[1] E. J. Moreau, E. Matutes, R. P. A'Hern et al., "Improvement of the chronic lymphocytic leukemia scoring system with the monoclonal antibody SN8(CD79b)," *American Journal of Clinical Pathology*, vol. 108, no. 4, pp. 378–382, 1997.

[2] M. Hallek, B. D. Cheson, D. Catovsky et al., "iwCLL guidelines for diagnosis, indications for treatment, response assessment, and supportive management of CLL," *Blood*, vol. 131, no. 25, pp. 2745–2760, 2018.

[3] K. R. Rai, A. Sawitsky, E. P. Cronkite, A. D. Chanana, R. N. Levy, and B. S. Pasternack, "Clinical staging of chronic lymphocytic leukemia," *Blood*, vol. 46, no. 2, pp. 219–234, 1975.

[4] J. L. Binet, A. Auquier, G. Dighiero et al., "A new prognostic classification of chronic lymphocytic leukemia derived from a multivariate survival analysis," *Cancer*, vol. 48, no. 1, pp. 198–206, 1981.

[5] A. J. Oloo and T. A. Ogada, "Chronic lymphocytic leukaemia (CLL): clinical study at Kenyatta national hospital (KNH)," *East African Medical Journal*, vol. 61, no. 11, pp. 797–801, 1984.

[6] K. A. Blum, D. Young, S. Broering et al., "Computed tomography scans do not improve the predictive power of 1996 national Cancer institute-sponsored working Group chronic lymphocytic leukemia response criteria," *Journal of Clinical Oncology*, vol. 25, no. 35, pp. 5624–5629, 2007.

[7] E. Viadana, I. D. J. Bross, and J. W. Pickren, "An autopsy study of the metastatic patterns of human leukemias," *Oncology*, vol. 35, no. 2, pp. 87–96, 1978.

[8] M. Barcos, W. Lane, G. A. Gomez et al., "An autopsy study of 1206 acute and chronic leukemias (1958 to 1982)," *Cancer*, vol. 60, no. 4, pp. 827–837, 1987.

[9] R. L. Siegel, K. D. Miller, and A. Jemal, "Cancer statistics," *A Cancer Journal for Clinicians*, vol. 68, no. 1, pp. 7–30, 2018.

[10] J. A. Hernández, K. J. Land, and R. W. Mckenna, "Leukemias, myeloma, and other lymphoreticular neoplasms," *Cancer*, vol. 75, no. Sl, pp. 381–394, 1995.

[11] J. F. Yamamoto and M. T. Goodman, "Patterns of leukemia incidence in the United States by subtype and demographic characteristics, 1997–2002," *Cancer Causes & Control*, vol. 19, no. 4, pp. 379–390, 2008.

[12] M. Sant, C. Allemani, C. Tereanu et al., "Incidence of hematologic malignancies in Europe by morphologic subtype: results of the HAEMACARE project," *Blood*, vol. 116, no. 19, pp. 3724–3734, 2010.

[13] K. Fischer, J. Bahlo, A. M. Fink et al., "Long-term remissions after FCR chemoimmunotherapy in previously untreated patients with CLL: updated results of the CLL8 trial," *Blood*, vol. 127, no. 2, pp. 208–215, 2016.

[14] P. A. Thompson, C. S. Tam, S. M. OBrien et al., "Fludarabine, cyclophosphamide, and rituximab treatment achieves long-term disease-free survival in IGHV-mutated chronic lymphocytic leukemia," *Blood*, vol. 127, no. 3, pp. 303–309, 2016.

7

Pure White Cell Aplasia and Immune Thrombocytopenia after Thymoma Resection: A Case Report and Review of the Literature

Michael Youssef,[1] Tyler W. Stratton,[2] Reid C. Gallant,[1] Christine Young,[3] Daniel Y. Li,[4] and Siavash Piran[5]

[1]*Faculty of Medicine, University of Toronto, Toronto, Canada*
[2]*Schulich School of Medicine & Dentistry, Western University, London, ON, Canada*
[3]*Department of Pharmacy, Trillium Health Partners, Mississauga, Ontario, Canada*
[4]*Department of Laboratory Medicine and Pathobiology, University of Toronto, Toronto, Canada*
[5]*Department of Medicine, Division of Hematology, University of Toronto, Toronto, Canada*

Correspondence should be addressed to Siavash Piran; siavash.piran@thp.ca

Academic Editor: Masayuki Nagasawa

We report a case of pure white cell aplasia (PWCA) postthymoma resection in a 74-year-old male presenting with a 2-week history of fevers, night sweats, and severe febrile neutropenia. His pure white cell aplasia was treated with intravenous immunoglobulin (IVIg), granulocyte colony-stimulating factor (G-CSF), prednisone, and cyclosporine with a mixed response. He also developed immune thrombocytopenia, which responded well to a short course of eltrombopag. With continued cyclosporine treatment, his platelet counts were stable after stopping eltrombopag. The patient's cyclosporine treatment was complicated by renal failure, resulting in cessation of cyclosporine. His PWCA and immune thrombocytopenia significantly worsened after stopping cyclosporine, and unfortunately, he died from multiorgan failure and sepsis.

1. Introduction

Thymoma is the most common neoplasm of the thymus and comprises 20% of mediastinal neoplasms, with an incidence in the US of 0.13 per 100,000 person-years [1, 2]. Patients with thymoma are commonly asymptomatic, although they may present with anterior mediastinal mass symptoms such as chest pain, dyspnea, and cough. Thymomas are classified histologically according to WHO classification of thymic tumours. This system classifies thymomas on the histological appearance of neoplastic cells into the following categories: spindle (type A), dendritic or stellate (type B1-3), or a combined appearance with both spindle and dendritic neoplastic cells (type AB). Type B thymomas are further subdivided into B1, B2, and B3 by evaluating the relative abundance of epithelial cells and lymphocytes [3]. Thymoma management includes surgical resection, radiation, or other systemic therapies e.g. chemotherapy [4, 5].

Thymomas are associated with various immune-mediated para-neoplastic syndromes like myasthenia gravis, Good's syndrome, and/or pure red cell aplasia [4, 6]. In contrast, PWCA is a rare manifestation that can present in patients with thymoma. In PWCA, myelopoiesis is absent or strongly inhibited, while erythropoiesis and megakaryocytopoiesis remain relatively normal [7, 8]. This presents in the form of severe neutropenia, which can thereby result in recurrent life-threatening infections. Many therapies have been used for the treatment of PWCA with varying successes including corticosteroids, cyclosporine, cyclophosphamide, alemtuzumab, G-CSF, high dose IVIg, or plasmapheresis [8–12]. Surgical removal of thymoma can also help eliminate PWCA in some cases [7, 13].

2. Case Presentation

A 74-year-old male was admitted to our hospital with severe febrile neutropenia and the Hematology service was consulted. His past medical history was significant for hypertension, obesity, dyslipidemia, type 2-diabetes, and venous stasis. His home medications included metformin and atorvastatin.

The patient had a mediastinal mass resected, which was found to be a Type B1 thymoma. Neutrophil counts prior to surgery were found to be normal (Table 1). The patient was discharged 4 days later and then returned to hospital with a history of fevers and night sweats. On presentation, he was febrile at 39.7°C and tachycardic with a pulse of 110. He had an undetectable neutrophil count of $<0.1 \times 10^9$/L and was started on broad-spectrum antibiotics (Table 1). A bone marrow aspirate and biopsy showed granulocytic hypoplasia (Figure 1) in keeping with a diagnosis of PWCA post-thymoma resection. A significantly reduced M: E ratio and mild megakaryocytic hyperplasia were also seen on bone marrow biopsy.

Based on laboratory investigations, the patient did not appear to have Good's Syndrome. At the onset of neutropenia, immunoglobulins were normal: IgA, 2.67 g/L; IgG, 12.90 g/L; IgM, 0.90 g/L. Peripheral blood flow cytometry demonstrated a normal number of T cells in peripheral blood with a CD4: CD8 ratio of 1 and normal CD19+ B cell population. Additionally, electromyography (EMG) did not show evidence of myasthenia gravis and serology for HIV, HBV, HCV, and TB was negative.

The patient was readmitted for a second time to the hospital with febrile neutropenia. He received IVIg 1 g/kg for 2 days as well as G-CSF 300 ug subcutaneously for 5 days (Figure 2). However, there was no response and the neutrophil count remained $<0.1 \times 10^9$/L. Therefore, the patient was started on cyclosporine 75 mg BID (Figure 2). Due to persistent severe neutropenia ($<0.1 \times 10^9$/L), the patient was started on prednisone 1 mg/kg once daily. The trough cyclosporine level was 147 ug/L 4 days after starting cyclosporine. The dose of cyclosporine was then increased to 100 mg BID (Figure 2). We used a target cyclosporine level of 200 to 400 ug/L. A second course of G-CSF was started. His neutrophil count normalized, however he developed severe thrombocytopenia (Figure 2).

The patient's thrombocytopenia was also thought to be immune-mediated and therefore he was started on eltrombopag 75 mg once daily (Figure 2). He responded well to eltrombopag, reaching a platelet count of 50×10^9/L. The patient's prednisone was tapered off. Eltrombopag was also tapered off and the patient was discharged home on only cyclosporine.

Despite cyclosporine treatment, he was readmitted to the hospital for the third time with febrile neutropenia undetectable neutrophil count in keeping with relapsed PWCA. He was then started on IVIg 1 g/kg for two days and supportive G-CSF with good response and his neutrophil count normalized (Figure 2). He was discharged home on cyclosporine 100 mg BID.

Although his cyclosporine level was in the target range of 200 to 400 ug/L, the patient developed worsening acute kidney injury. The cyclosporine dose was further reduced to 50 mg BID. However, his creatinine continued to rise despite a 50% reduction in his cyclosporine dose. At this point, the patient had been on cyclosporine for 5 months and a response was seen in his counts. As such, cyclosporine was discontinued due to worsening kidney function. Unfortunately, the patient's kidney function did not normalize and his counts dropped. He was started on dapsone 100 mg once daily followed by danazol 200 mg BID (Figure 2), which are both used for the management of refractory immune thrombocytopenia [14]. Dapsone and danazol were used as immunosuppressive therapies to target his immune cytopenias. However, his cytopenias continued to worsen and he was admitted to the hospital with weakness and febrile neutropenia. Despite treatment with dapsone, danazol, IVIg, and G-CSF his PWCA did not respond to any of these therapies and he died from sepsis and multiorgan failure.

3. Discussion

Thymomas are rare epithelial tumors that commonly present with paraneoplastic syndromes, with up to 50% of thymoma patients presenting with associated immunodeficiencies and autoimmune phenomena [15]. A recent systematic review reports estimates of common paraneoplastic syndromes in thymoma patients including myasthenia gravis (63%), pure red cell aplasia (7.7%) and hypogammaglobulinemia referred to as Good's syndrome (6%) [16]. However, PWCA is a rare disorder with only a few existing case reports. The etiology underlying PWCA remains elusive, although an autoimmune origin with dysregulated production of cytokines and antibody-mediated destruction of myelomonocytic precursor cells is speculated [7]. The severe neutropenia in these patients increases the risk of recurrent life-threatening infections and can even result in mortality. Our patient did not have any prior history of myasthenia gravis and his EMG testing was negative for any neuromuscular disorder. His blood work showed only PWCA and immune thrombocytopenia, with no evidence of hypogammaglobulinemia. Although most previous case reports have described PWCA at the time of thymoma diagnosis, our patient's first evidence of neutropenia first developed 2-weeks postthymectomy [17]. Here, we have reviewed and summarized several case reports for PWCA associated with thymoma (Table 2). However, to our knowledge, this is the first report of immune dysregulation with PWCA and immune thrombocytopenia post thymoma resection.

Each of the cases reported in Table 2 had the presence of thymoma and PWCA similar to our case presented here. In keeping with previous studies, the mean age was 62 (range of 36 to 76 years) with nine females and nine males [27]. Of the 18 cases examined, only 7 reported comorbidities including myasthenia gravis, autoimmune thyroiditis, type 1 diabetes, inflammatory bowel disease, clotting factor deficiencies or even hematological cancers like leukemia. In our case presented here, the patient had many more comorbid conditions than previous case reports.

The thymoma histology of cases examined in Table 2 varied widely, with type A being the most common. In our case report, the patient's thymoma type was classified as type B1. The WHO thymoma classification categories carry prognostic significance for patients. Reports show that those diagnosed with Type A and Type AB have 100% and 90% survival after 15 years, respectively. Types B1, B2, and B3

Table 1: Complete blood count values prethymectomy, postthymectomy, and at the onset of thrombocytopenia.

Value	Prethymectomy	Postthymectomy	At onset of thrombocytopenia	Ref. range
WBC	11.5*	3.4*	3.1*	$4.0–11.0 \times 10^9/L$
RBC	4.50	4.28	2.46*	$4.0–5.5 \times 10^{12}/L$
HGB	118*	114*	76*	135–170 g/L
HCT	0.364*	0.352*	0.227*	0.380–0.500 L/L
MCV	80.9	82.2	92.3	80–100 fL
MCH	26.2	26.6	30.9	25–34 pg
MCHC	324	324	335	300–365 g/L
RDW	16.9*	16.7*	21.1*	11.5–15.5%
PLT	231	164	11*	$150–400 \times 10^9/L$
Neutrophils	2.0	<0.1*	1.2*	$2.0–7.5 \times 10^9/L$

WBC: white blood cell; RBC: red blood cell; HGB: hemoglobin; HCT: hematocrit; MCV: mean corpuscular volume; MCH: mean corpuscular hemoglobin; MCHC: mean corpuscular hemoglobin concentration; RDW: red blood cell distribution width; PLT: platelet count.

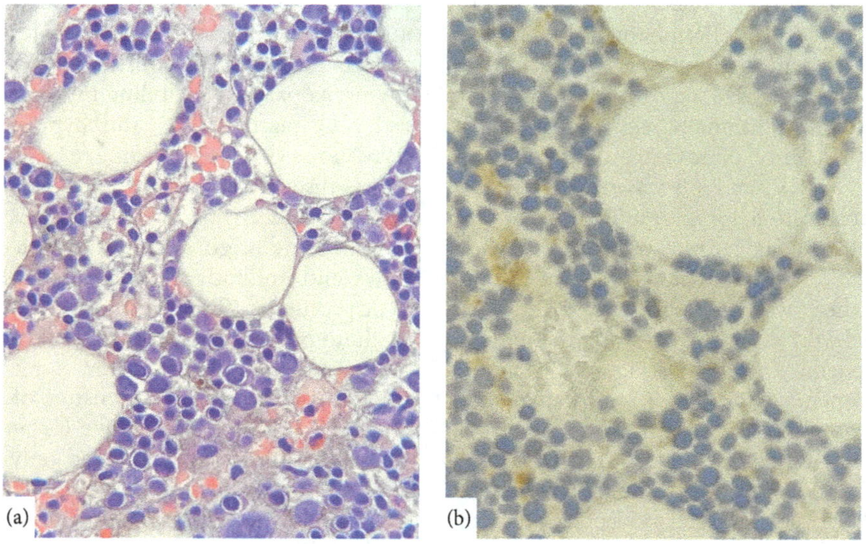

Figure 1: Granulocytic hypoplasia. Bone marrow core biopsy shows complete absence of granulocytic precursor elements on Hematoxylin/eosin staining (a) and confirmed by immunoperoxidase staining for myeloperoxidase (b). (40x objective).

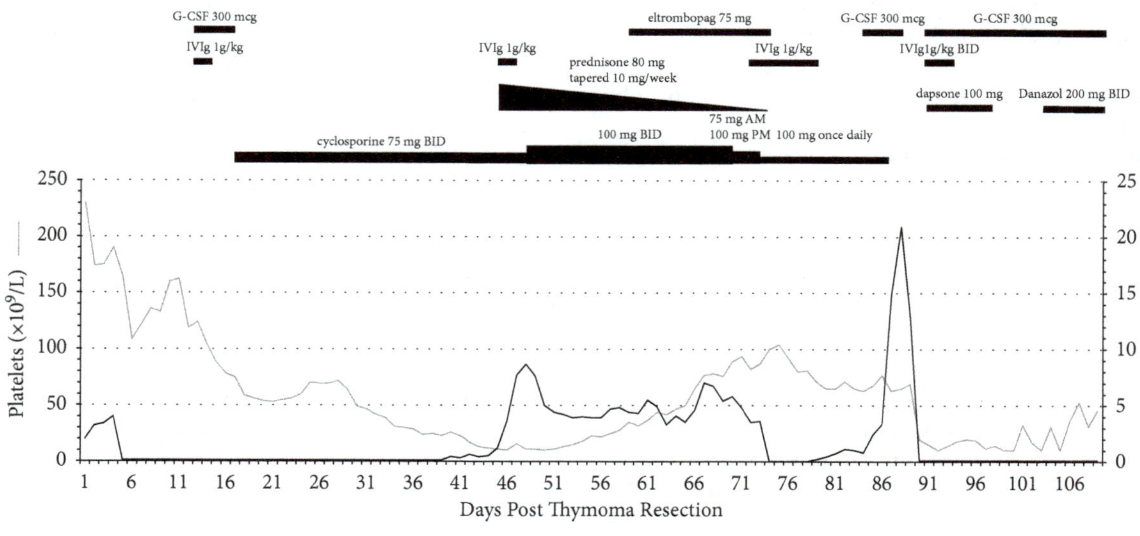

Figure 2: Trends in neutrophil and platelet counts following thymoma resection.

Table 2: Literature review of previous case reports for PWCA associated with thymoma. IVIg: Intravenous Immunoglobulins, G-CSF: Granulocyte Colony-Stimulating Factor.

Study	Ackland et al. 1988 [18]	Akinosoglou et al. 2014 [20]	Al-mohareb et al. 1992 [22]	Alvares et al. 2004 [21]	Degos et al. 1982 [8]	Desai et al. 2013 [23]	Fumeaux et al. 2003 [13]	Jethava et al. 2011 [24]
Patient age (gender)	70 (female)	70 (female)	70 (male)	59 (male)	52 (female)	73 (male)	76 (female)	45 (male)
Patient presentation	Neutropenia Pharyngeal candidiasis Hypogammaglobulinemia Sepsis (*Pseudomonas aeruginosa*) Recurrent upper respiratory infections	Fatigue Persistent fevers Disseminated Cryptococcosis	Fatigue Sweating Chest pain Productive cough Intermittent fevers	Fever Fatigue Aphthous oral ulcers	Mild anemia Agranulocytosis Hypogammaglobulinemia Severe recurrent infections (bacterial, mycotic, and parasitic)	Vomiting Dyspnea Dysphagia Atrial Fibrillation Abdominal Pain Oral candidiasis Productive cough	Fever Fatigue Diarrhea Weakness Weight loss Odynophagia Hyperglycemia	Hypoxia Dyspnea Oral ulcers Tachycardia Febrile neutropenia Factor XI deficiency Respiratory infection with lung nodules (*Aspergillus fumigatus*)
Comorbidities	Myasthenia gravis	Obesity Dyslipidemia	—	—	—	—	Autoimmune thyroiditis type 1 diabetes	Factor XI deficiency
Histology of thymoma (type)	Metastatic spindle cell thymoma	Spindle cell thymoma (type A)	Spindle cell thymoma (type A)	Spindle cell thymoma (type A)	Spindle cell thymoma (type A)	Thymic carcinoma (type C)	Malignant cortical thymoma (type B2)	Thymoma (type AB)
Management (chronological)	Broad spectrum antibiotics Pyridostigmine IVIg 0.4 g/kg/day	Broad spectrum antibiotics Amphotericin B G-CSF IVIg dexamethasone Acyclovir Fluconazole	Broad spectrum antibiotics Antifungal agents Antiviral medications	Broad spectrum antibiotics Antifungal agents G-CSF (5 μg/kg/day) thymectomy Plasmapheresis Campath-1H 100 mg Cyclosporin 150 mg bid Mycophenolate mofetil 500 mg bid	Thymectomy Plasmapheresis Prednisone 1.5 mg/kg/day Cyclophosphamide 2 mg/kg/day	—	IVIg 15 g/day G-CSF thymectomy Cyclosporin a 3 mg/kg/d (in two doses Prednisone 1 mg/kg/d	Broad spectrum IV antibiotics & antifungals IVIg 0.4 g/kg/d G-CSF cyclosporine A Thymectomy
Mortality outcome	Died	Survived	Died	Survived	Survived	n/a	Survived	Survived
Comments					Plasmapheresis Appeared to be the only effective treatment		IVIg and G-CSF were only effective when given with methylprednisone after thymectomy	
Study	Kobayashi et al. 2019 [25]	Mathieson et al. 1990 [19]	Okusu et al. 2016 [26]	Oyenuga et al. 2021 [17]	Uy et al. 2019 [7]	Yip et al. 1996 (1/2) [12]	Yip et al. 1996 (2/2) [12]	

Table 2: Continued.

Study	Ackland et al. 1988 [18]	Akinosoglou et al. 2014 [20]	Al-mohareb et al. 1992 [22]	Alvares et al. 2004 [21]	Degos et al. 1982 [8]	Desai et al. 2013 [23]	Fumeaux et al. 2003 [13]	Jethava et al. 2011 [24]
Patient age (gender)	63 (male)	36 (female)	72 (male)	64 (male)	65 (female)	51 (male)	52 (female)	
Patient presentation	Febrile neutropenia Hypogammaglobulinemia	Diarrhea Gingivitis Oral ulcers Abdominal pain Febrile neutropenia	Sore throat Myocarditis Oral candidiasis Febrile neutropenia Atrioventricular block Hypogammaglobulinemia Respiratory infection (*Pseudomonas aeruginosa*)	nasal congestion Cough Orthopnea Diverticulitis Gram-negative septic shock Recurrent colitis Hypogamma-globulinemia	Night sweats Oral candidiasis Febrile neutropenia Truncal morbilliform rash Hypogammaglobulinemia Lung nodules (likely respiratory fungal infections)	Night sweats Febrile neutropenia Hypogamma-globulinemia Upper respiratory tract infections	Lethargy Oral ulcers Sore throat Weight loss Oral candidiasis Febrile neutropenia	
Comorbidities	—	Myasthenia gravis	—	Inflammatory bowel disease	—	—	—	
Histology of thymoma (type)	Spindle cell thymoma (type A)	Thymoma (lymphoepithelial type)	Thymoma (type 2B)	Thymoma (type 2B)	Thymoma (mixed type a and B2)	Spindle cell thymoma (type A)	Spindle cell thymoma (type A)	
Management (chronological)	Oral garenoxacin (by primary care physician) G-CSF 5 μg/kg/d cyclosporin a 150 mg/d Thymectomy	Plasmapheresis Prednisolone 70 mg every other day Azathioprine 2.5 mg/kg/d	Antibiotic therapy IVIg	Thymectomy IVIg	IVIg G-CSF thymectomy Cyclosporin (target blood level 200–400 ng/mL)	Broad spectrum antibiotics Prednisone 100 mg/d G-CSF 150–600 μg/d IVIg	GM-CSF 5–10 μg/kg/d methylprednisolone 1 g/d Plasmapheresis Thymectomy IVIg 500 mg/kg/d cyclophosphamide 100 mg/d	
Mortality outcome	Survived	Survived	Died	Survived	Survived	Survived	Died	
Comments		Prednisone and azathioprine were the successful treatments	No specific treatment for PWCA since the patient developed AV block and shock			Thymectomy had no effect		

have been associated with 90%, 60% and 40% survival after 20 years, respectively [28]. However these estimates may differ in cases where patients with thymoma also develop PWCA.

A variety of different management options have been attempted in patients with PWCA and thymoma. A common approach involves immunosuppression with treatments including IVIg, cyclosporine, cyclophosphamide, azathioprine, corticosteroids, and mycophenolate mofetil (Table 1). Patients also commonly receive antibiotics, antifungals, and antivirals for comorbid infections. Additionally, G-CSF and alemtuzumab are often used to stimulate granulocyte or lymphocyte counts. Lastly, thymectomy and plasmapheresis have also been shown to raise granulocyte levels [8, 21].

Of the 18 cases with PWCA and thymoma examined here (including our case), 7 patients died. With our patient, treatment with IVIg, G-CSF, prednisone, and cyclosporine were unsuccessful. He ultimately died from sepsis and multiorgan failure, which illustrates the poor prognosis of PWCA. His age, comorbidities, and immune thrombocytopenia may have decreased his chance of survival. Despite this patient's poor clinical course, treatment with cyclosporine as a first-line therapy with concomitant use of G-CSF is still recommended. These two therapies were shown to be effective in previous case reports and initially restored our patient's granulocytic counts [29]. In the future, consideration should also be given to alternative immunosuppressive therapies such as rituximab, azathioprine or alemtuzumab, all of which were shown to have some effectiveness in treating PWCA [29, 30]. We also recommend long-term follow-up with thymoma patients given the high risk of relapse of PWCA as with our patient.

4. Conclusion

Our case report identifies a complex case of PWCA and immune thrombocytopenia postthymoma resection. This patient was treated with IVIg, G-CSF, prednisone, and cyclosporine with a mixed response. Our review of the literature and the current case highlights the high mortality rate observed in patients with PWCA. Future studies are needed to compare the clinical course of thymoma patients with and without PWCA to better understand the burden of disease and the utility of therapeutic intervention in management of PWCA.

Consent

Informed consent was obtained from the patient to publish this report.

Authors' Contributions

Siavash Piran is a Hematologist who obtained consent from the patient and prepared the case presentation section. Michael Youssef, Tyler W. Stratton, and Reid C. Gallant identified relevant case reports in the literature and conducted a literature review (Table 1). Together they completed the Abstract, Introduction, and Discussion sections of the manuscript. Daniel Y. Li is the pathologist who interpreted the patient's bone marrow biopsy results and provided the biopsy image. Christine Young provided details on the patient's medications administered throughout his hospital stay and outpatient clinic care. Michael Youssef, Tyler W. Stratton, and Reid C. Gallant contributed equally to this work.

References

[1] K. Harris, D. Elsayegh, B. Azab, H. Alkaied, and M. Chalhoub, "Thymoma calcification: is it clinically meaningful?" *World Journal of Surgical Oncology*, vol. 9, no. 1, p. 95, 2011.

[2] E. A. Engels, "Epidemiology of thymoma and associated malignancies," *Journal of Thoracic Oncology*, vol. 5, no. 10, pp. S260–S265, 2010.

[3] A. Marx, J. K. C. Chan, J.-M. Coindre et al., "The 2015 world health organization classification of tumors of the thymus: continuity and changes," *Journal of Thoracic Oncology*, vol. 10, no. 10, pp. 1383–1395, 2015.

[4] B. Sperling, J. Marschall, R. Kennedy, P. Pahwa, and R. Chibbar, "Thymoma: a review of the clinical and pathological findings in 65 cases," *Canadian Journal of Surgery Journal Canadien de Chirurgie*, vol. 46, no. 1, pp. 37–42, 2003.

[5] T. Luo, H. Zhao, and X. Zhou, "The clinical features, diagnosis and management of recurrent thymoma," *Journal of Cardiothoracic Surgery*, vol. 11, no. 1, p. 140, 2016.

[6] C. Bernard, H. Frih, F. Pasquet et al., "Thymoma associated with autoimmune diseases: 85 cases and literature review," *Autoimmunity Reviews*, vol. 15, no. 1, pp. 82–92, 2016.

[7] K. Uy, E. Levin, P. Mroz, F. Li, and S. Shah, "A rare complication of thymoma: pure white cell aplasia in good's syndrome," *Case Reports in Hematology*, vol. 2019, pp. 1–4, Article ID 1024670, 2019.

[8] L. Degos, A. Faille, M. Housset, L. Boumsell, C. Rabian, and T. Parames, "Syndrome of neutrophil agranulocytosis, hypogammaglobulinemia, and thymoma," *Blood*, vol. 60, no. 4, pp. 968–972, 1982.

[9] G. Marinone, B. Roncoli, and M. G. Marinone, "Pure white cell aplasia," *Seminars in Hematology*, vol. 28, no. 4, pp. 298–302, 1991.

[10] A. M. Risitano, C. Selleri, B. Serio et al., "Alemtuzumab is safe and effective as immunosuppressive treatment for aplastic anaemia and single-lineage marrow failure: a pilot study and a survey from the EBMT WPSAA," *British Journal of Haematology*, vol. 148, no. 5, pp. 791–796, 2010.

[11] S. Iida, T. Noda, S. Banno, M. Nitta, K. Takada, and M. Yamamoto, "Pure white cell aplasia (PWCA) with an inhibitor against colony-forming unit of granulocyte-macrophage (CFU-GM)," *Japanese Journal of Clinical Hematology*, vol. 31, no. 10, pp. 1726–1730, 1990.

[12] D. Yip, J. E. J. Rasko, C. Lee, H. Kronenberg, and B. O'Neill, "Thymoma and agranulocytosis: two case reports and literature review," *British Journal of Haematology*, vol. 95, no. 1, pp. 52–56, 1996.

[13] Z. Fumeaux, P. Beris, B. Borisch et al., "Complete remission of pure white cell aplasia associated with thymoma, autoimmune thyroiditis and type 1 diabetes," *European Journal of Haematology*, vol. 70, no. 3, pp. 186–189, 2003.

[14] A. Cuker and C. E. Neunert, "How I treat refractory immune thrombocytopenia," *Blood*, vol. 128, no. 12, pp. 1547–1554, 2016.
[15] R. F. Riedel and W. R. Burfeind, "Thymoma: benign appearance, malignant potential," *The Oncologist*, vol. 11, no. 8, pp. 887–894, 2006.
[16] J. Zhao, V. Bhatnagar, L. Ding et al., "A systematic review of paraneoplastic syndromes associated with thymoma: treatment modalities, recurrence, and outcomes in resected cases," *The Journal of Thoracic and Cardiovascular Surgery*, vol. 160, no. 1, pp. 306–314, 2020.
[17] M. Oyenuga, S. Shaikh, B. Harris, J. Sinha, and A. Lacasse, "Recurrent neutropenia and chronic diarrhea following thymectomy: the good, the bad, and the ugly," *Journal of Community Hospital Internal Medicine Perspectives*, vol. 11, no. 2, pp. 263–265, 2021.
[18] S. P. Ackland, M. E. Bur, S. S. Adler, M. Robertson, and J. M. Baron, "White blood cell aplasia associated with thymoma," *American Journal of Clinical Pathology*, vol. 89, no. 2, pp. 260–263, 1988.
[19] P. W. Mathieson, J. H. O'Neill, S. T. S. Durrant, S. J. Henderson, P. J. Green, and J. Newsom-Davis, "Antibody-mediated pure neutrophil aplasia, recurrent myasthenia gravis and previous thymoma: case report and literature review," *QJM: International Journal of Medicine*, vol. 74, no. 1, pp. 57–61, 1990.
[20] K. Akinosoglou, M. Melachrinou, D. Siagris et al., "Good's syndrome and pure white cell aplasia complicated by cryptococcus infection: a case report and review of the literature," *Journal of Clinical Immunology*, vol. 34, no. 3, pp. 283–288, 2014.
[21] C. L. Alvares, D. Svasti-Salee, M. Rowley, E. C. Gordon-Smith, and J. C. W. Marsh, "Remission induced by campath-1H for thymoma-associated agranulocytosis," *Annals of Hematology*, vol. 83, no. 6, pp. 398–400, 2004.
[22] F. Al-Mohareb, "Pure neutrophil aplasia associated with thymoma," *Annals of Saudi Medicine*, vol. 12, no. 6, pp. 571–574, 1992.
[23] P. C. Desai and P. Jones, "Pure white cell aplasia in a patient with thymic carcinoma," *Blood*, vol. 122, no. 8, p. 1340, 2013.
[24] Y. Jethava, J. Alamelu, S. Rangarajan, L. Lang-Lazdunski, J. van der Walt, and P. Fields, "Acquired agranulocytosis and factor XI deficiency in association with thymoma," *Journal of Clinical Oncology*, vol. 29, no. 20, pp. e604–e606, 2011.
[25] Y. Kobayashi, K. Ando, T. Hata et al., "Complete remission of pure white cell aplasia associated with thymoma after thymectomy and cyclosporine administration," *International Journal of Hematology*, vol. 109, no. 3, pp. 346–350, 2019.
[26] T. Okusu, T. Sato, Y. Ogata et al., "Good's syndrome accompanied by agranulocytosis following a rapid clinical course," *Internal Medicine*, vol. 55, no. 5, pp. 537–540, 2016.
[27] M. Zaman, A. Huissoon, M. Buckland et al., "Clinical and laboratory features of seventy-eight UK patients with Good's syndrome (thymoma and hypogammaglobulinaemia)," *Clinical and Experimental Immunology*, vol. 195, no. 1, pp. 132–138, 2018.
[28] Springer International Publishing, *TNM System Information. American College of Surgeons, Chicago, Illinois AJCC Cancer Staging Manual*, Springer International Publishing, New York, NY, USA, 8th edition, 2017.
[29] C. Roberto, A. Balerdi, L. I. Oleaga, M. Moreno, and J. Arzuaga-Mendez, "Pure white cell aplasia an exceptional condition in the inmunological conundrum of thymomas: responses to inmunosupresion and literature review," *Authorea Preparation*, pp. 1–5, 2021.
[30] G. Chakupurakal, R. J. A. Murrin, and J. R. Neilson, "Prolonged remission of pure white cell aplasia (PWCA), in a patient with CLL, induced by rituximab and maintained by continuous oral cyclosporin," *European Journal of Haematology*, vol. 79, no. 3, pp. 271–273, 2007.

8

Daratumumab, Lenalidomide and Dexamethasone (DRD), an Active Regimen in the Treatment of Immunosuppression-Associated Plasmablastic Lymphoma (PBL) in the Setting of Gorham's Lymphangiomatosis: Review of the Literature

Matthew Lee,[1] Beth A. Martin,[2] and Haifaa Abdulhaq[3]

[1]*UCSF Fresno, Department of Internal Medicine, Fresno, CA, USA*
[2]*Stanford University, Division of Hematology, Stanford, CA, USA*
[3]*UCSF Fresno, Division of Hematology and Oncology, Fresno, CA, USA*

Correspondence should be addressed to Haifaa Abdulhaq; haifaa.abdhulhaq@ucsf.edu

Academic Editor: Håkon Reikvam

Characterized by an aggressive course with a poor overall survival due to treatment refractoriness, plasmablastic lymphoma (PBL) is a rare variant of diffuse large cell B cell lymphoma. Gorham's lymphangiomatosis or Gorham–Stout disease (GSD) is a rare skeletal condition of unknown etiology characterized by progressive bone loss and nonmalignant proliferation of vascular and lymphatic channels within the affected bone. Neither disease has a standard of care. We present a 23-year-old HIV-negative woman with GSD, managed medically with octreotide and sirolimus, who developed PBL. After progressing on V-EPOCH (bortezomib, etoposide, vincristine, cyclophosphamide, doxorubicin, and prednisone), she was treated with daratumumab, lenalidomide, and dexamethasone (DRD) therapy and achieved complete remission after two cycles with progression after eight cycles. This is a report of treatment of PBL with DRD therapy. Clinical investigations of the DRD regimen in PBL in conjunction with other agents to improve both depth and durability of response are warranted.

1. Introduction

Plasmablastic lymphoma (PBL) is highly associated with a compromised immune system, with the majority of the cases found in HIV-positive individuals. HIV-negative disease occurs with a slight male predominance (male-to-female ratio of 1.7), a median age of 55 years, oral mucosal tropism, and is associated with a worse overall median survival [1–3]. Among this population, apparent immunocompetence exists in 80%, with the remainder having a concurrent lymphoproliferative or autoimmune disorder. Approximately 10% developed PBL after receiving a solid organ transplant [4, 5]. Importantly, Epstein–Barr virus (EBV) positivity is found in approximately half of HIV-negative cases. Both HIV and EBV-negative diseases are also associated with a decreased event-free survival [2, 3].

Plasmacytic differentiation, CD38+, high MYC expression secondary to translocation (8; 14), high Ki-67 activity, positive MUM-1, and absence of B cell markers such as CD20 are the key features of the histology of PBL [4, 6]. Distinguishing PBL from plasmablastic myeloma is difficult [7, 8]. PDL1 staining is positive in 25% of tumor cells, and PD1 staining is positive in the majority of infiltrating cells [2]. Currently, there is no standard treatment regimen for PBL. Dose-adjusted EPOCH or V-EPOCH is often utilized [9].

While the exact mechanism of GSD development is unknown, lymphangiogenic growth factors may be drivers [10, 11]. Although the majority of patients are younger than

40 years of age, no genetic predisposition has been found. GSD occurs in both genders and at all ages. Any bone can be involved with the most common sites being the hip and shoulders. The rarity of the disease and the limitation of treatment data to case series confine the standard of care to supportive surgical intervention and medical management. Medical therapy primarily utilizes inhibitors of lymphatic endothelial cell markers, such as sirolimus.

We present a case of PBL associated with sirolimus in a patient with GSD who achieved a complete response to treatment with daratumumab, lenalidomide, and dexamethasone.

1.1. Case Presentation. The patient was a 23-year-old Hispanic female in whom GSD was diagnosed at age 5 when she was found to have an absent left clavicle. Her manifestations of GSD were lymphedema of left upper extremity, resorption of the left clavicle, scapular head and humerus, chylothoraxes requiring chest tubes, and recurrent pericardial effusions requiring a window. Treatment with sirolimus and octreotide, for nearly 3 years, controlled lymphedema and effusions.

She developed pneumonia and hypoxic respiratory failure which required intubation. No oropharyngeal lesions were detected. CT scan of the chest, abdomen, and pelvis showed markedly enlarged supraclavicular, mediastinal, left axillary, and thoracic wall conglomerate, as well as enlargement of the thyroid with a significant mass effect on the trachea. Due to critical illness, biopsy was limited to a fine needle aspiration (FNA) of a left axillary lymph node and revealed sheets of cells with plasma cast and revealed sheets of cells with plasmablastic morphology. Immunohistochemical stains showed that the malignant cells were kappa restricted with MYC overexpression (>80%) and MUM-1 and CD 138 expression, Ki-67 > 90%. The cells were negative for CD20, CD30, CD3, ALK, BCL6, BCL2, and HHV8. Notably, EBV in situ hybridization was negative (Figure 1). PD1 and PDL1 stainings were not performed. By serology and PCR on blood, HIV, EBV, and human herpes virus 8 (HHV8) were negative.

Flow cytometry from FNA revealed an abnormal population of CD45-negative events, expressing bright CD38 and partial dim CD20. No definite surface light chain expression was detected. CD19, CD5, CD10, and any T cell antigens were not coexpressed.

Fluorescence in situ hybridization (FISH) was positive for MYC gene rearrangement t(8; 14) and negative for both BCL2 and BCL6 translocation.

PET/CT revealed hypermetabolic lymphadenopathy above and below the diaphragm, extensive conglomerate mass of the chest wall, left upper extremity, mediastinum, and left breast, and hypermetabolic involvement of the thyroid gland bilaterally with narrowing of the trachea. No bone lesions were found. SUV ranged from 4 to 12.8 with mean 9.4 and median 10.1 (Figure 2). Given the overall features of plasmablastic morphology and immunophenotype, nodal involvement without bone lesions, PBL was favored over plasmablastic myeloma.

Sirolimus was discontinued. Dose-adjusted V-EPOCH was initiated and was complicated by neutropenic fever despite high-dose granulocyte colony stimulating factor support. Cycle 2 of V-EPOCH was complicated by small bowel obstruction, prolonged neutropenia, and slow functional recovery. Repeat CT of the chest, abdomen, and pelvis revealed progression of disease in the small bowel and peritoneum. Treatment with lenalidomide, dexamethasone, and daratumumab as per the DRD regimen was initiated [12].

Repeat PET-CT after 2 cycles of DRD showed significant improvement in the size of the nodes and a metabolic complete response in all nodes (Deauville 2) (Figure 3). In addition, the DRD regimen controlled her GSD-associated lymphedema and effusions.

Autologous stem cell transplantation (ASCT) was considered. After 8 monthly cycles of DRD, PBL progressed. No IVIG was given. Standard dose carfilzomib was added to the regimen for one cycle without improvement. ICE (ifosfamide, carboplatin, and etoposide) regimen was initiated without improvement. She expired 13 months after diagnosis.

2. Discussion

This patient had two diseases that required active management: GSD and HIV-negative and EBV-negative immunosuppression-associated PBL. As stated above, both HIV-negative and EBV-negative statuses have been independently linked to worse overall survival [2, 3].

Plasmablastic lymphoma is a rare disease which makes up approximately 2% of HIV-associated lymphomas. The incidence of the disease is unknown, and it has been reported in patients of all ages.

Review of the database from eighteen Surveillance, Epidemiology, and End Results (SEER) registries showed median age at diagnosis was 52 years with male predominance (81.9%) and majority of patients were non-Hispanics (76.6%). Patients were slightly more frequently diagnosed with advanced stage (III-IV) (59.0%). Extranodal presentation was more common than nodal (54.8% vs. 45.2%). Oral and gastrointestinal (GI) sites were the most frequent primary extranodal locations (23% and 19.4%, respectively). Oral primary location was inversely associated with the presence of B symptoms and advanced Ann Arbor stage [13].

PBL in HIV-negative patients is more heterogeneous in sites of involvement with advanced clinical stage, B symptoms, and bone marrow involvement being less common (25%) than in HIV-positive patients.

The specific pathogenesis of PBL is not well understood, and the cell of origin is thought to be the plasmablast, an activated B cell that has undergone somatic hypermutation and class switching recombination and is in the process of becoming a plasma cell. Recent studies have identified the presence of *MYC* gene rearrangements in addition to the association with EBV infection as important pathogenic mechanisms [4].

EBV infection is associated with prevention of apoptosis in B cells by several mechanisms related to EBV antigens.

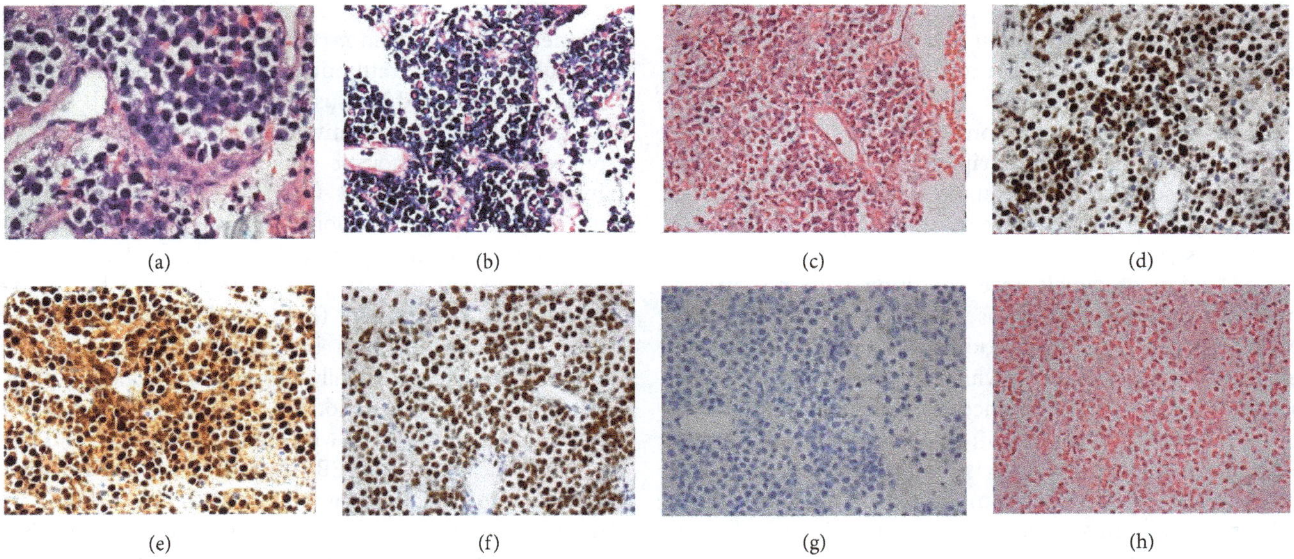

FIGURE 1: Pathology slides. (a) H&E stain of core biopsy. (b) High Kappa expression. (c) Negative lambda expression. (d) Positive cMYC expression. (e) Positive MUM-1 expression. (f) High Ki-67 expression. (g) Negative CD20 expression. (h) Negative EBER ISH.

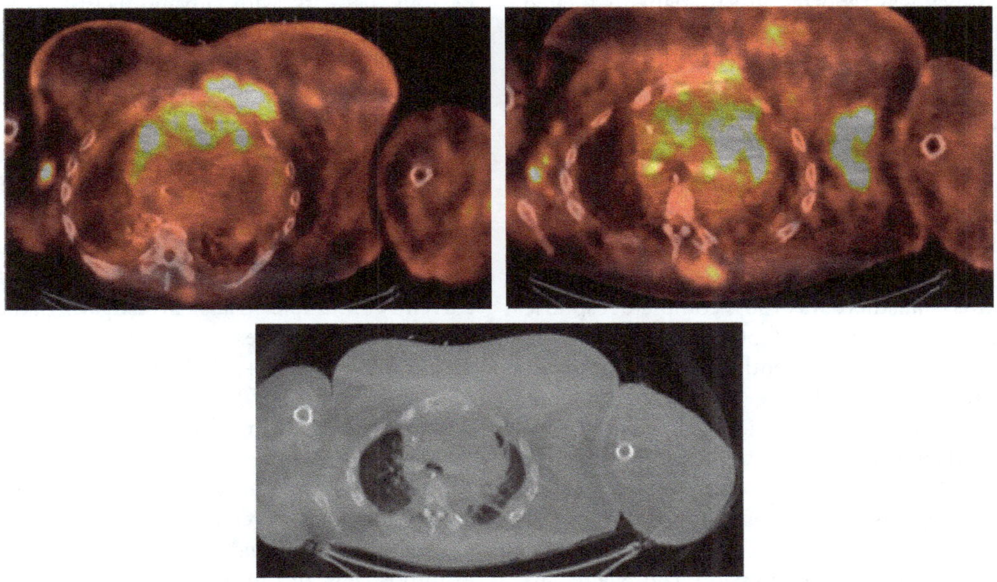

FIGURE 2: Initial PET/CT showing significant hypermetabolic activity above the diaphragm specifically located in the L axillary, mediastinal, and thoracic wall conglomerate.

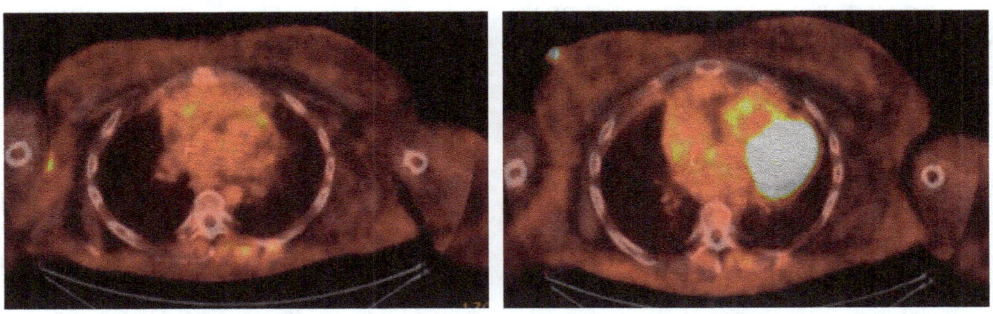

FIGURE 3: PET/CT after 2 rounds of DRD therapy showing significant improvement in hypermetabolic activity seen in previous imaging consistent with complete response (Deauville 2).

MYC dysregulation mediated by translocation or amplification may cause plasmablast development and prevent further differentiation. *MYC* translocations may allow PBL cells to escape apoptosis [4].

Finally, recurrent mutations in PRDM1, a gene that encodes the plasma cell transcription factor Blimp1 protein, have been described. These mutations in PRDM1 could alter the regulation of different targets, including *MYC*, in these lymphomas [13].

GSD is an extremely rare condition with no current consensus on management, as options are limited to case reports. One of the complications of the disease is the development of a chylothorax, which has a reported mortality rate of as high as 64% with medical management and 36% with surgical treatment [14, 15], and can result in significant morbidity if chronic drainage is required. Thalidomide is a known treatment for GSD complicated by the chylothorax and for multiple myeloma, thus making imides, including lenalidomide, a rational option [16–18].

PBL is a difficult condition to treat with a poor overall survival of 6–19 months and without standard treatment regimens [3, 19–21].

Improved survival was reported in PBL patients treated with chemotherapy recently. The 3-year and 5-year overall survival (OS) rates of treated PBL patients in SEER registries were 54% and 52.8%. HIV status did not affect survival outcomes in unadjusted and adjusted analyses [22].

In a study of 135 PBL patients reported by the Lymphoma Study Association (LYSA), 80% of patients received chemotherapy and their median OS was 32 months [23].

V-EPOCH has been associated with high complete response (CR) rates and improved overall survival [2, 19]. In a case series by Dittus et al., there was 100% complete response rate and 2-year overall survival of 50% with V-EPOCH therapy [24]. ASCT and, more recently, chimeric antigen-receptor T cell therapy (CAR-T) are considered for consolidation [25, 26]. Single agent lenalidomide has been effective in case reports of PBL throughout the literature, most recently by Ando et al. [27–29]. A recent review of 173 patients with PBL supports a wide range of therapies. None received daratumumab [30].

Surface signaling molecule expression can yield opportunities for utilization of antibody or cell-based therapeutics: CD19 (CAR-T), CD38 (daratumumab, isatuximab, and CAR-T directed to CD38 or CD138), CD 30 (brentuximab vedotin, and CAR-T directed to CD30), and PD1/PDL1/PDL2 (checkpoint inhibitors) [26].

The strong CD38+ expression that could be responsive to daratumumab, as well as the potential for dual activity of lenalidomide in PBL and GSD, supported the use of the DRD regimen in this patient.

To our knowledge, there are no reported cases of attaining a complete response of PBL with DRD therapy. Eight cases of use of daratumumab in the treatment of plasmablastic neoplasms have been published. In one HIV-negative patient with plasmablastic myeloma, three cycles of daratumumab and CHOP (cyclophosphamide, doxorubicin, vincristine, and prednisone) resulted in a partial response [31]. The second patient, who had HIV-positive PBL, progressed after 8 cycles of EPOCH and remitted after 3 cycles of combination of dexamethasone, cisplatin, cytarabine (DHAP regimen), bortezomib, and daratumumab. ASCT and maintenance lenalidomide resulted in a sustained remission [32]. The third case presents a HIV-negative patient who developed PBL from chronic lymphocytic leukemia transformation. The patient underwent therapy with daratumumab and CHOP with only a transient response, thus unable to proceed to allogenic stem cell transplant (alloSCT) [33]. The fourth case presents a female with HIV-negative disease who received multiple lines of treatment (daEPOCH, ASCT, and DHAP) before achieving CR with bortezomib, lenalidomide, and daratumumab and eventually proceeding to alloSCT with a prolonged disease-free period [34]. Raychaudhuri et al. were unable to induce remission with salvage carfilzomib and DRD in a HIV-negative and EBV-negative patient, eventually proceeding to CAR-T therapy [25]. Roche et al. found that daratumumab as a single agent was an ineffective salvage therapy in 3 patients with PBL [35]. A clinical trial of daratumumab with dose-adjusted EPOCH is underway for HIV-associated and non-HIV-associated PBL by the AIDS Malignancy Consortium [36]. Ricker et al. described a case series of four patients with advanced PBL who received daratumumab in combination with chemotherapy. All four subjects had CR and three had a durable response of at least 8 months (range 8–17 months) [37]. Table 1 provides a summary of cases of PBL treated with daratumumab.

CD30 is a viable target for PBL as positive expression has been found in approximately 30–50% of PBL cases [8]. Two case reports of brentuximab vedotin use both leading to impressive tumor reduction but also fatal outcome due to tumor lysis syndrome and comorbidities [38, 39]. There are currently multiple trials investigating the use of EBV cytotoxic lymphocytes expressing CD30 chimeric receptors in the use of CD30+ Hodgkin's and non-Hodgkin's lymphomas (e.g., NCT01192464 and NCT02917083), with Ramos et al. showing durable responses in patients with refractory NHL [40].

In a study by Laurent et al. on 82 patients with PBL, nearly all cases expressed PDL1 and PD1 in the immune infiltrate, and one-quarter of them strongly expressed PDL1 in tumor cells and in immune cells. PD1/PDL1 were more overexpressed in the microenvironment in EBV^{+}PBL [2]. As a result, immunotherapy is emerging as a treatment option for this disease. In a report of salvage therapy with single agent nivolumab in a patient with PDL1+ PBL, treatment was used as a successful bridge to allogeneic stem cell transplant [41]. In another report of chemoresistant EBV + PBL, one patient treated with tislelizumab and lenalidomide, the treatment resulted in CR with total overall survival of 18 months [42].

CD19 CAR-T therapy was described in a case report about a patient with relapsed PBL who had complete response with axicabtagene ciloleucel at 4 months with an undetectable CD-19+ count 2 months after administration. Unfortunately, the patient relapsed at 5 months with loss of CAR T cell activity [25].

Stem cell transplantation in PBL has been assessed as either consolidation in chemotherapy sensitive disease or as

TABLE 1: Summary of reported uses of daratumumab in PBL.

Reference	HIV status	EBV status	Stage	Lines of tx before Dara	Prior SCT	Dara regimen	Outcome
Suarez et al. [31]	—	—	IV	0	n/a	Dara + CHOP	PD
Chikeka et al. [32]	+	+	IV	1	n/a	Dara + V + DHAP	CR-ASCT
Marvyin et al. [33]	—	n/a		0		Dara + CHOP	PD
Kathrotiya et al. [34]	—	+	IV	2	ASCT	Dara + VR	CR-AlloSCT
Raychaudhari et al. [25]	—	—	IV	2	n/a	DRD + carfilzomib	PD-CAR-T
Roché et al. [35]	—	—	IV	4	ASCT	Dara alone	PD
Roché et al. [35]	—	+	II	2	n/a	Dara alone	PD
Roché et al. [35]	—	—	II	1	ASCT	Dara alone	PD
Ricker et al. [37]	—	+	IV	0	n/a	Dara + EPOCH	CR
Ricker et al. [37]	+	+	IV	0	n/a	Dara + EPOCH	CR
Ricker et al. [37]	—	+	IV	0	n/a	Dara + EPOCH	CR
Ricker et al. [37]	—	—	IV	0	n/a	Dara + EPOCH	PD

CHOP, cyclophosphamide, hydroxydaunorubicin, vincristine, and prednisone; V, bortezomib; DHAP, dexamethasone, cytarabine, and cisplatin; VR, bortezomib, rituximab; PD, progressive disease; CR, complete response.

salvage therapy [43]. There are multiple case series reporting favorable response to ASCT. Liu et al. reported 4 cases of HIV-negative PBL undergoing ASCT in CR1 with sustained remission [3]. Cattaneo et al. treated 24 patients with ASCT with 7 relapsing at 2 years [44]. Although the data are extremely limited, long-term survivorship has been reported in alloSCT for PBL. Hamadani and Devine achieved CR in a HIV + PBL patient [45]. As reported earlier by Kathrotiya et al., the patient has been disease-free for almost 3 years after undergoing haploidentical alloSCT [34]. Rong et al. achieved complete remission in a HIV-negative and EBV-negative patient for 4 years after salvage alloSCT [46].

3. Conclusion

Based on this patient's experience, the DRD regimen has a significant activity in treatment of both PBL and GSD. The response and drug mechanisms suggest noncross resistance. We speculate that maximizing immunocompetency as soon as possible, e.g., by minimizing intensive corticosteroids and myelosuppressive chemotherapies after initial deep remission, may be a beneficial strategy. Furthermore, given that the DRD regimen is not readily available as an emergency intervention in the inpatient setting, we anticipate that an EPOCH-based regimen will remain as the preferred upfront induction regimen. We believe that testing DRD regimen in conjunction with other therapeutics such as checkpoint inhibitors, cellular therapeutics such as CAR-T, and/or stem cell transplantation with curative intent in PBL is warranted.

Disclosure

The abstract was submitted and presented at the Society of Hematologic Oncology 2020 Annual Meeting.

Authors' Contributions

Beth A. Martin and Haifaa Abdulhaq contributed equally to the manuscript.

Acknowledgments

The authors acknowledge Calvin Chen, pathologist at Community Regional Medical Center in Fresno, CA, for providing photos of the slides.

References

[1] J. J. Castillo, E. S. Winer, D. Stachurski et al., "HIV-negative plasmablastic lymphoma: not in the mouth," *Clinical Lymphoma Myeloma and Leukemia*, vol. 11, no. 2, pp. 185–189, 2011.

[2] C. Laurent, B. Fabiani, C. Do et al., "Immune-checkpoint expression in Epstein-Barr virus positive and negative plasmablastic lymphoma: a clinical and pathological study in 82 patients," *Haematologica*, vol. 101, no. 8, pp. 976–984, 2016.

[3] J. J. Liu, L. Zhang, E. Ayala et al., "Human immunodeficiency virus (HIV)-negative plasmablastic lymphoma: a single institutional experience and literature review," *Leukemia Research*, vol. 35, no. 12, pp. 1571–1577, 2011.

[4] J. J. Castillo, M. Bibas, and R. N. Miranda, "The biology and treatment of Plasmablastic lymphoma," *Blood*, vol. 125, no. 15, pp. 2323–2330, 2015.

[5] M. Liu, B. Liu, B. Liu et al., "Human immunodeficiency virus-negative plasmablastic lymphoma: a comprehensive analysis of 114 cases," *Oncology Reports*, vol. 33, no. 4, pp. 1615–1620, 2015.

[6] C.-C. Chang, X. Zhou, J. J. Taylor et al., "Genomic profiling of plasmablastic lymphoma using array comparative genomic hybridization (aCGH): revealing significant overlapping genomic lesions with diffuse large B-cell lymphoma," *Journal of Hematology and Oncology*, vol. 2, no. 1, Article ID 47, 2009.

[7] A. Valera, O. Balagué, L. Colomo et al., "IG/MYC rearrangements are the main cytogenetic alteration in plasmablastic lymphomas," *American Journal of Surgical Pathology* vol. 34, no. 11, pp. 1636–1694, 2010.

[8] F. Vega, C.-C. Chang, L. J. Medeiros et al., "Plasmablastic lymphomas and plasmablastic plasma cell myelomas have nearly identical immunophenotypic profiles," *Modern Pathology*, vol. 18, no. 6, pp. 806–815, 2005.

[9] J. J. Castillo, T. Guerrero-Garcia, F. Baldini et al., "Bortezomib plus EPOCH is effective as frontline treatment in patients with plasmablastic lymphoma," *British Journal of Haematology*, vol. 184, no. 4, pp. 679–682, 2019.

[10] L. W. Gorham and A. P. Stout, "Massive Osteolysis acute spontaneous absorption of bone, phantom bone, disappearing bone," *The Journal of Bone and Joint Surgery*, vol. 37, no. 5, pp. 985–1004, 1955.
[11] S. Schulte-Merker, A. Sabine, and T. V. Petrova, "Lymphatic vascular morphogenesis in development, physiology, and disease," *Journal of Cell Biology*, vol. 193, no. 4, pp. 607–618, 2011.
[12] M. A. Dimopoulos, A. Oriol, H. Nahi et al., "Daratumumab, lenalidomide, and dexamethasone for multiple myeloma," *The New England Journal of Medicine*, vol. 375, no. 14, pp. 1319–1331, 2016.
[13] S. Montes-Moreno, N. Martinez-Magunacelaya, T. Zecchini-Barrese et al., "Plasmablastic lymphoma phenotype is determined by genetic alterations in *MYC* and *PRDM1*," *Modern Pathology*, vol. 30, no. 1, pp. 85–94, 2017.
[14] M. L. H. Tie, G. A. Poland, and E. C. Rosenow, "Chylothorax in Gorham's syndrome," *Chest*, vol. 105, no. 1, pp. 208–213, 1994.
[15] S. Y. Yoo, J. M. Goo, and J.-G. Im, "Mediastinal lymphangioma and chylothorax: thoracic involvement of Gorham's disease," *Korean Journal of Radiology*, vol. 3, no. 2, pp. 130–132, 2002.
[16] J. Hagendoorn, T. I. Yock, I. H. M. Borel Rinkes, T. P. Padera, and D. H. Ebb, "Novel molecular pathways in Gorham disease: implications for treatment," *Pediatric Blood and Cancer*, vol. 61, no. 3, pp. 401–406, 2013.
[17] A. Daneshvar Kakhaki, K. Khodadad, S. Pejhan et al., "Gorham's disease with chest wall involvement, a case report and a review of the literature," *Iranian Red Crescent Medical Journal*, vol. 16, no. 11, Article ID e12180, 2014.
[18] R. Pauzner, H. Mayan, A. Waizman, J. Rozenman, and Z. Farfel, "Successful thalidomide treatment of persistent chylous pleural effusion," *Annals of Internal Medicine*, vol. 146, no. 1, pp. 75-76, 2007.
[19] Y. Koizumi, T. Uehira, Y. Ota et al., "Clinical and pathological aspects of human immunodeficiency virus-associated plasmablastic lymphoma: analysis of 24 cases," *International Journal of Hematology*, vol. 104, no. 6, pp. 669–681, 2016.
[20] S. M. Horwitz, A. D. Zelenetz, L. I. Gordon et al., "NCCN guidelines insights: non-Hodgkin's lymphomas, version 3.2016," *Journal of the National Comprehensive Cancer Network*, vol. 14, no. 9, pp. 1067–1079, 2016.
[21] E. Campo, S. H. Swerdlow, N. L. Harris, S. Pileri, H. Stein, and E. S. Jaffe, "The 2008 WHO classification of lymphoid neoplasms and beyond: evolving concepts and practical applications," *Blood*, vol. 117, no. 19, pp. 5019–5032, 2011.
[22] J. A. Florindez, J. P. Alderuccio, I. M. Reis, and I. S. Lossos, "Survival analysis in treated plasmablastic lymphoma patients: a population-based study," *American Journal of Hematology*, vol. 95, no. 11, pp. 1344–1351, 2020.
[23] E. Tchernonog, P. Faurie, P. Coppo et al., "Clinical characteristics and prognostic factors of plasmablastic lymphoma patients: analysis of 135 patients from the LYSA group," *Annals of Oncology*, vol. 28, no. 4, pp. 843–848, 2017.
[24] C. Dittus, N. Grover, S. Ellsworth, X. Tan, and S. I. Park, "Bortezomib in combination with dose-adjusted EPOCH etoposide, prednisone, vincristine, cyclophosphamide, and doxorubicin induces long-term survival in patients with plasmablastic lymphoma: a retrospective analysis," *Leukemia and Lymphoma*, vol. 59, no. 9, pp. 2121–2127, 2018.
[25] R. Raychaudhuri, J. Qualtieri, and A. L. Garfall, "Axicabtagene ciloleucel for CD19+ plasmablastic lymphoma," *American Journal of Hematology*, vol. 95, no. 1, pp. E28–E30, 2020.
[26] T. A. Guerrero-Garcia and J. J. Castillo, "Plasmablastic lymphoma and primary effusion lymphoma," in *Novel Therapeutics for Rare Lymphomas*, pp. 101–118, 1st edn. Springer, Berlin, Germany, 2020.
[27] J. M. Schmit, J. DeLaune, M. Norkin, and A. Grosbach, "A case of plasmablastic lymphoma achieving complete response and durable remission after lenalidomide-based therapy," *Oncology Research and Treatment*, vol. 40, no. 1-2, pp. 46–48, 2017.
[28] W. D. Marrero, A. Cruz-Chacón, C. Castillo, and F. Cabanillas, "Successful use of bortezomib-lenalidomide combination as treatment for a patient with plasmablastic lymphoma," *Clinical Lymphoma Myeloma and Leukemia*, vol. 18, no. 7, pp. e275–e277, 2018.
[29] K. Ando, Y. Imaizumi, Y. Kobayashi et al., "Bortezomib- and lenalidomide-based treatment of refractory plasmablastic lymphoma," *Oncology Research and Treatment*, vol. 43, no. 3, pp. 112–116, 2020.
[30] N. F. Makady, D. Ramzy, R. Ghaly, R. R. Abdel-Malek, and K. S. Shohdy, "The emerging treatment options of plasmablastic lymphoma: analysis of 173 individual patient outcomes," *Clinical Lymphoma Myeloma and Leukemia*, vol. 21, no. 3, pp. e255–e263, 2021.
[31] J. A. Suarez-Londono, A. Rohatgi, C. Antoine-Pepeljugoski, and M. J. Braunstein, "Aggressive presentation of plasmablastic myeloma," *BMJ Case Reports*, vol. 13, no. 4, Article ID e234436, 2020.
[32] I. Chikeka, M. Grossman, C. Deng, A. T. Jacob, and S. Husain, "Plasmablastic lymphoma in an HIV patient with cutaneous presentation: a case of remarkable remission in a typically refractory disease," *JAAD Case Reports*, vol. 6, no. 3, pp. 161–165, 2020.
[33] K. Marvyin, E. B. Tjønnfjord, U. M. Breland, and G. E. Tjønnfjord, "Transformation to plasmablastic lymphoma in CLL upon ibrutinib treatment," *BMJ Case Reports*, vol. 13, no. 9, Article ID e235816, 2020.
[34] M. Kathrotiya, V. S. Radhakrishnan, S. J. Bhave et al., "Relapsed plasmablastic lymphoma in a HIV-negative patient: pushing the envelope," *Clinical Case Reports*, vol. 9, no. 2, pp. 873–877, 2021.
[35] P. Roché, G. Venton, Y. Berda-Haddad et al., "Could daratumumab induce the maturation of plasmablasts in plasmablastic lymphoma?-potential therapeutic applications," *European Journal of Haematology*, vol. 106, no. 4, pp. 589–592, 2021.
[36] C. R. Tan, S. K. Barta, S. Y. Lensing, and A. Noy, "A multicenter, open-label feasibility study of daratumumab with dose-adjusted EPOCH in newly diagnosed plasmablastic lymphoma: AIDS malignancy consortium 105," *Blood*, vol. 134, no. Supplement_1, p. 1595, 2019.
[37] E. C. Ricker, Y. K. Ryu, and J. E. Amengual, "Daratumumab plus chemotherapy induces complete responses in a consecutive series of four patients with plasmablastic lymphoma," *Blood*, vol. 138, no. Supplement 1, p. 4573, 2021.
[38] B. M. Holderness, S. Malhotra, N. B. Levy, and A. V. Danilov, "Brentuximab vedotin demonstrates activity in a patient with plasmablastic lymphoma arising from a background of chronic lymphocytic leukemia," *Journal of Clinical Oncology*, vol. 31, no. 12, pp. e197–e199, 2013.

[39] D. Pretscher, A. Kalisch, M. Wilhelm, and J. Birkmann, “Refractory plasmablastic lymphoma—a review of treatment options beyond standard therapy,” *Annals of Hematology*, vol. 96, no. 6, pp. 967–970, 2017.

[40] C. A. Ramos, N. S. Grover, A. W. Beaven et al., “Anti-CD30 CAR-T cell therapy in relapsed and refractory Hodgkin lymphoma,” *Journal of Clinical Oncology*, vol. 38, no. 32, pp. 3794–3804, 2020.

[41] M. Damlaj, M. Alzayed, B. Alahmari, A. Alhejazi, A. Alaskar, and M. Alzahrani, “Therapeutic potential of checkpoint inhibitors in refractory plasmablastic lymphoma,” *Clinical Lymphoma Myeloma and Leukemia*, vol. 19, no. 10, pp. e559–e563, 2019.

[42] L. Cheng, Q. Song, M. Liu et al., “Case report: successful management of a refractory plasmablastic lymphoma patient with tislelizumab and lenalidomide,” *Frontiers in Immunology*, vol. 12, Article ID 702593, 2021.

[43] M. M. Al-Malki, J. J. Castillo, J. M. Sloan, and A. Re, “Hematopoietic cell transplantation for plasmablastic lymphoma: a review,” *Biology of Blood and Marrow Transplantation*, vol. 20, no. 12, pp. 1877–1884, 2014.

[44] C. Cattaneo, H. Finel, G. McQuaker, E. Vandenberghe, G. Rossi, and P. Dreger, “Autologous hematopoietic stem cell transplantation for plasmablastic lymphoma: the European Society for Blood and Marrow Transplantation experience,” *Biology of Blood and Marrow Transplantation*, vol. 21, no. 6, pp. 1146-1147, 2015.

[45] M. Hamadani and S. M. Devine, “Reduced-intensity conditioning allogeneic stem cell transplantation in HIV patients with hematologic malignancies: yes, we can,” *Blood*, vol. 114, no. 12, pp. 2564–2566, 2009.

[46] C. Rong, L. Sheng, A. Wu, Y. Sun, and G. Ouyang, “Allogeneic hematopoietic stem cell transplantation in a patient with HIV-negative recurrent plasmablastic lymphoma,” *Medicine*, vol. 100, no. 7, Article ID e24498, 2021.

Extramedullary Manifestations of Chronic Myelomonocytic Leukemia: Do We Treat like an Acute Myeloid Leukemia?

Prasun Pudasainee,[1] **Bimatshu Pyakuryal**,[1] **Yogesh Subedi**,[2] **Jenisha Upadhyay**,[3] **and Subarna Adhikari**[3]

[1]*Department of Internal Medicine, Nepal Medical College, Kathmandu, Nepal*
[2]*Department of Internal Medicine, Institute of Medicine, Kathmandu, Nepal*
[3]*Mountain Medicine Society of Nepal, Kathmandu, Nepal*

Correspondence should be addressed to Prasun Pudasainee; ppudasainee1@gmail.com

Academic Editor: Salah Aref

Chronic myelomonocytic leukemia (CMML) is a relatively rare clonal hematologic disorder with features of myelodysplastic syndrome and myeloproliferative disease. Extramedullary leukemic involvement is rarely a presenting feature of CMML. As there are no clear guidelines in regard to the treatment of patients with extramedullary manifestations, its management is challenging. In this report, we discuss the management of our patient who presented with submandibular lymphadenopathy and gingivitis and was diagnosed with CMML.

1. Introduction

CMML is a malignant hematopoietic stem cell disorder with clinical and pathological features of both myelodysplastic syndrome and myeloproliferative neoplasms (MDS/MPN). The median age at diagnosis of CMML is 71 years and has a median survival of 14–22 months [1]. Extramedullary manifestations of CMML are uncommon and are seen in organs such as spleen, liver, skin, and lymph nodes. Here, we present a case of CMML with extramedullary manifestations of myeloid sarcoma (MS) of the lymph node and gingival infiltration.

2. Case Presentation

A 40-year-old male with no significant past medical history presented to his primary physician with swelling on the right side of his neck and gum bleeding for a few weeks. He complained of fatigue, night sweats, and weight loss (~25 lb) in the preceding two months. On examination, he had significant gum hypertrophy and mobile, nontender mass in the right submandibular area and right cheek. Lab results were significant for white blood cell count of 31,000/μL (4% neutrophils, 74% monocytes, and 0.5% immature granulocytes). Bone marrow biopsy revealed hypercellular bone marrow (95%) with MDS/MPN features, consistent with CMML-1. Cytogenetics showed 48XY, +6, del(11)(q23), +19(16)/50~53, idem, +4, +18[cp4]. JAK2 V617F mutation was negative. Fluorescence in situ hybridization (FISH) studies were normal and negative for platelet-derived growth factor receptor beta rearrangement PDGFRB (CEN)/ PDGFRB (TEL). Ultrasound-guided biopsy of right submandibular mass and fine-needle aspiration of right cheek mass were consistent with myeloid sarcoma (Figure 1).

After discussing in the multidisciplinary tumor board, it was decided to treat this case as acute myeloid leukemia (AML). Induction with idarubicin and cytarabine on 3 + 7 protocol was performed. A repeat bone marrow biopsy was hypercellular without evidence of CMML; cytogenetics and FISH were normal. The patient subsequently proceeded with matched related allogenic hematopoietic cell transplant (HCT). Conditioning regimen included targeted busulfan

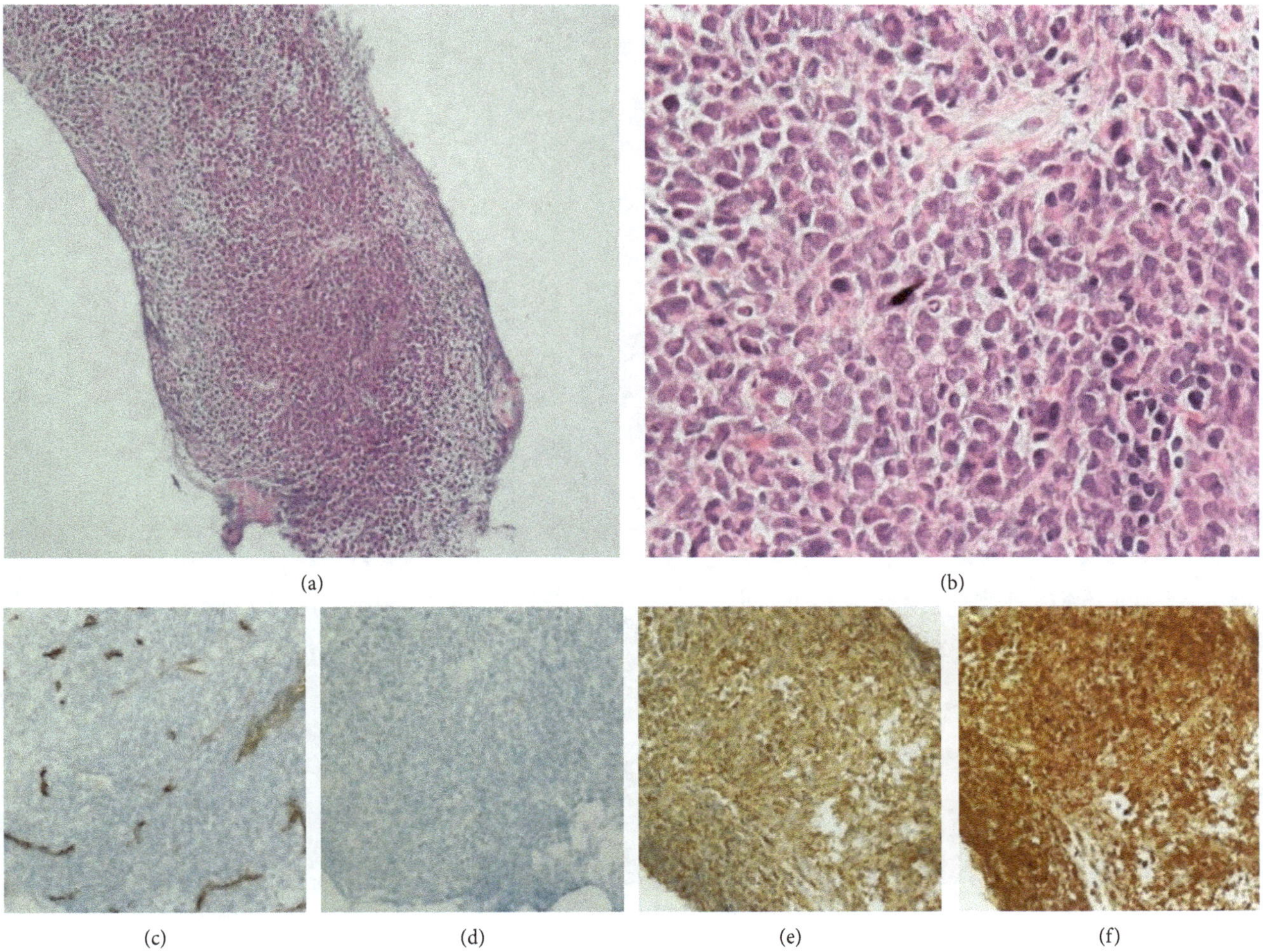

FIGURE 1: (a) Core needle biopsy of right submandibular mass. (b) Myeloid blast cells. (c) CD34 (+) blastic cells. (d) CD117 (+) blastic cells. (e) CD68 (+) blastic cells. (f) MPO (+) blastic cells.

and fludarabine. Graft-versus-host disease prophylaxis included tacrolimus and mycophenolate mofetil. The patient tolerated HCT fairly well, with only grade three mucositis and CMV reactivation. After five months of HCT, the patient developed skin rashes on the chest and right side of the abdomen. The biopsy of the skin was consistent with CMML (Figure 2).

Tacrolimus was discontinued. He received high-dose cytarabine salvage therapy followed by first donor lymphocyte infusion (DLI) at a 1×10^7 kg cell dose. Since he had side effects with cytarabine, he received 10 days of decitabine with the second dose of escalated DLI (8×10^7 kg cell dose). His second dose of DLI was given after five days of decitabine. However, the disease progressed with increased lymphadenopathy and new bony lesions. Despite three doses of DLI with decitabine, he developed large pleural effusion; analysis showed atypical hematopoietic cell population. Subsequently, he opted for hospice and died a week later.

3. Discussion

Myeloid sarcoma and gingival infiltration, although rare and described mostly with acute myeloid leukemia (AML), can be associated with CMML [2]. They may be the first manifestation of CMML, precede it by months or years, or represent the initial manifestation of relapse in a previously treated patient with CMML in remission. In our case, the patient presented with myeloid sarcoma and gingival infiltration at the time of CMML diagnosis, and subsequently had malignant pleural effusion with the progression of the disease. Myeloid sarcoma commonly involves skin, soft tissue, lymph nodes, bone, and periosteum [3]. Skin manifestations of AML can be nonspecific and may include pallor, petechiae or ecchymoses, neutrophilic dermatitis (Sweet syndrome), and infiltrative lesions such as leukemia cutis or myeloid sarcoma. Malignancy-associated Sweet's syndrome may occur in one of the three settings, either as paraneoplastic syndrome or drug-induced dermatosis or concurrently with leukemia cutis [4]. Pleural effusion secondary to malignant cell infiltration, similar to our case, has been reported rarely in AML [5]. CMML with extramedullary manifestations has a worse prognosis and needs aggressive treatment [6]. However, there are no randomized trials addressing the optimal management of CMML with extramedullary manifestations, and the data are limited to case reports and reviews. Thus, treatment is

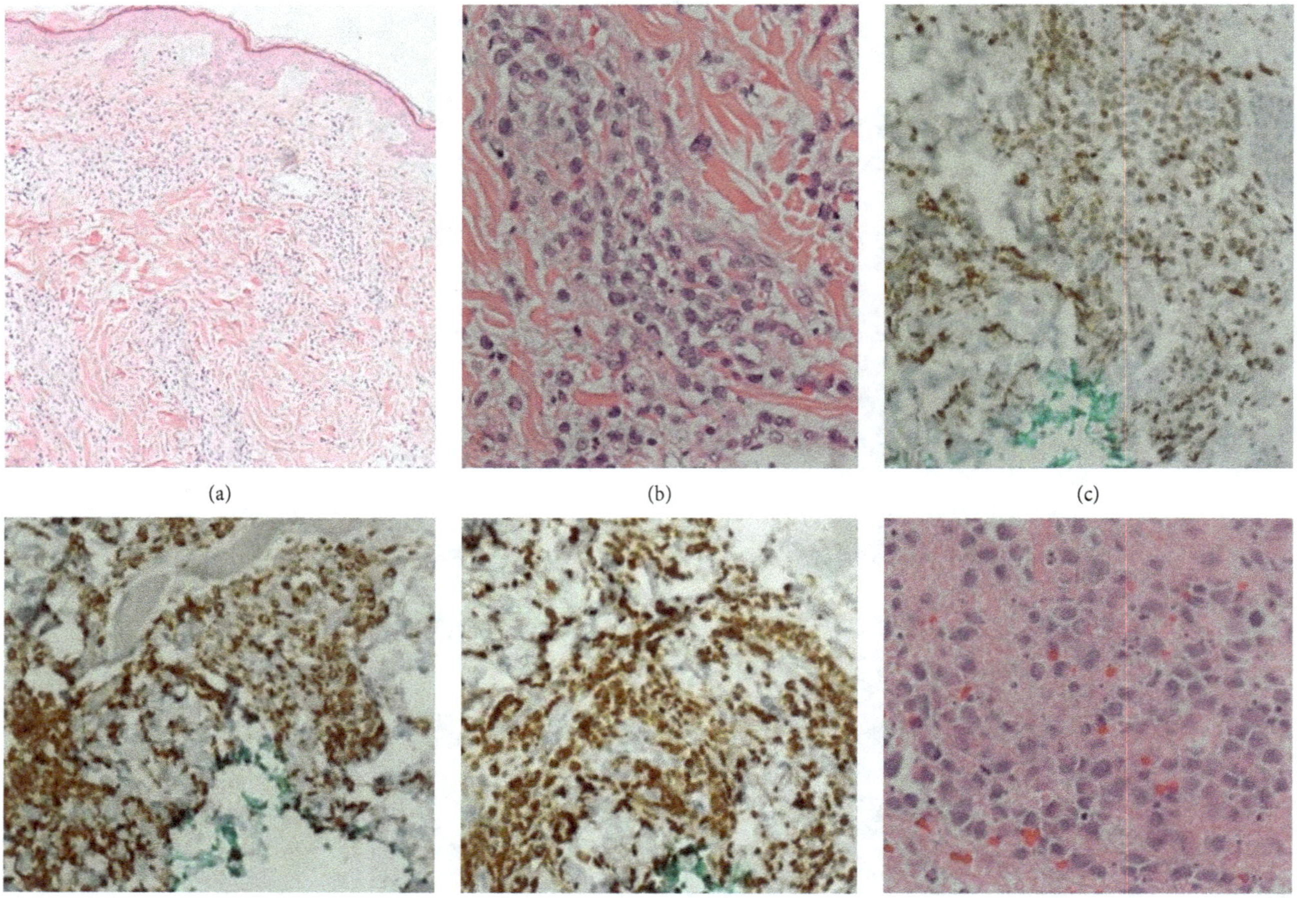

(a) (b) (c) (d) (e) (f)

Figure 2: (a) Punch biopsy of the skin rash. (b) Atypical monocytes consistent with chronic myelomonocytic leukemia. (c) CD68 (+) monocytes. (d) Lysosome (+) monocytes. (e) MPO (+) monocytes. (f) Pleural fluid aspirate with atypical hematopoietic cells.

usually at clinicians' discretion in these cases. Importantly, management depends on whether extramedullary manifestations are regarded as the progression of CMML or transformation into acute leukemia. If considered as a progression of CMML, the patient is initially treated with hypomethylating agents. HCT, which is the only potential cure, is attempted after remission [7]. However, if CMML with extramedullary manifestations is considered AML-equivalent, different management with AML-type chemotherapy followed by HCT is used [3]. In our patient, we decided to pursue AML-type treatment based on age, aggressive presentation, and multiple extramedullary manifestations.

4. Conclusions

Extramedullary manifestations with CMML have a poor prognosis. Management should be individualized and depending on the presentation it can either be treated as AML or progression of CMML.

References

[1] M. M. Patnaik, C. A. Hanson, J. M. Hodnefield et al., "Survival and prognosis in world health organization defined chronic myelomonocytic leukemia- a mayo clinic series of 227 patients," *American Society of Hematology*, vol. 120, no. 21, p. 3790, 2012.

[2] C. Campidelli, C. Agostinelli, R. Stitson, and S. A. Pileri, "Myeloid sarcoma: extramedullary manifestation of myeloid disorders," *American Journal of Clinical Pathology*, vol. 132, no. 3, pp. 426–437, 2009.

[3] R. L. Bakst, M. S. Tallman, D. Douer et al., "How I treat extramedullary acute myeloid leukemia," *Blood*, vol. 118, no. 14, pp. 3785–3793, 2011.

[4] U. Yanamandra, K. K. Sahu, A. Khadwal et al., "Recurrent sweet's syndrome in a case of AML," *Indian Journal of Hematology and Blood Transfusion*, vol. 32, no. S1, pp. 82–85, 2016.

[5] K. K. Sahu, R. Tyagi, A. D. Law et al., "Myeloid sarcoma: an unusual case of mediastinal mass and malignant pleural effusion with review of literature," *Indian Journal of Hematology and Blood Transfusion*, vol. 31, no. 4, pp. 466–471, 2015.

[6] K. Kawamoto, H. Miyoshi, N. Yoshida, J. Takizawa, H. Sone, and K. Ohshima, "Clinicopathological, cytogenetic, and prognostic analysis of 131 myeloid sarcoma patients," *The American Journal of Surgical Pathology*, vol. 40, no. 11, pp. 1473–1483, 2016.

[7] M. M. Patnaik and A. Tefferi, "Chronic myelomonocytic leukemia: 2016 update on diagnosis, risk stratification, and management," *American Journal of Hematology*, vol. 91, no. 6, pp. 631–642, 2016.

10

The Occurrence of Richter's Syndrome during Treatment with Obinutuzumab and Chlorambucil

Teng Fong Ng,[1,2] Benedict Carnley,[1,2] Celia Green,[2] Dominic Spagnolo,[2] and Michael F. Leahy[1,2]

[1]*Royal Perth Hospital, Perth, WA, Australia*
[2]*PathWest Laboratory Medicine, Perth, WA, Australia*

Correspondence should be addressed to Teng Fong Ng; ngtengfong.haem@gmail.com

Academic Editor: Sudhir Tauro

Chronic lymphocytic leukaemia is a slow-growing leukaemia of developing B-lymphocytes, which may transform to an aggressive lymphoma known as Richter's syndrome. While Richter's syndrome can present in untreated or relapsed-refractory cases, it may occur upon the commencement of less intensity treatment regimens. We present a case of Richter's syndrome following treatment with chlorambucil and obinutuzumab and review of available literature on the topic.

1. Background

Richter's syndrome (RS) is the development of an aggressive large cell lymphoma in the setting of the chronic lymphocytic leukaemia (CLL) or small lymphocytic leukaemia (SLL). RS was first described by Maurice Richter in 1928 as a "generalized reticular cell sarcoma" in a patient with CLL [1]. Clinically, RS is characterised by sudden clinical deterioration, marked increase in lymphadenopathy or splenomegaly, worsening "B" symptoms (i.e., fever, night sweats, weight loss), and increased serum lactate dehydrogenase (LDH) levels. RS occurs in approximately 2%–10% of CLL patients during the course of their disease [2–7]. The most common transformation is diffuse large B-cell lymphoma (DLBCL), but occasionally, CLL may transform into Hodgkin lymphoma [8]. Because of its dismal prognosis and aggressive nature, RS requires intensive chemo-immunotherapy with regimens such as R-CHOP and consolidation with haemopoietic stem cell transplantation.

2. Case Presentation

A 47-year-old Anglo-Saxon lady with chronic lymphocytic leukaemia, with weight loss, night sweats, and gradually progressive global lymphadenopathy, was commenced on treatment with a second-generation monoclonal anti-CD20 antibody obinutuzumab together with chlorambucil. The reduced intensity treatment is chosen as she has significant comorbidities which include ventricular septal defect, obesity, diabetes mellitus, chronic bronchitis, osteoarthritis limiting mobility, depression, recurrent migraine, and possibly tracheomalacia. Her pretreatment complete full blood count showed haemoglobin level of 158 g/L, elevated white cell count of 76×10^9/L with lymphocyte count of 68×10^9/L, and normal platelet count of 260×10^9/L. Serum lactate dehydrogenase was 280 U/L. The immunophenotype of her CLL is CD5+, CD19+, CD20+, CD23+, and CD200+, with lambda clonal restriction. Previous cytogenetic analysis was unremarkable, but molecular genetic analysis was not undertaken.

Cycle 1 of the 28-day protocol consisted of chlorambucil 0.5 mg/kg on day 1 and day 15, together with obinutuzumab 1000 mg on day 1-2 in split doses, day 8, and day 15. Subsequent 5 cycles have similar dosing of chlorambucil, but only one dose of obinutuzumab 1000 mg on day 1 is given [9]. On day 13 of cycle 1, 5 days after receiving obinutuzumab, she presented with dyspnoea, stridor, dysphagia, and increasing cervical lymphadenopathy. An urgent computed tomography scan demonstrated cervical and mediastinal lymphadenopathy resulting in tracheal compression (see Figure 1). Her serum LDH had increased from pretreatment

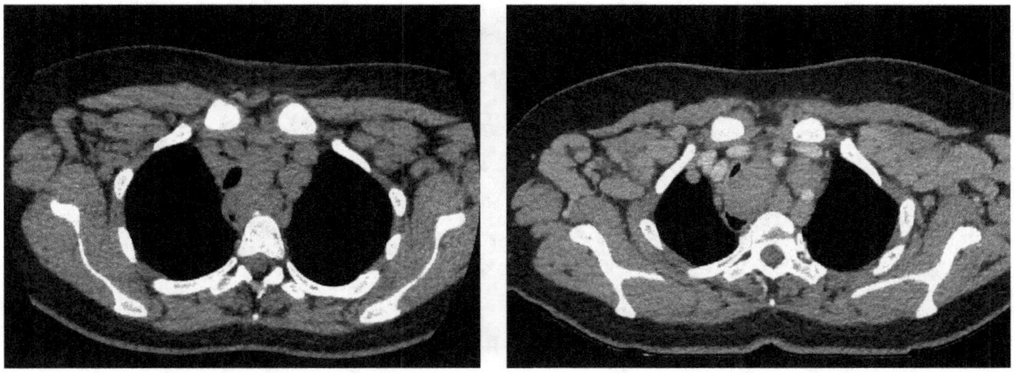

(a) (b)

FIGURE 1: Computed tomography of the chest showing the rapidly expanding mediastinal lymphadenopathy. The trachea was compressed with the narrow diameter of <1 cm. (a) Pretreatment. (b) Day 14 following commencement of treatment.

levels to 1260 U/L, but other tumour lysis markers remained unremarkable. Her peripheral blood lymphocyte count had declined to 0.3×10^9/L.

High dose intravenous dexamethasone was promptly commenced to attempt to reduce lymphadenopathy to alleviate the impending clinical airway compromise. In addition, the patient was empirically treated with antiherpetic treatment with intravenous high dose acyclovir as she had persistent herpes simplex labialis. This was due to concern of rapidly progressing herpetic lymphadenitis as a key differential diagnosis because there are case reports that has described similar presentation occurring during anti-CLL treatment [10, 11].

A percutaneous cervical lymph node biopsy was performed to obtained specimen for laboratorial analysis. Histologically, there was infiltration of skeletal muscle (there was no nodal tissue) by a confluent and sheet-like growth of centroblastoid cells accompanied by coagulative necrosis. The cells had large round to ovoid vesicular nuclei, one or more prominent nucleoli, often located on the nuclear membrane, and ample amphophilic or cleared cytoplasm. Mitoses were evident in any single high-power field and spotty apoptosis was present throughout. Based on paraffin section immunohistochemistry, the neoplastic cells were positive for CD20, CD5 (weak), CD23, CD43, BCL2 (>70%), and MUM1 and were lambda light-chain restricted; the Ki-67 proliferation index was approximately 70% (See Figure 2). The lymphoma was negative for CD10, CD30, cyclin D1, SOX11, C-MYC (<10% staining), BCL6, CD138, kappa light chain, HSV1/2, and EBER (by in situ hybridization). Interphase fluorescence in situ hybridization (FISH) studies on paraffin sections confirmed the presence of an IgH disruption but there was no disruption of BCL6 or MYC. Based on the Hans classifier, the features were those of an activated B-cell-like phenotype, with retained expression of the parent CLL markers CD5 (weak) and CD23, and not those of a double-expressor DLBCL (BCL2 high, MYC low). These large cells also exhibited similar lambda light-chain restriction which may imply a clonal relationship. Cytogenetic analysis did not identify ATM (11q22) or TP53 (17p13) deletions.

Following the histological diagnosis of RS, the patient was commenced on R-CHOP chemotherapy regimen, which resulted in reduction of lymphadenopathy and resolution of stridor and dyspnoea. Upon completion of 6 cycles, the patient achieved complete metabolic remission by a position emission tomography (PET) scan.

3. Discussion

RS may occur in CLL patients during the "watchful waiting" period before requiring any CLL treatment and can be a late event occurring following CLL treatment [5]. The incidence of RS increases with the number of prior therapies [12, 13]. Approximately, 50% cases of RS occur before the treatment of CLL [7]. However, there is little detail in reports in the literature about when during therapy. Most reports give a range that can start from 0 months which implied that RS occurs during the early period of treatment [7, 14].

Chlorambucil has been a long-standing alkylating agent used in the treatment of CLL since 1970s [15]. The risk of RS with treatment with chlorambucil alone is about 5%, observed in the prospective CALGB 9011 trial [16]. However, there is limited report of RS being precipitated by treatment with chlorambucil alone in the literature, which may be because the phenomenon is not highlighted in the relevant publications.

Recently, RS has been described during novel targeted treatments, notably the BCL2 inhibitor venetoclax [17]. Many of the RS cases developed shortly after starting treatment, suggesting unrecognised RS predates the initiation of the novel targeted therapy [18]. In the phase-1 venetoclax trial in heavily treated relapse-refractory CLL, 16% of patients on venetoclax develop RS and considered that as treatment failure and progressive disease [19]. The authors reported that RS appears to represent a mechanism of tumour escape from suppression by the inhibition of BCL2, particularly for patients with CLL with 17p deletion. RS was also observed in 8 of 25 patients with disease progression who were receiving ibrutinib monotherapy in an extended follow-up study [20].

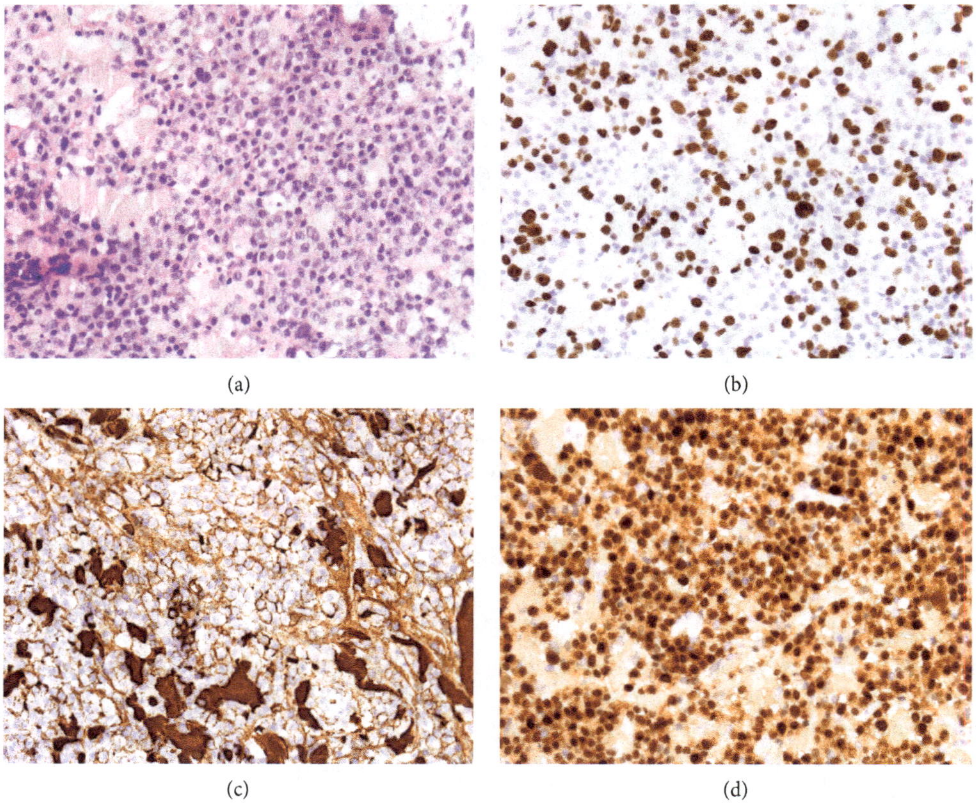

FIGURE 2: Sheets of large lymphocytes with centroblastic morphology ((a) haematoxylin and eosin stain), with positive immunohistochemistry for high Ki-67 index of 70%, CD20, and MUM1 (b)–(d), respectively.

There are some reports of the occurrence of RS in major clinical trials of treatment approaches using anti-CD20 monoclonal antibodies, but these rates are not well highlighted. In the CLL8 phase-3 trial investigating the efficacy of fludarabine and cyclophosphamide (FC) with 1st generation monoclonal anti-CD20 chimeric antibody rituximab, 13 out of 408 (3%) patients on the FC-rituximab treatment arm developed RS on long-term follow-up [21]. In the iLLUMUNATE trial, there were 2 out of 116 patients (2%) in the control arm treated with chlorambucil and obinutuzumab that developed RS as progression of disease [22]. In the CLL-BAG02 trial, 3 out of 66 patients (4.5%) experienced RS following treatment with bendamustine and obinutuzumab regimen [23]. The early trial of single agent ofatumumab had 1 case of RS in a patient that has been heavily treated with fludarabine and alemtuzumab [15]. In the phase-2 trial using bendamustine and ofatumumab in relapsed CLL patients, 3 out of 10 patients developed RS [16]. Of interest, 2 of these patients developed RS around cycle 2 of the treatment.

In our case, the chlorambucil and obinutuzumab combination seemed to have rapidly precipitated RS after the doses of both agents in a treatment naïve patient. This is similar timing to the 2 patients reported in the phase-2 bendamustine and ofatumumab trial [16]. In these cases, it is possible that the aggressive large cell clone may be present initially as a minor clone [24], and thus these patients do not exhibit the full clinical manifestations of RS until the commencement of the effective anti-CLL treatment. Our patient has limited clinical manifestations of RS including night sweats and weight loss, but pretreatment of serum lactate dehydrogenase is not markedly elevated till after the 2nd infusion of the anti-CD20 monoclonal antibody.

There is a possibility that the RS clone was clonally selected due to rapid cytoreduction of the treatment-sensitive CLL clones by chlorambucil and obinutuzumab. However, we do not have molecular studies to ascertain the origin of the RS in our case to determine whether it is clonally related or clonally unrelated. Rossi et al. have pointed out that the clonally related RS stems from a subclone cell that is present CLL initially, which become the dominant subclone during the clinical RS transformation as other CLL subclones reduce in proportion [25], whereas clonal unrelated RS is biologically different, characterised by a significantly higher mutation frequency. Interestingly, patients with clonally unrelated RS have a median survival of approximately 62 months, which is comparable to patients with de novo DLBCL [6]. On the contrary, the median survival of patients with clonally related RS is significantly shorter, ranging from 8 to 14 months [6]. Clonal dynamics monitoring of clonal unrelated RS has demonstrated clonal evolution, acquiring and selecting new mutations in response to treatment, and loss of cellular tumoral clone during progression [26].

In conclusion, this case spotlighted an uncommon phenomenon in CLL where RS can rapidly present following the commencement of the anti-CLL regimen. RS requires rapid histological confirmation and prompt treatment with intensive immunochemotherapy for large cell lymphoma in order to achieve a clinical response. We hope that this phenomenon can be reported distinctly in the future publications regarding RS.

References

[1] M. N. Richter, "Generalized reticular cell sarcoma of lymph nodes associated with lymphatic leukemia," *The American Journal of Pathology*, vol. 4, no. 4, pp. 285–292, 1928.

[2] F. R. Mauro, R. Foa, D. Giannarelli et al., "Clinical characteristics and outcome of young chronic lymphocytic leukemia patients: a single institution study of 204 cases," *Blood*, vol. 94, no. 2, pp. 448–454, 1999.

[3] P. D. Thornton, C. Bellas, A. Santon et al., "Richter's transformation of chronic lymphocytic leukemia: the possible role of fludarabine and the epstein-barr virus in its pathogenesis," *Leukemia Research*, vol. 29, no. 4, pp. 389–395, 2005.

[4] A.-M. Tsimberidou and M. J. Keating, "Richter syndrome: biology, incidence, and therapeutic strategies," *Cancer*, vol. 103, no. 2, pp. 216–228, 2005.

[5] K. Maddocks-Christianson, S. L. Slager, C. S. Zent et al., "Risk factors for development of a second lymphoid malignancy in patients with chronic lymphocytic leukaemia," *British Journal of Haematology*, vol. 139, no. 3, pp. 398–404, 2007.

[6] D. Rossi, V. Spina, C. Deambrogi et al., "The genetics of Richter syndrome reveals disease heterogeneity and predicts survival after transformation," *Blood*, vol. 117, no. 12, pp. 3391–3401, 2011.

[7] S. A. Parikh, K. G. Rabe, T. G. Call et al., "Diffuse large B-cell lymphoma (Richter syndrome) in patients with chronic lymphocytic leukaemia (CLL): a cohort study of newly diagnosed patients," *British Journal of Haematology*, vol. 162, no. 6, pp. 774–782, 2013.

[8] E. Campo, P. Ghia, E. Montserrat et al., "Chronic lymphocytic leukaemia/small lymphocytic lymphoma," in *WHO Classification of Tumours of Haematopoietic and Lymphoid Tissues*, S. H. Swerdlow, E. Campo, N. L. Harris et al., Eds., pp. 216–221, WHO, Geneva, Switzerland, 2017.

[9] V. Goede, K. Fischer, R. Busch et al., "Obinutuzumab plus chlorambucil in patients with CLL and coexisting conditions," *New England Journal of Medicine*, vol. 370, no. 12, pp. 1101–1110, 2014.

[10] D. Villa and B. Skinnider, "Herpes simplex virus lymphadenitis," *Blood*, vol. 123, no. 1, p. 12, 2014.

[11] R. Srivastava, D. Griswold, and M. O. Jamil, "Chronic lymphocytic leukaemia with necrotic herpetic adenitis: an elusive clinical condition," *BMJ Case Reports*, vol. 2018, 2018.

[12] L. E. Robertson, W. Pugh, S. O'Brien et al., "Richter's syndrome: a report on 39 patients," *Journal of Clinical Oncology*, vol. 11, no. 10, pp. 1985–1989, 1993.

[13] A. M. Tsimberidou, S. O'Brien, I. Khouri et al., "Clinical outcomes and prognostic factors in patients with Richter's syndrome treated with chemotherapy or chemoimmunotherapy with or without stem-cell transplantation," *Journal of Clinical Oncology*, vol. 24, no. 15, pp. 2343–2351, 2006.

[14] L. Fan, L. Wang, R. Zhang et al., "Richter transformation in 16 of 149 Chinese patients with chronic lymphocytic leukemia," *Leukemia & Lymphoma*, vol. 53, no. 9, pp. 1749–1756, 2012.

[15] W. G. Wierda, T. J. Kipps, J. Mayer et al., "Ofatumumab as single-agent CD20 immunotherapy in fludarabine-refractory chronic lymphocytic leukemia," *Journal of Clinical Oncology*, vol. 28, no. 10, pp. 1749–1755, 2010.

[16] C. Ujjani, P. Ramzi, E. Gehan, H. Wang, Y. Wang, and B. D. Cheson, "Ofatumumab and bendamustine in previously treated chronic lymphocytic leukemia and small lymphocytic lymphoma," *Leukemia & Lymphoma*, vol. 56, no. 4, pp. 915–920, 2015.

[17] M. A. Anderson, C. Tam, T. E. Lew et al., "Clinicopathological features and outcomes of progression of CLL on the BCL2 inhibitor venetoclax," *Blood*, vol. 129, no. 25, pp. 3362–3370, 2017.

[18] S. A. Parikh, N. E. Kay, and T. D. Shanafelt, "How we treat Richter syndrome," *Blood*, vol. 123, no. 11, pp. 1647–1657, 2014.

[19] A. W. Roberts, M. S. Davids, J. M. Pagel et al., "Targeting BCL2 with venetoclax in relapsed chronic lymphocytic leukemia," *New England Journal of Medicine*, vol. 374, no. 4, pp. 311–322, 2016.

[20] J. C. Byrd, R. R. Furman, S. E. Coutre et al., "Three-year follow-up of treatment-naïve and previously treated patients with CLL and SLL receiving single-agent ibrutinib," *Blood*, vol. 125, no. 16, pp. 2497–2506, 2015.

[21] K. Fischer, J. Bahlo, A.-M. Fink et al., "Extended follow up of the CLL8 protocol, a randomized phase-III trial of the German CLL study group (GCLLSG) comparing fludarabine and cyclophosphamide (FC) to FC plus rituximab (FCR) for previously untreated patients with chronic lymphocytic leukemia (CLL): results on survival, progression-free survival, delayed neutropenias and secondary malignancies confirm superiority of the FCR regimen," *Blood*, vol. 120, no. 21, p. 435, 2012.

[22] C. Moreno, R. Greil, F. Demirkan et al., "Ibrutinib plus obinutuzumab versus chlorambucil plus obinutuzumab in first-line treatment of chronic lymphocytic leukaemia (iLLUMINATE): a multicentre, randomised, open-label, phase 3 trial," *The Lancet Oncology*, vol. 20, no. 1, pp. 43–56, 2019.

[23] P. Cramer, J. V. Tresckow, J. Bahlo et al., "Bendamustine followed by obinutuzumab and venetoclax in chronic lymphocytic leukaemia (CLL2-BAG): primary endpoint analysis of a multicentre, open-label, phase 2 trial," *The Lancet Oncology*, vol. 19, no. 9, pp. 1215–1228, 2018.

[24] B. Timár, Z. Fülöp, E. Csernus et al., "Relationship between the mutational status of VH genes and pathogenesis of diffuse large B-cell lymphoma in Richter's syndrome," *Leukemia*, vol. 18, no. 2, pp. 326–330, 2004.

[25] D. Rossi, V. Spina, F. Forconi et al., "Molecular history of Richter syndrome: origin from a cell already present at the time of chronic lymphocytic leukemia diagnosis," *International Journal of Cancer*, vol. 130, no. 12, pp. 3006–3010, 2012.

[26] J. González-Rincón, S. Gómez, N. Martinez et al., "Clonal dynamics monitoring during clinical evolution in chronic lymphocytic leukaemia," *Scientific Reports*, vol. 9, no. 1, p. 975, 2019.

11

Prefibrotic Myelofibrosis Presenting with Multiple Cerebral Embolic Infarcts and the Rare *MPL* W515S Mutation

Stephen E. Langabeer,[1] **Lisa Lee Tokar,**[1] **Laura Kearney,**[1] **Cathal O'Brien,**[1] **Kowshika Thavarajah,**[2] **Aisling Barrett,**[3] **John McManus,**[2] **and Hilary O'Leary**[3]

[1]*Cancer Molecular Diagnostics, St. James's Hospital, Dublin D08 W9RT, Ireland*
[2]*Department of Medicine for the Elderly, University Hospital Limerick, Limerick V94 F858, Ireland*
[3]*Department of Haematology, University Hospital Limerick, Limerick V94 F858, Ireland*

Correspondence should be addressed to Stephen E. Langabeer; slangabeer@stjames.ie

Academic Editor: Pier Paolo Piccaluga

Acquired, activating mutations of *MPL* W515 are recognised driver mutations of the myeloproliferative neoplasms (MPN), namely, essential thrombocythemia and primary myelofibrosis. The most common mutation at this codon is W515L with several other mutations also described at a lower frequency. Of these less common mutations, *MPL* W515S has only been reported sporadically with limited information on clinicopathological associations. We describe the case of an elderly man with persistent thrombocytosis presenting with an ischemic cerebral event. Bone marrow biopsy showed evidence of prefibrotic myelofibrosis with targeted sequencing demonstrating the presence of the rare *MPL* W515S mutation. Thrombolytic and cytoreductive therapies resulted in a favorable outcome and follow-up. This case provides additional, necessary, and phenotypic data for the rare MPN-associated *MPL* W515S mutation.

1. Introduction

The most commonly acquired driver mutations of the Philadelphia chromosome-negative myeloproliferative neoplasms (MPN) of essential thrombocythemia (ET) and primary myelofibrosis (PMF) are those of *JAK2* V617F, *CALR* exon 9, and *MPL* exon 10. Identification of these mutations constitutes a major diagnostic criterion for disease diagnosis and classification [1]. *MPL* encodes the receptor for thrombopoietin with the first MPN-associated, *MPL* exon 10 mutation described as W515L swiftly followed by reports of several other mutations occurring at this particular tryptophan (Trp) codon in patients with both ET and PMF [2–4]. However, the W515 codon appears to be a hotspot for acquired mutations, and several other somatic and inherited variants of *MPL* (other than in exon 10) have also been annotated in familial and sporadic MPN [5–9].

Morphological comparison of *MPL*-mutated ET with *JAK2* V617F- and *CALR*-mutated ET has shown that *MPL*-mutated ET patients are older than those with other genotypes and have higher peripheral blood platelet counts and bone marrow megakaryocytes than *JAK2* V617F-mutated ET with histological features of prefibrotic myelofibrosis being rare [10]. Review of bone marrow histology of *MPL*-mutated PMF shows decreased vascularity and increased osteosclerosis [11]. Clinically, *MPL*-mutated MPN patients tend to have lower risk of thrombotic events than their *JAK2* V617F counterparts [12–14].

The W515S mutation was first described in *in vitro* as a spontaneously occurring point mutation in the intracellular domain of the protein after transfection of *c-mpl* into Ba/F3 cells that resulted in thrombopoietin-independent, constitutive activation of the receptor [15]. Isolated reports of *MPL* W515S in MPN patients exist in the literature, usually within a cohort, yet limited clinical and pathological associations regarding this specific mutation exist [16–19]. Of these four cases, two patients had annotated clinical histories and in whom no thrombotic episodes were observed.

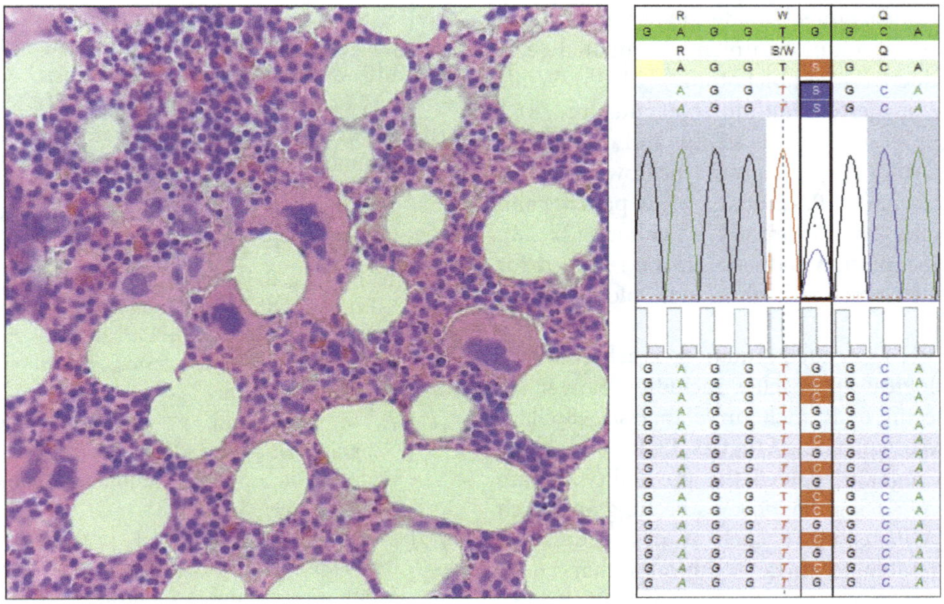

(a) (b)

FIGURE 1: (a) Bone marrow biopsy demonstrating megakaryocyte clustering with nuclear hypolobation and bulbous forms; (b) next-generation sequence analysis (Sequence Pilot, JSI Medical Systems, Ettenheim, Germany) identifying *MPL* p.W515S (c.1544G > C).

2. Case Report

A 71-year-old man with a persistent high platelet count for four years (range 483–797 × 10^9/L) presented with dense, right-sided weakness, aphasia, and a decreased level of consciousness. He was known to have hypercholesterolemia for which he was on atorvastatin. He was an ex-smoker for forty years and otherwise did not have any other vascular risk factors. Apart from thrombocytosis, blood count parameters including hemoglobin, hematocrit, white cell count, and white cell differential had always been normal. Initial computerized tomography (CT) scan showed an old, left occipital lobe infarction. CT angiogram did not show any large vessel occlusion. Magnetic resonance imaging scan confirmed multiple, left-sided, and embolic infarcts. Of note, a 72-hour Holter monitor excluded paroxysmal atrial fibrillation as a cause of cerebral ischemia. Standard stroke workup did not identify any other sources of cerebral embolic infarction. He was thrombolysed and subsequently commenced on low-dose aspirin 75 mg daily. He made an excellent recovery, the only residual deficit being that of slightly altered speech.

Following his discharge from the hospital, he was referred to the hematology service for investigation of the persistent thrombocytosis. Bone marrow aspirate was aparticulate. Bone marrow biopsy was hypercellular with increased numbers of megakaryocytes showing paratrabecular clustering and nuclear hypolobation as well as bulbous forms (Figure 1(a)); granulopoiesis and erythropoiesis looked normal with World Health Organization grade 1 reticulin fibrosis seen that are all features in keeping with a diagnosis of prefibrotic myelofibrosis. An International Prognostic Scoring System score of 1 predicted his median overall survival for more than 10 years [20]. Karyotypic analysis failed on the bone marrow aspirate; however, a next-generation sequencing approach identified p.(Trp515Ser), c.1544G > C mutation (NM_005373.2), usually referred to as *MPL* W515S, at an allele frequency of 35% in the patient's peripheral blood (Figure 1(b)). No *CALR* exon 9 or *JAK2* exon 12 or 14 mutations were identified.

In order to reduce the risk of further thrombotic events in the context of confirmed *MPL* W515S MPN, hydroxyurea 500 mg daily was introduced, resulting in the platelet count normalising within one month of starting this treatment and remaining to date within the normal range. Currently, the patient remains well and is fully capable of carrying out all daily activities. He has a persisting, slight speech impediment and remains on aspirin and hydroxyurea more than twelve months following the ischaemic cerebral event and has not had any bleeding sequelae.

3. Discussion

The Trp515 amino acid is located at the transmembrane-cytosolic junction of the MPL receptor controlling dimerization and activation [21]. This codon is recurrently mutated in MPN with the mutations W515L and W515K detected most frequently but with W5151R, W515A, and W515G also described [16, 22], whereas *MPL* W515S has only been sporadically reported in ET and PMF patients [16–19]. In a recent study of 17 active mutants resulting from substitutions at Trp515, W515S resulted in activation of the TpoR/JAK2/STAT5 transcriptional cascade in the absence of the ligand in a similar manner to that of other mutants described in MPN patients thus implicating its oncogenic potential [23].

As MPN are relatively rare, it is probable they represent an underdiagnosed cause of cerebral thrombosis. High clinical awareness is warranted to identify an underlying MPN in order that a prompt treatment is initiated (e.g., antiplatelet, cytoreductive, and phlebotomy) [24, 25]. While some studies have suggested routine screening for *JAK2* V617F in patients presenting with stroke and/or cerebral venous thrombosis (CVT) [26], given the lower risk of thrombosis in *CALR*- and *MPL*-mutated MPN patients and the near absence of these mutations in CVT cohorts [27, 28], wider evaluation of mutation status might be reserved for those patients with sustained abnormal blood count findings.

Detection of MPN-associated mutations is achieved by a number of technological approaches including Sanger sequencing, allele-specific PCR, melt curve analysis, capillary electrophoresis, pyrosequencing, digital PCR, and next-generation sequencing [29]. Given the possibility of rare mutations such as W515S, a diagnostic screening approach covering at least *MPL* exon 10 such as next-generation sequencing is preferable to those techniques that target individually the most prevalent mutations of *MPL* W515L and W515K.

Identification and reporting of such rare *MPL* mutations in conjunction with the clinical aspects in MPN patients allow for correct diagnosis, assessment of any genotype-phenotype relationship, and may provide information on any future therapeutic approaches in similar patients.

References

[1] D. A. Arber, A. Orazi, R. Hasserjian et al., "The 2016 revision to the world health organization classification of myeloid neoplasms and acute leukemia," *Blood*, vol. 127, no. 20, pp. 2391–2405, 2016.

[2] Y. Pikman, B. H. Lee, T. Mercher et al., "MPL W515L is a novel somatic activating mutation in myelofibrosis with myeloid metaplasia," *PLoS Medicine*, vol. 3, no. 7, p. e270, 2006.

[3] A. D. Pardanani, R. L. Levine, T. Lasho et al., "MPL515 mutations in myeloproliferative and other myeloid disorders: a study of 1182 patients," *Blood*, vol. 108, no. 10, pp. 3472–3476, 2006.

[4] R. Chaligné, C. Tonetti, R. Besancenot et al., "New mutations of MPL in primitive myelofibrosis: only the MPL W515 mutations promote a G1/S-phase transition," *Leukemia* , vol. 22, no. 8, pp. 1557–1566, 2008.

[5] J. D. Milosevic Feenstra, H. Nivarthi, H. Gisslinger et al., "Whole-exome sequencing identifies novel MPL and JAK2 mutations in triple-negative myeloproliferative neoplasms," *Blood*, vol. 127, no. 3, pp. 325–332, 2016.

[6] X. Cabagnols, F. Favale, F. Pasquier et al., "Presence of atypical thrombopoietin receptor (MPL) mutations in triple-negative essential thrombocythemia patients," *Blood*, vol. 127, no. 3, pp. 333–342, 2016.

[7] A. Angona, C. Fernández-Rodríguez, A. Alvarez-Larrán et al., "Molecular characterisation of triple negative essential thrombocythaemia patients by platelet analysis and targeted sequencing," *Blood Cancer Journal*, vol. 6, no. 8, p. e463, 2016.

[8] Y. C. Chang, H. C. Lin, Y. H. Chiang et al., "Targeted next-generation sequencing identified novel mutations in triple-negative myeloproliferative neoplasms," *Medical Oncology*, vol. 34, no. 5, 2017.

[9] S. Schulze, R. Stengel, N. Jaekel et al., "Concomitant and noncanonical JAK2 and MPL mutations in JAK2 V617F- and MPLW 515 L-positive myelofibrosis," *Genes, Chromosomes and Cancer*, vol. 58, no. 11, pp. 747–755, 2019.

[10] A. Alvarez-Larran, D. Martínez, L. Arenillas et al., "Essential thrombocythaemia with mutation in MPL: clinicopathological correlation and comparison with JAK2V617F-mutated and CALR-mutated genotypes," *Journal of Clinical Pathology*, vol. 71, no. 11, pp. 975–980, 2018.

[11] W. J. Wong, R. P. Hasserjian, G. S. Pinkus et al., "JAK2, CALR, MPL and ASXL1 mutational status correlates with distinct histological features in Philadelphia chromosome-negative myeloproliferative neoplasms," *Haematologica*, vol. 103, no. 2, pp. e63–e68, 2018.

[12] A. M. Vannucchi, E. Antonioli, P. Guglielmelli et al., "Characteristics and clinical correlates of MPL 515W>L/K mutation in essential thrombocythemia," *Blood*, vol. 112, no. 3, pp. 844–847, 2008.

[13] N. Gangat, E. A. Wassie, T. L. Lasho et al., "Mutations and thrombosis in essential thrombocythemia: prognostic interaction with age and thrombosis history," *European Journal of Haematology*, vol. 94, no. 1, pp. 31–36, 2015.

[14] M. C. Finazzi, A. Carobbio, F. Cervantes et al., "CALR mutation, MPL mutation and triple negativity identify patients with the lowest vascular risk in primary myelofibrosis," *Leukemia*, vol. 29, no. 5, pp. 1209-1210, 2015.

[15] M. Abe, K. Suzuki, O. Inagaki, S. Sassa, and H. Shikama, "A novel MPL point mutation resulting in thrombopoietin-independent activation," *Leukemia*, vol. 16, no. 8, pp. 1500–1506, 2002.

[16] W. Ma, X. Zhang, X. Wang et al., "MPL mutation profile in JAK2 mutation-negative patients with myeloproliferative disorders," *Diagnostic Molecular Pathology*, vol. 20, no. 1, pp. 34–39, 2011.

[17] J. Tao, X. Zghang, J. Lancet et al., "Concurrence of B-lymphoblastic leukemia and myeloproliferative neoplasm with copy neutral loss of heterozygosity at chromosome 1p harbouring a MPL W515S mutation," *Cancer Genetics*, vol. 2017, no. 10-12, pp. 489–494, 2014.

[18] A. Tefferi, T. L. Lasho, K. H. Begna et al., "A pilot study of the telomerase inhibitor imetelstat for myelofibrosis," *New England Journal of Medicine*, vol. 373, no. 10, pp. 908–919, 2015.

[19] A. Beucher, M. Dib, C. Orvain et al., "Next generation sequencing redefines a triple negative essential thrombocythaemia as double-positive with rare mutations on JAK 2 V617 and MPL W515 hotspots," *British Journal of Haematology*, vol. 186, no. 5, pp. 785–788, 2019.

[20] P. Guglielmelli, A. Pacilli, G. Rotunno et al., "Presentation and outcome of patients with 2016 WHO diagnosis of prefibrotic and overt primary myelofibrosis," *Blood*, vol. 129, no. 24, pp. 3227–3236, 2017.

[21] J.-P. Defour, M. Itaya, V. Gryshkova et al., "Tryptophan at the transmembrane-cytosolic junction modulates thrombopoietin receptor dimerization and activation," *Proceedings of the National Academy of Sciences*, vol. 110, no. 7, pp. 2540–2545, 2013.

[22] J. Z. Gong, J. R. Cook, T. C. Greiner et al., "Laboratory practice guidelines for detecting and reporting JAK2 and MPL mutations in myeloproliferative neoplasms," *The Journal of Molecular Diagnostics*, vol. 15, no. 6, pp. 733–744, 2013.

[23] J.-P. Defour, I. Chachoua, C. Pecquet, and S. N. Constantinescu, "Oncogenic activation of MPL/thrombopoietin receptor by 17 mutations at W515: impli-

cations for myeloproliferative neoplasms," *Leukemia*, vol. 30, no. 5, pp. 1214–1216, 2016.

[24] A. Artoni, P. Bucciarelli, and I. Martinelli, "Cerebral thrombosis and myeloproliferative neoplasms," *Current Neurology and Neuroscience Reports*, vol. 14, no. 11, 2014.

[25] M. I. Stefanou, H. Richter, F. Härtig et al., "Recurrent ischaemic cerebrovascular events as presenting manifestations of myeloproliferative neoplasms," *European Journal of Neurology*, vol. 26, no. 6, pp. 903–e64, 2019.

[26] M. Lamy, P. Palazzo, P. Agius et al., "Should we screen for janus kinase 2 V617F mutation in cerebral venous thrombosis?" *Cerebrovascular Diseases*, vol. 44, no. 3-4, pp. 97–104, 2017.

[27] I. Martinelli, V. De Stefano, A. Carobbio et al., "Cerebral vein thrombosis in patients with philadelphia-negative myeloproliferative neoplasms an european leukemia net study," *American Journal of Hematology*, vol. 89, no. 11, pp. E200–E205, 2014.

[28] E. Verger, I. Crassard, B. Cassinat, and S. Bellucci, "Low incidence of CALR gene mutations in patients with cerebral venous thrombosis without overt chronic myeloproliferative neoplasm," *Thrombosis Research*, vol. 136, no. 4, pp. 839-840, 2015.

[29] S. E. Langabeer, H. Andrikovics, J. Asp et al., "Molecular diagnostics of myeloproliferative neoplasms," *European Journal of Haematology*, vol. 95, no. 4, pp. 270–279, 2015.

12

Persistent Mixed Donor Chimerism following Double Umbilical Cord Transplantation in a Patient with T-Cell Prolymphocytic Leukemia

Ronak H. Mistry[1] **Elizabeth O. Hexner,**[2] **and James K. Mangan**[2]

[1]*Department of Internal Medicine, Pennsylvania Hospital of the University of Pennsylvania, 800 Spruce Street, Philadelphia, PA 19107, USA*
[2]*Abramson Cancer Center, Perelman Center for Advanced Medicine, University of Pennsylvania, 34th Street and Civic Center Boulevard, 12th Floor South Pavilion, Philadelphia, PA 19104, USA*

Correspondence should be addressed to James K. Mangan; jkm3476@yahoo.com

Academic Editor: Takashi Sonoki

T-cell prolymphocytic leukemia (T-PLL) is a rare and aggressive postthymic T-cell neoplasm with an associated survival time of 1 year when left untreated. Current standard of care for T-PLL is with alemtuzumab, followed by allogeneic or autologous stem cell transplant. Little is found in the literature about alternative donor transplantation in T-PLL. Here, we present the case of a patient treated with double umbilical cord blood transplantation, which resulted in initial complete remission. An unusual outcome of this case is that coengraftment of both cords was established. After 16 months, the patient had relapse of the disease, unfortunately, prompting treatment with alemtuzumab and pentostatin, which resulted in remission once again. Here, we report a unique phenomenon whereby single-cord dominance occurred after treatment with these agents, suggesting that anti-T-cell therapy after transplant may help achieve single-unit dominance. A second relapse of the disease occurred six months thereafter, ultimately resulting in the patient's death, highlighting the aggressive nature of this disease.

1. Introduction

T-cell prolymphocytic leukemia (T-PLL) is a rare postthymic T-cell neoplasm, accounting for approximately 2% of all leukemia cases, with a greater incidence in males beginning in their sixth decade [1]. Typically, untreated T-PLL is associated with a survival of less than 1 year [2]. The aggressive nature of this disease, and its rarity, presents both diagnostic and therapeutic challenges to physicians [2]. Current standard of care for T-PLL includes the use of alemtuzumab (Campath-1H), a humanized IgG1 antibody specific for the CD52 antigen which is highly expressed on normal and malignant lymphocytes [1, 3]. Thereafter, postremission therapy with either autologous or allogeneic stem cell transplant (SCT) has been associated with disease-free and long-term survival, with a median overall survival of 48 months for both allogeneic and autologous SCT, compared to 20 months for those patients who received alemtuzumab alone [1]. There is a paucity of data on alternative donor transplantation in T-PLL. A Japanese group reported the first case of an umbilical cord blood transplant for T-PLL in 2005 [4]; however, we cannot find subsequent reports of umbilical cord blood transplants for this disease. Accordingly, we report here a second case of umbilical cord transplantation used for T-PLL, employing two umbilical cord units this time. Double umbilical cord blood transplant (dUCBT) is increasingly utilized in adults as it appears to improve outcomes, though almost inevitably only one cord blood unit engrafts, a phenomenon known as single-unit dominance [5]. This case is notable for successful engraftment and complete remission that lasted 16 months despite the presence of residual disease at the time of reduced-intensity transplant. An unusual feature of this case was persistent coengraftment of both umbilical cord units, which can be associated with relapse [6]. Persistent coengraftment is rare in dUCBT and has been reported in a small number of case reports [7]. Following relapse 16 months after transplant, a second remission was achieved with a repeat course of alemtuzumab and pentostatin, which lasted 6 months before relapse occurred again. Unbalanced and dynamic coengraftment endured until frank relapse, when the unit contributing less was no longer detectable. This case illustrates the tenuous nature of complete remissions which involve coengraftment after dUCBT. It also demonstrates that dUCBT can result in complete remissions in T-PLL, though the prognosis of patients remains grim with or without allogeneic SCT. We present details of our case below.

2. Case Presentation

A 59-year-old female presented to the local emergency department with reports of fatigue and shortness of breath. The patient was observed to have a WBC >400,000/μL, in addition to pitting edema at the ankles and scattered petechiae. Peripheral smears indicated a marked leukocytosis with atypical blast-like cells. A bone marrow biopsy showed extensive involvement with a T-cell lymphoproliferative disorder with the following immunophenotypes: CD2+, CD4+, CD5+, CD7+, cytoplasmic CD3+, and CD52+, with loss of membrane-associated CD3. Fluorescence in situ hybridization (FISH) indicated a loss of the TCL1 locus, consistent with cyotgenetics showing monosomy 14, as well as numerous other abnormalities (complex and monosomal karyotype), including an addition of 22q. CT imaging indicated splenomegaly and multiple enlarged lymph nodes. Collectively, these findings were diagnostic of T-PLL. This patient was started on intravenous alemtuzumab on a Monday, Wednesday, Friday regimen, initially with a dose escalation of 3 mg on day 1, 10 mg on day 3, and 30 mg on day 5. She continued on 30 mg intravenous alemtuzumab three times weekly for 12 weeks, consistent with current treatment protocols [3].

After four weeks of therapy, the anticipated decrease in WBC was not observed. Therefore, pentostatin was added at 4 mg/m^2 per week, as previously described [8]. With the addition of pentostatin, bone marrow biopsy indicated complete morphologic and cytogenetic remission. An allogeneic SCT was planned, but since she had neither a related nor a suitable unrelated donor, umbilical cord blood grafts were selected. The grafts were both HLA matched at 5/6 loci. A pretransplant bone marrow biopsy demonstrated a normocellular marrow with trilineage hematopoiesis and 5–10% residual T-PLL cells. Shortly thereafter, the patient underwent reduced intensity dUCBT, conditioned with fludarabine, cyclophosphamide, and total body irradiation [9]; cyclosporine and mycophenolate mofetil were used for graft-versus-host disease (GVHD) prophylaxis. She received 4.2×10^7 total nucleated cells/kg (TNC/kg) from cord 1 (female) and 2.4×10^7 TNC/kg from cord 2 (male). Neutrophil engraftment occurred on day +18, and no signs or symptoms of GVHD ensued. One year after transplantation, a biopsy showed a normocellular marrow (40%) with trilineage hematopoiesis and no overt signs of residual or recurrent T-PLL. Chimerism

Table 1: Postengraftment analysis following double UCB transplantation, prior to relapse.

Time post-UCB transplant		Donor 1 (female) (%)	Donor 2 (male) (%)
Day +35	Whole blood	48	40
	T-cell subset	>90	<10
Day +141	Whole blood	68	30
	T-cell subset	67	17
Day +251	Whole blood	70	27
	T-cell subset	56	23
12 months	Whole blood	72	21
	T-cell subset	49	44
21 months	Whole blood	95	5
	T-cell subset	79	13

studies indicated 68% donor 1 and 30% donor 2. A summary of her engraftment analysis is provided in Table 1.

Sixteen months after transplant, she began to experience increased fatigue and developed new leukocytosis. Flow cytometry confirmed a second relapse of the disease. Soon thereafter, retreatment with alemtuzumab and pentostatin began. The patient became profoundly cytopenic following her alemtuzumab and pentostatin therapy. Bone marrow biopsy in mid-October confirmed a third remission, with 99% donor cells, though again with both grafts represented 80% donor 1 and 19% donor 2. She remained in complete remission with incomplete platelet recovery; the percentage of donor 1 increased to 95% and percentage of donor 2 dropped to 5% during this time. Unfortunately, however, after a remission that lasted six months, the patient relapsed for a third time and was refractory to attempts at salvage therapy. She expired after surviving for 29 months following her transplant.

3. Discussion

The phenomenon of single-unit dominance has been well described [5]. It is thought to be mediated by rejection of one graft by T cells in the dominant graft [10], though predicting which cord will predominate is not possible [7]. Coengraftment and mixed donor/recipient chimerism have been associated with relapse [6]. Following successful treatment of relapse after dUCBT with alemtuzumab and pentostatin, no recipient chimerism was detectable, while donor 1 engraftment peaked at 95%, but donor 2 still persisted (5%). It is interesting that posttransplant therapy with alemtuzumab and pentostatin brought the patient closer to achieving single-unit dominance, which raises the possibility that anti-T-cell therapy after transplant may promote single-unit dominance and potentially protect against relapse. There is clinical evidence supporting the idea that the presence of specific T-cell populations after transplant can mediate the dominance of one cord blood unit over the other, and preclinical data demonstrating that depletion of immune cell fractions within a graft strongly influences coengraftment [10]. Additional research will be needed to fully elucidate the mechanisms of single-unit dominance after dUCBT and to learn whether immune manipulation in a way that promotes single-unit dominance can reduce relapse risk. This case does illustrate, however, that dUCBT is feasible for T-PLL, and postremission dUCBT should be considered for patients with T-PLL who lack available suitably matched related or unrelated donors. This patient remained relatively responsive to salvage therapies even after relapsing following dUCBT and survived for 12 months following her initial posttransplant relapse and 29 months after transplant. This exceeds the anticipated survival for patients treated with alemtuzumab-based therapies alone without transplant, particularly given detectable residual disease at the time of transplant and treatment with a reduced intensity conditioning regimen.

References

[1] A. Collignon, A. Wanquet, E. Maitre, E. Cornet, X. Troussard, and T. Aurran-Schleinitz, "Prolymphocytic leukemia: new insights in diagnosis and in treatment," *Current Oncology Reports*, vol. 19, no. 4, 2017.

[2] M. Damlaj, N. H. Sulai, J. L. Oliveira et al., "Impact of alemtuzumab therapy and route of administration in T-prolymphocytic leukemia: a single-center experience," *Clinical Lymphoma Myeloma and Leukemia*, vol. 15, no. 11, pp. 699–704, 2015.

[3] A. Österborg, R. Foà, R. F. Bezares et al., "Management guidelines for the use of alemtuzumab in chronic lymphocytic leukemia," *Leukemia*, vol. 23, no. 11, pp. 1980–1988, 2009.

[4] T. E. Tanimoto, A. Hirano, K. Nagafuji et al., "Mismatched unrelated cord blood transplantation in a patient with T-cell prolymphocytic leukemia," *Leukemia*, vol. 19, no. 4, pp. 679–681, 2005.

[5] N. S. Majhail, C. G. Brunstein, and J. E. Wagner, "Double umbilical cord blood transplantation," *Current Opinion in Immunology*, vol. 18, no. 5, pp. 571–575, 2006.

[6] P. Ramirez, J. E. Wagner, T. E. DeFor et al., "Factors predicting single-unit predominance after double umbilical cord blood transplantation," *Bone Marrow Transplantation*, vol. 47, no. 6, pp. 799–803, 2012.

[7] H. Hashem and H. M. Lazarus, "Double umbilical cord blood transplantation: relevance of persistent mixed-unit chimerism," *Biology of Blood and Marrow Transplantation*, vol. 21, no. 4, pp. 612–619, 2015.

[8] J. Mercieca, E. Matutes, C. Dearden, K. MacLennan, and D. Catovsky, "The role of pentostatin in the treatment of T-cell malignancies: analysis of response rate in 145 patients according to disease subtype," *Journal of Clinical Oncology*, vol. 12, no. 12, pp. 2588–2593, 1994.

[9] J. N. Barker, "Rapid and complete donor chimerism in adult recipients of unrelated donor umbilical cord blood transplantation after reduced-intensity conditioning," *Blood*, vol. 102, no. 5, pp. 1915–1919, 2003.

[10] C. H. J. Lamers, R. Wijers, C. A. M. van Bergen et al., "CD4+ T-cell alloreactivity toward mismatched HLA class II alleles early after double umbilical cord blood transplantation," *Blood*, vol. 128, no. 17, pp. 2165–2174, 2016.

13

Monoclonal Gammopathy of Renal Significance with Progression to Multiple Myeloma in a Patient with ASIA-MO Syndrome

David Alejandro Vargas Gutiérrez,[1] Karina Ivonne Arias Callejas,[2] Edwin Pavel Palacios Ruiz,[3] Priscila Joseline Pérez Vinueza,[1] Juan Diego Muñoz Vega,[4] Ana Karen G. Mejía Geraldo,[5] and Ingrid Salinas Zaldívar[3]

[1]*Department of Rheumatology, Instituto Nacional de Rehabilitación Luis Guillermo Ibarra Ibarra, CDMX, Mexico*
[2]*Department of Rheumatology, Instituto Nacional de Cardiología Ignacio Chávez, CDMX, Mexico*
[3]*Department of Internal Medicine, Hospital General de México: "Dr. Eduardo Liceaga", CDMX, Mexico*
[4]*Department of Hematology, Hospital General Mexico: "Dr. Eduardo Liceaga", CDMX, Mexico*
[5]*Department of Pathological Anatomy, Hospital General Mexico: "Dr. Eduardo Liceaga", CDMX, Mexico*

Correspondence should be addressed to Ingrid Salinas Zaldívar; salinaszaldivar@hotmail.com

Academic Editor: Kostas Konstantopoulos

Background. Autoimmune/inflammatory syndrome induced by adjuvants is a disease associated with an unregulated hyperactivity of the immune system and may also be associated with a high frequency of hematologic malignancies. *Report.* This is a case of a female with ASIA-MO syndrome secondary to infiltration of mineral oil for aesthetic purposes and presented with multiple episodes of urolithiasis resulting in renal impairment of her left kidney confirmed by scintigraphy and ending in unilateral nephrectomy. Retrospective renal piece analysis confirmed tubulointerstitial infiltration with light chains and plasma cells. Paraffin fixation prevented subsequent immunofluorescence analysis for better follow-up of the patient. *Conclusion.* The presence of positive immunofixation kappa chains explained the sudden deterioration of renal function with monoclonal gammopathy of renal significance which concluded in an association between diseases, such as multiple light chain myeloma, as a final diagnosis.

1. Introduction

This case report presents a patient with end-stage renal disease and hypercalcemia of unknown etiology alongside with a long-standing inflammatory state.

Therefore, hypercalcemia malignancy suspicion was intensified by identifying parathormone (PTH) suppression, in addition to light-chain screening with a positive monoclonal gammopathy and a bone biopsy with 60% of clonal plasma cells receiving a diagnosis of multiple myeloma with an ominous outcome.

Because of the absence of risk factors for a young female with end-stage renal disease, multiple etiologies were subjected to analysis such as monoclonal gammopathy of renal significance (MGRS), amyloidosis, and nephrocalcinosis, among others.

As a consequence, it was decided to review the surgical piece postmortem with light-chain deposit, tubular damage, and light-chain proximal tubulopathy (LCPT) as the main findings.

2. Case Presentation

This is a case of a 38-year-old female from the Mexico City with a history of infiltration of mineral oil in the mammary region back in 2001, which conditioned the development of subcutaneous nodules, thickening of the skin, and hyperpigmentation. This lesion spread throughout the anterior chest and abdomen, resulting in mechanical lumbar discomfort.

Her condition began one year before her first hospital admission with multiple episodes of urinary tract infection (UTI) secondary to urolithiasis which required left nephrostomy with subsequent clinical improvement. She was diagnosed with renal lithiasis, along with hypercalciuria (urinary calcium 322 mg/dl), CaU/CrU = 0.33, and phosphorus excretion fraction of 21%, and it was initially managed with thiazide diuretic (hydrochlorothiazide).

However, 6 months later, fever returned together with a fall in the glomerular filtration rate (GFR) of 44 ml/min/1.73 m^2 CKD-EPI (Chronic Kidney Disease Epidemiology Collaboration) (Table 1), but also proteinuria in the subnephrotic range (960 mg/24 hours), albuminuria of 53 mg/24 hours, and urinary sediment with granular casts, without dysmorphia or acanthocytes. Blood tests reported hypoalbuminemia (3.2 mg/dl) and total serum protein of 7.8 mg/dl. Renal USG showed bilateral loss of the medullary cortex relationship and a left kidney size of 9.6 cm*4.4 cm*45.2 cm (without pyelocaliceal dilation or any anatomy abnormalities); however, it did describe stranding of the perinephric fat on the right kidney as a sign of pyelonephritis.

As part of the febrile syndrome workout, immunological tests were performed such as antinuclear and antineutrophil cytoplasm antibodies; both were negative. After a myeloproliferative syndrome was suspected, the BMA smear was labeled as normocellular without the presence of blasts, with plasma cells <7%, and with negative myelocultures. Treatment with empirical antimicrobials showed improvement in the infection and fever of unknown origin.

Unfortunately, 3 months later, the renal function continued to deteriorate, requiring renal scintigraphy, reaching a GFR of 10.1 ml/min in the left kidney and 61 ml/min in the right one, determining renal exclusion. Due to recurrent pyelonephritis and the exclusion mentioned above, a left nephrectomy was performed. Despite this approach, 3 months later, the patient presented with pallor, palpitations, fatigue, nausea, and persistent vomiting, and blood work reported acidosis and a high anion gap (16), accompanied by azotemia, normocytic normochromic anemia (hemoglobin 7 mg/dl), and moderate hypercalcemia (corrected calcium 12.7 mg/dl).

She required hemodialysis, IV fluids, diuretic therapy, and blood transfusion with clinical improvement. Despite this, hypercalcemia persisted with PTH suppression (1.8 pg/ml). Consequently, the analysis was redirected for independent PTH hypercalcemia, ruling out 25-hydroxycholecalciferol toxicity (24 ng/dl) (she actually had this deficiency). Phase-contrast CT showed a large-volume granulomatous disease with extensive infiltration which included the anterior and posterior mediastinum, pelvis, and spleen. Moreover, evidence of splenomegaly in the absence of tumor disease and lytic lesions is found in the L4 posterior wall (Figure 1). Abnormally high concentrations of $\beta 2$ microglobulin (B2M) (5.6 mg/L) were found, which could also be found not only in lymphoproliferative disorders but in renal failure as well (41). Serum immunoglobulin was normal, but high values of serum-free kappa light chains (FLCs) (102 mg/L) and the lambda chain (9.1 mg/L) were additionally with a κ/λ ratio (11.2) as synonymous to monoclonality. Urinary and serum protein electrophoresis was analyzed without evidence of any gamma monoclonality.

Urinary protein immunofixation electrophoresis (IFE) showed tubular protein positivity with a monoclonal kappa band peak along with anemia, hypercalcemia, and renal function impairment of unknown etiology pointing to plasma cell dyscrasia. Bone biopsy showed clonal plasma cells (immunohistochemistry with 60% positive plasma cells for CD38).

Then, MGRS evolving into MM was concluded, and chemotherapy sessions were scheduled. However, by yielding a poor result, association of ASIA-MO and kidney disease reflected in the death of the patient, even before we could start the procedure.

In conclusion, a postmortem histopathological of the renal piece reported the presence of interstitial nephritis with the plasma cell infiltrate with positive immunohistochemistry for light-chain kappa in the interstitium and LCPT (Figure 2).

3. Discussion

3.1. Monoclonal Gammopathy of Renal Significance and LCPT. Paraprotein originates from monoclonal immunoglobulins or their light chains, characterized by the expression of a single light chain, κ or λ, also called monoclonal protein or M protein. The most common is the low-level nonmalignant paraprotein monoclonal gammopathy of undetermined significance (MGUS) [1].

Approximately 1% of asymptomatic MGUS (IgG or IgA) will progress to MM, which could later become light-chain MM or AL amyloidosis. Currently, this "indolent" state is considered premalignant, although it has been questioned since cloned plasma cells may occasionally be responsible for serious organ damage through tissue toxicity by M protein [2].

MGRS is defined as a plasma or lymphoplasmocytic clonal cell disorder with secretion and deposit of monoclonal immunoglobulins or their fractions in the renal parenchyma with toxic effects by several mechanisms [3].

This kidney injury phenomenon was replicated in animal models where Bence Jones proteins were administered intravenously or by intraperitoneal infusion, resulting in deposit-associated nephropathy which supports the theory that MM presence is not always required [4].

In chronic glomerular injury, tubular cells lose integrity with an increase in proinflammatory cytokines. Moreover, patients with higher amounts of urinary protein >20 KDa presented poor response rates to both glucocorticoid and cyclophosphamide treatments than patients with proteinuria <20 KDa alone (30% vs. 80%) such as light chains [5].

MGUS development is multifactorial. The most accepted theory states 2 essential hits in the development of premalignant and malignant lesions; the first one is an abnormal response to antigenic stimulation, mediated by an

Table 1: Laboratory and clinical findings in a chronological order.

Parameters	Initial 03/06/2016	Nephrectomy 01/08/2017	Reentry for impairment 01/04/2018
Urea (mg/dl)	36	51	290
Creatinine (mg/dl)	1.5	2	7.1
Uric acid (mg/dl)	7.1	8.5	6
Total proteins (mg/dl)	5.2	7.7	6.9
Albumin (mg/dl)	1.5	2.17	2.3
Corrected calcium (mg/dl)	10.9	12.7	13.2
Phosphorus (mg/dl)	3.6	3.2	4
WBC (cel/L)	15,000	6.5	7.6
Neutrophils (cel/L)	13,300	4.8	5.3
Hemoglobin (g/dl)	10.4	9	7
MCV (fL)	90	83	96
MCH (pg)	32	30	33
Platelets (109/L)	410	373	348

WBC: white blood cell, MCV: mean corpuscular volume, and MCH: mean corpuscular hemoglobin.

aberrant expression of TLRs, and the second one is determined by overexpression of IL-6r and IL-1r secondary to persistent inflammatory processes as observed in our patient, which promoted the development of primary cytogenetic abnormalities. The development of MM manifestations from premalignant states such as MGUS or SMM requires a second DNA lesion or loss of cell cycle surveillance and repairing systems such as chromosome 16 methylation, MYC abnormalities, and RAS and p53 mutations [6].

Therefore, symptoms of MM could be initially noticed after nephrectomy, expressed by low levels of plasma cells with dysplasia [7]. A high incidence of malignant tumors is observed in CKD due to the chronic increase in cytokines and growth factors caused by hyperazotemia, low renal clearance of proinflammatory cytokines, and oxidative stress [8]. Furthermore, high levels of sialic acid are present in the monoclonal immunoglobulins of MGUS and MM [9], and this was observed in the analysis of 2817 CKD patients in a hospital in Turkey, with the report of malignancy on 6.7% of patients (188) and 2.6% of MM [10].

In multiple myeloma, the serum level of β2M has been widely studied as a biomarker of renal function in humans and murine models; however, it can increase its production and its presence as a free molecule in hematological and solid neoplasms. Part of this is the main determinant in the International Staging System (ISS), which predicts not only the prognosis but also the progression of asymptomatic disease (HR 3.30; $P = 0.002$); despite this, it is important to take into account that renal insufficiency can elevate β2M levels and therefore complicates determination of the exact origin of an elevated serum level [11].

While kidney damage in the presence of intact immunoglobulin molecules is limited to the glomerulus, incomplete light and heavy chains can affect all renal compartments, but tubulointerstitial lesions are caused by any of the light chains (most often kappa). Light chains are internalized by tubular epithelial cells; when this tubular reabsorption capacity is exceeded, the intracellular protein gradient saturates, resisting degradation with the generation of ROS, sustained inflammation, and apoptosis of epithelial cells.

LCPT is an uncommon form of renal disease associated with progressive renal failure dysproteinemia with the presence or absence of inclusion. It presents with a normal glomerulus along the first needle-shaped rhomboidal or rectilinear eosinophilic inclusions (periodic acid-Schiff (PAS) negative) by light microscopy, and LCPT without inclusion and vacuolar changes or excessive drops, necrosis of epithelial cells with displacement, detachment, and apical blisters are common findings with 13%–77% [12, 13].

3.2. ASIA-MO.

ASIA is a disorder associated with unregulated hyperactivity of the immune system with the infiltration of exogenous substances as a main characteristic. The initial criteria proposed in 2011 by Shoenfeld and Agmon-Levin to classify patients with autoimmune manifestations with preexisting conditions together with adjuvants have generated controversy. Despite that, the so-called ASIA associated with mineral oil (ASIA-MO) was added recently to this classification and defined as the infiltration of modeling substances for aesthetic purposes. Mineral oils (MOs) are saturated hydrocarbons of variable, linear, and branched ring chain structures of carbon. The MO acts as an adjuvant capable of accelerating, prolonging, or increasing an autoimmune response [14].

High incidence of systemic manifestations of autoimmune-type phenomena, such as carbon-rich mineral oils and silicone, has shown to promote animal model expansion of the adaptive immune response, producing ASIA-MO-like syndromes [15].

Isolated cases of ASIA-associated breast cancer reported with the highest frequency of hematologic malignancies such as non-Hodgkin lymphoma [16, 17]. Anaplastic large-cell lymphoma associated with breast implants is a recent clinical entity with 80 cases identified worldwide and four associated deaths. In 2016, the WHO classified this subtype as a recognized entity and emphasized the importance of foreign material removal surgery as a prophylactic measure [18]. The cytogenetic and biochemical study of 3 patients with breast anaplastic lymphoma and breast implants was

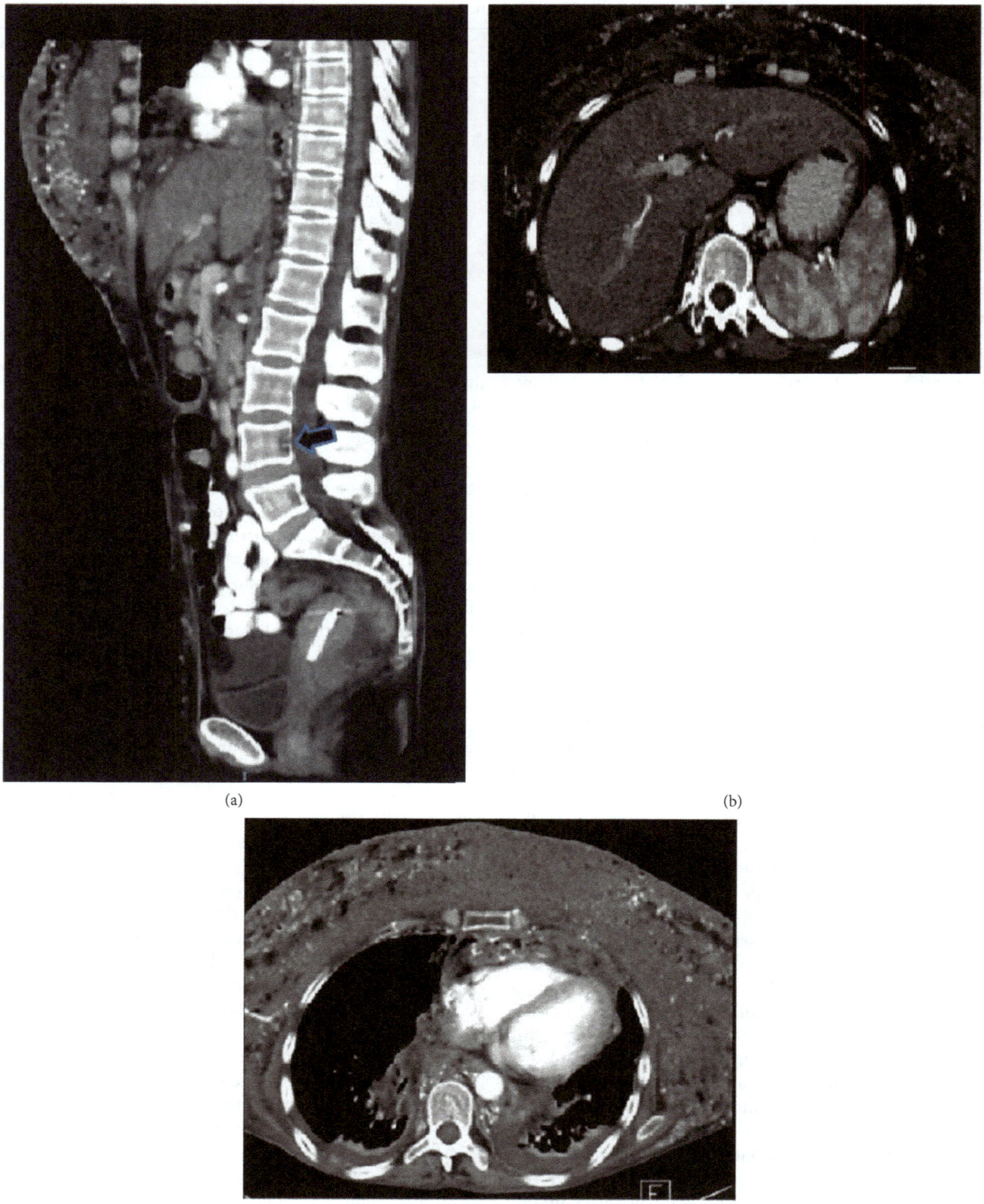

(a) (b) (c)

Figure 1: Computed axial tomography (contrast phase). (a) Sagittal section shows an increase in soft tissue volume in the mammary region of the L4 vertebral body. A hypodense lesion with continuity loss is seen at the posterior vertebra wall suggestive of erosive injury (arrow). (b) Cross section at the abdomen shows the spleen with granular characteristics and heterogeneity of its content. (c) In the thorax, abundant granular tissue is observed not only at the rib cage but also in the anterior and posterior mediastinum, secondary to the substance dissemination and infiltration.

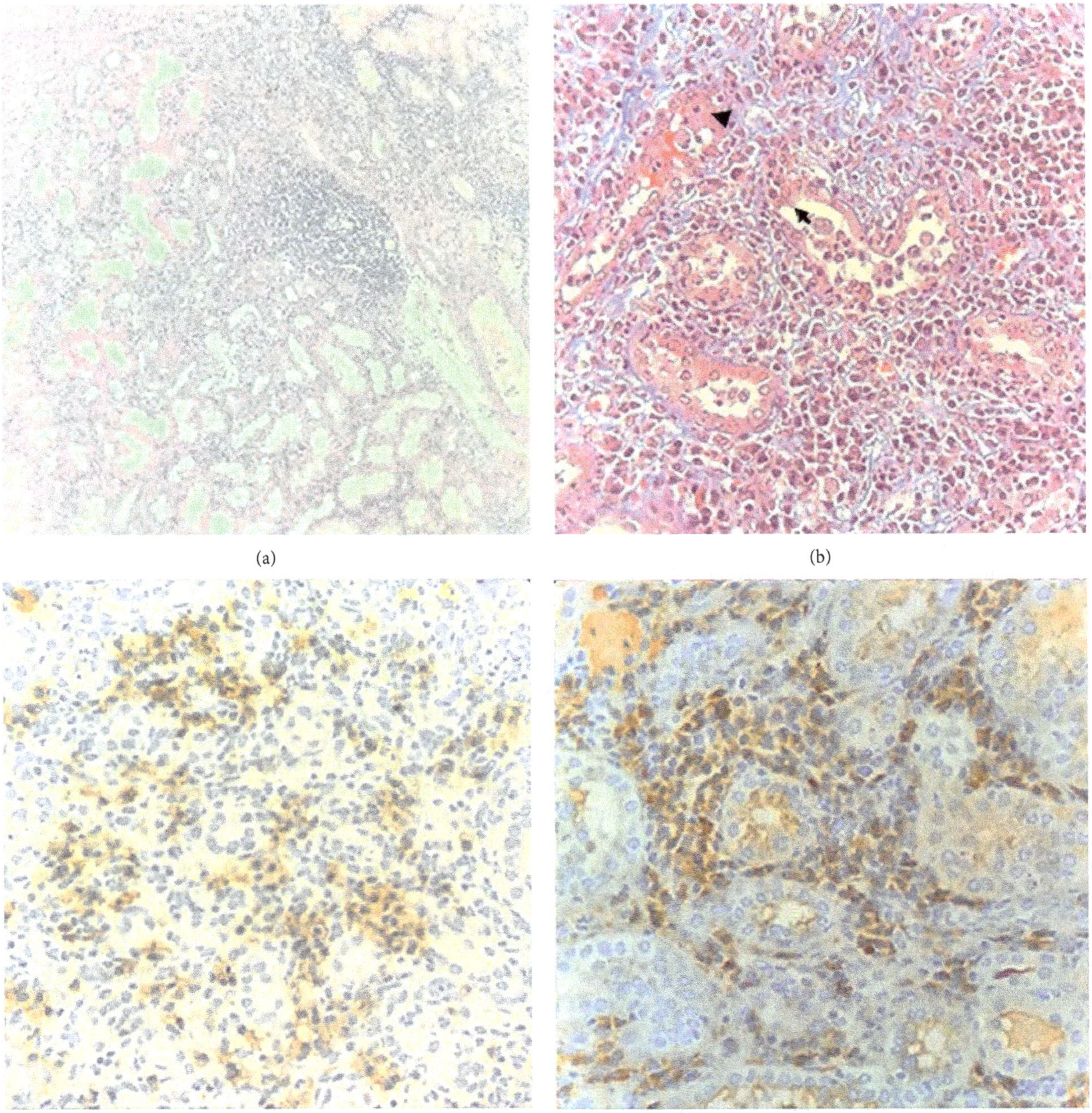

(a) (b) (c) (d)

FIGURE 2: Renal biopsy immunohistochemistry. (a) In the microphotograph with HyE, we can observe part of the medulla composed by tubules with acute tubular necrosis and disappearance of nuclei in a few cells. The interstitium is altered by the presence of the chronic lymphoplasmacytic infiltrate, arranged by cumulus in some areas, but also the presence of slight fibrosis. (b) Masson staining shows interstitial thickening secondary to the lymphoplasmacytic infiltrate reaching the proximal contoured tubules giving an irregularity in its contour. As a paramount feature, the presence of eosinophilic inclusions (arrowhead) in the cytoplasm of the epithelium covering these tubules is seen and also the desquamation of this epithelium which is compatible with LCPT (arrow). Blue staining confirms the presence of slight fibrosis. (c) Immunohistochemical staining for CD138 (plasma cell biomarker) was performed with a significant reaction at the membrane level highlighting the abundant presence of plasma cells. (d) Reaction to kappa light chains (brown staining) shows variable positivity inside the cytoplasm of plasma cells at the interstitium, which represents its monoclonality.

described by Lechner et al., showing an increase in STAT3 signaling related to the autocrine production of IL-6, a mechanism shared with the development of MM [19]. In contrast, a study by Karlson et al. found little evidence for MGUS risk in patients with breast implants [20].

Anderson and Potter demonstrated the molecular association of plasma cell neoplasms and ASIA-MO in BALB/c susceptible murine models with pristane intraperitoneal induction as an enhancer of the innate immune system with arthritis, lupus-related autoantibodies, and IgA-secreting plasma cell neoplasms as a result [21, 22]. However, it also relates to the granulomatous reaction at the site of application with limited tissue antigen clearance, granulomatous body strange reaction, and a proinflammatory state [23]. Other studies observed small plasmocytomas within 3 weeks of subsequent infiltration with kappa or lambda polypeptides which induce nephrosis [24].

3.3. Diagnostic Approach. Low levels of vitamin 25 (OH) D, related to the CKD, and hypercalcemia of malignancy contributed to decreased reabsorption and higher excretion of calcium. In this particular case, the presence of granulomatous disease in thoracic visceral sites was demonstrated by CT with ASIA-MO-induced spread and initial inflammation in both breasts.

Granulomatous pathologies in the breast are complex problems that require an exhaustive study to identify various causes, including infectious etiologies such as mycobacterial infection (*M. tuberculosis*). In this patient, IGRAs screening was negative. Other autoimmune etiologies of granulomatous mastitis are sarcoidosis, which represents 1% of these disorders, and GPA. The first was ruled out because it did not present classic sarcoid conditions in other sites and vitamin D levels were low. GPA was ruled out since it did not show evidence of epithelial proliferative lesions of the glomerulus, and ANCA antibody titers were reported negative. Finally, hematological neoplasms such as lymphoma were ruled out given that during its evolution, it did not present B symptoms, although no biopsy of granulomatous or ganglion tissue was performed [25]. Finally, systemic amyloidosis AA or AL was ruled out in the absence of nephrotic phenotype, and the biopsy was Congo red negative.

Another mechanism carrying tubular damage is the presence of hypercalcemia with hypercalciuria but also with precipitation of calcium crystals and lesions of the epithelium affected by episodes of lithiasis. Bataille et al. evaluated osteoclast-mediated bone resorption in 87 bone biopsies from patients with MGUS, 45% of whom presented some degree of bone resorption and 52% of whom were classified as high-risk patients which progressed to MM compared to 4% of the low-risk group [26]. Low-grade bone resorption through premalignant or malignant neoplasms of plasma cells reflected at the urinary level by hypercalciuria since compensation mechanisms manage to mitigate the increase in calcium plasma levels as observed in our case report [27].

Autoimmune diseases along with chronic inflammatory conditions are reported to be associated with an increased risk of MGUS [28]. Malignant transformation is associated with the presence of heavy-chain IgA, high levels of ESR, high percentage of plasma cells in the bone marrow, and osteoporosis [29]. A case-control study involving men and women diagnosed with MM and MGUS over a period of 40 years found an increased risk of MGUS (OR = 2.1; 95% CI, and 1.9–2.4) in patients with all subcategories of autoimmune diseases characterized by chronic inflammation (OR = 1.4; 95% CI, 1.2–1.5) [30].

Yang et al. describe 41 patients with rheumatic diseases and a positive screening for monoclonal gammopathies, the most common associated finding being Sjogren's syndrome (SSj). Disease activity was an independent risk factor for the development of monoclonal gammopathy, and its presence was associated with an OR of 17.5 (95% CI: 1.5–197) for MM. Similar findings in other autoimmune diseases such as rheumatoid arthritis, systemic lupus erythematosus, and inflammatory myopathies with MM or MGUS had an RR of 2.29 with a prevalence of MGUS up to 42%. Here, chronic B cell activation and antibody production develop a chronic immune environment with pro-oncogene mutations [31].

Chronic inflammatory nephropathy previously reported by pathologists was a light-chain nephropathy; hence, immunohistochemistry was performed with kappa chain findings and changes suggestive of LCPT. Despite the current awareness of ASIA-MO syndrome, there is still skepticism that this could explain why this patient was not clearly diagnosed or treated for 18 years; as a consequence, disease activity could become a possible explanation.

4. Conclusion

This is an interesting case because it describes the possible association between both pathologies in which chronic inflammation becomes a substrate triggered by ASIA as an epigenetic factor aimed at monoclonal paraproteinemia, tubular injury, and acute inflammation, where the nephrectomy played a second hit which contributed to the final manifestation of MM. There are not enough studies in the field, and there is much heterogeneity which makes it difficult to analyze this or any other case. We suggest that more studies should be analyzed in the future, and hopefully, prospective studies will be conducted to determine the relationship between these two pathologies.

Abbreviations

ASIA: Autoimmune/inflammatory syndrome induced by adjuvants
ASIA-MO: ASIA associated with mineral oil
BMA: Bone marrow aspirate
B2M: *β*2 Microglobulin
CKD-EPI: Chronic Kidney Disease Epidemiology Collaboration
CT: Computed tomography
DAMPs: Molecular patterns associated with damage
DC: Dendritic cells
ESR: Erythrocyte sedimentation rate
FLCs: Free light chains
GFR: Glomerular filtration rate
IFE: Immunofixation electrophoresis
IL-6r: Interleukin 6 receptor
LCPT: Light-chain proximal tubulopathy
MGRS: Monoclonal gammopathy of renal significance
MGUS: Monoclonal gammopathy of undetermined significance
MM: Multiple myeloma
PAS: Periodic acid-Schiff
PTH: Parathormone

ROS: Reactive oxygen species
SSj: Sjogren's syndrome
SMM: Smoldering multiple myeloma
TLRs: TOLL-like receptors
UTI: Urinary tract infection.

Consent

Written informed consent was obtained from the patient for publication of this case report and any accompanying images.

Authors' Contributions

David Alejandro Vargas Gutiérrez was responsible for medical data recollection, patient interview, follow-up and description of the case, composition, and bibliography research. Karina Ivonne Arias Callejas contributed to medical data recollection, sample and image recollection, composition, bibliography, research, and case reviewing. Edwin Pavel Palacios Ruiz carried out case reviewing, composition, and renal expertise contributions and bibliography research. Juan Diego Muñoz Vega performed hematology expertise contributions and bibliography research. Priscila Joseline Pérez Vinueza was responsible for translation, case reviewing, composition, and bibliography research. Ana Karen G. Mejía Geraldo took part in pathology sample description and expertise assessment and bibliography research. Ingrid Salinas Zaldívar performed the first translation, case reviewing, composition, and bibliography research.

Acknowledgments

The authors express their gratitude to the patient's family for allowing them to collect data, which will contribute to clinical information and future research.

References

[1] L. Cook and D. H. Macdonald, "Management of paraproteinaemia," *Postgraduate Medical Journal*, vol. 83, no. 978, pp. 217–223, 2007.

[2] N. W. C. J. Van de Donk, T. Mutis, P. J. Poddighe, H. M. Lokhorst, and S. Zweegman, "Diagnosis, risk stratification and management of monoclonal gammopathy of undetermined significance and smoldering multiple myeloma," *International Journal of Laboratory Hematology* vol. 38, no. Suppl 1, pp. 110–122, 2016.

[3] N. Leung, F. Bridoux, V. Batuman et al., "The evaluation of monoclonal gammopathy of renal significance: a consensus report of the International Kidney and Monoclonal Gammopathy Research Group," *Nature Reviews Nephrology*, vol. 15, no. 1, pp. 45–59, 2019.

[4] C. Sirac, G. A. Herrera, P. W. Sanders et al., "Animal models of monoclonal immunoglobulin-related renal diseases," *Nature Reviews Nephrology*, vol. 14, no. 4, pp. 246–264, 2018.

[5] G. D'Amico and C. Bazzi, "Pathophysiology of proteinuria," *Kidney International*, vol. 63, no. 3, pp. 809–825, 2003.

[6] S. K. Kumar, V. Rajkumar, R. A. Kyle et al., "Multiple myeloma," *Nature Reviews Disease Primers*, vol. 3, Article ID 17046, 2017 20.

[7] J. Tecklenborg, D. Clayton, S. Siebert, and S. M. Coley, "The role of the immune system in kidney disease," *Clinical and Experimental Immunology*, vol. 192, no. 2, pp. 142–150, 2018.

[8] C. Musolino, A. Allegra, V. Innao, A. G. Allegra, G. Pioggia, and S. Gangemi, "Inflammatory and anti-inflammatory equilibrium, proliferative and antiproliferative balance: the role of cytokines in multiple myeloma," *Mediators of Inflammation*, vol. 2017, Article ID 1852517, 12 pages, 2017.

[9] A. Bosseboeuf, S. Allain-Maillet, N. Mennesson et al., "Pro-inflammatory state in monoclonal gammopathy of undetermined significance and in multiple myeloma is characterized by low sialylation of pathogen-specific and other monoclonal immunoglobulins," *Frontiers in Immunology*, vol. 8, Article ID 1347, 2017.

[10] K. Cengiz, "Increased incidence of neoplasia in chronic renal failure (20-year experience)," *International Urology and Nephrology*, vol. 33, no. 1, pp. 121–126, 2002.

[11] C. P. Argyropoulos, S. S. Chen, Y. H. Ng et al., "Rediscovering beta-2 Microglobulin as a biomarker across the spectrum of kidney diseases," *Frontiers of Medicine*, vol. 473 pages, 2017.

[12] S. G. Sharma, S. M. Bonsib, D. Portilla, A. Shukla, A. B. Woodruff, and N. Gokden, "Light chain proximal tubulopathy: expanding the pathologic spectrum with and without deposition of crystalline inclusions," *ISRN Pathology*, vol. 2012, Article ID 541075, 6 pages, 2012.

[13] A. Jain, R. Haynes, J. Kothari, A. Khera, M. Soares, and K. Ramasamy, "Pathophysiology and management of monoclonal gammopathy of renal significance," *Blood Advances*, vol. 3, no. 15, pp. 2409–2423, 2019.

[14] V. Borba, A. Malkova, N. Basantsova et al., "Classical examples of the concept of the ASIA syndrome," *Biomolecules*, vol. 10, no. 10, Article ID 1436, 2020.

[15] S. Janz, B. Rassmann, F. Raabe, and H. Storch, "[Histologic studies of paraproteinemic nephropathy in BALB/c mice with mineral oil-induced plasmacytoma]," *Zeitschrift für Urologie und Nephrologie*, vol. 82, no. 12, pp. 671–678, 1989.

[16] R. Ameratunga, D. Gillis, M. Gold, A. Linneberg, and J. M. Elwood, "Evidence refuting the existence of autoimmune/autoinflammatory syndrome induced by adjuvants (ASIA)," *Journal of Allergy and Clinical Immunology: In Practice*, vol. 5, no. 6, pp. 1551–1555, 2017.

[17] O. Vera-Lastra, G. Medina, M. P. Cruz-Domínguez et al., "Autoimmune/inflammatory syndrome induced by mineral oil: a health problem," *Clinical Rheumatology*, vol. 37, no. 6, pp. 1441–1448, 2018.

[18] S. A. McIntosh and K. Horgan, "Breast cancer following augmentation mammoplasty-a review of its impact on prognosis and management," *Journal of Plastic, Reconstructive & Aesthetic Surgery*, vol. 60, no. 10, pp. 1127–1135, 2007.

[19] O. Moling, A. Piccin, M. Tauber et al., "Intravascular large B-cell lymphoma associated with silicone breast implant, HLA-DRB1*11:01, and HLA-DQB1*03:01 manifesting as macrophage activation syndrome and with severe

neurological symptoms: a case report," *Journal of Medical Case Reports*, vol. 10, no. 1, 254 pages, 2016.

[20] A. Chacko and T. Lloyd, "Breast implant-associated anaplastic large cell lymphoma: a pictorial review," *Insights Imaging*, vol. 9, no. 5, pp. 683–686, 2018.

[21] M. G. Lechner, C. Megiel, C. H. Church et al., "Survival signals and targets for therapy in breast implant-associated ALK-- anaplastic large cell lymphoma," *Clinical Cancer Research*, vol. 18, no. 17, pp. 4549–4559, 2012.

[22] E. W. Karlson, M. Tanasijevic, S. E. Hankinson et al., "Monoclonal gammopathy of undetermined significance and exposure to breast implants," *Archives of Internal Medicine*, vol. 161, no. 6, pp. 864–867, 2001.

[23] P. N. Anderson and M. Potter, "Induction of plasma cell tumours in BALB-c mice with 2, 6, 10, 14-tetramethylpentadecane (pristane)," *Nature*, vol. 222, no. 5197, pp. 994-995, 1969.

[24] M. Potter, "A resumé of the current status of the development of plasma-cell tumors in mice," *Cancer Research*, vol. 28, no. 9, pp. 1891–1896, 1968.

[25] R. M. Jales, P. N. Pereira, R. F. Stelini, and L. Moro, "Systemic granulomatous diseases associated with multiple palpable masses that may involve the breast: case presentation and an approach to the differential diagnosis," *Case Report of Medicine*, vol. 2014, Article ID 146956, 8 pages, 2014.

[26] M. A. Khalighi, W. Dean Wallace, and M. F. Palma-Diaz, "Amyloid nephropathy," *Clinical Kidney Journal*, vol. 7, no. 2, pp. 97–106, 2014.

[27] R. Bataille, D. Chappard, and M. F. Basle, "Quantifiable excess of bone resorption in monoclonal gammopathy is an early symptom of malignancy: a prospective study of 87 bone biopsies," *Blood*, vol. 87, no. 11, pp. 4762–4769, 1996.

[28] A. W. Smith and C. L. Mcilwaine, "Hypercalciuria," *British Medical Journal*, vol. 1, no. 5436, pp. 671-672, 1965 13.

[29] E. Terpos, D. Christoulas, M. Gavriatopoulou, and M. A. Dimopoulos, "Mechanisms of bone destruction in multiple myeloma," *European Journal of Cancer Care*, vol. 26, no. 6, 2017.

[30] N. W. van de Donk, A. Palumbo, H. E. Johnsen et al., "The clinical relevance and management of monoclonal gammopathy of undetermined significance and related disorders: recommendations from the European Myeloma Network," *Haematologica*, vol. 99, no. 6, pp. 984–996, 2014.

[31] M. E. González García, C. Fernández Alvarez, V. Robles Marinas et al., "[A series of 618 cases of monoclonal gammopathies of undetermined significance: predictive factors of disappearance of monoclonal component or evolution to malignant gammopathies]," *Revista Clinica Espanoia*, vol. 208, no. 6, pp. 288–294, 2008.

14

Venetoclax and Decitabine for T/Myeloid Mixed-Phenotype Acute Leukemia Not Otherwise Specified (MPAL NOS)

Heather Klocke,[1] Zhao Ming Dong,[1,2] Craig O'Brien,[1] Nicholas Burwick,[1,3] Robert E. Richard,[1,3] Daniel Y. Wu,[1,4,5] Thomas R. Chauncey,[1,4,5] and Solomon A. Graf[1,4,5]

[1]*Veterans Affairs Puget Sound Health Care System, Seattle, WA, USA*
[2]*Department of Pathology, University of Washington Medicine, Seattle, WA, USA*
[3]*Division of Hematology, University of Washington Medicine, Seattle, WA, USA*
[4]*Division of Medical Oncology, University of Washington Medicine, Seattle, WA, USA*
[5]*Clinical Research Division, Fred Hutch Cancer Research Center, Seattle, WA, USA*

Correspondence should be addressed to Solomon A. Graf; grafsa@uw.edu

Academic Editor: Sudhir Tauro

T/myeloid mixed-phenotype acute leukemia not otherwise specified (MPAL NOS) is an uncommon and aggressive leukemia without well-established treatment guidelines, particularly when relapsed. Venetoclax plus a hypomethylating agent offers a promising option in this situation since studies support its use in both acute myeloid and, albeit with fewer data to date, acute T-cell-lymphoblastic leukemias. We report the successful eradication of T/myeloid MPAL NOS relapsed after allogeneic stem cell transplant with venetoclax plus decitabine. A consolidative allogeneic stem cell transplant from a second donor was subsequently performed, and the patient remained without evidence of disease more than one year later. Further investigation is indicated to evaluate venetoclax combined with hypomethylating agents and/or other therapies for the management of T/myeloid MPAL NOS.

1. Introduction

Mixed-phenotype acute leukemia (MPAL) is characterized by leukemic blasts expressing antigens of more than one lineage to such a degree that it is not possible to assign one lineage with certainty. MPAL and acute undifferentiated leukemia (which shows no lineage-specific antigen) constitute a group of acute leukemias of ambiguous lineage. MPAL are uncommon, accounting for <5% of acute leukemias [1, 2]. MPAL T/myeloid NOS (T/myeloid MPAL) fulfills criteria for both T-cell and myeloid lineage without specific genetic abnormalities such as BCR-ABL1 or KMT2A rearrangement and is one of 5 MPAL subtypes recognized by 2016 World Health Organization classification [3]. T/myeloid MPAL is considered a high-risk acute leukemia, and limited data guide its management at diagnosis and relapse [4]. Venetoclax plus a hypomethylating agent (HMA) was approved for use by the Food and Drug Administration in November 2018 for older or relatively frail patients with newly diagnosed acute myeloid leukemia (AML) [5]. We report here the first, to our knowledge, successful application of venetoclax plus HMA for relapsed T/myeloid MPAL.

2. Case Report

A previously healthy 65-year-old man presented to an outside hospital with fatigue, folliculitis, easy bruising, vision changes, and decreased hearing. He had a normal coagulation screen; however, he was found to have cytopenias with a white blood cell count of 5.5 K/μL that included approximately 50% blast forms, hemoglobin of 10.0 g/dL, and platelet count of 78 K/μL. Marrow showed 70–80% blasts positive for CD34, terminal deoxynucleotidyl transferase (TdT), CD3, myeloperoxidase (MPO), and CD5, and negative for PAX-5 and c-Kit (Figure 1). Flow cytometry (FC) demonstrated the blasts to express markers specific for myeloid (cytoplasmic MPO) and T-lymphoid (cytoplasmic CD3) lineages. Blasts were also positive for CD5, CD7, CD10, CD34, CD11b, CD33, and TdT on FC. Cytogenetics were normal, and no abnormalities were identified on 200 interphase cells examined by fluorescence in-situ hybridization: specifically, analysis showed no evidence of 3q21.3q26.2 translocation or inversion, deletion 5q31, monosomy 7, deletion 7q31, RUNX1T1-RUNX1 translocation, KMT2A rearrangement, CBFB rearrangement, or PML/RARA translocation. Next generation sequencing identified the following mutations: DNMT3A c.2206C > T (variant allele frequency (VAF) 43.9%); DNMT3A c.1755dup (VAF 36.5%); IDH1 c.394C > T (VAF 44.0%); CBL c.1227 + 2T > C (VAF 51.6%); and NOTCH 1 c.5023_5025del (VAF 13.9%). Together, findings established the diagnosis of T/myeloid MPAL. Cerebrospinal fluid was negative by cytology and FC.

Induction treatment was given with 3 half cycles (1A, 1B, and 2A) of cyclophosphamide, vincristine, doxorubicin, and dexamethasone alternating with methotrexate and cytarabine (hyper-CVAD) and intrathecal (IT) prophylaxis [6]. This achieved a complete remission (CR), with bone marrow biopsy after cycle 1A, showing no evidence of disease by morphology or FC and no circulating blasts in the peripheral blood. He was transferred to our facility for consideration of consolidation stem cell transplantation. A repeat bone marrow exam was performed and demonstrated continued remission. The patient proceeded to a matched related donor allogeneic stem cell transplantation (allo-SCT) from his brother with reduced intensity conditioning (RIC) (fludarabine 30 mg/m^2 daily for 3 consecutive days (Flu) and 200 cGy total body irradiation (TBI)) with tacrolimus and mycophenolate mofetil graft versus host disease (GvHD) prophylaxis [7]. Marrow on day 28 posttransplant showed morphologic remission with 0.06% blasts by FC. Markers used to detect MRD by FC included CD45, CD34, CD38, CD48, CD56, CD71, CD117, CD123, CD5, CD7, CD33, cCD3, sCD3, CD4, CD8, CD13, CD14, CD15, CD16, CD19, CD64, and HLA-DR. A repeat marrow one week later showed an increase in blasts to 0.1% by FC, and chimerism analysis showed donor CD3 of 40%, CD33 of 85%, and CD56 of 71%. His immunosuppression was tapered and completely discontinued on day 47, and he received donor-lymphocyte infusion with pentostatin on day 50 posttransplant. At day 18 post DLI blasts had increased to 6% by FC; by morphology, a population of 5% TDT + CD34+ blasts were shown. The patient was next treated with one cycle of intensive reinduction using cladribine, cytarabine, filgrastim, and mitoxantrone (CLAG-M) [8] plus vincristine and dexamethasone. This was complicated by neutropenic sepsis requiring prolonged intensive care, but the patient made a full recovery, and restaging bone marrow biopsy showed a CR by morphology and FC. A second allogeneic stem cell transplant was planned, but shortly beforehand, the patient developed grade 2 GvHD of the skin and was treated successfully with oral corticosteroids. Given that he was still in CR by FC and hoping the GvHD would correspond to increased graft versus leukemia, the 2nd transplant was postponed. Unfortunately, repeat bone marrow exam approximately 3 months later confirmed low-level relapse detectable by FC. Reinduction with 2 cycles of CLAG-M plus vincristine and dexamethasone (with mitoxantrone omitted from the 2nd cycle) was again administered but associated with substantially increased toxicity to the patient's functional status and a prolonged length of recovery. CR by morphology and FC was briefly achieved before disease was identified at a level of 0.9% by FC on day 441 posttransplant.

At this juncture, the patient was >1-year post-allo-SCT with relapsed T/myeloid MPAL despite several rounds of high-intensity chemotherapy. He was reasonably fit, evidenced by his regular exercise bicycling regimen, but had shown declining tolerance of successive cytotoxic chemotherapy regimens. He had no clinically active GvHD. Given the paucity of published data to inform this clinical scenario, we presented 3 options for management that included (1) directly pursuing a 2nd allo-SCT using a different donor; (2) additional conventional multiagent chemotherapy; or (3) venetoclax plus HMA. He began venetoclax 400 mg by mouth daily and decitabine 20 mg/m^2 intravenous daily on days 1–5 in 28 day cycles. No dose ramp-up of venetoclax was given in the setting of low disease burden. Because of grade 4 neutropenia and grade 4 thrombocytopenia, venetoclax was stopped on day 25. Both cell lines recovered by day 35, and a bone marrow exam at that time showed CR by morphology and FC. A 2nd cycle was given, with venetoclax dose-reduced to 100 mg daily. A full 28 days of venetoclax was administered with recovery of neutrophils and platelets on day 37. Other than cytopenias, the regimen was well tolerated. He proceeded to a 2nd SCT from a matched unrelated donor allograft with Flu/TBI RIC and cyclosporine, mycophenolate mofetil, and sirolimus GvHD prophylaxis [9]. Engraftment of neutrophils occurred on day 19 after transplantation, and no grade >1 GvHD has been observed to date. At his most recent follow-up 1 year after his 2nd allo-SCT he remains in CR by morphology and FC with CD3, CD33, and CD56 compartments entirely of donor origin.

3. Discussion

Relapsed T/myeloid MPAL, including after allo-SCT, carries a poor prognosis with no established treatment protocols. Generally, strategies are extrapolated from studies of more common acute leukemias [4]. Consolidative second allo-SCT can be beneficial to select patients with relapsed AML [10]. In our case, a 2nd allo-SCT was considered a reasonable approach if CR without detectable disease could be achieved since the patient had a good functional status, few comorbidities, and a different matched donor. Venetoclax, an inhibitor of the antiapoptotic protein BCL-2, is a generally well-tolerated oncolytic with synergistic antileukemic activity when combined with an HMA [5]. Though limited prospective data detail the regimen's use in the relapsed AML setting, it appears to have significant activity, with CR rates as high as 40% in a retrospective analysis of 219 patients

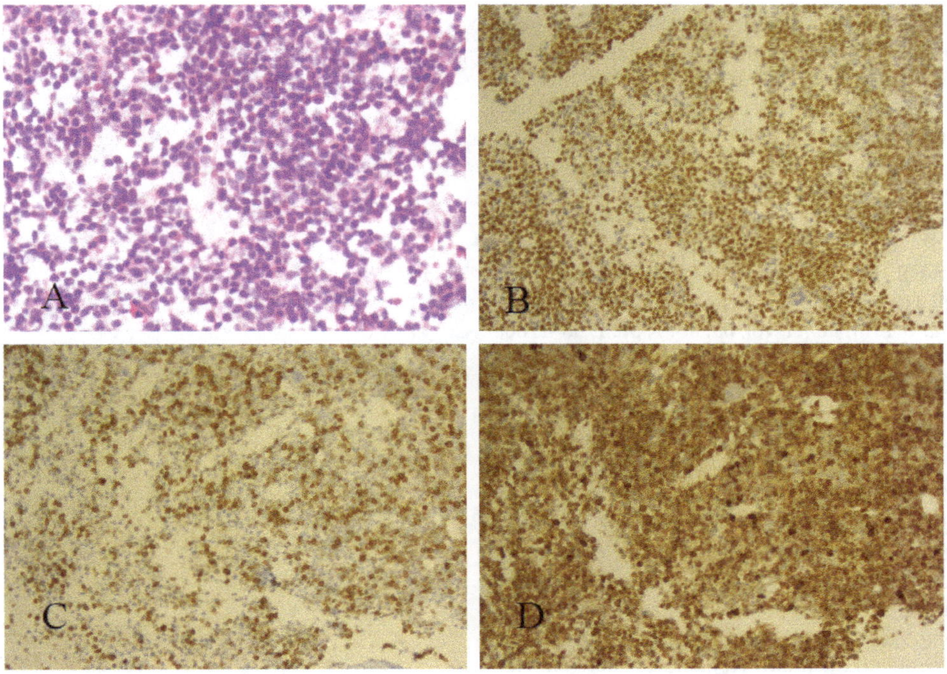

FIGURE 1: Bone marrow biopsy with T/myeloid mixed-phenotype acute leukemia as demonstrated by H&E stain with 80% blasts. (a) 200x and immunohistochemical stains for terminal deoxynucleotidyl transferase. (b) DAB, 200x, cytoplasmic CD3 with anti-CD3 (2GV6) rabbit monoclonal antibody against the epsilon chain. (c) DAB, 200x, and myeloperoxidase. (d) DAB, 200x.

with relapsed AML, myelodysplastic syndrome, or blastic plasmacytoid dendritic cell neoplasm [11]. Still fewer data exist on the use of venetoclax plus HMA in relapsed T-cell leukemias [12]. A series of 12 patients with relapsed T-cell leukemia treated with venetoclax plus various chemotherapies (included an HMA in 3) was recently published and showed an impressive response rate of 60% [13]. In addition, emerging data from recent and ongoing clinical trials have shown promising outcomes with venetoclax and an HMA in cases of acute myeloid leukemia with an IDH1/2 mutation; this may have particular relevance to our case in which a mutation in IDH1 was detected at diagnosis [14].

4. Conclusion

To our knowledge, this is the first report of venetoclax plus HMA for relapsed T/myeloid MPAL. The regimen was a successful bridge to 2nd allo-SCT and well-tolerated aside from prolonged cytopenias in the setting of repeated prior cytotoxic chemotherapy regimens. Regimens for MPAL are typically designed to treat both myeloid and lymphoid lineages; therefore, based on publications of retrospective series to date, venetoclax plus HMA offers a promising novel approach to this clinically challenging entity [11, 13]. Future research is required to further explore this strategy and combine venetoclax with other agents active in T/myeloid MPAL.

Disclosure

The contents of this paper do not represent the views of the U.S. Department of Veterans Affairs or the United States Government.

References

[1] W. van den Ancker, M. Terwijn, T. M. Westers et al., "Acute leukemias of ambiguous lineage: diagnostic consequences of the WHO 2008 classification," *Leukemia*, vol. 24, no. 7, pp. 1392–1396, 2010.

[2] J. H. Kurzer and O. K. Weinberg, "Acute leukemias of ambiguous lineage," *Surgical Pathology Clinics*, vol. 12, no. 3, pp. 687–697, 2019.

[3] D. A. Arber, A. Orazi, R. Hasserjian et al., "The 2016 revision to the World Health Organization classification of myeloid neoplasms and acute leukemia," *Blood*, vol. 127, no. 20, pp. 2391–2405, 2016.

[4] O. Wolach and R. M. Stone, "Optimal therapeutic strategies for mixed phenotype acute leukemia," *Current Opinion in Hematology*, vol. 27, no. 2, pp. 95–102, 2020.

[5] C. D. DiNardo, K. W. Pratz, A. Letai et al., "Safety and preliminary efficacy of venetoclax with decitabine or azacitidine in elderly patients with previously untreated acute myeloid leukaemia: a non-randomised, open-label, phase 1b study," *The Lancet Oncology*, vol. 19, no. 2, pp. 216–228, 2018.

[6] H. M. Kantarjian, S. O'Brien, T. L. Smith et al., "Results of treatment with hyper-CVAD, a dose-intensive regimen, in adult acute lymphocytic leukemia," *Journal of Clinical Oncology*, vol. 18, no. 3, p. 547, 2000.

[7] Y. Nieto, N. Patton, T. Hawkins et al., "Tacrolimus and mycophenolate mofetil after nonmyeloablative matched-sibling donor allogeneic stem-cell transplantations conditioned with fludarabine and low-dose total body irradiation," *Biology of Blood and Marrow Transplantation*, vol. 12, no. 2, pp. 217–225, 2006.

[8] A. B. Halpern, M. Othus, E. M. Huebner et al., "Phase I/II trial of cladribine, high-dose cytarabine, mitoxantrone, and G-CSF with dose-escalated mitoxantrone for relapsed/refractory

acute myeloid leukemia and other high-grade myeloid neoplasms," *Haematologica*, vol. 104, no. 4, pp. e143–e146, 2019.

[9] B. M. Sandmaier, B. Kornblit, B. E. Storer et al., "Addition of sirolimus to standard cyclosporine plus mycophenolate mofetil-based graft-versus-host disease prophylaxis for patients after unrelated non-myeloablative haemopoietic stem cell transplantation: a multicentre, randomised, phase 3 trial," *The Lancet Haematology*, vol. 6, no. 8, pp. e409–e418, 2019.

[10] B. Gyurkocza, R. Storb, T. R. Chauncey, D. G. Maloney, B. E. Storer, and B. M. Sandmaier, "Second allogeneic hematopoietic cell transplantation for relapse after first allografts," *Leukemia & Lymphoma*, vol. 60, no. 7, pp. 1758–1766, 2019.

[11] J. P. Bewersdorf, S. Giri, R. Wang et al., "Venetoclax as monotherapy and in combination with hypomethylating agents or low dose cytarabine in relapsed and treatment refractory acute myeloid leukemia: a systematic review and meta-analysis," *Haematologica*, vol. 60, 2020.

[12] L. T. Rahmat, A. Nguyen, H. Abdulhaq, S. Prakash, A. C. Logan, and G. N. Mannis, "Venetoclax in combination with decitabine for relapsed T-cell acute lymphoblastic leukemia after allogeneic hematopoietic cell transplant," *Case Reports in Hematology*, vol. 2018, 2018.

[13] G. Richard-Carpentier, E. Jabbour, N. J. Short et al., "Clinical experience with venetoclax combined with chemotherapy for relapsed or refractory T-cell acute lymphoblastic leukemia," *Clinical Lymphoma, Myeloma & Leukemia*, vol. 18, 2019.

[14] C. D. DiNardo, C. R. Rausch, C. Benton et al., "Clinical experience with the BCL2-inhibitor venetoclax in combination therapy for relapsed and refractory acute myeloid leukemia and related myeloid malignancies," *American Journal of Hematology*, vol. 93, no. 3, pp. 401–407, 2018.

15

A Case of Parathyroid Adenocarcinoma and Hyperparathyroidism, When "CRAB" Symptoms are Not due to a Plasma Cell Myeloma

Habib Moshref Razavi[1,2] **and Reza Alaghehbandan**[2,3]

[1]*Division of Hematopathology, Department of Pathology and Laboratory Medicine, University of British Columbia, Vancouver, British Columbia, Canada*
[2]*Fraser Health Authority, Royal Columbian Hospital, Department of Laboratory Medicine, New Westminster, British Columbia, Canada*
[3]*Division of Anatomical Pathology, Department of Pathology and Laboratory Medicine, University of British Columbia, Vancouver, British Columbia, Canada*

Correspondence should be addressed to Habib Moshref Razavi; habib.moshrefrazavi@fraserhealth.ca

Academic Editor: Alessandro Gozzetti

A previously well 49-year-old patient presented to our hospital with symptomatic hypercalcaemia complaining of polyuria and polydipsia, as well as abdominal and lower back pain (serum/ionized calcium at 3.66 milli mole/l and 1.90 milli moles/l). At admission, he had a normocytic anemia (Hb, 99 g/L) and acute kidney injury (creatinine at 161 μM). His parathyroid hormone (PTH) levels were at 67.6 pico moles/l. A plain X-ray of the lumbar spine showed the presence of a lytic lesion in the L4 vertebrae. CT and MRI confirmed this to be a destructive lesion. A subsequent pan CT scan showed a 2.8 cm complex nodule in the left lobe of the thyroid posteriorly. Excisional biopsy of the resected mass was associated with an infiltrative cellular parathyroid neoplasm with solid and nested architectural growth pattern admixed with hemorrhage and focal calcifications. The tumor showed lymphovascular and perineural invasion. At the time of workup and despite the absence of a positive SPEP/UPEP, a bone marrow biopsy was requested to rule out multiple myeloma. His normocellular bone marrow biopsy showed marked paratrabecular fibrosis and extensive bony remodelling but no metastatic invasion. The diagnosis of a metastatic parathyroid carcinoma was made. He is subsequently considered for palliative radiotherapy to the primary tumor bed and the lumbar spine. In addition, a role for immunotherapy with ipilimumab and nivolumab in context of clinical trials is envisioned and he is being considered for enrollment.

1. Introduction

Primary hyperparathyroidism, although usually asymptomatic, can routinely be discovered on biochemical evaluation. One manifestation of primary hyperparathyroidism, parathyroid/hypercalcemic crisis, is defined as calcium levels greater than 3.75 milli moles/l with signs and symptoms of acute calcium intoxication [1]. Parathyroid carcinoma is a rare event [2, 3]. This diagnosis should be considered in patients with primary hyperparathyroidism, who present with a hyperparathroid crisis, or in those who present with a neck mass. Although the classic features of tissue diagnosis include a trabecular pattern, presence of mitotic figures, thick fibrous bands, and capsular and vascular invasion, the two criteria upon which a more definitive diagnosis of parathyroid cancer is reached include local invasion of contiguous structures (such as vascular or neural invasion) and/or invasion of lymph nodes/distant metastases [4–6]. Treatment for this incurable disease includes medical management starting with correction of hypercalcaemia with hydration and bisphosphonates. Cases of refractory hypercalcaemia are treated with calcimimetics such as cinacalcet or the potent inhibitor of bone resorption denosumab [7, 8]. The mainstay of therapy however includes surgical resection including palliative debulking of metastatic disease. In cases of widespread metastatic disease not amenable to surgery, chemotherapy and adjuvant palliative radiation of bone metastases or locoregional disease play a role. However, patients in this stage generally have many comorbidities and an overall poor prognosis [2]. Here, the case of a patient with hypercalcaemia, renal failure, anemia, and lytic lesions (CRAB) is described. This constellation of these symptoms evoked the diagnosis of plasma cell myeloma, which was not diagnosed in the described case.

2. Case Report

The case of a 49-year-old patient with several years of lower back pain with acute exacerbation is described. His past medical history is notable for epilepsy associated with childhood head trauma. Following a prior left frontal lobe resection of brain scar tissue in 1996, this condition has since resolved. He has a 45 pack-year history of smoking, and until October of 2019, he had been a heavy drinker, consuming up to 15 drinks per day. He works on a boat yard. He reported a 40 pounds weight loss over the previous couple of years. His family history is significant for maternal history of lung cancer. His father had skin cancer. On admission to our hospital, the patient reported some constipation, polyuria, and polydipsia. He denied any flushing, diaphoresis, or presence of renal stones. A routine CBC and chemistry panel showed a normocytic anemia (99 g/l) and much elevated calcium levels (serum/ionized calcium at 3.66 milli moles/l and 1.90 milli moles/l). He also had an acute kidney injury (creatinine at 161 μmoles/l). His serum phosphorous was low at 0.6 mmol/l. His 24-hour urine calcium level was increased at 13 mmol/day. His PTH was markedly elevated at 67.6 pico moles/l. Given his lower back pain and CRAB features, a spine X-ray as well as a lumbar CT were done, which showed lytic lesions in the L4 vertebral body (Figure 1). The biochemical correlate, his bone-specific alkaline phosphatase, was accordingly elevated at 170 U/l. His physical examination showed normal vital signs and no physical evidence of lymphadenopathy or splenomegaly. However, palpation of the thyroid revealed a 2 cm nodule on the left lobe. A pan CT showed a 2.8 cm × 2.6 cm complex left lobe thyroid nodule concerning for malignancy (Figure 2). The CT scan also confirmed lytic lesions at L4, as well as more lesions in C6-C7 and 9th ribs. A parathyroid scan done showed increased uptake at the mid and inferior aspect of the left thyroid bed posteriorly. A renal ultrasound showed mild echogenic changes bilaterally, but no hydronephrosis. A fine needle aspiration biopsy of the thyroid mass showed the presence of follicular-like epithelial clusters arranged in papillary and microfollicular architecture. The aspirated cells were stained for synaptophysin and chromogranin and were negative for TTF1 and thyroglobulin immunostains which in context of clinical findings suggested the presence of cellular parathyroid tissue. A parathyroidectomy was attempted. Upon exposure of the thyroid gland, a fibrous tumor with obvious macroscopic invasion of the esophagus, trachea, and left lobe of the thyroid gland was identified and resected. Tumor histology showed an infiltrative cellular parathyroid neoplasm with solid and nested architectural growth pattern admixed with hemorrhage and focal calcifications. The tumor also showed evidence of lymphovascular and perineural invasions consistent with features of a parathyroid carcinoma. In light of CRAB symptoms and in order to rule out a plasma cell myeloma and/or any other bone marrow intrinsic etiology, a bone marrow biopsy was requested. His normocellular bone marrow biopsy showed marked paratrabecular fibrosis (Figure 3). Increased osteoclastic activity showed surface bone excavation and trabecular tunneling. This stemmed from enlarging Howship lacunae, which effectively bisected the trabeculae (Figure 4). CD34 immunoperoxidase for blasts and CD3 (pan T) and CD20 (B) immunoperoxidase stains for T and B lymphocytes respectively were noncontributory. In addition, CD138, kappa and lambda stains showed polytypic plasma cells (Figure 5). Upon diagnosis, the patient was managed with fluids and cinacalcet as well as a one-time dose of bisphosphonates (pamidronate disodium 60 mg I.V.). He was a candidate for palliative radiation to his L4 lesion. There was also a consideration for enrollment in a phase II trial of immunotherapeutic agents ipilimumab and nivolumab which is not available in Canada. This trial is ongoing in the United States. However, unfortunately, the patient has as of this writing been unable to enroll due to traveling restrictions during the worldwide COVID-19 pandemic.

3. Discussion

Parathyroid carcinoma is a rare disease. In >90% of cases, it manifests with hyperparathyroidism [9]. The consequences of hyperparathyroidism reflects its physiological role of calcium metabolism including calcium resorption from the bone by way of PTHR1 receptor as well as renal activation of vitamin D and increased intestinal calcium uptake [10]. Pathophysiological consequences of overt hyperparathyroidism may present with renal, musculoskeletal, and neurological abnormalities such as nephrolithiasis/nephrocalcinosis, bone pain, and osteopenia, as well as anxiety and depression. Rarely, patients with parathyroid carcinoma present with clinical outcomes of life-threatening hypercalcaemia including renal failure, cardiac arrhythmias, and coma [11, 12]. Diagnosis requires a high index of suspicion. However, presence of some risk factors is informative. These include albumin-corrected hypercalcaemia (>3 milli moles/l), PTH levels being more than 3 times the upper limit of normal, presence of a neck mass at more than 3 cm along with neck pain and hoarseness as well as imaging evidence of infiltration and/or calcification on a neck ultrasound [13]. Accurate diagnosis is paramount for treatment regimens as pathological correlates such as parathyroid adenoma and hyperplasia exist and have markedly different clinical outcomes [14]. Features when present that are diagnostic of parathyroid carcinoma include unequivocal vascular invasion by the tumor, perineural invasion, gross invasion into adjacent anatomic structures, and distant metastases [15, 16]. Worrisome but nondiagnostic features include the

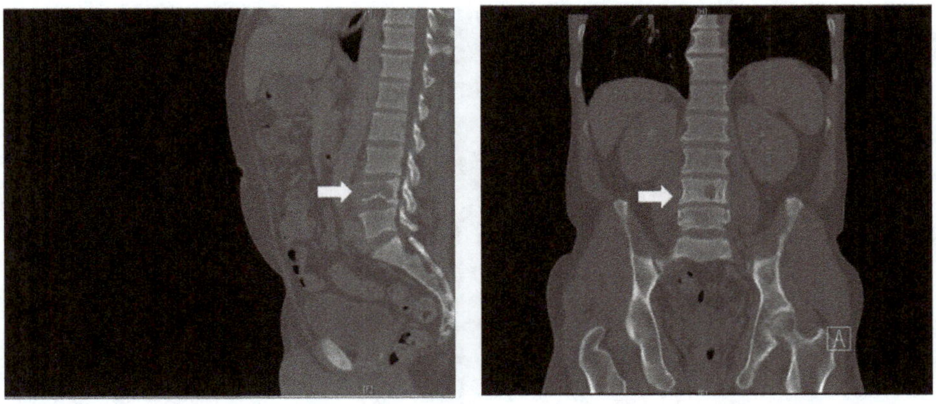

(a) (b)

FIGURE 1: Lumbar CT, left sagittal (a) and coronal (b) planes. A destructive lesion causing pathological fracture of the L4 vertebral body with mild adjacent soft tissue thickening. No abnormal soft tissue in the spinal canal was identified.

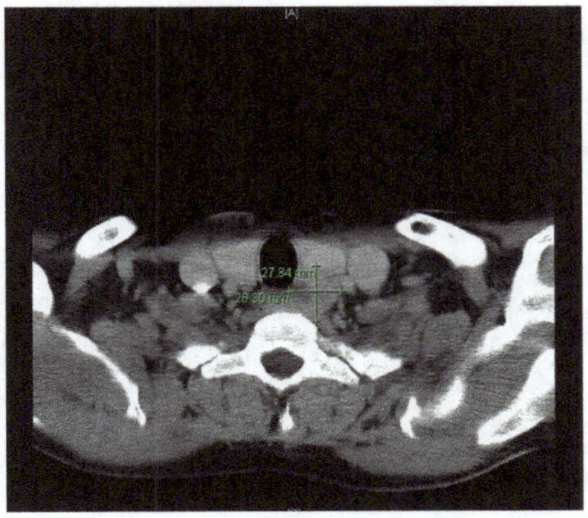

FIGURE 2: CT neck, transverse plane. A 2.8 × 2.6 cm complex nodule in the left lobe of the thyroid. On further examination by way of a thyroid ultrasound, the lesion was further characterized and described as an echo poor mass showing lobulated margins and coarse internal calcification, highly suspicious for malignancy.

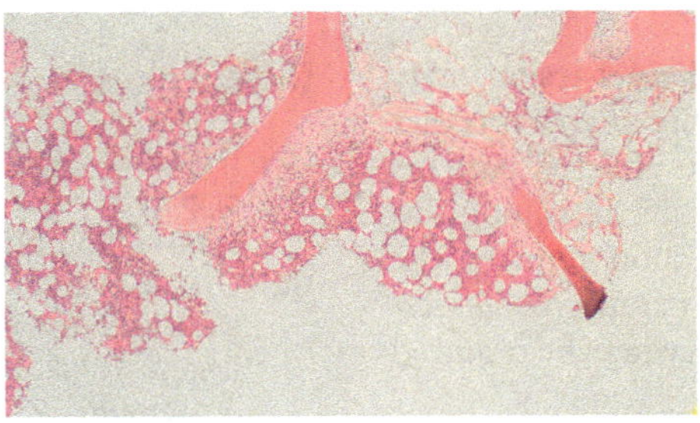

FIGURE 3: Bone marrow trephine biopsy, H&E × 10. Bony trabecular remodelling and paratrabecular fibrosis are present. The bone marrow biopsy is otherwise normocellular and shows trilinear hematopoiesis.

presence of coagulative necrosis, increased mitotic activity (>5/50 high power field), nuclear atypia, presence of macronucleoli, and presence of broad fibrous bands. In most cases, diagnosis is reached by morphology with clinical correlation. However, a panel of biomarkers such as galectin-3, parafibromin, p27, Rb, APC, Bcl-2a, p53, and MIB-1/Ki67 proliferation index may be helpful in borderline cases [17].

Bony and skeletal changes have been attributed to primary and secondary hyperparathyroidism. In fact, bony remodelling due to renal osteodystrophy and/or hyperparathyroidism secondary to intestinal malabsorption and/or gastric bypass surgery is indistinguishable to changes attributed to primary hyperparathyroidism. Enhanced activation of both osteoclasts and osteoblasts results in bone resorption by way of enlarging Howship lacunae, trabecular

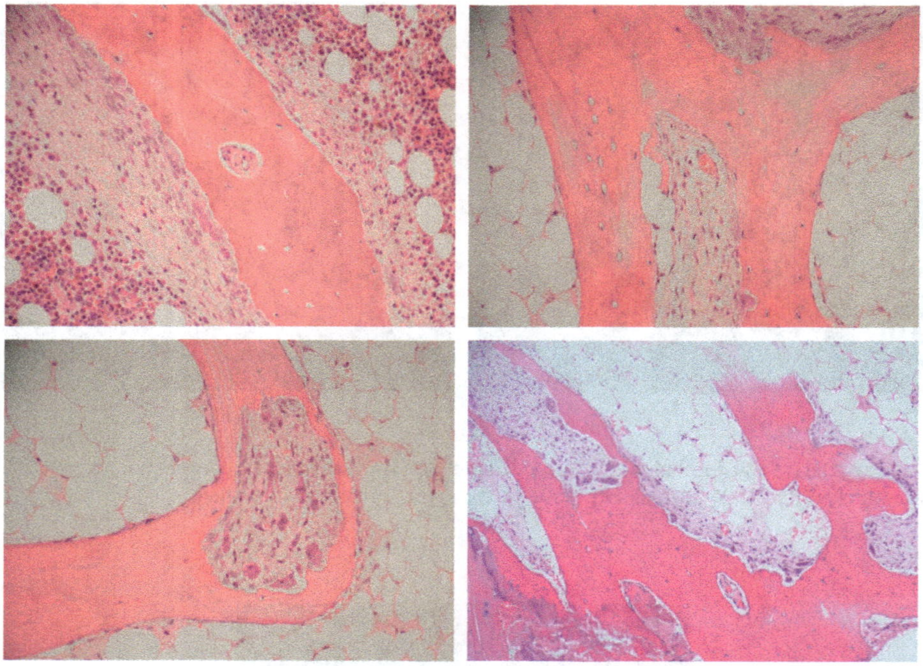

FIGURE 4: Enlarging Howship lacunae populated by osteoclasts. These enlarge and transect the bone marrow trabeculae forming swaths of intertrabecular fibrosis (lower row, right panel).

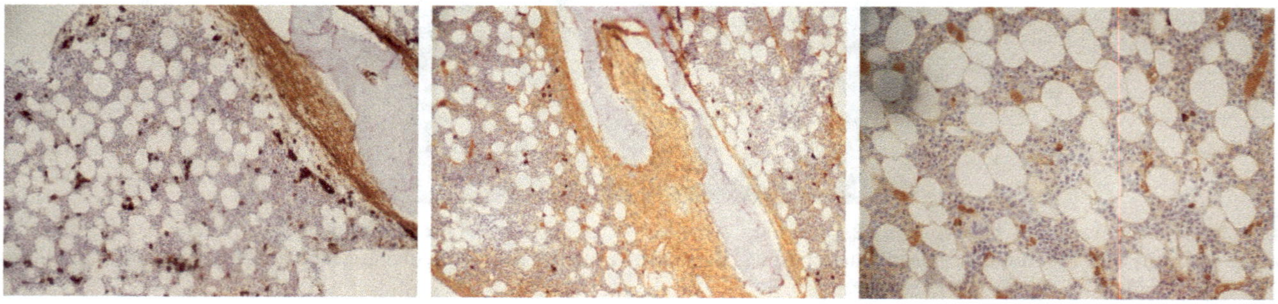

FIGURE 5: CD 138 and kappa and lambda stains show presence of polytypic plasma cells.

transection, and paratrabecular fibrosis. Larger lesions may cause the presence of fibrosis in an entire intertrabecular space [18, 19]. Therefore, at least in part, afflicted patients present with a hypoproliferative trilinear hematopoiesis manifesting as cytopenias. Surgical resection remains the mainstay of therapy and if by biopsy a parathyroid carcinoma is diagnosed, further revision surgery may be required for optimal disease control.

In conclusion, here we present a case of a patient with hypercalcaemia, renal dysfunction, anemia, and bony lytic lesions, initially evoking the diagnosis of plasma cell myeloma. However, a bone marrow biopsy as part of an extensive workup showed bone marrow manifestation of primary hyperparathyroidism associated with a hypoproliferative hematopoiesis. While the prognosis of metastatic parathyroid carcinoma remains poor, enhanced understanding of the disease mechanism has provided possible molecular targets such as cyclin D1, beta catenin, and calcium sensing receptors (CaSR) which may offer better outcomes.

References

[1] J. I. Lew, C. C. Solorzano, and G. L. Irvin, "Long-term results of parathyroidectomy for hypercalcemic crisis," *Archives of Surgery*, vol. 141, no. 7, pp. 696–699, 2006.

[2] C. H. Wei and A. Harari, "Parathyroid carcinoma: update and guidelines for management," *Current Treatment Options in Oncology*, vol. 13, no. 1, pp. 11–23, 2012.

[3] A. Ozolins, Z. Narbuts, A. Vanags et al., "Evaluation of malignant parathyroid tumours in two European cohorts of patients with sporadic primary hyperparathyroidism," *Langenbeck's Archives of Surgery*, vol. 401, no. 7, pp. 943–951, 2016.

[4] A. Schantz and B. Castleman, "Parathyroid carcinoma. A study of 70 cases," *Cancer*, vol. 31, no. 3, pp. 600–605, 1973.

[5] L. Bondeson, K. Sandelin, and L. Grimelius, "Histopathological variables and DNA cytometry in parathyroid carcinoma," *The American Journal of Surgical Pathology*, vol. 17, no. 8, pp. 820–829, 1993.

[6] C. E. Quinn, J. Healy, A. H. Lebastchi et al., "Modern experience with aggressive parathyroid tumors in a high-volume

New England referral center," *Journal of the American College of Surgeons*, vol. 220, no. 6, pp. 1054–1062, 2015.

[7] M. T. Collins, M. C. Skarulis, J. P. Bilezikian et al., "Treatment of hypercalcemia secondary to parathyroid carcinoma with a novel calcimimetic agent," *The Journal of Clinical Endocrinology & Metabolism*, vol. 83, no. 3, p. 1083, 1998.

[8] D. Karuppiah, G. Thanabalasingham, and B. Shine, "Refractory hypercalcaemia secondary to parathyroid carcinoma: response to high-dose denosumab," *The European Journal of Endocrinology*, vol. 171, no. 1, pp. K1–K5, 2014.

[9] W. D. Fraser, "Hyperparathyroidism," *The Lancet*, vol. 374, no. 9684, pp. 145–158, 2009.

[10] F. M. Hannan, E. Kallay, W. Chang et al., "The calcium-sensing receptor in physiology and in calcitropic and non-calcitropic diseases," *Nature Reviews Endocrinology*, vol. 15, no. 1, pp. 33–51, 2018.

[11] A. Al-Kurd, M. Mekel, and H. Mazeh, "Parathyroid carcinoma," *Surgical Oncology*, vol. 23, no. 2, pp. 107–114, 2014.

[12] W. T. Kassahun and S. Jonas, "Focus on parathyroid carcinoma," *International Journal of Surgery*, vol. 9, no. 1, pp. 13–19, 2011.

[13] K. Duan and O. Mete, "Parathyroid carcinoma: diagnosis and clinical implications," *Turkish Journal of Pathology*, vol. 31, pp. 80–97, 2015.

[14] B. M. Erovic, D. P. Goldstein, D. Kim et al., "Parathyroid cancer: outcome analysis of 16 patients treated at the princess Margaret hospital," *Head & Neck*, vol. 35, no. 1, pp. 35–39, 2013.

[15] S. J. Johnson, "Changing clinicopathological practice in parathyroid disease," *Histopathology*, vol. 56, no. 7, pp. 835–851, 2010.

[16] O. Mete and S. L. Asa, "Pathological definition and clinical significance of vascular invasion in thyroid carcinomas of follicular epithelial derivation," *Modern Pathology*, vol. 24, no. 12, pp. 1545–1552, 2011.

[17] A. Shifrin, V. Li Volsi, S. Shifrin-Douglas et al., "Primary and metastatic parathyroid malignancies: a rare or under-diagnosed condition?" *The Journal of Clinical Endocrinology & Metabolism*, vol. 100, pp. E478–E481, 2015.

[18] A. E. Broadus, "Primary hyperparathyroidism," *Journal of Urology*, vol. 141, no. 3, pp. 723–728, 1989.

[19] M. V. DeVita, L. L. Rasenas, M. Bansal et al., "Assessment of renal osteodystrophy in hemodialysis patients," *Medicine*, vol. 71, pp. 284–290, 1993.

16

Acute Laryngeal Dyspnea as the First Presentation of Mantle Cell Lymphoma: A Case Report and Review of the Literature

Mounir Ababou,[1] **Hicham El Maaroufi**,[1] **Adnane Hammani**,[1] **Selim Jennane**,[1] **El Mehdi Mahtat**,[1] **Mohammed Mikdame**,[2] **and Kamal Doghmi**[1]

[1]*Department of Clinical Hematology, Military Hospital Mohammed V, Mohammed V University, Rabat, Morocco*
[2]*Faculty of Medicine and Pharmacy of Rabat, Mohammed V University, Rabat, Morocco*

Correspondence should be addressed to Mounir Ababou; mounir.3b@gmail.com

Academic Editor: Kostas Konstantopoulos

Introduction. Acute laryngeal dyspnea is a life-threatening emergency, and the causes in adults are most often laryngeal tumors or inflammatory edema. Lymphoma of the larynx and especially the mantle cell type is extremely rare. *Case Presentation.* We report a case of a 43-year-old woman with no particular pathological history. She presented with progressive dyspnea which has evolved towards an inspiratory bradypnea that worsened until she ultimately required an emergency tracheotomy. Biopsies revealed mantle cell lymphoma. The patient has been staged IVB MIPI 6, and she was treated by immunochemotherapy followed by ASCT. The therapeutic evaluation shows a complete remission, 18 months after, and the patient was always disease free. *Conclusion.* The laryngeal localization of the mantle cell lymphoma is extremely rare; it may present catastrophically with acute airway obstruction. The diagnosis is mostly histological, hence the interest of deep biopsy. Given its rarity, the therapeutic strategy must be discussed case by case in a multidisciplinary consultation meeting.

1. Introduction

Acute laryngeal dyspnea is a life-threatening emergency, and the causes in adults are most often laryngeal tumors or inflammatory edema [1]. Laryngeal lymphoma is extremely rare, accounting for less than 1% of laryngeal tumors [2]. Less than 100 cases have been reported in the literature, including some cases of laryngeal mantle cell lymphoma [3–5]. Because of its rarity, we want to show to the medical community the clinical presentation of mantle cell lymphoma of the larynx which can be an emergency while discussing possible therapeutic choices by reviewing the literature.

2. Case Presentation

We report a case of a 43-year-old woman with no particular pathological history. She presented with progressive dyspnea which has evolved towards an inspiratory bradypnea that worsened until she ultimately required an emergency tracheotomy. Laryngoscopic examination showed an obstructive mass in the right infraglottic area. A punch biopsy of larynx tumor and excision of left cervical adenopathy were performed. The anatomopathological and immunohistochemical examination revealed a blastoid variant of mantle cell lymphoma CD20+, CD5+, cycline-D1+, LCA+, BCL6+/−, MUM1+/−, CD3−, CD30−, ALK−, and Ki67 at 90%. The patient reported general signs such as weight loss and nocturnal sweats in the last six months. The ECOG (Eastern Cooperative Oncology Group) performance status was 2, and the clinical examination revealed a tumoral syndrome made of bilateral cervical lymphadenopathy. Blood test showed leukocytosis at 11300/mm^3 with hyperlymphocytosis at 6200/mm^3 predominantly of small mature lymphocytes and a high LDH level at 779 U/l (the upper normal level limit of the laboratory is 245U/l). The rest of the biological assessment was normal. The 18-FDG positron emission tomography (PET) scan showed an over

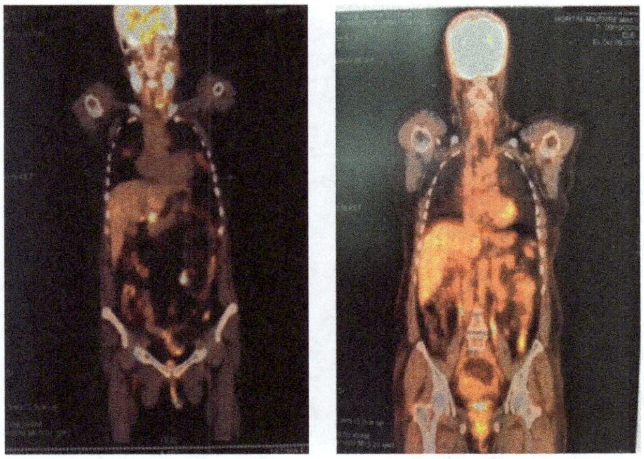

(a) (b)

FIGURE 1: (a) PET/CT at diagnosis showed hyperpathological lymph node metabolism over and under the diaphragmatic involvement. (b) PET/CT after treatment showed a complete metabolic remission.

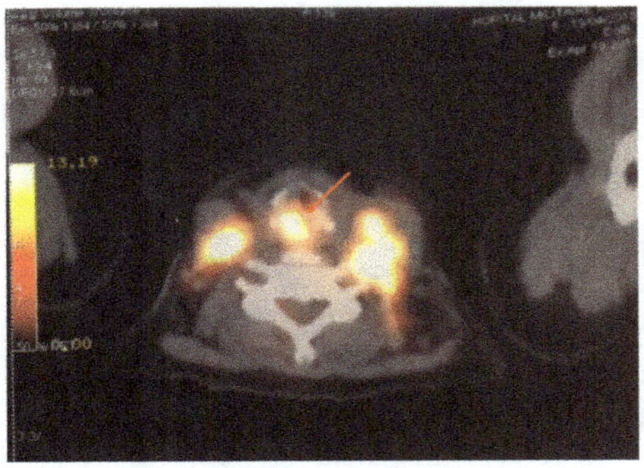

FIGURE 2: PET/CT at diagnosis showed pathological laryngeal hypermetabolism with cricoid cartilage involvement (red arrow).

and under diaphragmatic lymph node involvement and bilateral pathological pulmonary nodules (Figure 1(a)). A pathological laryngeal hypermetabolism with cricoid cartilage involvement (SUVmax = 15) was noticed (Figure 2), and bone marrow biopsy was negative. The patient has been staged IVB (Ann Arbor Classification), and the Mantle Cell Lymphoma International Prognostic Index (MIPI) score was 6 (high-risk group). She was treated by immunochemotherapy with 4 cycles of R-DHAOx (rituximab, high-dose aracytine, oxaliplatin, and dexamethasone), followed by autologous hematopoietic stem cell transplantation (ASCT). The therapeutic evaluation by PET scan shows a complete remission (Figure 1(b)), and it was decided to continue with maintenance therapy with rituximab every 2 months, but it was refused by the patient. At the last visit, 18 months of ASCT, the patient was always disease free.

3. Discussion

Acute laryngeal dyspnea is a life-threatening emergency, and the causes in adults are most often laryngeal tumors or inflammatory edema [1]. Laryngeal lymphoma in adults is uncommon, accounting for less than 1% of all cases of laryngeal malignancies. Less than 100 cases have been reported in the literature [2]. Mantle cell lymphoma (MCL) is rare and very aggressive; this subtype presents 5% of all non-Hodgkin's lymphomas [6]. Extranodal involvement in mantle cell lymphoma is common in the bone marrow, the gastrointestinal tract, and Waldeyer's ring [7]. The larynx involvement is extremely rare. In our literature review, some cases of laryngeal MCL were reported [3–5] (Table 1). Laryngeal lymphoma presents clinically in a similar fashion to squamous cell carcinoma, with symptoms such as hoarseness, dyspnea, a foreign body sensation in the throat, or stridor. Uncommonly, it may present catastrophically with acute airway obstruction requiring immediate surgical intervention as in our case [8]. Systemic symptomatology is unusual, since laryngeal lymphomas tend to remain localized for prolonged periods, although more aggressive forms tend to spread earlier [9]. There is no consensus on the treatment of MCL, and for young patients (<65 years) in good general condition, the first-line therapeutic strategy is based on the use of induction immunochemotherapy containing cytarabine followed by consolidation with intensive chemotherapy and autologous stem cell transplantation [10]. We opted for this strategy in our case. MCL is considered incurable with current therapies and has historically been associated with a poor prognosis. However, increased understanding of the disease biology has led to the development of promising novel therapies in recent years [11].

4. Conclusion

Mantle cell lymphoma (MCL) is a rare and very aggressive subtype of non-Hodgkin's lymphoma with poor prognosis. The laryngeal localization is extremely rare, and it may present catastrophically with acute airway obstruction. The diagnosis is mostly histological, hence the interest of deep biopsy. Given its rarity, the therapeutic strategy must be

Table 1: Case reports of mantle cell lymphoma of the larynx.

Article	Year of publication	Age	Sex	Clinical presentation	Tracheotomy	Laryngeal localization	B Symptoms	Ann arbor stage at diagnosis	Therapy	Outcome for MCL	Status on date of publication
Our case	2020	43	F	Inspiratory bradypnea	Yes	Right infraglottic	Yes	IVB	R-DHAOX + ASCT	CR	Alive
K.L.Groom et al. [4]	2011	60	M	Progressive hoarseness	No	Left anterior false vocal cord	NA	NA	NA	NA	NA
S.Naciri [3]	2012	70	M	Progressive laryngeal respiratory distress	Yes	Subglottic	No	IIA	R-CHOP	NA	Died
Y. Ç. Kumbul et al. [5]	2019	76	M	Progressive nasal obstruction	No	Midline nasopharyngeal + left aryepiglottic fold	NA	NA	R-CHOP + radiotherapy	CR	Alive

MCL: mantle cell lymphoma; R-DHAOX: rituximab, dexamethasone, aracytine, oxaliplatin; R-CHOP: rituximab, cyclophosphamide, doxorubicine, vincristine, prednisone; CR: complete remission; NA: not available.

discussed case by case in a multidisciplinary consultation meeting.

Consent

Written informed consent was obtained from the patient for publication of this case report and any accompanying images.

Authors' Contributions

MA and AH collected data and drafted the manuscript. HM, EM, and SJ reviewed the literature. KD revised the manuscript. All authors read and approved the final manuscript.

Acknowledgments

The authors would like to thank the entire medical and paramedical team of the Clinical Hematology department of the Military Hospital Mohammed V in Rabat, for the enormous work they performed.

References

[1] A. Cros and Y. Hervé, "Acute laryngeal dyspnea," *Revue du Praticien*, vol. 53, no. 9, pp. 985–988, 2003.

[2] H.-P. Horny and E. Kaiserling, "Involvement of the larynx by hemopoietic neoplasms," *Pathology-Research and Practice*, vol. 191, no. 2, pp. 130–138, 1995.

[3] S. Naciri et al., "Mantle cell lymphoma of the larynx: primary case report," *Journal of Medical Case Reports*, vol. 6, no. 1, p. 201, 2012.

[4] K. L. Groom, D. S. Ruhl, and J. C. Sniezek, "Mantle cell lymphoma presenting as a saccular cyst," *Otolaryngology-Head and Neck Surgery*, vol. 146, no. 1, pp. 173-174, 2012.

[5] Y. Ç. Kumbul, M. Tüz, S. Bircan, H. Yasan, M. Sivrice, and V. Akin, "Synchronous mantle cell lymphoma of larynx and nasopharynx," *Turkish Journal of Geriatrics*, vol. 22, no. 4, pp. 504–508, 2019.

[6] S. H. Swerdlow, E. Campo, S. A. Pileri et al., "The 2016 revision of the World Health Organization classification of lymphoid neoplasms," *Blood*, vol. 127, no. 20, pp. 2375–2390, 2016.

[7] H. Samaha, C. Dumontet, N. Ketterer et al., "Mantle cell lymphoma: a retrospective study of 121 cases," *Leukemia*, vol. 12, no. 8, pp. 1281–1287, 1998.

[8] C. P. Azzopardi, J. Degaetano, A. Betts et al., "Laryngeal lymphoma: the high and low grades of rare lymphoma involvement sites," *Case Report in Medicine*, vol. 2014, 2014.

[9] K. Markou, J. Goudakos, J. Constantinidis, I. Kostopoulos, V. Vital, and A. Nikolaou, "Primary laryngeal lymphoma: report of 3 cases and review of the literature," *Head and Neck Journal for the Sciences and Specialties of the Head and Neck*, vol. 32, no. 4, pp. 541–549, 2010.

[10] R. Le Calloch, M. Voldoire, and S. Le Gouill, "Mantle cells lymphoma: standards and news," *Hématologie*, vol. 21, no. 3, pp. 169–176, 2015.

[11] J. T. Romancik and J. B. Cohen, "Management of older adults with mantle cell lymphoma," *Drugs Aging*, vol. 37, no. 7, pp. 469–481, 2020.

17

Rapid Response in a Patient with Relapsed/Refractory Multiple Myeloma Treated with BRAF/MEK Inhibitors

Steve Biko Otieno,[1,2,3] Syed Nasir,[1,3] Alva Weir,[1,2] and Robert Johnson[1,3]

[1]*The University of Tennessee Health Science Center, Department of Hematology/Oncology, 19 S. Manassas, Memphis, TN 38103, USA*
[2]*The Veterans Affairs Medical Center, 1030 Jefferson Ave, Memphis, TN 38104, USA*
[3]*The West Cancer and Research Institute, 7945 Wolf River Blvd, Germantown, TN 38138, USA*

Correspondence should be addressed to Steve Biko Otieno; sotieno@uthsc.edu

Academic Editor: Kostas Konstantopoulos

Patients with relapsed and refractory multiple myeloma have a poor prognosis. The mitogen-activated protein kinase (MAPK) pathway has been implicated in the pathogenesis of multiple myeloma. Several mutations in this pathway can lead to its constitutive activation leading to oncogenesis. One such mutation is BRAFV600E which is a therapeutic target in the treatment of melanoma, lung cancer, colon cancer, thyroid cancer, and hairy cell leukemia. BRAFV600E-directed therapy currently does not have approval in multiple myeloma. It has been proposed that this mutation leads to proteasome inhibitor resistance. About 4–10% of multiple myeloma cases harbor the BRAFV600E mutation. Herein, we report a case of a patient with relapsed and refractory multiple myeloma who had a progression-free survival (PFS) of 8.5 months on BRAF-targeted therapy.

1. Background

Multiple myeloma is a malignancy caused by neoplastic proliferation of atypical plasma cells that can cause hypercalcemia, renal failure, bone lesions, and anemia [1]. It is generally considered incurable with patients eventually requiring salvage therapy. Several drug classes have been shown to be effective in myeloma treatment and include proteasome inhibitors, immunomodulatory imide drugs (IMiDs), CD38 inhibitors, alkylating agents, histone deacetylase inhibitors, nuclear protein export inhibitors, anthracyclines, and steroids. Patients can also undergo autologous stem cell transplant. All these treatment options have improved overall survival in multiple myeloma [2]. However, some patients still develop relapsed and refractory disease despite these lines of treatment or are not good candidates for some of these therapies due to toxicities or comorbidities. There is therefore a need to expand the therapeutic armamentarium against multiple myeloma in the relapsed and refractory setting. Molecular analysis of multiple myeloma has revealed that about 4–10% of myeloma cases harbor BRAF mutations [3]. BRAF-directed therapy is used in melanoma, thyroid cancer, colon cancer, and hairy cell leukemia. While there are no approved BRAF-directed therapies in multiple myeloma, a few cases of off-label use have been reported [4–6].

We report a case of a patient with relapsed and refractory myeloma harboring the BRAFV600E mutation who was treated off-label with combination of BRAF and MEK inhibition with a gratifying response.

2. Case Report

The patient is a 68-year-old male with a past medical history notable for prostate cancer, in remission, who initially presented with high fevers, cough, and congestion. A computed tomography (CT) scan of his chest, abdomen, and pelvis showed a 4 centimeter (cm) lytic lesion within the manubrium and lytic lesions in the thoracic spine with the largest being a 1.4 cm T6 lesion and a 1.1 cm lucent T4 lesion. Also noted was a 1.1 cm lucent right iliac lesion. A subsequent positron emission tomography (PET) scan done a week later showed diffuse hypermetabolic lesions throughout the axial skeleton with prominent lesions in the manubrium, right ilium, cervical, thoracic and lumbar spines, sacrum, bilateral scapulae, and humeri. Multiple myeloma was suspected.

A protein electrophoresis revealed two M-bands 0.13 grams per deciliter (g/dL) and 3.37 g/dL (normal reference 0). Immunofixation showed IgG lambda light chain restriction. Kappa-free light chains were 1.9 milligrams per deciliter (mg/dL), and lambda-free chains were 124 mg/dL with a kappa to lambda ratio of 0.02 (reference range 0.26–1.65). Evaluation of immunoglobulins showed IgG of 7641 mg/dL (reference range 700–1600), IgA of 71 mg/dL (reference range 70–400), and IgM of 55 mg/dL (reference range 40–230). 24-hour urine protein was 5 grams with M protein comprising 90% of total urine protein. Calcium was 9 mg/dL (reference range 8.4–10.2). Antinuclear antibody (ANA), rheumatoid factor (RF), human immunodeficiency virus (HIV), and hepatitis B and C were all negative.

The lytic sternal lesion was biopsied, and a bone marrow biopsy was also done. The bone marrow biopsy revealed a 90–100% hypercellular marrow with IgG lambda-restricted plasma cells comprising 80% of the bone marrow cellularity. Cytogenetics showed a complex karyotype. Fluorescence *in situ* hybridization (FISH) showed del13q, 12p, 12q, 16q, and 22q and gain of 1q, 5, 6p, 7, 9, 15q, and Xq. Next generation sequencing showed BRAFV600E mutation with a 12% variant frequency and increased stainable iron. Congo red stain was negative. He was diagnosed with ISS stage III, high-risk multiple myeloma.

He was initially treated with lenalidomide-bortezomib-dexamethasone (RVd) regimen but was primary refractory with disease progression noted within 1 month. His case was discussed in the tumor board, and it was recommended the he should be started on a combination of dexamethasone, cisplatin, doxorubicin, cyclophosphamide, and etoposide (D-PACE). However, the patient declined this therapy. He was instead treated with pomalidomide, daratumumab, and dexamethasone. He had primary progression and was switched to pomalidomide, carfilzomib, and dexamethasone and had a response for 8 months before progression. His case was again reviewed, and it was decided to try a BRAF/MEK inhibitor combination. He started treatment with cobimetinib 60 mg daily on days 1–21 of a 28-day cycle and vemurafenib 960 mg twice a day for 28 days in a 28-day cycle. The patient was seen in clinic on weeks 5, 9, 13, 16, 25, and 37 after initiation of treatment. Progression was noted in week 37. His therapy was changed to selinexor.

He tolerated therapy well. His only complaint was mild fatigue and occasional nausea controlled with antiemetics. His M protein levels and kappa/lambda ratio were as shown in Figure 1. His kappa/lambda light chain ratio normalized in 5 weeks. He had a PFS of 8.5 months.

3. Discussion

Multiple myeloma is generally considered incurable with most patients eventually requiring multiple lines of salvage therapy. Some patients can have limited treatment options due to toxicity or comorbidities. There is therefore a need for new treatment options.

The BRAF protein is part of the MAPK pathway, and BRAF mutations lead to constitutive activation of this pathway. BRAF mutation-directed therapies are used in solid malignancies including melanoma, colon cancer, and thyroid cancer. In B-cell malignancies, this mutation is found mainly in hairy cell leukemia where it is targeted for therapy in the relapsed refractory setting [7]. However, this mutation is rare in hematologic malignancies in general [8, 9]. About 4–10% of multiple myeloma cases harbor the BRAFV600E mutation [3]. While there are no completed large randomized clinical trials of BRAF inhibitors in multiple myeloma, a few cases of off-label use of BRAF inhibitors have been reported [4–6].

The patient in this case report progressed despite multiple lines of treatment. With a few cases of response to BRAF-directed therapy reported in multiple myeloma patients harboring BRAFV600E mutations, off-label treatment was deemed to be rational and reasonable for this patient. Studies in melanoma have demonstrated that targeting BRAF using a single-agent BRAF inhibitor eventually leads to acquired resistance through a variety of pathways, one of them being activation of the downstream MEK protein [10]. Combination therapy with BRAF inhibitors and MEK inhibitors has been shown to have better outcomes [10]. Extrapolating from these data in melanoma studies, we decided to treat with a combination of the BRAF inhibitor vemurafenib and the MEK inhibitor cobimetinib.

Since the optimal dose in myeloma is still unknown, we decided to treat at doses used in melanoma. The patient achieved a rapid response with the light chain ratio normalizing in 5 weeks and with the patient achieving a partial response in 5 weeks with a PFS of 8.5 months. Our case adds to the list of case reports that suggest that treatment of multiple myeloma harboring BRAFV600E mutations with BRAF/MEK inhibitors is a reasonable treatment option.

BRAF mutations are usually a poor prognostic indicator in other malignancies [11, 12]. In multiple myeloma, the prognostic significance is unclear. However, the study by Andrulis et al. reported a clinically more aggressive phenotype characterized with decreased OS in patients with BRAFV600E, and the study by Rustan et al. did not show any relation to a poor prognosis when compared to BRAF wild type. These differences may be due to different patient populations and small sample sizes [4, 13].

Shirazi et al. linked activating RAS and RAF mutations to enhanced proteasome assembly and capacity, thereby conferring proteasome inhibitor resistance in established myeloma cell lines. [14] This resistance was overcome by combination of BRAF and MEK inhibitors [14]. The initial bone marrow for our patient showed a BRAFV600E

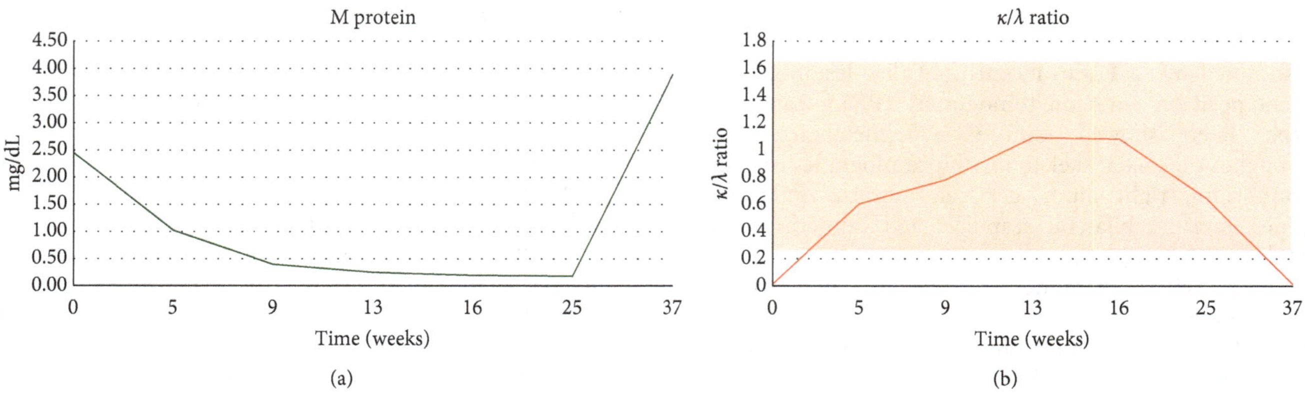

Figure 1: Response to treatment. (a) M protein levels after initiation of treatment with vemurafenib and cobimetinib at 0, 5, 9, 13, 16, 25, and 37 weeks. (b) Changes in kappa/lambda ratio at 0, 5, 9, 13, 16, 25, and 37 weeks. The beige box shows the normal range of the kappa/lambda ratio.

mutation with a variant frequency of 12% suggesting that it was a significant subclone but likely not the dominant clone. It is reasonable to surmise that the initial therapies conferred a growth advantage to BRAFV600E clone. Unfortunately, we do not have another biopsy to confirm if this clone had expanded prior to the BRAF inhibitor therapy.

Two clinical trials to assess the effectiveness of BRAF/MEK inhibition in relapsed/refractory multiple myeloma, NCT02834364 and NCT03091257, are currently recruiting. The results of these trials should provide further insight into the targeting of the MAPK pathway in treatment of multiple myeloma.

4. Conclusion

This case report suggests that targeting of the MAPK pathway through BRAF/MEK inhibition may be an additional therapeutic option in relapsed/refractory multiple myeloma.

Consent

Verbal consent was obtained from the patient, and a written consent will be obtained at the future clinic visit.

Authors' Contributions

Steve Biko Otieno, MD, PhD, wrote the article and made the figure. Sayed Nasir, MD; Alva Weir, MD; and Robert Johnson, MD, reviewed the article and provided comments.

References

[1] A. Palumbo and K. Anderson, "Multiple myeloma," *New England Journal of Medicine*, vol. 364, no. 11, pp. 1046–1060, 2011.

[2] R. Fonseca, S. Abouzaid, M. Bonafede et al., "Trends in overall survival and costs of multiple myeloma, 2000–2014," *Leukemia*, vol. 31, pp. 1915–1921, 2017.

[3] A. Danu, S. Cotteret, L. Lacroix et al., "BRAF V600E targetable mutation in relapsed/refractory multiple myeloma (R/R mm) patients: a high incidence in R/R mm detected using cell sorting screening," *Blood*, vol. 128, p. 5638, 2016.

[4] M. Andrulis, N. Lehners, D. Capper et al., "Targeting the BRAF V600E mutation in multiple myeloma," *Cancer Discovery*, vol. 3, no. 8, pp. 862–869, 2013.

[5] U. J. M. Mey, C. Renner, and R. von Moos, "Vemurafenib in combination with cobimetinib in relapsed and refractory extramedullary multiple myeloma harboring the BRAF V600E mutation," *Hematological Oncology*, vol. 35, no. 4, pp. 890–893, 2017.

[6] J. P. Sharman, J. Chmielecki, D. Morosini et al., "Vemurafenib response in 2 patients with posttransplant refractory BRAF V600E-mutated multiple myeloma," *Clinical Lymphoma Myeloma and Leukemia*, vol. 14, no. 5, pp. e161–e163, 2014.

[7] E. Tiacci, J. H. Park, L. De Carolis et al., "Targeting mutant BRAF in relapsed or refractory hairy-cell leukemia," *New England Journal of Medicine*, vol. 373, no. 18, pp. 1733–1747, 2015.

[8] N. Ping, Q. Wang, Q. Wang et al., "Absence of BRAF V600E mutation in hematologic malignancies excluding hairy-cell leukemia," *Leukemia & Lymphoma*, vol. 53, no. 12, pp. 2498-2499, 2012.

[9] A. P. Trifa, R. A. Popp, A. Cucuianu et al., "Absence of BRAF V600E mutation in a cohort of 402 patients with various chronic and acute myeloid neoplasms," *Leukemia & Lymphoma*, vol. 53, no. 12, pp. 2496-2497, 2012.

[10] K. B. Kim, R. Kefford, A. C. Pavlick et al., "Phase II study of the MEK1/MEK2 inhibitor trametinib in patients with metastatic BRAF-mutant cutaneous melanoma previously treated with or without a BRAF inhibitor," *Journal of Clinical Oncology*, vol. 31, no. 4, pp. 482–489, 2013.

[11] L. Ny, M. Nyakas, M. Hernberg et al., "BRAF mutation as a prognostic marker for survival in malignant melanoma: a systematic review and meta-analysis," *Journal of Clinical Oncology*, vol. 36, no. 15, Article ID e21566, 2018.

[12] A. D. Roth, S. Tejpar, M. Delorenzi et al., "Prognostic role of KRAS and BRAF in stage II and III resected colon cancer: results of the translational study on the PETACC-3, EORTC 40993, SAKK 60-00 trial," *Journal of Clinical Oncology*, vol. 28, no. 3, pp. 466–474, 2010.

[13] E. H. Rustad, H. Y. Dai, H. Hov et al., "BRAF V600E mutation in early-stage multiple myeloma: good response to broad acting drugs and no relation to prognosis," *Blood Cancer Journal*, vol. 5, no. 3, p. e299, 2015.

[14] F. Shirazi, R. J. Jones, R. K. Singh et al., "Activating KRAS,NRAS, andBRAFmutants enhance proteasome capacity and reduce endoplasmic reticulum stress in multiple myeloma," *Proceedings of the National Academy of Sciences*, vol. 117, no. 33, pp. 20004–20014, 2020.

18

Treatment of T-Cell Prolymphocytic Leukemia with Central Nervous System Involvement using Intrathecal Alemtuzumab Administration

Jinichi Mori,[1] Kumi Oshima,[1,2] Satoshi Kimura,[3] and Takayuki Ikezoe[3]

[1]*Department of Hematology, Jyoban Hospital, Tokiwa Foundation, Fukushima, Japan*
[2]*Patient Safety Division, QI Center, St. Luke's International Hospital, Tokyo, Japan*
[3]*Department of Hematology, Fukushima Medical University, Fukushima, Japan*

Correspondence should be addressed to Jinichi Mori; jinichimori@gmail.com

Academic Editor: Vincent Ribrag

T-cell prolymphocytic leukemia (T-PLL) is a rare hematologic cancer with a dismal prognosis. Although a small number of patients have central nervous system (CNS) involvement, a standard treatment approach for these patients has not been established. Herein, we present a case of T-PLL with CNS involvement that was treated with a higher dose of intrathecal alemtuzumab than that previously reported. A 66-year-old man who had T-PLL with CNS involvement was admitted to our hospital. Intravenously administered alemtuzumab, a monoclonal antibody against the CD52 antigen, successfully reduced leukemia cells in peripheral blood; however, intrathecal treatment with methotrexate, cytarabine, and prednisone had a limited effect on the CNS involvement. Therefore, we intrathecally injected alemtuzumab as an experimental treatment. Although we escalated the dose of intrathecal alemtuzumab up to 5 mg, no adverse reaction was noted; however, this treatment did not completely clear the leukemia cells from the patient's cerebrospinal fluid (CSF). We performed whole brain and whole spinal irradiation therapies and subsequently performed allogeneic transplantation from a human leukocyte antigen-matched sibling donor with a conditioning regimen containing total body irradiation. At 21 days after transplantation, leukemia cells remained in his CSF. Although intrathecal alemtuzumab did not eliminate the CNS-invading leukemia cells, it was well-tolerated in our case. Further accumulation of similar cases is needed to determine the benefits and safety of intrathecal alemtuzumab administration.

1. Introduction

T-cell prolymphocytic leukemia (T-PLL), a rare hematologic cancer, is associated with poor patient prognosis; the overall 3-year survival rate is 40% after allogeneic hematopoietic stem-cell transplantation (HSCT) in patients who have previously received conventional chemotherapies [1]. Induction therapy with alemtuzumab, a humanized monoclonal antibody against the CD52 antigen, and subsequent allogeneic HSCT may promote longer survival; however, overall, the 4-year survival rate remains at 56% [2]. Few reports have described central nervous system (CNS) involvement, a dismal prognostic factor, in patients with T-PLL [3–5]. For transplantation candidates, pre-HSCT control of CNS involvement is needed to achieve improved transplantation outcomes, as in other types of leukemia [6]; however, a standard treatment approach for cases of T-PLL with CNS involvement does not exist. To date, only one previous report has demonstrated a case where 3 mg of intrathecal alemtuzumab was safely administered; however, the efficacy of this treatment was not evaluated in that case. Here, we present a case of T-PLL with CNS involvement that was treated with up to 5 mg of intrathecal alemtuzumab, but was not eliminated.

2. Case Presentation

A 66-year-old man was diagnosed with T-PLL in 2011. At the time of diagnosis, he was asymptomatic and had a peripheral white blood cell (WBC) count of 17,600 μL, including an abnormal lymphocyte count of 15,000 μL. Thus, his attending physician chose an observant waiting approach. The patient's lymphocyte count gradually increased and reached 30,000–40,000 μL in 2018. He developed night sweats, fatigue, low-grade fever, and headaches. Computed tomography revealed hepatosplenomegaly, and in 2019, he was moved to our hospital to initiate treatment. At the time of the transfer, his WBC count was 52,600 μL, including a lymphocyte count of 46,800 μL. Microscopic examination of the blood smear revealed small-to-medium-sized lymphocytes that featured irregularly shaped nuclei and condensed chromatin (Figure 1).

The lymphocytes exhibited a post-thymic T-cell phenotype (Tdt$^-$, CD1$^-$, CD5$^+$, CD2$^+$, and CD7$^+$) and harbored chromosomal abnormalities (add(15)(q24) and del(7)(p?)). As the patient was experiencing headaches, we performed a cerebrospinal fluid (CSF) examination and found leukemic lymphocytes carrying the same pattern of surface antigens as those in the peripheral blood. As the initial chemotherapy (fludarabine and cyclophosphamide) caused tumor lysis syndrome, we discontinued the treatment and started administering intravenous alemtuzumab after the resolution of the tumor lysis syndrome. Following these changes, the patient's lymphocyte count dropped sharply (Figure 2).

We concurrently treated the CNS involvement with a dose of intrathecal methotrexate and followed it by intrathecal therapy containing methotrexate, cytarabine, and prednisone weekly. However, the number of CNS-invading leukemic cells reached the lowest point after the fourth intrathecal injection, and the number of leukemic cells in the patient's CSF increased. Once we received approval from our institutional review board, we initiated an experimental treatment with intrathecal alemtuzumab injections. The patient did not experience any adverse reactions to the intrathecal alemtuzumab injections. To eliminate the leukemia cells in the patients' CSF, we increased the intrathecal alemtuzumab dose to 5 mg; however, the cells did not completely disappear. We performed whole brain and whole spinal irradiation therapies and subsequently performed allogeneic transplantation from an HLA-matched sibling donor with a conditioning regimen containing total body irradiation. At 21 days after transplantation, 23 leukemia cells μL remained in his CSF. The patient is currently receiving best supportive care.

3. Discussion

We demonstrated here a patient with T-PLL and CNS involvement that was treated with intrathecal alemtuzumab. This treatment unfortunately did not clear the CNS-invading leukemia cells but allowed us to bridge to allogeneic transplantation without any adverse reactions. To the best of our knowledge, this is the first report of a case in which the efficacy and tolerance to intrathecal

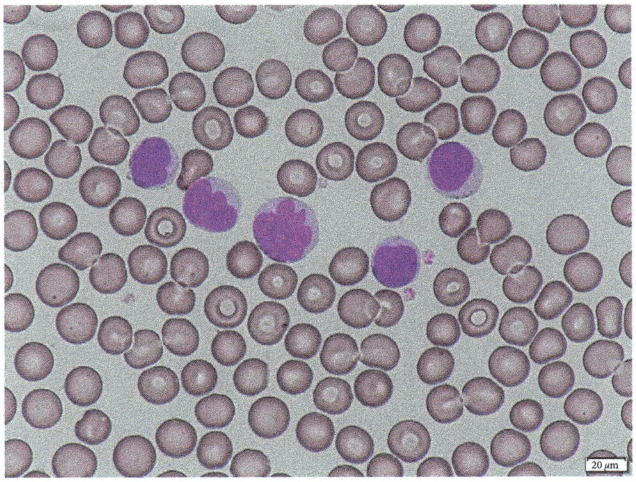

Figure 1: Microscopic image of leukemic lymphocytes in the peripheral blood smear.

alemtuzumab injections were evaluated. In a previous report by Alsawah et aL, the authors claimed successful treatment with 3 mg of intrathecal alemtuzumab for CNS involvement that was refractory to prior treatment with intrathecal cytarabine and methotrexate and whole brain irradiation [7]. However, when intrathecal alemtuzumab administration was initiated in their case, the patient's CSF leukemic cell count was 1 μL, limiting the evaluation of the treatment efficacy. In contrast, in our case, the patient had a CSF leukemic cell count of 3 μL at the initiation of intrathecal alemtuzumab treatment. Unfortunately, our patient's CNS involvement did not resolve, despite the use of a higher dose (5 mg) of intrathecal alemtuzumab than that previously reported.

Several *in vitro* studies have demonstrated that alemtuzumab exerts its antitumor effect by both complement-dependent cytotoxicity (CDC) and antibody-dependent cellular cytotoxicity (ADCC) [8–10]. Although the effect *in vivo* has not been studied extensively, a preclinical study using human CD52 transgenic mice showed that ADCC plays a crucial role in the elimination of CD52-positive lymphocytes [11]. The study also demonstrated that intravenous administration of alemtuzumab cleared CD52-positive lymphocytes from the peripheral blood but not from certain organs (spleen and thymus) that contain fewer ADCC effector cells, such as neutrophils, natural killer cells, and macrophages. In our patient, intrathecally injected alemtuzumab might have provoked weak CDC and no ADCC in the CSF, which had complement levels that were 100–200-fold lower than those in the serum and extremely few ADCC effector cells. Thus, we speculate that this resulted in the lack of a significant response to the CNS-invading T-PLL cells [12].

Although the efficacy of intrathecal alemtuzumab therapy was limited in our case, it was well-tolerated even at a dose of 5 mg. Further information from similar cases is needed to determine the benefits and safety of this treatment.

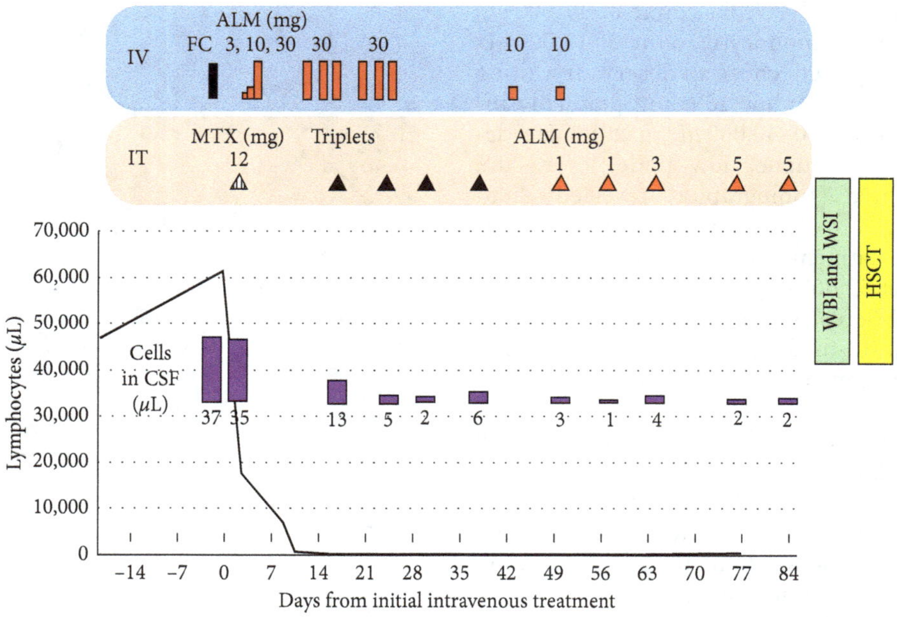

Figure 2: Treatment time course for the leukemia and central nervous system involvement. ALM: alemtuzumab; CSF: cerebrospinal fluid; FC: fludarabine and cyclophosphamide; HSCT: hematopoietic stem-cell transplantation; IT: intrathecal treatment; IV: intravenous treatment; MTX: methotrexate; WBI: whole brain irradiation; and WSI: whole spine irradiation. Triplets consist of 15 mg of methotrexate, 40 mg of cytarabine, and 20 mg of prednisolone.

Consent

We obtained written informed consent for the experimental procedure and publication of the research results.

References

[1] S. Yamasaki, H. Nitta, E. Kondo et al., "Effect of allogeneic hematopoietic cell transplantation for patients with T-prolymphocytic leukemia: a retrospective study from the Adult Lymphoma Working group of the Japan society for hematopoietic cell transplantation," *Annals of Hematology*, vol. 98, no. 9, pp. 2213–2220, 2019.

[2] B. R. Dholaria, E. Ayala, L. Sokol et al., "Allogeneic hematopoietic cell transplantation in T-cell prolymphocytic leukemia: a single-center experience," *Leukemia Research*, vol. 67, pp. 1-5, 2018.

[3] F. Brito-Babapulle, D. Huang, P. Lavender, D. Galton, and D. Catovsky, "Regression of intracerebral lesions in T prolymphocytic leukaemia treated with intravenous deoxycoformycin," *European Journal of Haematology*, vol. 40, no. 2, pp. 185–187, 1988.

[4] L. Garderet, H. Bittencourt, A. Kaliski et al., "Treatment of T-prolymphocytic leukemia with nonmyeloablative allogeneic stem cell transplantation," *European Journal of Haematology*, vol. 66, no. 2, pp. 137–139, 2001.

[5] U. Y. Malkan, G. Gunes, O. Yayar, H. Demiroglu, A. Yesilirmak, and A. Uner, "A T-cell prolymphocytic leukemia case with central nervous system involvement," *International Journal of Clinical and Experimental Medicine*, vol. 8, no. 8, pp. 14207–14209, 2015.

[6] S. Ikegawa, N. Doki, S. Kaito et al., "Central nervous system involvement at the time of allogeneic hematopoietic stem cell transplantation is associated with a poor outcome in patients with acute myeloid leukemia," *Pathology & Oncology Research*, vol. 23, no. 2, pp. 433–437, 2017 Apr.

[7] F. Alsawah, L. Benitez, S. Choi et al., "Intrathecal alemtuzumab: a potential treatment of refractory leptomeningeal T-cell prolymphocytic leukemia," *Blood Advances*, vol. 3, no. 21, pp. 3333–3336, 2019.

[8] C. S. Zent, C. R. Secreto, B. R. LaPlant et al., "Direct and complement dependent cytotoxicity in CLL cells from patients with high-risk early-intermediate stage chronic lymphocytic leukemia (CLL) treated with alemtuzumab and rituximab," *Leukemia Research*, vol. 32, no. 12, pp. 1849–1856, 2008.

[9] J. Golay, M. Manganini, A. Rambaldi, and M. Introna, "Effect of alemtuzumab on neoplastic B cells," *Haematologica*, vol. 89, no. 12, pp. 1476–1483, 2004.

[10] R. I. Cruz, F. J. Hernandez-Ilizaliturri, S. Olejniczak et al., "CD52 over-expression affects rituximab-associated complement-mediated cytotoxicity but not antibody-dependent cellular cytotoxicity: preclinical evidence that targeting CD52 with alemtuzumab may reverse acquired resistance to rituximab in non-Hodgkin lymphoma," *Leukemia & Lymphoma*, vol. 48, no. 12, pp. 2424–2436, 2007.

[11] Y. Hu, M. J. Turner, J. Shields et al., "Investigation of the mechanism of action of alemtuzumab in a human CD52 transgenic mouse model," *Immunology*, vol. 128, no. 2, pp. 260–270, 2009.

[12] M. Trbojević-Cepe, V. Brinar, M. Pauro, Z. Vogrinc, and N. Stambuk, "Cerebrospinal fluid complement activation in neurological diseases," *Journal of the Neurological Sciences*, vol. 154, no. 2, pp. 173–181, 1998.

19

Efficacy of Venetoclax and Dexamethasone in Refractory IgM Primary Plasma Cell Leukemia with t(11;14) and TP53 Mutation: A Case Report and Literature Review

Salimah Valliani,[1] **Mir Ali**,[1] **Omar Mahmoo**,[1] **Sanjay Hinduja**,[1] **Calvin K. Chen**,[2] **Lloyd Damon**,[3] **and Haifaa Abdulhaq**[1]

[1]*University of California San Francisco-Fresno (UCSF Fresno), Fresno, California, USA*
[2]*Community Regional Medical Center (CRMC), Fresno, California, USA*
[3]*University of California San Francisco (UCSF), San Francisco, California, USA*

Correspondence should be addressed to Salimah Valliani; svalliani@fresno.ucsf.edu

Academic Editor: Sudhir Tauro

Primary plasma cell leukemia (pPCL) is an uncommon disease. IgM multiple myeloma (MM) is an infrequent subtype that accounts for less than 1 percent of MM cases. IgM pPCL is quite rare with only a few cases published to date. We describe a case of a patient with IgM pPCL who initially presented with hyperviscosity syndrome requiring urgent plasma exchange. His bone marrow biopsy demonstrated t(11;14). He progressed on proteasome inhibitors, immunomodulating agents, and other chemotherapy medications but later achieved very good partial response (VGPR) to venetoclax and dexamethasone. Given the poor prognosis of pPCL, further studies using venetoclax alone or in combination with other novel agents as first-line treatment options are warranted particularly in patients with t(11;14).

1. Background

Plasma cell leukemia (PCL) is an aggressive variant of multiple myeloma (MM). The diagnostic criteria initially proposed required more than 20% circulating plasma cells and an absolute plasma cell count greater than 2×10^9/L in peripheral blood. The International Myeloma Working Group considers one of the above two criteria to be sufficient for diagnosis [1]. Primary PCL (pPCL) is a terminology used for a patient who meets the above criteria at initial diagnosis with no prior history of MM. pPCL accounts for only 1-2% of cases at initial diagnosis of multiple myeloma [2]. Secondary PCL is a leukemic transformation of relapsed or refractory MM.

IgM-subtype of MM occurs in only 0.8% of MM cases [3]. Waldenstrom's disease is the more common presentation for an IgM monoclonal lymphoproliferative neoplasm. However, patients who have elevated serum IgM monoclonal protein along with features of multiple myeloma including clonal plasma cells in the marrow and lytic bone lesions should be diagnosed as IgM MM [3]. IgM pPCL is a particularly rare entity with only a handful of cases reported. pPCL has a poor prognosis even with the utilization of novel agents. pPCL is known to have a high incidence of cytogenetic and molecular abnormalities such as 17p deletion, TP53 mutation, and 1q gain. t(11;14) is present in 15–20% of MM patients, while reported in up to 50% of patients with pPCL.

Overexpression of BCL-2 and other antiapoptotic proteins is a hallmark of tumor cell survival in MM [4]. Venetoclax, a selective, oral, BCL-2 inhibitor, has shown activity in relapsed and refractory multiple myeloma, specifically in patients with t(11;14) [5]. Few cases have reported the activity of venetoclax in PCL, but none reported in IgM pPCL. We describe a case of IgM pPCL with t(11;14) that demonstrated excellent response to venetoclax and dexamethasone (ven/dex) combination.

2. Case Presentation

A 58-year-old man with no known hematologic disease presented with fatigue, lethargy, and increased drowsiness for a few weeks. He also had episodes of confusion, headache, and epistaxis. A review of symptoms was negative for fever, night sweats, or weight loss. His past medical history included Hurthle cell thyroid carcinoma, which was treated with surgery and radioiodine therapy. The patient was initially admitted to an outside hospital for altered mental status. His symptoms were attributed to *E. coli* sepsis and suspected hepatic encephalopathy. He was treated with intravenous antibiotics with partial improvement in symptoms. He was discharged but subsequently readmitted and transferred to our facility within a few days with worsening mental status. He continued to have intermittent epistaxis and hemoptysis. On physical examination, he was noted to be somnolent. Blood crusting was noted on his nose. Initial laboratory data at our institution were as follows: hemoglobin, 8 gm/dl; platelet count, 60,000/μl; and white blood cell count, 15,600/μl. A complete metabolic panel showed creatinine, 0.6 mg/dL; BUN, 13 mg/dl; calcium, 9.2 mg/dl (10.2 when corrected for albumin); total protein, 12.2 g/dl; albumin, 2.6 g/dL; alkaline phosphate, 75 μ/l; AST, 8 μ/l; ALT, 14 μ/l; and total bilirubin, 0.2 mg/dl. Serum viscosity was elevated at 4.22. Serum protein electrophoresis and immunofixation showed an IgM-kappa monoclonal protein with M protein of 7.3 gm/dL and IgM of 10,000 mg/dL. Bone survey and computed tomography scan (CT scan) findings were consistent with multiple lytic lesions in the vertebrae (Figure 1) and hepatosplenomegaly. Magnetic resonance imaging (MRI) brain was unremarkable. Bone marrow biopsy showed >90% kappa-restricted plasma cells, which were CD 138 positive by immunohistochemistry (Figures 2 and 3). Fluorescence in situ hybridization (FISH) was positive for t(11; 14) CCND1/IGH and 13q del. MYD88 mutation by polymerase chain reaction (PCR) analysis was negative. Cytogenetics showed complex karyotype with del [6] (q25), add [1] (p13), del [7] (q13q23), add [8] (q24), del [9] (q22q34), t(11;14) (q13; q32), −13, −16, and add [10] (q13). Next-generation sequencing on bone marrow biopsy by Foundation One Heme showed IGH-CCND1 rearrangement and a TP53 mutation. Peripheral blood flow cytometry demonstrated 54.3% plasmacytoid B-cells/plasma cells with CD 20 positive and partially positive for CD 19 and HLA/DR. Peripheral smear showed 55% plasma cells leading to the diagnosis of IgM pPCL (Figure 4).

The patient was initially treated with daily plasmapheresis for five days, which decreased the IgM levels from >10,000 mg/dl to 2758 mg/dl with significant improvement in his symptoms of headache, confusion, and epistaxis. He was then started on combination chemotherapy with bortezomib, dexamethasone, cisplatin, adriamycin, cyclophosphamide, and etoposide (VD-PACE). Following the first cycle of VD-PACE, IgM increased steeply to 8568 mg/dl. Given the aggressive nature of the disease, treatment was changed to hyper-CAD (fractionated cyclophosphamide, doxorubicin, and dexamethasone) plus carfilzomib. Prior data show that the combination of proteasome inhibitors and hyper-CAD is effective in refractory multiple myeloma cases and can often serve as a bridge to subsequent treatment [7]. IgM level dropped to 5798 mg after one cycle. However, treatment was stopped after one cycle as the patient developed an acute decrease in cardiac ejection fraction. Treatment was changed to daratumumab, lenalidomide, cyclophosphamide, and dexamethasone after two months of initial diagnosis. After three cycles, IgM decreased from 5000 mg/dL to 2500 mg/dL, and bone marrow plasma cells decreased to 30%. With three additional cycles, IgM plateaued at 2400, and a repeat bone marrow biopsy showed an increase of plasma cells to 50%. He was then switched to ven/dex after eight months of initial diagnosis. He received venetoclax at 400 mg daily and dex at 40 mg weekly. He achieved a very good partial response (VGPR) within two months. IgM level decreased to 200 mg/dL, M protein to 0.2 gm/dL, and bone marrow plasma cells to 3%, with no peripheral plasma cells (Figures 5 and 6). The patient was evaluated for autologous hematopoietic cell transplantation (AuHCT) after achieving VGPR. However, mobilization failed despite the use of cyclophosphamide, granulocyte colony-stimulating factor, and plerixafor. The patient continued ven/dex for fifteen months and tolerated treatment well. The only drug-related adverse event has been grade 1 thrombocytopenia. His IgM levels have remained <100 mg/dl with no detectable serum M protein, but immunofixation continues to demonstrate the IgM-kappa monoclonal protein.

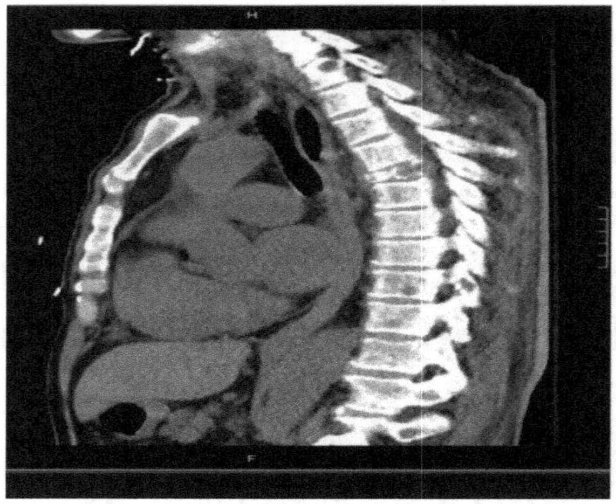

Figure 1: CT scan showing lytic bone lesions.

3. Discussion

Primary plasma cell leukemia has unique pathophysiologic and clinical features that predispose for poor prognosis. pPCL has lower expression of the bone marrow adhesion molecule CD56 expression [11] and downregulation of CXCR4, leading to impaired retention of plasma cells within the bone marrow and increased circulating plasma cells. There is overexpression of CD27 in pPCL, which causes activation of NFkB, leading to higher antiapoptotic activity. There is also a high incidence of molecular and cytogenetic

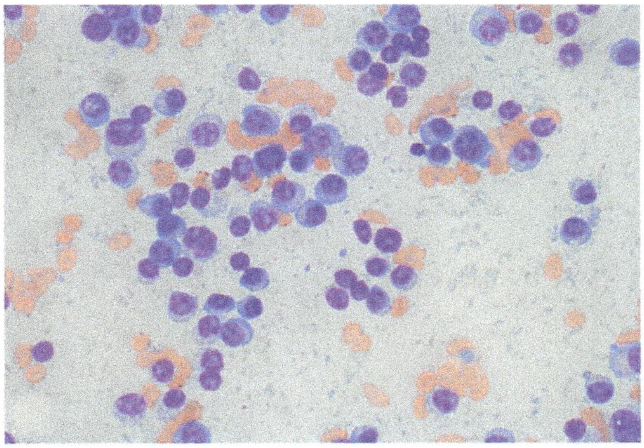

FIGURE 2: Plasma cells in bone marrow aspirate smear.

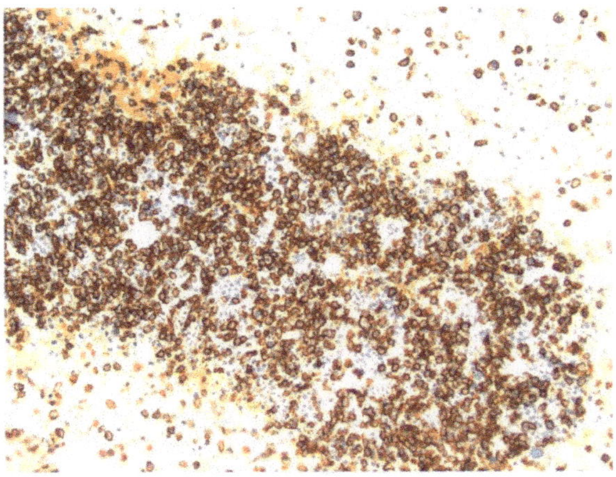

FIGURE 3: Bone marrow CD 138 IHC stain.

abnormalities, including del 13q, del 17q, 1q gain, TP53 mutation, and hypodiploidy [8]. These features lead to the common findings of cytopenias and increased frequency of extramedullary disease with hepatosplenomegaly, which was noted in our patient. Our patient also had TP53 mutation, which is associated with poor prognosis [9].

In our patient, IgM MM was favored over Waldenstrom macroglobulinemia (WM) due to the presence of bone lytic lesions and t(11;14). Furthermore, the absence of MYD88 mutation favored the diagnosis of IgM MM as this mutation is present in more than 90% of cases of lymphoplasmacytic lymphoma (LPL)/WM [6]. Our patient had symptoms of hyperviscosity with blurred vision and confusion at presentation along with elevated IgM levels. His symptoms improved after plasmapheresis. The overlapping symptoms between LPL/WM and IgM MM can provide a diagnostic challenge. IgM MM is an infrequent subtype that accounts for only 0.8% of MM [3]. As per the Center for International Blood and Marrow Transplant Research (CIBMTR), among 3578 MM patients who received AuHCT over 10 years (1995–2005), only 11 patients had IgM multiple myeloma. This exhibits the rarity of the disease [12]. A retrospective study from the Mayo Clinic

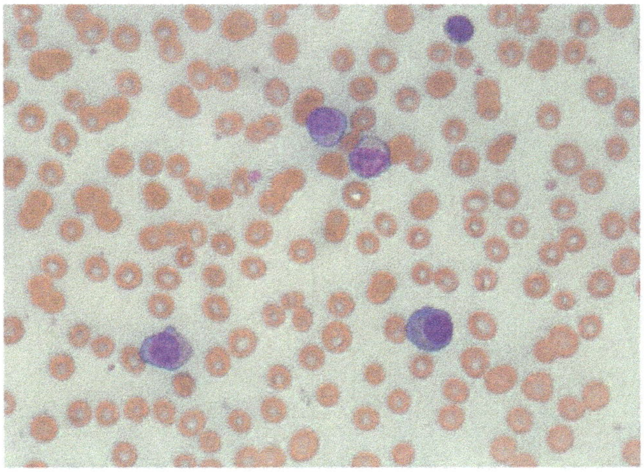

FIGURE 4: Circulating plasma cells in peripheral blood smear.

database looked at the prognosis of patients diagnosed with IgM MM. Twenty-one patients met the diagnostic criteria of 10% or more plasma cells on bone marrow biopsy, plus the presence of lytic bone lesions and or t(11;14) [3]. These patients had a median overall survival of 30 months, like myeloma population, but shorter than WM. Furthermore, we identified only three cases of IgM PCL reported in the literature. One patient had a durable response to multiagent chemotherapy along with rituximab, but the other two patients responded only briefly before progressing and eventually expiring [13–15]. None of the cases reported using venetoclax as a treatment modality.

Primary PCL has a poor prognosis compared to non-pPCL MM. Based on the SEER database review from 2006–2009, the median overall survival (OS) was around 12 months, even in the era of treatment with novel agents [2]. Primary PCL patients have high early mortality with 15% of deaths reported within a month of diagnosis. They usually present with a higher R-ISS (Revised International Staging system) stage. The treatment goal in primary plasma cell leukemia is focused on the rapid institution of therapy to achieve cytoreduction to reverse and or prevent complications. Treatment options include a combination of novel agents and chemotherapy to achieve a deep response. Retrospective data in pPCL have also shown a clear benefit of consolidation with AuHCT [16].

Few prospective studies evaluated various treatment options in pPCL. In an IFM study [17], bortezomib-based treatment led to improved overall survival (OS) of 36 months and a median progression-free survival (PFS) of 15 months. The overall response rate (ORR) was 72% with 37% response rate for very good partial response (VGPR) + complete response (CR). A GEMIMA study used lenalidomide and dexamethasone, which showed OS of 28 months and PFS of 14 months [18]. Both studies have also demonstrated the benefit of maintenance of bortezomib or lenalidomide, respectively, after AuHCT. Patients who responded to first-line therapy had OS of 26 months compared to 4.2 months in nonresponders. Response criteria in pPCL are MM with the addition of no plasma cells

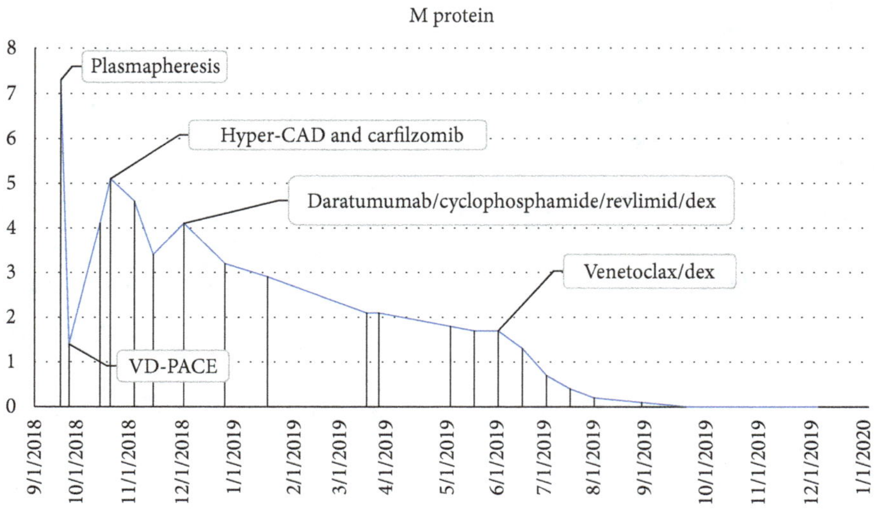

Figure 5: Serum monoclonal proteins.

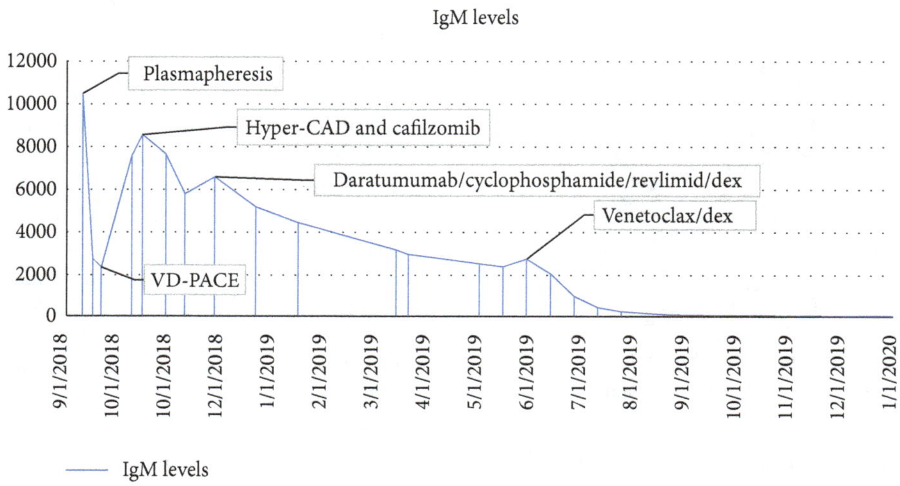

Figure 6: Ig M levels.

seen in peripheral blood and the absence of extramedullary disease [1]. Our patient had rapid progression on bortezomib- and carfilzomib-based therapies signaling a short survival expectation.

Daratumumab, an anti-CD38 monoclonal antibody, is effective in relapsed refractory MM [19] and should be explored in pPCL. The EMN12 trial of carfilzomib, lenalidomide, and dexamethasone in pPCL showed deep hematologic responses after 4 cycles (≥VGPR in 80% and ≥CR in 33%) [20]. Our patient had a partial response with daratumumab, lenalidomide, and dexamethasone, but this response was not persistent.

Venetoclax is a potent Bcl-2 inhibitor which showed efficacy in relapsed and refractory MM. It has been demonstrated in vitro as well as in vivo that a subgroup of plasma cells is Bcl-2 dependent and thus sensitive to venetoclax. This subset is restricted to those with t(11;14). It is associated with high Bcl-2, and low Bcl-X_L and Mcl-1 mRNA expression, resulting in higher sensitivity to Bcl-2 inhibition [21].

A phase I trial evaluated the response of venetoclax in patients with relapsed refractory MM, the majority of who were refractory to both bortezomib and lenalidomide. The ORR was 21% with VGPR in 15% of patients. ORR and ≥VGPR among patients with t(11;14) group were 40% and 27%, respectively. Median time to progression (TTP) in patients with t(11;14) was 6.6 months compared with 1.9 months in the group without t(11;14) [5]. The randomized phase 3 BELLINI trial showed improvement in PFS with the addition of venetoclax to bortezomib and dexamethasone (22.4 vs 11.5 months), but the trial was suspended due to increased deaths in venetoclax arm. Patients with t(11;14) receiving venetoclax had 95% ORR, including ≥VGPR in 75%, CR or stringent (sCR) in 55%, and minimal residual disease- (MRD-) negativity in 25% versus 47%, 27%, 7%, and 0% with placebo, respectively. There was also a trend towards improvement in OS in patients with t(11;14) [22].

Few case reports described the activity of venetoclax in PCL. In one case, a patient with IgG lambda pPCL with t(11;

14) relapsed six months after undergoing an AuHCT. The patient had an excellent response to venetoclax at the dose of 1200 mg daily in 21-day cycles and achieved MRD negativity after nine cycles. He continued to be on treatment at the time of publication [10]. Another case described a patient with lambda light chain pPCL with t(11;14) and TP53 mutation who failed to respond to initial induction treatment with combination chemotherapy consisting of VD-PACE. This patient was treated with a combination of venetoclax, daratumumab, and dexamethasone and achieved a sCR two months after initiating treatment with negative MRD. Venetoclax was dosed at 300 mg daily, and the patient continues to have stringent complete response (sCR) after 10 months of initiation of the treatment [23]. A third case described a patient with kappa light chain-restricted pPCL with del 17p and t(11;14) who had VGPR with carfilzomib, lenalidomide, and dexamethasone and proceeded to AuHCT. She relapsed on day +30 and was treated with bortezomib (days: 1, 4, 8, and 11), venetoclax (800 mg/day), and weekly dexamethasone. After just one cycle, she had dramatic suppression of light chains, and bone marrow evaluation was negative for MRD. The patient continued to be on treatment at the time of publication [24].

Our case highlights the efficacy of venetoclax in pPCL with t(11;14), similar to the above cases but is unique in that it was the rare IgM subtype of pPCL and it was associated with TP53 mutation. The patient achieved a very good partial response with normalization of quantitative IgM protein and disappearance of serum M-protein and plasma cells from peripheral blood. Bone marrow biopsy after two cycles showed only 3% kappa-restricted plasma cells. The patient continues to be on ven/dex after 15 months without significant side effects with IgM level <100 mg/dl showing the durability of response.

This case raises the prospect of evaluating venetoclax as a first-line treatment of pPCL with t(11;14), alone or in combination with other novel agents such as daratumumab and/or lenalidomide. Given the rarity of the disease, it may be challenging to enroll patients in prospective studies to evaluate the above question.

4. Conclusions

Our case demonstrates the efficacy of ven/dex in an aggressive and refractory pPCL patient with t(11;14) and TP53 mutation and, in this case, IgM-subtype. Given the poor prognosis of pPCL, further studies incorporating venetoclax in combination with other novel agents in the treatment of this disease particularly in the first-line setting are warranted.

Consent

Written informed consent was obtained from the patient for publication of this case report and accompanying images.

Authors' Contributions

All authors contributed to the acquisition of data, drafting, and editing the manuscript and to clinical management of the patient.

References

[1] C. Fernández de Larrea, R. A. Kyle, R. A. Kyle et al., "Plasma cell leukemia: consensus statement on diagnostic requirements, response criteria and treatment recommendations by the International Myeloma Working Group," *Leukemia*, vol. 27, no. 4, pp. 780–791, 2013.

[2] W. I. Gonsalves, S. V. Rajkumar, R. S. Go et al., "Trends in survival of patients with primary plasma cell leukemia: a population-based analysis," *Blood*, vol. 124, no. 6, pp. 907–912, 2014.

[3] S. R. Schuster, S. V. Rajkumar, A. Dispenzieri et al., "IgM multiple myeloma: disease definition, prognosis, and differentiation from Waldenstrom's macroglobulinemia," *American Journal of Hematology*, vol. 85, no. 11, pp. 853–855, 2010.

[4] L. Scarfò and P. Ghia, "Reprogramming cell death: BCL2 family inhibition in hematological malignancies," *Immunology Letters*, vol. 155, no. 1-2, pp. 36–39, 2013.

[5] S. Kumar, J. L. Kaufman, C. Gasparetto et al., "Efficacy of venetoclax as targeted therapy for relapsed/refractory t(11;14) multiple myeloma," *Blood*, vol. 130, no. 22, pp. 2401–2409, 2017.

[6] D. Rossi, "Role of MYD88 in lymphoplasmacytic lymphoma diagnosis and pathogenesis," *Hematology*, vol. 2014, no. 1, pp. 113–118, 2014.

[7] M. M. Saraceni, E. Scott, R. T. Maziarz et al., "Modified hyperCVAD versus bortezomib-hyperCAD in patients with relapsed/refractory multiple myeloma," *Clinical Lymphoma Myeloma and Leukemia*, vol. 18, no. 1, pp. e77–e84, 2018.

[8] L. Chiecchio, G. P. Dagrada, H. E. White et al., "Frequent upregulation of MYC in plasma cell leukemia," *Genes, Chromosomes and Cancer*, vol. 48, no. 7, pp. 624–636, 2009.

[9] W. J. Chng, T. Price-Troska, N. Gonzalez-Paz et al., "Clinical significance of TP53 mutation in myeloma," *Leukemia*, vol. 21, no. 3, pp. 582–584, 2007.

[10] T. Jelinek, J. Mihalyova, M. Kascak et al., "Single-agent venetoclax induces MRD-negative response in relapsed primary plasma cell leukemia with t(11;14)," *American Journal of Hematology*, vol. 94, no. 1, pp. E35–E37, 2019.

[11] C. Pellat-Deceunynck, S. Barillé, G. Jego et al., "The absence of CD56 (NCAM) on malignant plasma cells is a hallmark of plasma cell leukemia and of a special subset of multiple myeloma," *Leukemia*, vol. 12, no. 12, pp. 1977–1982, 1998.

[12] D. E. Reece, D. H. Vesole, S. Shrestha et al., "Outcome of patients with IgD and IgM multiple myeloma undergoing autologous hematopoietic stem cell transplantation: a retrospective CIBMTR study," *Clinical Lymphoma Myeloma and Leukemia*, vol. 10, no. 6, pp. 458–463, 2010.

[13] S. Oka, T. Yokote, T. Akioka et al., "Successful treatment of multi-agent chemotherapy with rituximab for IgM plasma cell leukemia," *Leukemia Research*, vol. 30, no. 12, pp. 1581–1583, 2006.

[14] S. Chhabra, S. Jain, A. Fowler et al., "IgM myeloma with plasma cell leukemia: case report and literature review," *Annals of Clinical and Laboratory Science*, vol. 47, no. 5, pp. 611–619, 2017.

[15] R. Costello, D. Sainty, R. Bouabdallah et al., "Primary plasma cell leukaemia: a report of 18 cases," *Leukemia Research*, vol. 25, no. 2, pp. 103–107, 2001.
[16] M. B. Drake, S. Iacobelli, A. van Biezen et al., "Primary plasma cell leukemia and autologous stem cell transplantation," *Haematologica*, vol. 95, no. 5, pp. 804–809, 2010.
[17] B. Royer, S. Minvielle, M. Diouf et al., "Bortezomib, doxorubicin, cyclophosphamide, dexamethasone induction followed by stem cell transplantation for primary plasma cell leukemia: a prospective phase II study of the intergroupe francophone du myélome," *Journal of Clinical Oncology*, vol. 34, no. 18, pp. 2125–2132, 2016.
[18] P. Musto, V. Simeon, M. C. Martorelli et al., "Lenalidomide and low-dose dexamethasone for newly diagnosed primary plasma cell leukemia," *Leukemia*, vol. 28, no. 1, pp. 222–225, 2014.
[19] M. A. Dimopoulos, A. Oriol, H. Nahi et al., "Daratumumab, lenalidomide, and dexamethasone for multiple myeloma," *New England Journal of Medicine*, vol. 375, no. 14, pp. 1319–1331, 2016.
[20] N. W. C. J. Van De Donk, B. van der Holt, F. H. Schjesvold et al., "Treatment of primary plasma cell leukemia with carfilzomib and lenalidomide-based therapy: results of the first interim analysis of the phase 2 EMN12/HOVON129 study," *Blood*, vol. 134, no. 1, p. 693, 2019.
[21] E. A. Punnoose, J. D. Leverson, F. Peale et al., "Expression profile of BCL-2, BCL-XL, and MCL-1 predicts pharmacological response to the BCL-2 selective antagonist venetoclax in multiple myeloma models," *Molecular Cancer Therapeutics*, vol. 15, no. 5, pp. 1132–1144, 2016.
[22] S. Kumar, *A Phase 3 Study of Venetoclax or Placebo in Combination with Bortezomib and Dexamethasone in Patients with Relapsed/refractory Multiple Myeloma EHA24*, European Hematology Association Library, Brussels, Belgium, 2019.
[23] S. Nalghranyan, A. P. Singh, and C. Schinke, "The combination of venetoclax, daratumumab and dexamethasone for the treatment of refractory primary plasma cell leukemia," *American Journal of Hematology*, vol. 95, no. 2, pp. E34–E35, 2020.
[24] W. I. Gonsalves, F. K. Buadi, and S. K. Kumar, "Combination therapy incorporating Bcl-2 inhibition with Venetoclax for the treatment of refractory primary plasma cell leukemia with t(11;14)," *European Journal of Haematology*, vol. 100, no. 2, pp. 215–217, 2018.

20

Diagnosis Dilemma of Angioimmunoblastic T-Cell Lymphoma in Tuberculosis Endemic Region

S. A. Touré, M. Seck, A B. Diallo, E. H. D. Niang, M. Keita, M. F. Dabo, B. F. Faye, and S. Diop

Hematology Department, Cheikh Anta Diop University, Dakar, Senegal

Correspondence should be addressed to S. A. Touré; touresonia90@yahoo.fr

Academic Editor: Kostas Konstantopoulos

Angioimmunoblastic T-cell lymphoma (AITL) is a rare hematologic malignancy recognized in the WHO 2016 classification as a clinical and histological entity. It is a very poorly described disease in Africa due to its rarity and diagnostic difficulties, particularly differential diagnosis with tuberculosis. Here, we report a 57-year-old man who presented with fever, weight loss, and lymphadenopathies. The diagnosis of tuberculosis was carried out based on lymph node fine needle aspiration showing the image of tuberculous adenitis and CT images in favor of necrotic lymphadenopathies. The presence of autoantibodies and the failure of tuberculosis treatment led us to perform a biopsy with immunostaining that confirmed pathological features of AITL. The patient was treated by CHOP-based chemotherapy, and complete remission was achieved. This case highlights the difficulty of recognizing AITL and the importance of considering other potential differential diagnoses of tuberculosis in the endemic region.

1. Introduction

AITL represents only 1%-2% of all non-Hodgkin lymphoma (NHL) cases, but nearly 1 in 5 cases of peripheral T-cell lymphoma (PTCL) is diagnosed per year. AITL clinical course is characterized by multiple relapses and a fatal outcome in the majority of patients. AITL, previously named angioimmunoblastic lymphadenopathy with dysproteinemia, immunoblastic lymphadenopathy, or lymphogranulomatosis *X*, is now a well-established subtype of PTCL, recognized by the 2008 WHO classification of lymphoid neoplasms with expansion in the 2016 revision [1, 2].

AITL is a very poorly described disease in Africa due to its rarity and diagnostic difficulties. The nonspecificities of clinical symptoms and its possible association with infectious diseases and autoimmune manifestations can also delay the diagnosis. Tuberculosis is an endemic disease in Africa, and tuberculosis patients may present similar signs as AITL. Here, we report a case of AITL who was first diagnosed as multifocal tuberculosis and was finally confirmed as AITL and who achieved a good outcome after chemotherapy.

2. Case Report

A 57-year-old man was received in our department with a long acting fever, which had been developing for 3 months, weight loss, and profuse night sweats. He was a smoker (pack years were 10) and had neither regular medication nor a particular medical antecedent. Physical examination showed a poor performance status (PS = 4/5), clinical anemia, and diffuse lymphadenopathies at different sites: cervical, axillary, and inguinal. Pain and inflammatory swelling were also found particularly on knees, elbows, and interphalangeal joints. Pulmonary examination showed a diminution of vocal fremitus and the presence of coarse precipitations on the left side. Physical examination also revealed a 7 cm subcutaneous nodule, located in the anterior face of the right arm.

Blood count results showed hyperleukocytosis associated with anemia and thrombocytopenia (HB: 9.1 g/dl, MCV: 94 fl, WBC: 22600/mm3 with neutrophils: 53% and lymphocytes: 36%, and PLQ: 34400/mm3). Antinuclear autoantibodies were positive, and rheumatoid factors were high: 62 IU/ml. No bone marrow involvement was found after cytological examination.

A thoraco-abdominopelvic CT scan was performed and showed the presence of mediastinal and abdominal lymphadenopathies with necrotic centers and bilateral basal pneumopathy (Figure 1).

Diagnosis of multifocal tuberculosis was retained based on clinical symptoms and cytological examination of lymph node sample obtained by fine needle aspiration showing aspect of tuberculous adenitis and CT imaging.

Antituberculosis (TB) treatment (rifampicin, isoniazid, pyrazinamide, and ethambutol) was administered for two months, but it did not reduce clinical signs. A lymph node biopsy was then performed, and pathological analysis revealed a diffuse lymphomatous proliferation consisting of large atypical cells with clarified nuclei and immunostaining showed a lymphoid proliferation consistent with the diagnosis of AITL : EBV+, CD3+, CD5+, CD2+, CD4+, CD278+, CXCL13+, PD1a+/−, CD10+, and Ki67+. The time from the onset of signs to definitive diagnosis of AITL was 5 months. The patient was diagnosed at an advanced stage and was classified as IPI3 (Ann Arbor: IIIBb, PS: 4, and lactate dehydrogenase: 680 U/L).

Pretherapeutic evaluation revealed hyperuricemia and polyclonal gammaglobulinemia; all other results were normal (serology of HIV, hepatitis B and C, ionogram, urea, creatininemia, 24 hours proteinuria, alanine aminotransferase, aspartate aminotransferase, bilirubinemia, C-reactive protein, prothrombin time, activated partial thromboplastin time, fibrinemia, fasting blood glucose, and cardiac ultrasound).

Chemotherapy according to CHOP protocol (cyclophosphamide: 750 mg/m^2, hydroxydaunorubicin: 50 mg/m^2, vincristine: 1.4 mg/m^2, and prednisone: 40 mg/m^2), applied every 21 days, was performed. After 8 cycles of CHOP, complete remission was achieved with normalization of clinical and biological anomalies. A relapse occurred 5 months later, and treatment consisted of 2 additional CHOP cures followed by 2 COP cures. A complete clinical and radiological remission was achieved again. Currently, one year after stopping treatment, the patient remains with no clinical symptoms; biological and morphological explorations are normal. Considering complications during treatment, febrile neutropenia was noted after the first treatment, and the patient was treated with G-CSF and antibiotics (3rd generation cephalosporin + gentamicin) for a duration of 10 days. Other complications were alopecia and nail hyperchromy.

3. Discussion

AITL afflicts advanced-age individuals with a median age between 60 and 65 years and is slightly predominant in men [3]. It accounts for only 1-2% of NHL and 15–20% of peripheral T lymphoma (PTL) cases. Its incidence is low, with 0.05 new cases diagnosed per 100,000 patients in the United States per year. The incidence of the disease is highest in Europe (29% of all PTL cases), followed by Asia (18%) and North America (16%); the reasons for this heterogeneity in different parts of the world are unexplained [3, 4].

AITL is a neoplasm characterized by intense inflammatory and immune reactions, as evidenced by its clinical, pathologic, cellular, and biologic properties. Because tumor cells phenotypically resemble T follicular helper (Tfh) cells, they are considered to function similarly to some extent to nonneoplastic Tfh cells seen in reactive follicular hyperplasia.

Tuberculosis (TB) is an airborne infectious disease caused by organisms of the *Mycobacterium tuberculosis* complex. Although primarily a pulmonary pathogen, *M. tuberculosis* can cause disease in almost any part of the body. Tuberculosis remains the leading cause of death from an infectious disease among adults worldwide, with more than 10 million people becoming newly sick from tuberculosis each year. T-helper 1 (Th1) responses are a major component of protective immunity because they clearly limit bacterial expansion. CD4$^+$ T cells are well known to be required for immunity to Mtb, and recruitment of T cells is necessary for containment of Mtb within granulomas.

In sub-Saharan Africa, any case of AITL has been found when searching in the literature. This low prevalence and reporting are mainly due to the difficulties of confirming such diagnosis, especially with the lack of human and logistical resources on histopathology.

Our presented case was on advanced disease, and thus presented with many symptoms such as weight loss, long acting fever, and lymphadenopathies, mimicking an infectious disease. These B symptoms, associated with lymphadenopathies, are not only the most common clinical findings in AITL but are also characteristics of tuberculosis. The reactive follicular hyperplasia seen in AITL may give the appearance of adenitis that may have caused the diagnosis of tuberculosis on lymph node cytology.

The present case was described in an advanced stage of the disease and presented many symptoms such as weight loss, long acting fever, and lymphadenopathies, mimicking an infectious disease. The presence of pulmonary symptoms and aspect of tuberculosis adenitis on the lymph node fine needle aspiration were also to diagnosing tuberculosis. Nevertheless, we cannot rule out an association between the two diseases.

The association between tuberculosis and lymphoma is not trivial and is possible even in the absence of HIV infection. The lymphoma-induced immunodeficiency is a suitable situation for TB infection, particularly in endemic countries and in patients with a history of proven TB. It is a source of diagnostic wandering, with clinical and morphological data similar in both conditions [5]. An immunohistochemical study of all sites accessible for punctures and biopsies can make up for a diagnostic delay that could permanently compromise the prognosis [6].

The positivity of antinuclear autoantibodies and rheumatoid factors support the idea considering AITL as an immunologically functional disease. Hypergammaglobulinemia and the positive Coombs test were reported, respectively, among 50% and 33% of the patients in a large population of 157 AILT cases reported in France [7]. An improved understanding of the interactions between

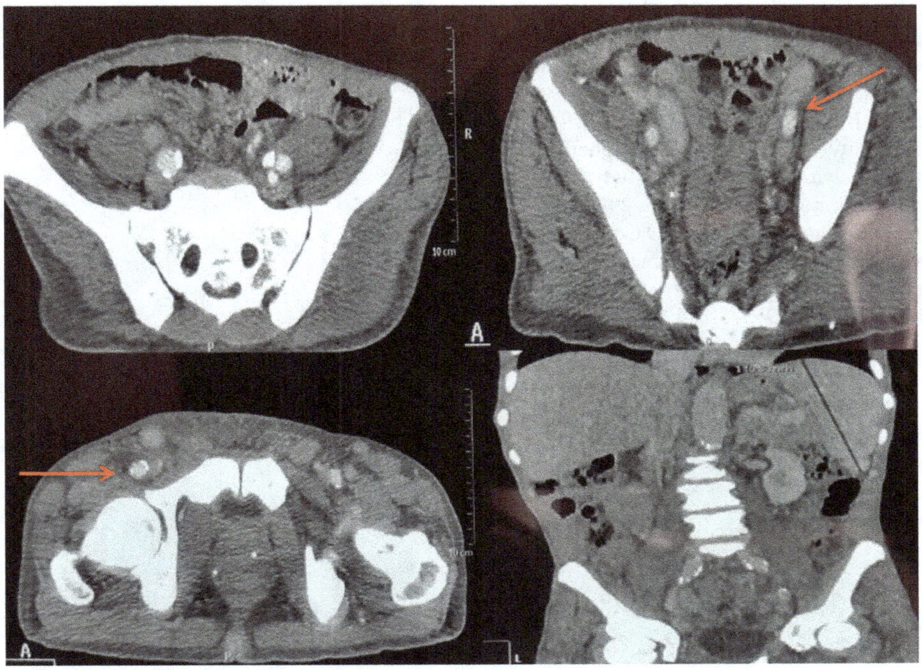

Figure 1: Multiple mediastinal and abdominal lymphadenopathies with central necrosis.

neoplastic cells and microenvironment in AITL would offer the possibility of identifying immunomodulatory approaches for rationale design of future treatments.

Concerning the treatment, the patient received 8 cycles of CHOP, followed by 2 additional ones and 2 cycles of COP before obtaining a durable complete remission.

Even if this remission still persists one year after the end of treatment, it is highly likely that a relapse will occur in the near future. The recurrent nature of AITL is known, and a new line of treatment should therefore to be considered [8].

Furthermore, it has been described that patients with relapsed or refractory AITL have always been a challenge for physicians. The median and survival or relapse rates are only a few months [9], as in the case of our studied patient who relapsed for the first time after 5 months.

Given the aggressiveness of the disease and the poor results obtained with chemotherapy, autologous SCT should be proposed for the treatment of these patients in first remission [10]. Relapsed and refractory patients should be enrolled in clinical trials, as new approaches and drugs are needed [11, 12].

4. Conclusion

The systematic practice of biopsy with immunostaining should facilitate the diagnosis of AITL, especially in a context where diseases such as tuberculosis with clinical and paraclinical similarities may delay this diagnosis.

References

[1] S. H. Swerdlow, E. Campo, S. A. Pileri et al., "The 2016 revision of the world health organization classification of lymphoid neoplasms," *Blood*, vol. 127, no. 20, pp. 2375–2390, 2016.

[2] J. O. Armitage, "The aggressive peripheral T-cell lymphomas: 2017," *American Journal of Hematology*, vol. 92, no. 7, pp. 706–715, 2017.

[3] P. L. Broccoli and P. L. Zinzani, "Angioimmunoblastic T-cell lymphoma," *Hematology/oncology clinics of North America*, vol. 31, no. 2, pp. 223–238, 2017.

[4] N. P. C. Zing, T. Fischer, J. Zain, M. Federico, and S. T. Rosen, "Peripheral T-cell lymphomas: incorporating new developments in diagnostics, prognostication, and treatment into clinical practice-part 1: PTCL-NOS, FTCL, AITL, ALCL," *Oncology (Williston Park)*, vol. 32, no. 7, pp. e74–e82, 2018.

[5] K. Antel, C. Levetan, Z Mohamed et al., "The determinants and impact of diagnostic delay in lymphoma in a TB and HIV endemic setting," *BMC Cancer*, vol. 19, no. 1, p. 384, 2019 A.

[6] N. Mourad, N. Mounier, J. Brière et al., "Clinical, biologic, and pathologic features in 157 patients with angioimmunoblastic T-cell lymphoma treated within the groupe d'Etude des Lymphomes de l'Adulte (GELA) trials," *Blood*, vol. 111, no. 9, pp. 4463–4470, 2008.

[7] K. Fukumoto, T. B. Nguyen, S. Chiba, and M. Sakata-Yanagimoto, "Review of the biologic and clinical significance of genetic mutations in angioimmunoblastic T-cell lymphoma," *Cancer Science*, vol. 109, no. 3, pp. 490–496, 2017.

[8] K. Mosalpuria, R. G. Bociek, and J. M. Vose, "Angioimmunoblastic T-cell lymphoma management," *Seminars in Hematology*, vol. 51, no. 1, pp. 52–58, 2014.

[9] A. J. Moskowitz, M. A Lunning, and S. M. Horwitz, "How I treat the peripheral T-cell lymphomas," *Blood*, vol. 123, no. 17, pp. 2636–2644, 2014.

[10] P. Reimer, T. Rüdiger, E. Geissinger et al., "Autologous stem-cell transplantation as first-line therapy in peripheral T-cell lymphomas: results of a prospective multicenter study," *Journal of Clinical Oncology*, vol. 27, no. 1, pp. 106–113, 2009.
[11] F. Ellin, M. Jerkeman, J. Törnqvist, T. Brudin, and T. Relander, "Impact of comorbidity on survival in peripheral T-cell lymphomas: a swedish lymphoma registry study," *Hematological Oncology*, vol. 36, no. 1, pp. 159–165, 2018.
[12] E. Marchi, O. A. O'Connor, and O. A. O'Connor, "Novel agents in the treatment of relapsed or refractory peripheral T-cell lymphoma," *Hematology/Oncology Clinics of North America*, vol. 31, no. 2, pp. 359–375, 2017.

21

Prolonged Response of a Patient with Relapsed Acute Myeloid Leukemia to a Novel Oral Bromodomain Extraterminal Inhibitor (BETi)

Meilen Chang Muñoz,[1] Jennifer A. Murphy,[2,3] Johannes E. Wolff,[4] and Brian A. Jonas[1,3]

[1]*Department of Internal Medicine, University of California Davis, School of Medicine, Sacramento, CA, USA*
[2]*Department of Pharmacy Services, University of California Davis Medical Center, Sacramento, CA, USA*
[3]*University of California Davis Comprehensive Cancer Center, Sacramento, CA, USA*
[4]*AbbVie Inc., North Chicago, IL, USA*

Correspondence should be addressed to Brian A. Jonas; bajonas@ucdavis.edu

Academic Editor: Kostas Konstantopoulos

Acute myeloid leukemia (AML) is an aggressive clonal bone marrow cancer characterized by high rates of relapse and mortality. A middle-aged woman with AML relapsed twice after achieving complete remission with induction therapy and subsequent salvage therapy. She was then enrolled in a clinical trial with the bromodomain extraterminal inhibitor (BETi) mivebresib and achieved complete remission with incomplete count recovery (CRi) with monotherapy. Subsequently, she relapsed and was transitioned to combination therapy with mivebresib plus venetoclax and achieved CR again. The patient required eltrombopag to decrease platelet dependence in both arms of the trial and exhibited less myelosuppression with the combination therapy. The exceptional response to mivebresib demonstrated by this patient underscores the therapeutic potential of mivebresib.

1. Introduction

Acute myeloid leukemia (AML) is an aggressive and heterogeneous bone marrow cancer driven by genetic and epigenetic alterations. It is the second most common type of adult leukemia making up approximately 30% of all cases and is the leading cause of leukemia-related deaths [1, 2]. Risk factors for development of AML include age >65, male gender, smoking, prior treatment with chemotherapy or radiation, certain environmental exposures, and history of antecedent myeloid disorder, such as myelodysplastic syndrome [3, 4]. The 5-year overall survival rate ranges from 40–50% in younger patients to 20–30% in older patients who receive high-intensity chemotherapy [5]. Relapse rates vary from 30–35% in patients aged <60 with favorable risk factors, up to 90% in patients aged >60 with adverse risk factors [6]. If the disease relapses, salvage therapy may be offered to achieve remission again, but survival in the relapsed setting is very poor [7]. Given the poor outcomes seen with AML, especially in the relapsed setting, it is imperative to find new strategies to improve remission and overall survival rates.

Bromodomain (BRD) and extraterminal (BET) proteins are a family of proteins that recognize acetylated lysine residues on histones to promote chromosome remodeling, histone modification or recognition and control transcription machinery to upregulate gene expression driving oncogenesis [8, 9]. Preclinical studies demonstrate that BET inhibitors (BETis) have antiproliferative activity and trigger a strong apoptotic response in cell lines derived from hematologic malignancies through the downregulation of MYC [10]. Thus, BET proteins have been identified as key targets for leukemia therapy [11, 12]. Mivebresib is a potent oral BETi that has recently entered phase I clinical trials [13]. It functions in a variety of mechanisms including G1 cell cycle arrest, induction of apoptosis, and potentially targeting

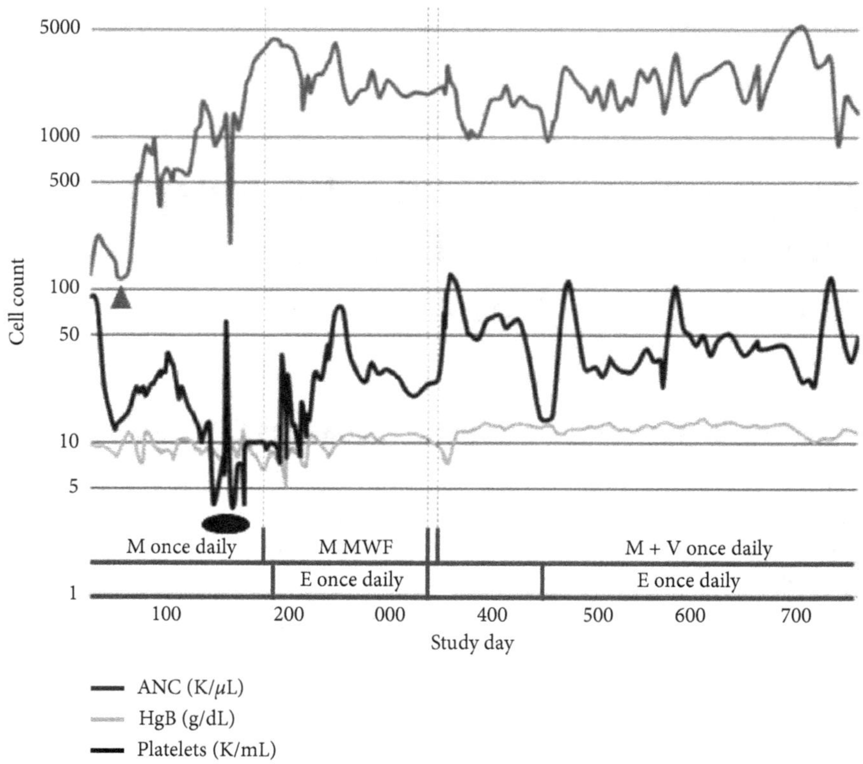

FIGURE 1: Absolute neutrophil count (ANC), hemoglobin (Hgb), and platelet counts throughout mivebresib mono- or combination therapy with venetoclax. ANC was less than 100/μL during days 1 to 84, corresponding to cycles 1 to 3 of monotherapy (as denoted by grey triangle), and recovered to greater than 1,000/μL, thereafter. Hgb generally remained between 7 and 12 g/dL throughout all treatment modalities. Platelets remained less than 10,000/μL between days 140 and 190, corresponding to cycles 4 and 6 of monotherapy (as denoted by black oval), and then increased to 15,000 to 120,000/μL for the duration of the trial. M = mivebresib; V = venetoclax; E = eltrombopag.

the tumor microenvironment to provide additional therapeutic benefit. Another agent that has demonstrated high response rates and encouraging remission durations in AML is venetoclax, an oral B-cell lymphoma-2 (BCL-2) inhibitor that can activate apoptosis in malignancies [14]. Venetoclax is approved in combination with a hypomethylating agent (HMA) or low-dose cytarabine (LDAC) backbone in older patients with newly diagnosed AML or those who are not candidates for intensive chemotherapy [15, 16].

Like other systemic therapies, mivebresib and venetoclax cause myelosuppression that can lead to transfusion dependence. Allogeneic blood transfusions are associated with transfusion-related organ injury and sepsis, hemolytic transfusion reactions [17], platelet-refractory alloimmunization [18], and increased graft-versus-host disease after allogeneic hematopoietic stem cell transplantation [19] and hinder finding a suitable stem cell donor. Hence, bone marrow growth factors have been used to promote blood count recovery and decrease transfusion dependency. For example, eltrombopag is a potent thrombopoietin receptor agonist that has been studied for use in AML among other diseases characterized by thrombocytopenia [20].

In this study, we report the exceptional clinical response of a patient with multiply relapsed AML who was treated with mivebresib as monotherapy and subsequently after relapse with mivebresib in combination with venetoclax and eltrombopag. Complete remission with incomplete count recovery (CRi) was achieved with monotherapy, and after relapse she achieved a second CRi with combination therapy.

2. Case Description

A 60-year-old woman with no significant past medical history presented with *de novo* AML discovered on routine CBC. She presented with night sweats, bruising, and pancytopenia. The initial bone marrow biopsy revealed 66% myeloblasts, 30–40% cellularity, normal karyotype, and negative molecular studies. She achieved complete remission (CR) with 7 + 3 induction therapy and proceeded with 4 cycles of high-dose cytarabine consolidation. She remained in remission for nearly 20 months when a surveillance bone marrow biopsy revealed relapsed disease. She subsequently underwent salvage reinduction and achieved a second CR. The patient declined allogenic hematopoietic stem cell transplant in favor of consolidation therapy with intermediate-dose cytarabine. She remained in CR for approximately 10 months without additional therapy before relapsing for a second time.

The patient subsequently elected to enroll in a phase I clinical trial of mivebresib for relapsed or refractory AML (NCT02391480) and was treated with mivebresib monotherapy. Her disease did not initially respond with an increase in marrow blasts from 21% to 40% after the first cycle,

Table 1: Clinical course, including bone marrow, molecular, and peripheral blood responses.

Day	Circulating blasts (%)	BM blast morphology (%)	MLFS achieved	MRD flow blasts (%)	Cytogenetics	Molecular	ANC (K/μL)	Hgb (g/dL)	Plt (K/μL)	ELN response
Screening mono (M)	6	21	N/A	Not done	46,XX [20]	STAG2 R213Efster12 (VAF 18%)	0.12	10.6	95	N/A
C2D1M	3	40	No	Not done	46,XX [18]	Not done	0.12	8	13	Resistant disease
C3D1M	0	11	No	Not done	Failed	Not done	0.76	7.5	23	Resistant disease
C5D1M	0	8	No	Not done	46,XX [20]	Not done	1.2	9	12	Resistant disease
C6D1M	0	4	Yes	20.1	46,XX [20]	Not done	1.34	8.9	4	CRi
C7D1M	0	4	Yes	10.8	46,XX [20]	Not done	3.3	8.2	10	CRi
C9D1M	0	8	No	12.1	46,XX [20]	Not done	2.5	10.9	28	Morphologic relapse
C10D1M	0	4	Yes	Not done	46,XX [20]	Not done	3.1	8.6	43	CRi
C11D1M	0	8	No	13.5	46,XX [20]	STAG2 R213Efster12 (VAF 6.6%), WT1 K467Ter (VAF 7.4%)	2.7	11.4	33	Morphologic relapse
C13D1M	0	14	No	26.3	46,XX [20]	Not done	1.9	10.6	24	Resistant disease
Screening combo (C)	Not reported	8	N/A	Not done	46,XX [20]	Not done	>1.0	9.3	29	N/A
C2D1C	0	2	Yes	0.99	46,XX [20]	Not done	1.1	11.9	51	CRi
C3D1C	0	2	Yes	0.64	46,XX [20]	Not done	1.8	12.8	68	CRi
C5D1C	0	1	Yes	0.35	46,XX [20]	None detected	1.3	12	20	CRi
C7D1C	0	2	Yes	0.14	46,XX [20]	Not done	1.5	12.2	30	CRi
C9D1C	0	1	Yes	0.34	46,XX [20]	Not done	3.5	12.9	104	CR
C11D1C	0	N/A	N/A	0.9	46,XX [20]	None detected	3	13.7	51	CRi
C13D1C	0	6	No	5.3	46,XX [20]	Not done	4.4	13.3	42	Morphologic relapse
C14D1C	0	4	Yes	5.5	46,XX [20]	KMT2A I3423V (VUS, VAF 50.6%)	2.9	10.2	24	CRi
C15D1C	0	10	No	10.7	46,XX [20]	Not done	1.4	11.5	50	Morphologic relapse
EOT marrow deferred							2.6	11.7	75	

BM, bone marrow; MLFS, morphologic leukemia-free state; MRD, measurable residual disease; VAF, variant allele frequency; ANC, absolute neutrophil count; Hgb, hemoglobin; Plt, platelet; ELN, European LeukemiaNet; CRi, complete remission with incomplete count recovery; CR, complete remission; N/A, not applicable; EOT, end of treatment; VUS, variant of uncertain significance.

but this was followed by a decrease to 11% after cycle 2 and eventual CRi, due to ongoing thrombocytopenia, by the end of cycle 5. The patient first developed thrombocytopenia during cycle 2 and became transfusion dependent by cycle 5 (Figure 1 and Table 1). Eltrombopag 50 mg daily was added during cycle 7, and mivebresib was modified from 1.5 mg daily to 3 mg MWF during cycle 8 resulting in decreased transfusion requirements (Figure 2). Eltrombopag was increased to 100 mg daily, eliminating transfusion dependency, but the patient remained thrombocytopenic. Prior to the start of cycle 13 of mivebresib monotherapy, the patient relapsed with 14% blasts. She then discontinued mivebresib monotherapy and, after a washout period, was enrolled in a drug combination cohort of the study. The patient initially achieved CRi after cycle 1 of treatment with mivebresib and venetoclax (target dose 800 mg) before improving to CR after cycle 8 (Table 1). Eltrombopag was held during the early cycles of combination therapy as she maintained a platelet count greater than 50,000/μL. However, during cycle 4 of mivebresib and venetoclax, the patient developed leukopenia and thrombocytopenia and eltrombopag was resumed. Platelet counts remained greater than 20,000/μL and eventually improved to greater than 100,000/μL with eltrombopag, mivebresib, and venetoclax. In contrast,

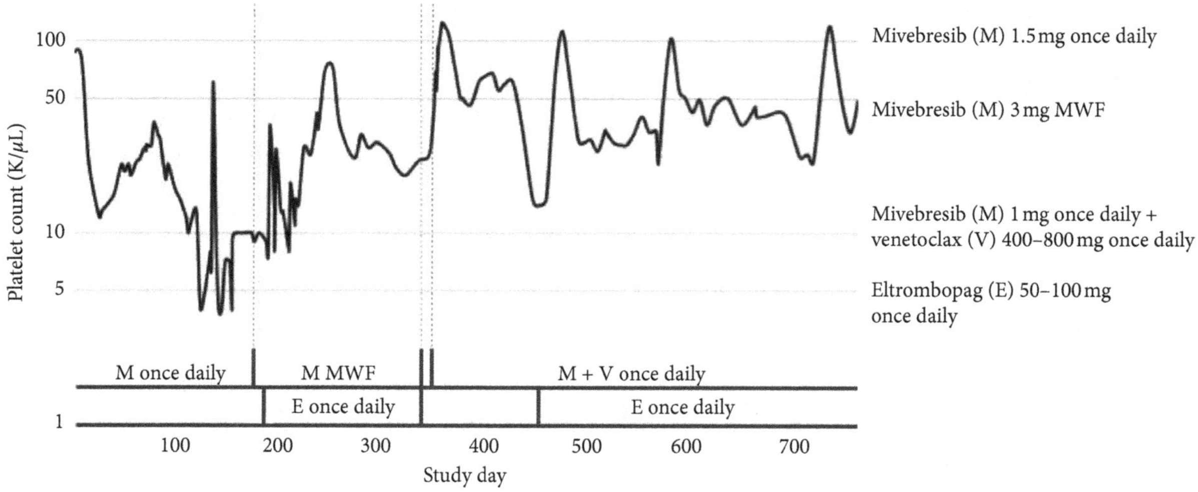

Figure 2: Platelet count response to therapy. Platelets decreased to less than 10,000/μL with mivebresib 1.5 mg once daily monotherapy. Platelets increased to greater than 10,000/μL with a change in mivebresib dosing to 3 mg MWF and increased further to greater than 50,000/μL with the addition of eltrombopag. Platelet counts remained greater than 15,000/μL and up to 120,000/μL with the combination mivebresib and venetoclax and sustained with eltrombopag.

platelet counts generally had previously remained below 30,000/μL with eltrombopag and mivebresib monotherapy.

Pretrial genomic screening revealed a STAG2 R213Efster12 mutation with 18% variant allele frequency (VAF) (Table 1). Genomics performed during cycle 11 of monotherapy revealed persistence of STAG2 mutation with a decrease in VAF to 6.6% and a new mutation WT1 K467Ter (VAF 7.4%). Genomics performed during cycle 5 of combination therapy did not detect any mutations. However, a KMT2A I3432V (VAF 50.6%) variant of unknown significance was detected after cycle 13, and the patient relapsed soon thereafter.

3. Discussion

AML comprises ~30% of all adult leukemia cases, and relapse rates can be as high 90% in elderly patients with adverse risk factors. High relapse rates necessitate novel systemic therapies with longer remission durations. New targets have been identified that can induce apoptosis in malignant cells, including BET and BCL-2 proteins. Mivebresib is a pan-inhibitor of the BET proteins that is currently in phase I clinical trials. In this case, mivebresib was initially used as a monotherapy per protocol with the patient achieving CRi after completion of cycle 5. Given that the patient continued to experience severe thrombocytopenia and transfusion dependence, which prevented the patient from achieving CR, as defined by <5% blasts by morphology in a cellular marrow with recovery of both neutrophils and platelets, eltrombopag was added as a supportive measure. This resulted in decreased transfusion dependency, but the thrombocytopenia persisted. At disease relapse, mivebresib monotherapy was discontinued, and after a washout period, combination therapy with venetoclax and mivebresib was started. The patient once again achieved CRi during cycle 2 before improving to a CR after cycle 8. Response was maintained for approximately 11 months until cycle 13 when there was morphologic relapse.

Interestingly, platelet counts were not as low with combination therapy as with monotherapy, and the patient sustained only mild to moderate thrombocytopenia with the addition of eltrombopag to venetoclax and mivebresib. She did not require any platelet transfusions with this combination regimen. Possible explanations for this observation include a deeper response to the combination therapy resulting in improved count recovery, response related to the venetoclax component alone, or that combination therapy may have resulted in a more effective response to eltrombopag potentially attributable to a synergistic effect between the three drugs.

Studies demonstrate that eltrombopag stimulates thrombopoiesis via the JAK-STAT signaling cascade [21]. This same pathway regulates expression of the apoptosis regulatory genes BCL-2 [22] and MYC [23]. Given that venetoclax is a BCL-2 inhibitor and mivebresib downregulates MYC expression, we can hypothesize that venetoclax and mivebresib downregulate the apoptotic pathway in platelets, allowing the cell proliferation pathway to predominate. Additional studies are required to explore these potential mechanisms of response and synergy.

In addition, we can consider the contribution of STAG2 deficiency on incomplete count recovery. STAG2 is a part of the cohesin multimeric protein complex responsible for cohesion of sister chromatids, transcription regulation, and homologous DNA repair [24]. Preliminary data suggest that loss of STAG2 can lead to dysregulated transcription in AML [25]. Considering that our patient initially expressed a STAG2 mutation, it is conceivable that STAG2 deficiency globally prevented appropriate transcription, inevitably inhibiting effective platelet production. Once this mutation resolved in the setting of combination therapy, we posit that eltrombopag-induced platelet production was more efficient. Given resolution of this mutation with combination therapy, we can also consider the potential for STAG2 to be a predictive marker for response to mivebresib-based therapy.

4. Conclusion

In this case study of an exceptional responder, mivebresib as monotherapy and in combination with venetoclax conferred an 18-month survival supporting the potential clinical activity of this novel BETi in relapsed or refractory AML. In combination with mivebresib and/or venetoclax, eltrombopag also led to decreased transfusion dependence, which can augment quality of life, decrease healthcare costs, and reduce platelet alloimmunization. Primary data analyses of all patients in the AML cohorts investigated in this trial, including safety and clinical efficacy, will be described elsewhere.

Authors' Contributions

MCM, JAM, JW, and BAJ were responsible for conception and design; MCM, JAM, and BAJ were involved in analysis and interpretation of data; MCM, JAM, JW, and BAJ were responsible for writing, review, and/or revision of the manuscript.

Acknowledgments

The authors wish to thank our patient for participating in the AbbVie-sponsored clinical trial (NCT02391480) and Nichole Mahaffey, PhD, for assistance with the data. The trial was approved by the UC Davis Institutional Review Board (#984817). This case study did not have funding support. The case belongs to a clinical study (NCT02391480), and the case is eligible to be published as an isolated case report. The clinical trial the patient participated in was funded by AbbVie.

References

[1] A. Redaelli, J. M. Lee, J. M. Stephens, and C. L. Pashos, "Epidemiology and clinical burden of acute myeloid leukemia," *Expert Review of Anticancer Therapy*, vol. 3, no. 5, pp. 695–710, 2003.

[2] R. L. Siegel, K. D. Miller, and A. Jemal, "Cancer statistics, 2020," *CA: A Cancer Journal for Clinicians*, vol. 70, no. 1, pp. 7–30, 2020.

[3] S. A. Speer, J. C. Semenza, T. Kurosaki et al., "Risk factors for acute myeloid leukemia and multiple myeloma: a combination of GIC and case-control studies," *Journal of Environmental Health*, vol. 64, no. 7, pp. 8–15, 2002.

[4] S. S. Strom, R. Oum, K. Y. Elhor Gbito, G. Garcia-Manero, and Y. Yamamura, "De novo acute myeloid leukemia risk factors," *Cancer*, vol. 118, no. 18, pp. 4589–4596, 2012.

[5] H. Kantarjian, "Acute myeloid leukemia-major progress over four decades and glimpses into the future," *American Journal of Hematology*, vol. 91, no. 1, pp. 131–145, 2016.

[6] C. Röllig, M. Bornhäuser, C. Thiede et al., "Long-term prognosis of acute myeloid leukemia according to the new genetic risk classification of the European leukemianet recommendations: evaluation of the proposed reporting system," *Journal of Clinical Oncology*, vol. 29, no. 20, pp. 2758–2765, 2011.

[7] D. A. Breems, W. L. J. Van Putten, P. C. Huijgens et al., "Prognostic index for adult patients with acute myeloid leukemia in first relapse," *Journal of Clinical Oncology*, vol. 23, no. 9, pp. 1969–1978, 2005.

[8] G. Borthakur, J. E. Wolff, I. Aldoss et al., "First-in-human study of ABBV-075 (mivebresib), a pan-inhibitor of bromodomain and extra terminal (BET) proteins, in patients (pts) with relapsed/refractory (RR) acute myeloid leukemia (AML): preliminary data," *Journal of Clinical Oncology*, vol. 36, no. 15, p. 7019, 2018.

[9] G. M. Borthakur, O. Odenike, I. Aldoss et al., "Biomarker modulation by mivebresib (ABBV-075) +/− venetoclax in relapsed/refractory acute myeloid leukemia," *Blood*, vol. 134, no. 1, p. 539, 2019.

[10] M. H. Bui, X. Lin, D. H. Albert et al., "Preclinical characterization of BET family bromodomain inhibitor ABBV-075 suggests combination therapeutic strategies," *Cancer Research*, vol. 77, no. 11, pp. 2976–2989, 2017.

[11] A. Alqahtani, K. Choucair, M. Ashraf et al., "Bromodomain and extra-terminal motif inhibitors: a review of preclinical and clinical advances in cancer therapy," *Future Science OA*, vol. 5, no. 3, Article ID FSO372, 2019.

[12] G. Andrieu, A. C. Belkina, and G. V. Denis, "Clinical trials for BET inhibitors run ahead of the science," *Drug Discovery Today: Technologies*, vol. 19, pp. 45–50, 2016.

[13] S. A. Piha-Paul, J. C. Sachdev, M. Barve et al., "First-in-human study of mivebresib (ABBV-075), an oral pan-inhibitor of bromodomain and extra terminal proteins, in patients with relapsed/refractory solid tumors," *Clinical Cancer Research*, vol. 25, no. 21, p. 6309, 2019.

[14] B. A. Jonas and D. A. Pollyea, "How we use venetoclax with hypomethylating agents for the treatment of newly diagnosed patients with acute myeloid leukemia," *Leukemia*, vol. 33, no. 12, pp. 2795–2804, 2019.

[15] C. D. DiNardo, K. Pratz, V. Pullarkat et al., "Venetoclax combined with decitabine or azacitidine in treatment-naive, elderly patients with acute myeloid leukemia," *Blood*, vol. 133, no. 1, pp. 7–17, 2019.

[16] A. H. Wei, S. A. Strickland, J.-Z. Hou et al., "Venetoclax combined with low-dose cytarabine for previously untreated patients with acute myeloid leukemia: results from a phase Ib/II study," *Journal of Clinical Oncology*, vol. 37, no. 15, pp. 1277–1284, 2019.

[17] E. C. Vamvakas and M. A. Blajchman, "Transfusion-related mortality: the ongoing risks of allogeneic blood transfusion and the available strategies for their prevention," *Blood*, vol. 113, no. 15, pp. 3406–3417, 2009.

[18] E. Delaflor-Weiss and P. D. Mintz, "The evaluation and management of platelet refractoriness and alloimmunization," *Transfusion Medicine Reviews*, vol. 14, no. 2, pp. 180–196, 2000.

[19] S. Hosoba, E. K. Waller, N. Shenvi et al., "Peritransplantation red blood cell transfusion is associated with increased risk of graft-versus-host disease after allogeneic hematopoietic stem cell transplantation," *Biology of Blood and Marrow Transplantation*, vol. 24, no. 5, pp. 973–982, 2018.

[20] M. Mittleman, U. Platzbecker, B. Afanasyev et al., "Eltrombopag for advanced myelodysplastic syndromes or acute myeloid leukaemia and severe thrombocytopenia (ASPIRE): a

randomised, placebo-controlled, phase 2 trial," *The Lancet Hematology*, vol. 5, no. 1, pp. e34–e43, 2018.

[21] K. P. Garnock-Jones and S. J. Keam, "Eltrombopag," *Drugs*, vol. 69, no. 5, pp. 567–576, 2009.

[22] P. Sepúlveda, A. Encabo, F. Carbonell-Uberos, and M. D. Miñana, "BCL-2 expression is mainly regulated by JAK/STAT3 pathway in human CD34+ hematopoietic cells," *Cell Death & Differentiation*, vol. 14, no. 2, pp. 378–380, 2007.

[23] A. Lollies, S. Hartmann, M. Schneider et al., "An oncogenic axis of STAT-mediated BATF3 upregulation causing MYC activity in classical Hodgkin lymphoma and anaplastic large cell lymphoma," *Leukemia*, vol. 32, no. 1, pp. 92–101, 2018.

[24] A. Kon, L.-Y. Shih, M. Minamino et al., "Recurrent mutations in multiple components of the cohesin complex in myeloid neoplasms," *Nature Genetics*, vol. 45, no. 10, pp. 1232–1237, 2013.

[25] J. S. Smith, S. G. Craig, F. G. Liberante et al., "Chronic loss of STAG2 leads to altered chromatin structure contributing to de-regulated transcription in AML," 2019, https://www.biorxiv.org/content/10.1101/856195v1.

22

PML-RARA Fusion Transcripts Detectable 8 Months prior to Promyelocytic Blast Crisis in Chronic Myeloid Leukemia

Stephanie Wolanin,[1] Robert K. McCall,[2] Mark J. Pettenati,[1] Michael W. Beaty,[1] Giovanni Insuasti-Beltran,[1] Bayard L. Powell,[3] and Stacey S. O'Neill[1]

[1] *Wake Forest Baptist Medical Center, Department of Pathology, Winston-Salem, NC, USA*
[2] *Molecular Pathology Laboratory Network, Maryville, TN, USA*
[3] *Wake Forest Baptist Comprehensive Cancer Center, Section on Hematology and Oncology, Winston-Salem, NC, USA*

Correspondence should be addressed to Stacey S. O'Neill; soneill@wakehealth.edu

Academic Editor: Sudhir Tauro

Promyelocytic blast crisis arising from chronic myeloid leukemia (CML) is rare. We present a 40-year-old male who developed promyelocytic blast crisis 17 months after CML diagnosis, confirmed by the presence of the *t*(15;17) and *t*(9;22) translocations in the leukemic cells. Preserved nucleic acids from routine *BCR-ABL1* testing provided a unique opportunity to evaluate clonal progression over time. Retrospective analysis demonstrated *PML-RARA* fusion transcripts were first detectable 8 months prior to blast crisis presentation. A review of 21 cases of promyelocytic blasts crisis published in the literature reveals a male predominance with earlier age at onset as compared to females. Interestingly, TKI therapy during chronic phase did not impact the time interval between diagnosis and promyelocytic blast crisis. Treatment with standard acute promyelocytic leukemia regimens provides more favorable outcomes with complete molecular remission. Although rare, it is important to consider a promyelocytic blast crisis when evaluating for transformation of CML due to its effective treatment with specific therapies.

1. Introduction

Chronic myeloid leukemia (CML) is a myeloproliferative neoplasm defined by the presence of a translocation between chromosomes 9 and 22 leading to the *BCR-ABL1* gene fusion product. The aberrant fusion protein leads to abnormal activation of multiple cellular signaling pathways including JAK/STAT, PI3K/AKT, and Ras/MEK that promote cell growth and survival [1, 2]. Without therapy, progression from chronic phase to accelerated and blast phase is typical. Small molecule tyrosine kinase inhibitors (TKIs) that selectively inhibit the *BCR-ABL1* fusion protein have dramatically prolonged survival of CML patients from an average of 3 years to greater than 8 years and decreased the annual rate of progression to blast crisis from 20% to less than 1% per year [1, 3–5]. While fewer patients continue on to develop blast crisis, the prognosis in blast crisis remains poor, with death generally 3-4 months after diagnosis in pre-TKI era and 7–11 months with TKI therapy [4, 6].

Blast crisis in CML derives from the myeloid lineage in 70% of cases, with the majority of the remaining cases having a lymphoid origin [4]. Rare forms of blast crisis have been described including megakaryocytic, erythroid, monoblastic, eosinophilic, basophilic, and biphenotypic [4]. Promyelocytic blast crisis is a rare variant with <25 cases reported in the literature. Herein, we present a case of CML with promyelocytic blast crisis and review of the literature.

2. Case Presentation

The patient is a 40-year-old male with a past medical history significant for classic Hodgkin lymphoma treated with 4 cycles of doxorubicin, bleomycin, vinblastine, and dacarbazine (ABVD) and adjuvant radiation therapy. Approximately seven years after achieving a complete remission, the patient was noted to have asymptomatic leukocytosis (white blood count $44 \times 10^3/\mu L$) during routine follow-up (Table 1). A differential count revealed prominent neutrophilia with maturational left shift and basophilia. No circulating blasts were identified. Hemoglobin and platelets were within normal ranges.

A bone marrow biopsy performed at that time revealed a hypercellular marrow (greater than 95%) with a marked myeloid hyperplasia with maturational left shift and increased myeloid to erythroid ratio. There was no increase in blasts or myelofibrosis. Routine cytogenetics demonstrated presence of the *t*(9;22)(q34;q11.2) translocation in all cells; no other chromosomal abnormalities were detected (Table 1). Fluorescent in situ hybridization (FISH) was positive for *BCR-ABL1* fusion events in 96% of interphase nuclei. Quantitative real-time polymerase chain reaction (RT-PCR) performed on the peripheral blood was positive for p210 *BCR-ABL1* fusion transcripts, with an international scale percent ratio (IS%) of 93.869% (Table 2). Together, the findings supported the diagnosis of chronic myeloid leukemia, *BCR-ABL1*-positive, in chronic phase. The patient was initially treated with imatinib 400 mg daily for 5 months and then reduced for low neutrophils to 300 mg daily for seven months. However, a major molecular response defined as IS% ≤0.1% [7] was not achieved, and therapy was changed to dasatinib 100 mg daily approximately a year after diagnosis secondary to increasing *BCR-ABL1* transcripts by RT-PCR testing. His dose of dasatinib was reduced to 60 mg daily for cytopenias just prior to his diagnosis of blast crisis.

Seventeen months after the initial CML diagnosis, routine laboratory evaluation revealed pancytopenia with circulating immature myeloid cells (Table 1). Clinically, the patient was asymptomatic without splenomegaly or evidence of bleeding. Peripheral blood smear review demonstrated 44% immature cells with rare Auer rods, concerning promyelocytic blast crisis. Coagulation studies showed no definitive evidence of disseminated intravascular coagulation.

Flow cytometric analysis of peripheral blood demonstrated an immature myeloid population comprising 42% of all cells with expression of CD13, CD33, CD64, CD4, CD117 (dim), CD38, CD45, and cytoplasmic MPO and without expression of CD34, HLA-DR, or CD11c. The bone marrow revealed a mildly hypercellular marrow largely replaced by promyelocytes (67% by manual aspirate differential count; Figure 1). Morphologically, the promyelocytes had a classic appearance with "sliding-plate" nuclei, course cytoplasmic granules, occasional nucleoli, and Auer rods.

Routine cytogenetic analysis demonstrated an abnormal cell line containing *t*(9;22)(q34;q11.2) with a simultaneous *t*(15;17)(q22;q21) translocation involving 18 of 20 metaphases examined (Figure 2); the two remaining cells showed a normal male karyotype. FISH was positive for the *BCR-ABL1* and *PML-RARA* fusions in 41% and 47% of interphase nuclei, respectively. Quantitative RT-PCR performed on peripheral blood revealed a p210 *BCR-ABL1* IS% of 49.667% (Table 2). Quantitative RT-PCR for the common breakpoints associated with the *PML-RARA* fusion including bcr1 (long form) and bcr3 (short form) was positive for bcr3 (short form) with a fusion to control ratio of 0.2029 in peripheral blood and 0.2909 in bone marrow; bcr1 was negative in both.

With the aggregate evaluation, a diagnosis of chronic myeloid leukemia in promyelocytic blast phase was rendered. Induction treatment with all-*trans* retinoic acid (ATRA) and arsenic trioxide (ATO) was initiated using the regimen developed by Lo-Coco et al. with arsenic trioxide 0.15 mg/kg intravenously daily and all-*trans* retinoic acid 45 mg per square meter divided into twice daily oral doses [8]; treatment was continued until blood count recovery (42 days). Dasatinib was restarted on day 4 of induction therapy after tolerance, and a stable QTc was confirmed. Dasatinib was held on days 14–16 for pulmonary edema but restarted with aggressive fluid management; it was discontinued prior to discharge on day 42 when repeat imaging showed pulmonary edema, bilateral pleural effusions, and a moderate pericardial effusion. Two weeks after discharge, he was started on nilotinib 300 mg daily, followed in another two weeks by initiation of outpatient consolidation therapy with ATRA 14 days on and 14 days off for seven cycles plus ATO 5 days per week for 4 weeks on and 4 weeks off for four cycles (same doses as induction [8]). The ATRA dose was decreased to 50% beginning with cycle 2 for headaches. Nilotinib was increased to 300 mg twice daily after completion of ATRA and ATO consolidation but was reduced two weeks later after the patient developed rash and dizziness. He is currently on a dose of 150 mg in the morning and 300 mg in the evening. The side effects observed are commonly noted with the individual agents and do not suggest increased toxicities with the combination of a TKI with ATRA and ATO. Fluid retention including pleural and pericardial effusions is well described with dasatinib, and headaches are a common toxicity of ATRA, frequently requiring dose reduction and even discontinuation. His QTc remained stable throughout induction and consolidation therapy.

The patient had a complete morphologic and molecular remission of the promyelocytic blast crisis in less than three months, and RT-PCR for *PML-RARA* transcripts remains undetectable 26 months after diagnosis. With respect to the p210 *BCR-ABL1* transcripts, the patient reached a major molecular response 7 months after diagnosis of blast crisis but has not achieved a complete molecular response to date.

Since we had been following the patient over time for the p210 *BCR-ABL1* fusion transcript by PCR, we had the unique opportunity to retrospectively evaluate the nucleic acids from peripheral blood samples for the *PML-RARA* fusion product. Analysis of multiple samples demonstrated that the *PML-RARA* bcr3 fusion product was first detectable 8 months prior to the onset of promyelocytic blast crisis (Table 2; Figure 3). The *PML-RARA* transcript level remained at a relatively stable low level for several months leading up to blast crisis diagnosis. Of note, the p210 *BCR-ABL1* transcript trend paralleled the *PML-RARA* transcripts in the progression to blast phase.

3. Discussion

Therapies that target the *BCR-ABL1* fusion tyrosine kinase have dramatically improved survival in CML; however,

TABLE 1: Peripheral blood, bone marrow, and conventional cytogenetic findings over time.

Time relative to CML diagnosis	Peripheral blood				Bone marrow		Conventional cytogenetics
	WBC ($\times10^3/\mu$L)	Hemoglobin (g/dL)	Platelets ($\times10^3/\mu$L)	Promyelocytes (%)	Cellularity	Promyelocytes (%)	
−7 years	7.2	14.9	200	0	Normocellular	<1	46, *XY* [20]
0	44	14.8	225	0	>95%	1	46, *XY*, *t*(9;22)(q34; q11.2) [20]
10 months	3	13.2	106	0	N/A*	1	46, *XY*, *t*(9;22)(q34; q11.2) [1]/46, XY [19]
17 months	2	12.8	56	44	70%	67	46, *XY*, *t*(9;22)(q34; q11.2), *t*(15;17)(q22; q21) [18]/46, *XY* [2]

*The trephine biopsy was suboptimal and unable to be accessed for cellularity. Reference ranges: WBC 4.8–10.8 × $10^3/\mu$L, hemoglobin 14.0–18.0 g/dL, platelets 160–360 × $10^3/\mu$L. CML, chronic myeloid leukemia; WBC, white blood count; N/A, not applicable.

TABLE 2: Quantitative RT-PCR analysis of fusion transcripts in peripheral blood over time.

Months after CML diagnosis	p210 *BCR-ABL1* (IS%)	*PML-RARA* (bcr3 F/C ratio)	WBC ($\times10^3/\mu$L)
0	93.869	0	44
1	49.315	ND	3.7
2	15.427	ND	2.6
3	1.085	ND	1.9
5	2.678	ND	2.3
6	1.594	ND	2.6
8	0.691	0	3.7
9	0.567	0.0003	3.2
12	0.879	0.0057	2.3
14	1.174	0.0031	2.7
17*	45.328	0.2029	1.7
19	0.107	0	2.5
21	0.138	0	3.8
24	0.070	0	2.9
27	0.074	0	3.5
30	0.104	0	4.1
33	0.045	0	4.2
36	0.081	0	4.8

*Blast crisis diagnosis. CML, chronic myeloid leukemia; IS%, international scale percent ratio; F/C, fusion to control; WBC, white blood count; ND, not done.

transformation to blast crisis remains a significant cause of mortality. Though fewer patients now develop blast crisis, the prognosis after blast transformation is still poor, with death generally 7–11 months after diagnosis with TKI therapy as compared to 3-4 months in the pre-TKI era [4, 6]. Herein, we describe an unusual variant of blast crisis in which the *PML-RARA* fusion characteristic of acute promyelocytic leukemia (APL) is acquired during progression of the disease and summarize a review of 21 cases of promyelocytic blast crisis of CML in the literature [9–28].

Promyelocytic blast crisis is molecularly analogous to de novo APL, which requires demonstration of the *PML-RARA* fusion by routine cytogenetics, fluorescence in situ hybridization, and/or molecular testing [29]. In our review of the literature, evidence of the *t*(15;17) translocation or *PML-RARA* fusion was provided in 16 of the 21 cases of promyelocytic blast crisis (Table 3). Two additional cases had aberrations in chromosome 17 including an iso(17q) and +17, with a normal chromosome 15 [22, 28]; FISH testing was not performed in either of these cases. Reports of cryptic translocations have been seen in APL cases with iso(17q) [30], raising the possibility that an undetected cryptic translocation may have been present in the case with iso(17q). Additionally, rare APL cryptic translocations have been documented that are negative by karyotype and FISH. In such cases, evidence of the *PML-RARA* fusion is only detectable by PCR and sequence analysis [31]. Other variant translocations including RARβ are difficult to detect by routine karyotype [32]. Although uncommon, APL cases without *t*(15;17) may have complex translocations involving chromosomes 15 and 17 and a nontraditional chromosome partner, resulting in a submicroscopic insertion of *RARA* into *PML* [30]. In 3 of the reviewed cases, the promyelocytic blast crisis diagnosis was based on morphologic, immunophenotypic, and/or flow cytometric findings alone; no disease-defining cytogenetic or molecular results were reported [20, 21, 24]. For the purpose of this review, all cases were considered promyelocytic blast crisis of CML, even in the absence of defining reported cytogenetic/molecular evidence.

Review of the 21 promyelocytic blast crisis cases documented in the literature reveals a male predominance, with a

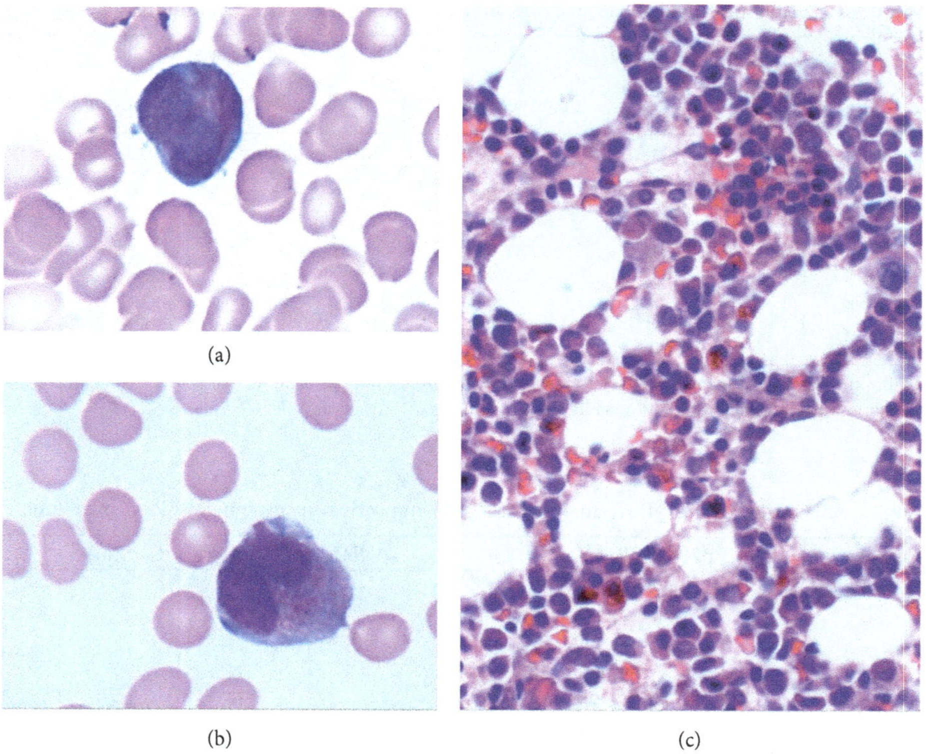

FIGURE 1: Bone marrow at diagnosis of promyelocytic blast crisis. Promyelocytes with multiple Auer rods (a) and sliding plate nuclear morphology (b) in bone marrow aspirate smears. The bone marrow clot section demonstrates a mildly hypercellular bone marrow with increased promyelocytes (c).

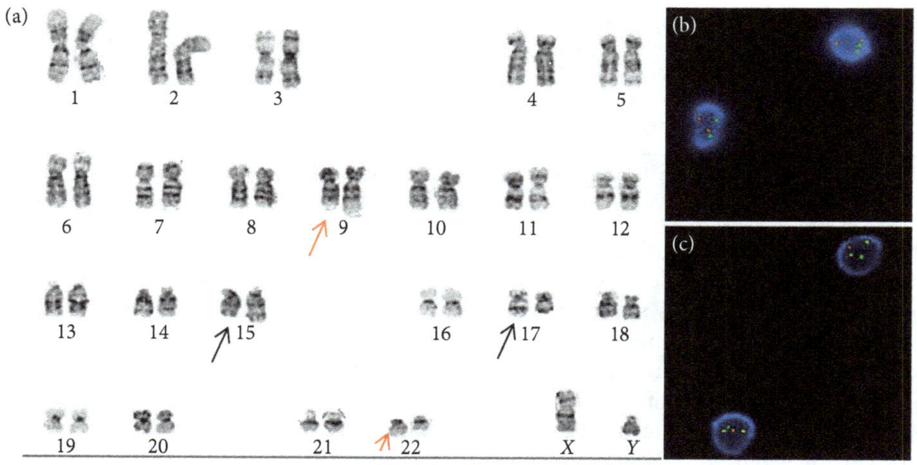

FIGURE 2: Cytogenetic findings at the time of promyelocytic blast crisis. (a) Conventional karyotype demonstrating *t*(15;17) (black arrows) and *t*(9;22) (red arrows) translocations. (b) FISH probes positive for the *PML-RARA* fusion. (c) FISH probes positive for the *BCR-ABL1* fusion (dual-color, dual-fusion probes).

male-to-female ratio of 3.2 : 1. This finding is keeping with male predominance in CML [29]. In addition, men developed blast crisis at an earlier average age (38 years ± 17) as compared to women (64 years ± 22 years) (two-tailed p value of 0.0127). The interval of time between initial CML diagnosis and promyelocytic blast crisis was less than 1 year in 33% of cases, including two patients who presented with promyelocytic blast crisis at CML diagnosis, 1–5 years in 52% of cases, and greater than 5 years in 14% of cases (average 30 months). This interval of time to promyelocytic blast crisis is similar to the reported time of development of nonpromyelocytic blast crisis (3 years) [4].

Many of the CML promyelocytic blast crisis reports in the literature were published prior to the discovery of TKIs, and accordingly, only 5 of the 19 patients who carried a diagnosis of CML at the time of blast phase were receiving

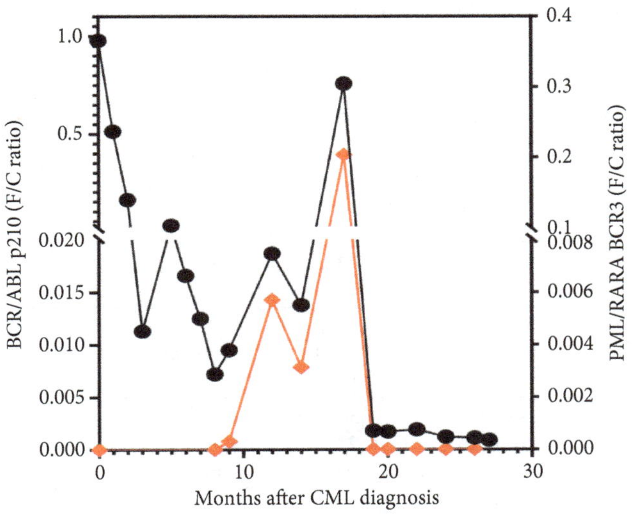

FIGURE 3: *BCR-ABL1* and *PML-RARA* fusion products over time. CML, chronic myeloid leukemia; F/C, fusion to control ratio.

TKI therapy and only one patient was on second-generation TKI therapy. Interestingly, there was no significant difference in time from initial CML diagnosis to promyelocytic blast crisis in patients with and without TKI therapy in this cohort, and the interval ranged from 4 months to 7 years for patients receiving TKI therapy as compared to 10 months to 8 years for patients who were not on TKI therapy (two-tailed p value of 0.4964). The data in this cohort suggest that TKI therapy does not prolong the time before progression to promyelocytic blast crisis.

Survival data and/or response to treatment were provided in 16 of the 21 cases. Nine patients died during or within 3 months of the promyelocytic blast crisis diagnosis. Death in these nine patients was primarily due to infection or bleeding events. Survival of patients with promyelocytic blast crisis overall was poor, with only 4 cases resulting in full remission. Such poor outcomes are in contrast to de novo APL in which 90% of patients with the traditional *t*(15;17) are alive and disease-free after 5 years [33]. In our literature review, the treatment regimen was provided for 7 of the 9 patients with survival ≤3 months, and only one patient received APL-specific therapy (e.g., ATRA and ATO). In contrast, 3 of 4 of the patients with complete remission were treated with ATRA; the remaining patient had no documentation of the characteristic *t*(15;17) or *PML-RARA* transcripts [24]. Overall, the data suggest that APL-specific treatment is most successful in achieving remission of promyelocytic blast crisis with documented characteristic cytogenetic/molecular changes.

Herein, we present a unique evaluation of the clonal development of promyelocytic blast crisis in a patient with CML on TKI therapy. At 9 months after initial diagnosis of chronic phase CML, the appearance of low-level *PML-RARA* transcripts was identified by RT-PCR. *PML-RARA* transcripts remained at a stable low level for several months before showing a dramatic increase 8 months after initial detection. In conjunction with this elevation in transcript levels, a marked increase in promyelocytes was appreciated by peripheral blood and bone marrow morphologic evaluation. These findings were consistent with overt promyelocytic blast crisis occurring 17 months after the initial CML diagnosis. With standard APL treatment and continued TKI therapy, the patient has achieved complete molecular remission of the promyelocytic blast crisis. To our knowledge, this is the first report demonstrating the time course of molecular acquisition of *PML-RARA* during chronic phase CML and progression to blast crisis.

Also, of note, is our patient's history of treated classic Hodgkin lymphoma approximately 7 years prior to the diagnosis of CML. This raises the possibility that the CML may be a therapy-related myeloid neoplasm. Although there is an unusual manifestation of a therapy-related myeloid neoplasm, documented cases are present in the literature [34–36]. No additional cytogenetic changes were present at the time of CML chronic phase diagnosis or blast phase to give additional insight into this possibility.

Although therapy-related CML is rare, therapy-related APL (t-APL) is well documented and is most commonly associated with DNA topoisomerase II inhibitor administration [37, 38]. *In vitro* studies have elucidated the mechanism as chemotherapeutic drug-induced DNA topoisomerase II cleavage of double-stranded DNA at the *PML* and *RARA* breakpoint hotspots seen in APL [39]. In our patient, the history of doxorubicin administration for classic Hodgkin lymphoma raises the possibility of a therapy-related *PML-RARA* translocation. In a systemic review, the peak incidence of t-APL following completion of DNA topoisomerase II inhibitor treatment was 2 years, with 95% of cases occurring within 8 years [37]. Our patient presented with promyelocytic blast crisis approximately 8.6 years after completion of ABVD therapy for classic Hodgkin lymphoma. Although this is a long interval, a therapy-related process cannot be excluded. Interestingly, more than one-third of cases in this systematic review were incidentally found on laboratory testing during routine clinical follow-up [37], analogous to our patient. Treatment and outcomes in t-APL are similar to de novo APL [37, 40].

In summary, promyelocytic blast crisis in CML is rare, occurring more commonly in younger males with relatively few cases documented in the literature. Analogous to de novo APL, the *t*(15;17) translocation leads to the aberrant *PML-RARA* fusion protein, and treatment with standard APL regimens provides better outcome in these patients. While the power of this study is limited due to the relatively few published cases available, no previous comprehensive reviews have been published on this subject. Additional studies on these rare cases to further investigate the pathophysiologic mechanisms behind the development of promyelocytic clones, as well as the nidus for the evolution of blast crisis, are warranted. Quantitative RT-PCR has become a routine, highly sensitive tool used not only in the initial diagnosis of APL and CML but also in monitoring patients for treatment response. Since many of these patients are followed by routine *BCR-ABL1* PCR studies for months or years before progression to promyelocytic blast crisis, preserved extracted nucleic acids leading up to the blast crisis are often available, providing a unique opportunity to evaluate clonal development and progression.

Table 3: Summary of 21 reported cases of promyelocytic blast crisis in CML.

Sex	Age (years)	Treatment during CML chronic phase	Interval between CML diagnosis and blast crisis	Treatment during promyelocytic blast phase	Conventional cytogenetic results	Survival (after blast crisis onset)/outcome	Reference
F	82	Imatinib	2 years	ND	ND‡	ND	[9]
M	22	N/A	Concurrent	ATRA, chemotherapy, allogeneic SCT	46, *XY*, *t*(9;22)(q34; q11) [5], 47, *XY*, *t*(9;22), +8, *t*(15;17)(q22;q11-21) [4]‡	118 days after allogeneic SCT	[10]
M	31	Cytosine arabinoside, 6-thioguanine#	27 months	ND	46, *XY*, *t*(9;22) [40%], 46, *XY*, *t*(9;22), *t*(15;17)(q15;q21) [60%]	3 months	[11]
F	69	Imatinib	13 months	ATRA, idarubicin, Ara-C, imatinib, ATO	46, *XX*, *t*(9;22)(q34; q11.2), *t*(15;17)(q22; q12) [19], 46, *XX* [1]$‡	Complete molecular response	[12]
F	85	None#	10 months	None	46, *XX*, *t*(9;22), *t*(15;17)(q22;q21) [100%]	2 days	[13]
M	78	Imatinib, dasatinib	7 years	ATRA, ATO	46, *XY*, *t*(9;22)(q34; q11.2), *t*(15;17)(q24; q21) [100%]$‡	2 months	[14]
M	32	Imatinib	6 months	ATRA, imatinib	46, *XY*, *t*(9;22)(q34; q11), *t*(15;?;17)(q22;?;q21) [100%]$‡	Complete remission	[15]
M	37	Misulban#	10 months	Daunorubicin, cytosine arabinoside	46,(9;22), *t*(15;17) [26], 46, *t*(9;22) [5]*	ND	[16]
F	52	Hydroxyurea#	3 years	Mitoxantrone, etoposide	*t*(9;22)(q34;q11.2), *t*(15;17)(q24;q11.2–12) [9]*	6 weeks	[17]
M	55	Hydroxyurea#	2 years	ATRA, mitoxantrone, cytosine arabinoside, etoposide	*t*(9;22)(q34;q11.2), *t*(15;17)(q22;q11.2–12) [2]*	ND	[17]
M	60	ND#	3 years	Cytarabine, mitoxantrone, etoposide, idarubicine, 6-thioguanine	46, *XY*, *t*(9;22)(q34; q11)[40%], 46, *XY*, *t*(9;22)(q34;q11), *t*(15;17)(q22;q21) [60%]$	3 weeks	[18]
M	50	ND#	3 years	ND	46, *XY*, *t*(9;12;22)(q34;q22;q11) [43.8%], 46, *XY*, *t*(9;12;22)(q34; q22;q11), *t*(15;17)(q22; q12–21) [56.2%]	ND	[19]
M	30	Busulfan#	10 months	N^4-Behenoyl-1-β-D-arabinofuranosyl-cytosine, daunorubicin, 6-mercaptopurine, prednisone	46, *XY*, *t*(9;22)(q34; q11) [25%], 46, *XY*, *t*(9;22)(q34;q11), *t*(3; 21)(q12;q22) [75%]◊	5 months	[20]
F	32	Busulfan#	8 years	Doxorubicin	74, *XX*, *t*(9;22), *t*(9;22)($3n\pm$)◊	1 month	[21]
M	3	Busulfan, alpha-2a interferon, hydroxyurea, cytarabine#	3.5 years	"Chemotherapy"	Hypodiploidy, *t*(9;22), iso(17q)*◊	2 months	[22]
M	38	ND#	25 months	Aziridinyl-benzoquinone	46, *XY*, *t*(9;22)(q34; q11) [4], 46, *XY*, *t*(15;17), *t*(9;22) [4], 45, *X*, -*Y*, *t*(15;17), *t*(9;22) [2]	1 month	[23]

Table 3: Continued.

Sex	Age (years)	Treatment during CML chronic phase	Interval between CML diagnosis and blast crisis	Treatment during promyelocytic blast phase	Conventional cytogenetic results	Survival (after blast crisis onset)/outcome	Reference
M	26	N/A	Concurrent	Cytarabine, arabinoside, daunorubicin, dasatinib, allogeneic SCT	*t*(9;22)*†	Complete molecular remission	[24]
M	31	Hydroxy-carbamide, imatinib	4 months	ATRA, ATO, dasatinib, idarubicin, cytarabine, allogeneic SCT	ND$‡	Complete molecular remission	[25]
M	27	Natural interferon-*α*	4 years	ND	51, *XY*, +der(1) *t*(1;17)(p11;q11), +7, +8, +8, *t*(9;22)(q34; q11), 22q-‡	ND	[26]
M	38	Allopurinol, busulfan	25 months	ND	46, *XY*, *t*(9;22)(q34: q11) [4], 46, *XY*, *t*(15;17)(q22;q12?), *t*(9;22) (q34;q11) [6]	47 days	[27]
M	48	ND#	6 years	ATRA	46, *XY* [6]/48, *XY*, +17, +der(1)*t*(1;?)(p13;?), *t*(9;22)(q34;q11) [14]◊	>87 days	[28]

*Full karyotype information not provided. #Publication date prior to 2001. †FISH studies negative for *PML-RARA* fusion. $FISH studies positive for *PML-RARA* fusion. ◊FISH and RT-PCR testing not performed. ‡RT-PCR positive for *PML/RARA* fusion. ND, no data provided; N/A, not applicable; ATRA, all-trans retinoic acid; ATO, arsenic trioxide; SCT, stem-cell transplantation.

References

[1] B. Chereda and J. V. Melo, "Natural course and biology of CML," *Annals of Hematology*, vol. 94, no. 2, pp. S107–S121, 2015.

[2] D. Perrotti, G. Silvestri, L. Stramucci, J. Yu, and R. Trotta, "Cellular and molecular networks in chronic myeloid leukemia: the leukemic stem, progenitor and stromal cell interplay," *Current Drug Targets*, vol. 18, no. 4, pp. 377–388, 2017.

[3] L. Gorkin and H. Kantarjian, "Generic imatinib—impact on frontline and salvage therapy for CML," *Nature Reviews Clinical Oncology*, vol. 13, no. 5, pp. 270–272, 2016.

[4] Y. Shi, A. J. Rand, J. H. Crow, J. O. Moore, and A. S. Lagoo, "Blast phase in chronic myelogenous leukemia is skewed toward unusual blast types in patients treated with tyrosine kinase inhibitors," *American Journal of Clinical Pathology*, vol. 143, no. 1, pp. 105–119, 2015.

[5] A. Hochhaus, G. Saglio, T. P. Hughes et al., "Long-term benefits and risks of frontline nilotinib vs imatinib for chronic myeloid leukemia in chronic phase: 5-year update of the randomized ENESTnd trial," *Leukemia*, vol. 30, no. 5, pp. 1044–1054, 2016.

[6] P. Jain, H. M. Kantarjian, A. Ghorab et al., "Prognostic factors and survival outcomes in patients with chronic myeloid leukemia in blast phase in the tyrosine kinase inhibitor era: cohort study of 477 patients," *Cancer*, vol. 123, no. 22, pp. 4391–4402, 2017.

[7] A. Hochhaus, M. Baccarani, R. T. Silver et al., "European leukemianet 2020 recommendations for treating chronic myeloid leukemia," *Leukemia*, vol. 34, no. 4, pp. 966–984, 2020.

[8] F. Lo-Coco, G. Avvisati, M. Vignetti et al., "Retinoic acid and arsenic trioxide for acute promyelocytic leukemia," *New England Journal of Medicine*, vol. 369, no. 2, pp. 111–121, 2013.

[9] F. Angriman, M. N. G. Acevedo, M. S. Rossi et al., "Promyelocytic blastic crisis in chronic myeloid leukemia during imatinib treatment," *Turkish Journal of Hematology*, vol. 32, no. 2, pp. 193-194, 2015.

[10] K. Matsue, K. Yamada, M. Takeuchi, and T. Tabayashi, "Rapid improvement of disseminated intravascular coagulation by donor leukocyte infusions in a patient with promyelocytic crisis of chronic myelogenous leukemia after reduced-intensity stem cell transplantation from an HLA 2-antigen-mismatched mother," *International Journal of Hematology*, vol. 77, no. 4, pp. 408–411, 2003.

[11] A. C. Louwagie, C. Mecucci, A. Criel, A. Van Hoof, and H. Van Den Berghe, "Variant translocation *t*(15q; 17q) accompanying a promyelocytic accelerated phase of Ph-positive chronic myeloid leukemia," *Cancer Genetics and Cytogenetics*, vol. 28, no. 2, pp. 349–352, 1987.

[12] M. Kashimura and K. Ohyashiki, "Successful imatinib and arsenic trioxide combination therapy for sudden onset promyelocytic crisis with *t*(15; 17) in chronic myeloid leukemia," *Leukemia Research*, vol. 34, no. 8, pp. e213–e214, 2010.

[13] J.-L. Laï, P. Fenaux, M. Zandecki et al., "Promyelocytic blast crisis of Philadelphia-positive thrombocythemia with translocations (9; 22) and (15; 17)," *Cancer Genetics and Cytogenetics*, vol. 29, no. 2, pp. 311–314, 1987.

[14] T. A. Colvin, P. Vachhani, S. Sait, V. Neppalli, and E. S. Wang, "All-trans-retinoic-acid and arsenic trioxide induced remission in promyelocytic blast crisis," *Leukemia Research Reports*, vol. 10, pp. 16–19, 2018.

[15] H. J. Chung, H. S. Chi, Y. U. Cho et al., "Promyelocytic blast crisis of chronic myeloid leukemia during imatinib treatment," *Annals of Clinical and Laboratory Science*, vol. 38, no. 3, pp. 283–286, 2008.

[16] R. Berger, A. Bernheim, M.-T. Daniel, and G. Flandrin, "*t*(15; 17) in a promyelocytic form of chronic myeloid leukemia

blastic crisis," *Cancer Genetics and Cytogenetics*, vol. 8, no. 2, pp. 149–152, 1983.
[17] N. S. Rosenthal, D. Knapp, and D. C. Farhi, "Promyelocytic blast crisis of chronic myelogenous leukemia: a rare subtype Associated with disseminated intravascular coagulation," *American Journal of Clinical Pathology*, vol. 103, no. 2, pp. 185–188, 1995.
[18] M. P. Scolnik, M. F. Palacios, S. H. Acevedo et al., "Promyelocytic blast crisis of chronic myelogenous leukaemia with translocations (9; 22) and (15; 17)," *Leukemia & Lymphoma*, vol. 31, no. 1-2, pp. 231–236, 1998.
[19] P. R. Kadam, A. A. Merchant, and S. H. Advani, "Cytogenetic findings in patients with acute promyelocytic leukemia and a case of CML blast crisis with promyelocytic proliferation," *Cancer Genetics and Cytogenetics*, vol. 50, no. 1, pp. 109–117, 1990.
[20] R. Abe, T. Shichishima, M. Kawaguchi, T. Uchida, and S. Kariyone, "Promyelocytic crisis of chronic myelogenous leukemia without *t*(15; 17)," *Cancer Genetics and Cytogenetics*, vol. 21, no. 2, pp. 175–179, 1986.
[21] A. Mijovic, Z. Rolovic, A. Novak, L. Biljanovic-Paunovic, and D. Tomin, "Chronic myeloid leukemia associated with pure red cell aplasia and terminating in promyelocytic transformation," *American Journal of Hematology*, vol. 31, no. 2, pp. 128–130, 1989.
[22] H. Ören, Ö. Düzovalı, E. Yüksel, M. Sakızlı, and G. I·rken, "Development of acute promyelocytic leukemia with isochromosome 17q after BCR/ABL positive chronic myeloid leukemia," *Cancer Genetics and Cytogenetics*, vol. 109, no. 2, pp. 141–143, 1999.
[23] S. Misawa, E. Lee, C. Schiffer, Z. Liu, and J. Testa, "Association of the translocation (15; 17) with malignant proliferation of promyelocytes in acute leukemia and chronic myelogenous leukemia at blastic crisis," *Blood*, vol. 67, no. 2, pp. 270–274, 1986.
[24] R. K. Bobba and D. C. Doll, "Promyelocytic blast crisis of chronic myelogenous leukemia," *Blood*, vol. 120, no. 19, p. 3873, 2012.
[25] B. Cai, W. Yang, Y. Zhao et al., "Successful management with an effective induction regimen followed by allogeneic hematopoietic stem cell transplantation for promyelocytic blast crisis of chronic myelogenous leukemia," *Annals of Hematology*, vol. 91, no. 4, pp. 621–623, 2012.
[26] M. Amano, A. Togawa, S. Tsurugano et al., "Rearrangement of retinoic acid receptor alpha and PML in promyelocytic blast crisis of Ph1 chromosome positive chronic myelocytic leukemia with normal copies of chromosome 15," *Blood*, vol. 81, no. 9, pp. 2469-2470, 1993.
[27] D. E. Hogge, S. Misawa, C. A. Schiffer, and J. R. Testa, "Promyelocytic blast crisis in chronic granulocytic leukemia with 15; 17 translocation," *Leukemia Research*, vol. 8, no. 6, pp. 1019–1023, 1984.
[28] P. Wiernik, J. Dutcher, E. Paietta et al., "Treatment of promyelocytic blast crisis of chronic myelogenous leukemia with all trans-retinois acid," *Leukemia*, vol. 5, no. 6, pp. 504–509, 1991.
[29] S. H. Swerdlow, E. Campo, N. L. Harris et al., *WHO Classification of Tumours of Haematopoietic and Lymphoid Tissues*, IARC, Lyon, France, 2017.
[30] Y. Tang, Y. Wang, L. Hu et al., "Acute promyelocytic leukemia with cryptic *t*(15; 17) on isochromosome 17: a case report and review of literature," *International Journal of Clinical and Experimental Pathology*, vol. 8, no. 11, pp. 15294–15300, 2015.
[31] M. J. Kim, S. Y. Cho, M.-H. Kim et al., "FISH-negative cryptic PML-RARA rearrangement detected by long-distance polymerase chain reaction and sequencing analyses: a case study and review of the literature," *Cancer Genetics and Cytogenetics*, vol. 203, no. 2, pp. 278–283, 2010.
[32] T. Osumi, S.-I. Tsujimoto, M. Tamura et al., "Recurrent RARB translocations in acute promyelocytic leukemia lacking RARA translocation," *Cancer Research*, vol. 78, no. 16, pp. 4452–4458, 2018.
[33] J. Adams and M. Nassiri, "Acute promyelocytic leukemia: a review and discussion of variant translocations," *Archives of Pathology & Laboratory Medicine*, vol. 139, no. 10, pp. 1308–1313, 2015.
[34] R. C. Aguiar, "Therapy-related chronic myeloid leukemia: an epidemiological, clinical and pathogenetic appraisal," *Leukemia & Lymphoma*, vol. 29, no. 1-2, pp. 17–26, 1998.
[35] N. Iriyama, M. Tokuhira, T. Takaku et al., "Incidences and outcomes of therapy-related chronic myeloid leukemia in the era of tyrosine kinase inhibitors: surveillance of the CML cooperative study group," *Leukemia Research*, vol. 54, pp. 55–58, 2017.
[36] F. Bauduer, L. D. Jensen, N. Dastugue, and J.-P. Marolleau, "Chronic myeloid leukemia as a secondary neoplasm after anti-cancer radiotherapy: a report of three cases and a brief review of the literature," *Leukemia & Lymphoma*, vol. 43, no. 5, pp. 1057–1060, 2002.
[37] A. Rashidi and S. I. Fisher, "Therapy-related acute promyelocytic leukemia: a systematic review," *Medical Oncology*, vol. 30, pp. 625–634, 2013.
[38] F. Lo-Coco, S. K. Hasan, P. Montesinos, and M. A. Sanz, "Biology and management of therapy-related acute promyelocytic leukemia," *Current Opinion in Oncology*, vol. 25, no. 6, pp. 695–700, 2013.
[39] A. R. Mistry, C. A. Felix, R. J. Whitmarsh et al., "DNA topoisomerase II in therapy-related acute promyelocytic leukemia," *New England Journal of Medicine*, vol. 352, no. 15, pp. 1529–1538, 2005.
[40] S. Kayser, J. Krzykalla, M. A. Elliott et al., "Characteristics and outcome of patients with therapy-related acute promyelocytic leukemia front-line treated with or without arsenic trioxide," *Leukemia*, vol. 31, no. 11, pp. 2347–2354, 2017.

23

T-Cell Large Granular Lymphocytic Leukemia with Extremely Rare Immunophenotype (CD4/CD8 Double-Positive) Followed by Multiple Myeloma Diagnosis

Dina Soliman,[1,2,3] Sherin Sallam,[2] Susanna Akiki,[1,2] Deena Mudawi,[4] and Feryal Ibrahim[1]

[1]*Department of Laboratory Medicine and Pathology, National Center for Cancer Care and Research, Hamad Medical Corporation, Doha, Qatar*
[2]*Weill Cornell Medicine, Doha, Qatar*
[3]*Department of Clinical Pathology, National Cancer Institute, Cairo University, Cairo, Egypt*
[4]*Department of Hematology and Medical Oncology, National Center for Cancer Care and Research, Hamad Medical Corporation, Doha, Qatar*

Correspondence should be addressed to Dina Soliman; dsoliman@hamad.qa

Academic Editor: Gergely Feher

T-cell large granular lymphocytic leukemia is characterized by clonal expansion of a $CD3^+/CD57^+$ subpopulation, which are typically $CD8^+$ positive cytotoxic T- cells, and can only be diagnosed if there is a persistent, greater than 6 months, elevation of LGL in the blood (usually $2–20 \times 10^9$/L), in the absence of an identifiable cause. T-LGLL has been associated with reactive conditions such as autoimmune diseases and viral infections and has also been reported in association with hematologic and non-hematologic malignancies. We report a case of asymptomatic CD4/CD8 double-positive T-LGLL. Flow cytometry on peripheral blood revealed a subpopulation of CD4/CD8 double-positive T cells expressing CD57 and cTIA. Clonality was established by flow cytometric analysis of T-cell receptor *V(â)* region repertoire which showed that >70% of the cells failed to express any of the tested *V(â)* regions. Clonality was further confirmed by PCR with the detection of clonal TCR beta and TCR gamma gene rearrangements. Six months later, she presented with persistent lower back pain and diagnosed with IgG kappa multiple myeloma. CD4/CD8 double-positive T-large granular leukemia is the first case reported in the literature. This rare phenotype is either underreported or a truly rare clinical entity. More studies are warranted to characterize the pathogenesis and clinical characteristics of this group of patients and to further assess the relationship between multiple myeloma and T-LGLL as a cause-and-effect relationship or simply related to the time at which diagnosis has been made.

1. Case Presentation

A 54-year-old female, with no known chronic illnesses, was referred under the care of the hematology team after the incidental finding of thrombocytopenia and lymphocytosis in her routine laboratory workup. The patient had no abnormal bleeding or ecchymosis. She also denied any fever, weight loss, or skin rash. At that time, her platelet count was 65,000/μL.

Complete blood count (CBC) revealed mild leukocytosis (WBC count of $12,600 \times 10^3$/uL; n:4–10) with absolute lymphocytosis (7.3×10^3/uL) and no neutropenia. Her initial workup showed high total protein at 95 gm/L (66–78), normal albumin at 4.3 g/dL, and normal beta-2-microglobulin (2.09 mg/L) with mildly elevated LDH at 258 U/L (135–214). Her calcium level was normal (2.36 mmol/L), with normal electrolytes and normal liver and kidney function tests.

The peripheral blood (PB) smear showed mild anemia with increased rouleaux formation. There was lymphocytosis composed of small mature-looking lymphocytes mixed with some large granular forms, some of which showed irregular nuclear contours (Figure 1(a)). Lymphocytosis is persistent and slowly progressive for more than 11 months of duration (Figure 1(b)). Flow cytometry done on the PB (Figure 1(c)) showed 37% T cells, including a subpopulation of CD57-positive cells (NK-T cells) comprising approximately 17%. There was a subpopulation of CD4/CD8 double-positive T cells (10%) expressing CD57 and cTIA and showing a dim expression of CD4 and CD7. Flow cytometric analysis of T-cell receptor *V(â)* region repertoire performed on CD4/CD8 double-positive population (on PB) (Figure 1(d)) showed that more than 70% of the cells failed to express any of the tested *V(â)* regions, a finding that is suggestive of T-cell clonality.

Six months after her initial presentation, the patient presented with persistent lower back pain. On physical examination, there was tenderness at the lumbosacral junction with no distal nerve deficit. MRI showed an old fracture of the L1 body and a large Schmorl's node-like lesions within the superior end plates L3 and L4. CT thorax, abdomen, and pelvis showed evidence of an infiltrative bone marrow (BM) disease.

MRI whole spine showed heterogeneous marrow signal pattern of the visualized bones with multiple osseous lesions possibly indicative of an infiltrative myelomatous deposits. FDG PET showed multiple small lytic lesions.

Serum protein electrophoresis was performed as part of the myeloma workup and revealed hypogammaglobulinemia and a monoclonal band typed as IgG kappa 28.8 g/l in size. The kappa : lambda ratio was 43.595 with the kappa free light chains at 352.68 mg/L and the lambda free light chains at 8.09 mg/L. 24-hour urinary protein was negative for Bence Jones protein.

BM examination was performed, and PB showed persistent lymphocytosis with no neutropenia. BM aspirate smear (Figure 2(a)) revealed ~18% myeloma plasma cells with a few atypical binucleate forms and rare immature forms with plasmablastic morphology. BM biopsy was infiltrated by many myeloma plasma cells with kappa light chain restriction. BM involvement by myeloma cells was uneven, roughly estimated by 30–60% of cellularity. Flow cytometry on BM aspirate (Figure 2(b)) showed a population of monotypic plasma cells ~5% expressing CD45, CD38, and CD138 with cytoplasmic kappa light chain restriction and aberrant expression of CD56 and CD117. The plasma cells were negative for CD19 with no significant expression of CD20. LGL included a population of CD4/CD8 double-positive cells (~2% of total cells) showing a dimmer expression of CD4 and CD7 (similar to the population detected earlier on peripheral blood) (Figure 2(b), red arrow). Flow cytometric analysis of T-cell receptor *V(â)* region repertoire on CD4/CD8 double-positive population (on PB) was repeated and showed persistent clonal population.

Cytogenetic analysis revealed a normal karyotype. FISH testing for the following genes was normal: RB1/CEP10: 13q14, TP53/CEP17 : 17p13.1/17p11.1-q11.1, and IGH: 14q32.

This concluded a diagnosis of plasma cell myeloma associated with a persistent increase in clonal large granular lymphocytes (CD4/CD8-positive) indicating T-large granular lymphocytic leukemia (T-LGLL).

T-cell receptor (TCR) gene rearrangement molecular genetics studies were performed and confirmed the presence of clonal TCR beta and TCR gamma gene rearrangements: TCR beta DBJ-C : clonal (175 bp and 305 bp) and TCR gamma VGJ-B : clonal (204 bp).

The patient was started on bortezomib-based therapy regimen, VRd (Velcade® one dose (cycle 1, day 1), lenalidomide 25 mg for 3 days, and dexamethasone pulse for 4 days), followed by stem cell mobilization and high-dose melphalan and autologous stem cell transplantation (tandem).

2. Discussion

This is a rather unusual case of asymptomatic T-LGLL with a unique immunophenotype incidentally discovered upon workup for lymphocytosis, followed by multiple myeloma diagnosed 6 months after T-LGLL diagnosis.

T-cell large granular lymphocytic leukemia is characterized by the clonal expansion of a $CD3^+/CD57^+$ subpopulation, referred to as large granular lymphocytes which are morphologically distinct, larger than small mature lymphocytes with mature nuclear chromatin and moderate-to-abundant cytoplasm and fine or course azurophilic granules. T-LGLL is typically characterized by CD8+ positive cytotoxic T cells and characterized clinically by neutropenia, anemia, and/or thrombocytopenia with modest persistent lymphocytosis [1].

According to the most recent WHO classification of hematologic disorders (2016), T-LGLL can only be diagnosed if there is a persistent, greater than 6 months, elevation of LGL in the blood (usually $2–20 \times 10^9/L$), in the absence of an identifiable cause. It is usually a disorder of mature CD2+, CD3+, CD8+, CD57+, and alpha-beta TCR-positive cytotoxic T cells. CD4+/alpha-beta TCR-positive cases are uncommon variants. Gamma-delta TCR-positive cases, with 60 percent of them expressing CD8 and the remainder being CD4/CD8-negative, are also uncommon variants. T-LGLL that is CD4/CD8 double-positive is not documented [2].

T-LGLL is a relatively rare malignancy and accounts for 2–5% of chronic lymphoproliferative diseases in the US [1]. It appears more frequently in the elderly, with a median age of diagnosis at 60 years and median survival of more than 10 years [3]. It has been hypothesized that T-LGLL arises in a setting of sustained immune stimulation which could explain the frequent association of T-LGLL with autoimmune disorders, including rheumatoid arthritis and inclusion body myositis [4–6].

CD4/CD8 dual-positive T cells are a developmental stage of T-cell maturation/differentiation within the thymus. The interaction of T-cell receptor with antigens bound to major histocompatibility complex (MHC) molecules causes the dual-positive T cell to commit to either CD4 (helper and regulatory) or CD8 (cytotoxic and suppressor). Besides mature single-positive CD4+ or CD8+ lymphocytes, extrathymic CD4+/CD8+ double-positive T cells are present

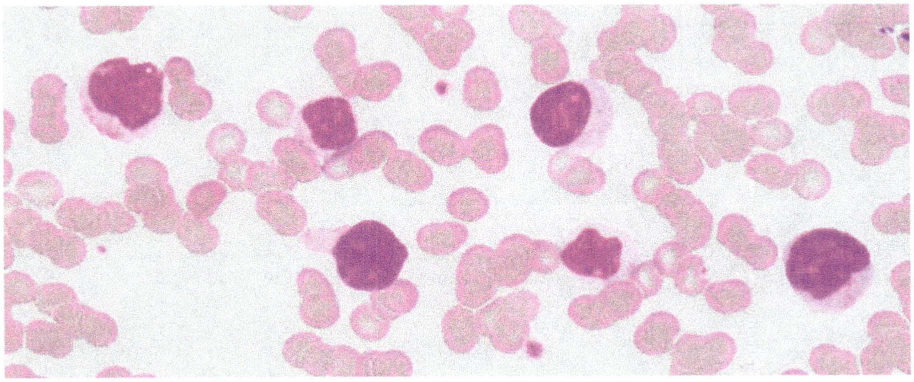

(a)

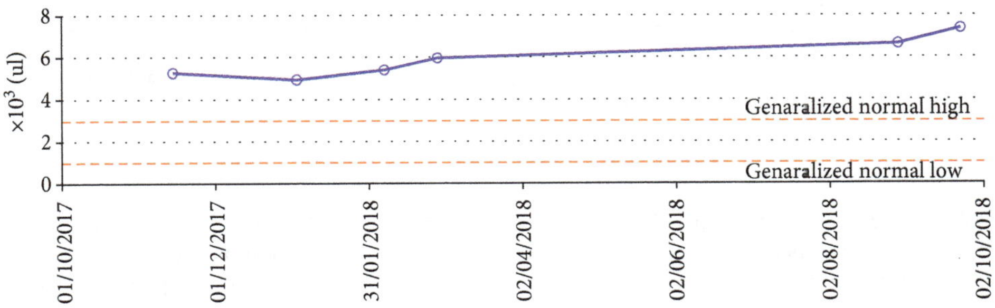

(b)

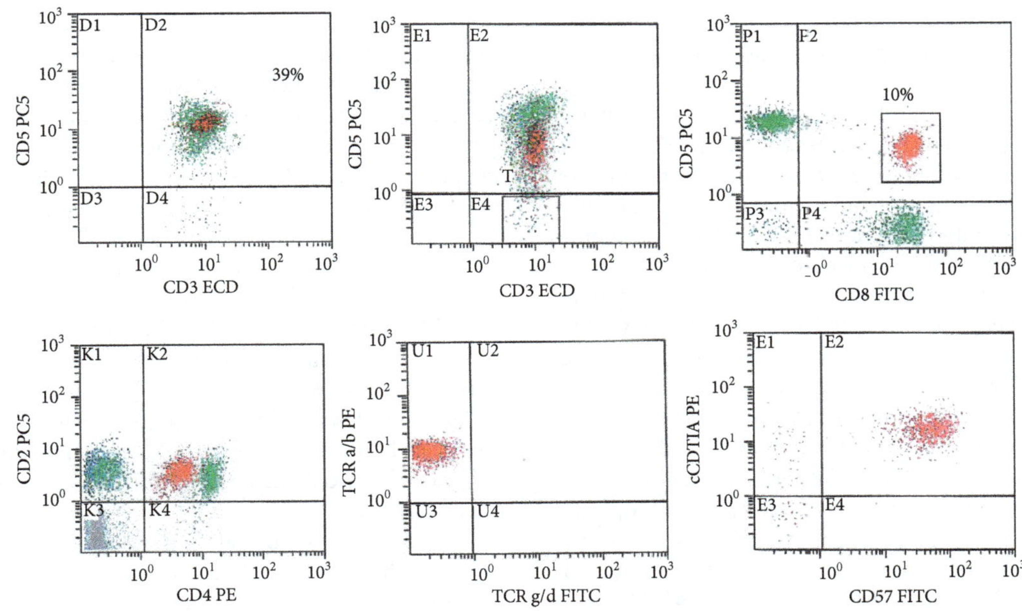

(c)

Figure 1: Continued.

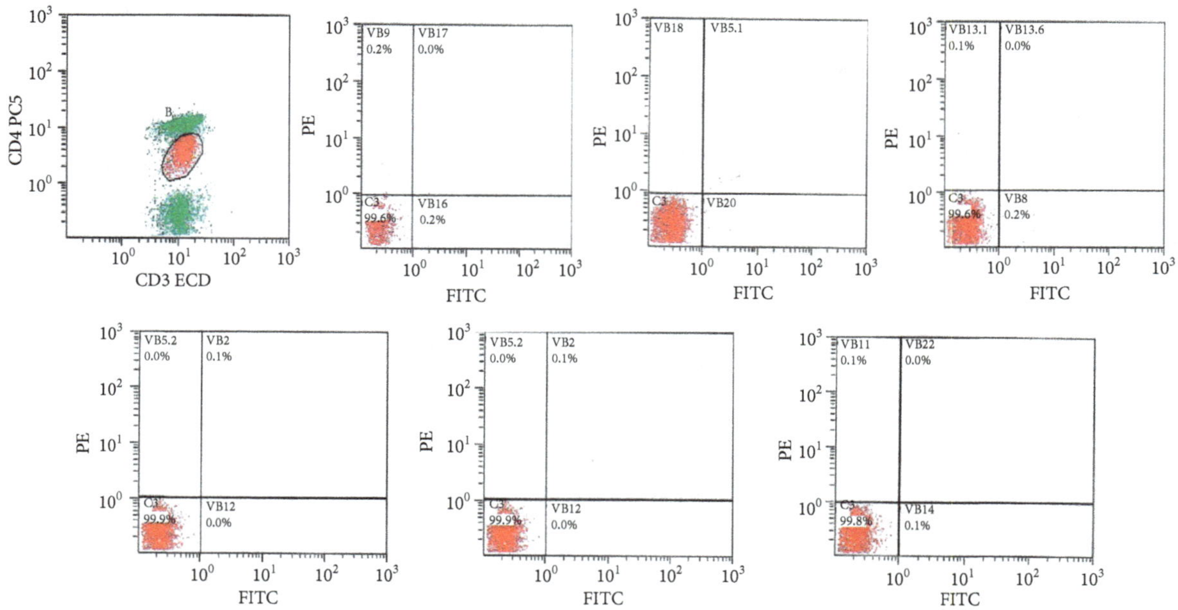

(d)

Figure 1: Peripheral blood smear (Wright's stain, 100x) shows increased large granular lymphocytes, some of which showed irregular nuclear contours (a). Lymphocytosis is persistent and slowly progressive for more than 11 months of duration (b). Flow cytometry done on the PB (c) showing 37% T cells, including a subpopulation of CD4/CD8 double-positive T cells (10%) expressing TCR alpha/beta, CD57, and cTIA, and a showing dim expression of CD4 and CD7. FCM on PB for T-cell receptor $V(\beta)$ region repertoire on CD4/CD8 double-positive population shows more than 70% of the cells fails to express any of the tested $V(\beta)$ regions, suggestive of clonal population of T-LGLL ($CD3^+/CD4^+/CD8^+/CD57^+$) (d).

in a small percentage in the peripheral blood of healthy humans [7].

On the contrary, multiple myeloma (MM) is a different hematologic neoplasm of B-cell lineage, characterized by the clonal proliferation of plasma cells in the bone marrow resulting in accumulation of monoclonal immunoglobulin. It usually presents with hypercalcemia, renal failure, anemia, and bony lesions [8]. There is a well-documented association between T-LGLL leukemia and B-cell neoplasms, in general, and plasma cell neoplasms, in particular. Upon review of the literature, a total of 42 patients with a diagnosis of T-LGLL and a plasma cell neoplasm were found [9–13]. The majority of these cases had a concomitant diagnosis of both T-LGLL and a plasma cell neoplasm or had a plasma cell neoplasm diagnosis followed by T-LGLL. Interestingly, in the largest case series of patients diagnosed with T-LGL and a plasma cell disorder by Sidiqi et al., all reported 22 cases, who had T-LGLs, showed the classic immunophenotype (CD8+ positive cells) [12]. Not a single case of CD4/CD8 dual-positive T-LGLL was reported.

The detection of an expanded population of LGL after MM treatment was previously described. In one study by Hashiguchi et al., a patient with MM received lenalidomide as part of a clinical trial. They noted an expansion in peripheral LGL from 8% prior to initiating lenalidomide to 25–40% after. The study proposed a beneficial immunomodulatory effect of increasing NK/T cells in patients with MM [14]. This is particularly important because MM patients have been shown to demonstrate a deficit in NK/T-cell counts and activity [15]. In one study, none of the 12 patients diagnosed with T-LGLL and MGUS progressed to MM [13]. This has raised the possibility that the T-LGL clonal expansion represents an immune response to MGUS and suggests a potential role in tumor surveillance [16].

In addition to posttreatment proliferation of LGL, there have also been descriptions of proliferation after bone marrow transplant for refractory MM. Wolniak et al. noted the proliferation of LGL after BM transplant in 20 patients with MM and concluded that this proliferation is a reactive response to the autologous BM transplant [17]. Based on the studies by Hashiguchi et al. and Wolniak et al., and the other studies that described the development of MM in the setting of T-cell LGL or vice versa, it is clear that the relationship between the two disorders is complicated and needs further studies [14, 17].

It has been shown that CD4-positive T-LGLL and CD4/CD8 double-negative T-LGLL are rarely reported in the literature [18, 19]. CD4/CD8 double-positive T-LGLL (as the case reported here) is even more rare. On a similar note, Mizuki et al. studied 8 cases of CD4+/CD8+ chronic T-lymphoproliferative disorders and have found that the dual-positive T cells expressed IL-4 mRNA and produced large amounts of IL-4, suggesting that they are derived from peripheral CD4+ cells rather than immature T cells that escaped the thymus. Of note, none of these cases were T-LGLL [20]. On the other hand, for other types of leukemia such as the adult T-cell leukemia/lymphoma associated with HTLV1, the dual-positive phenotype has been extensively

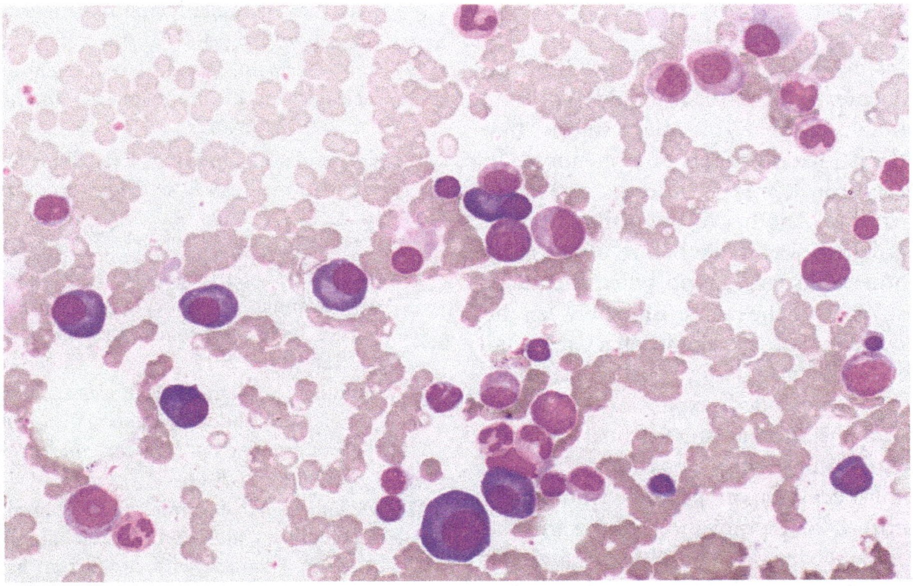

(a)

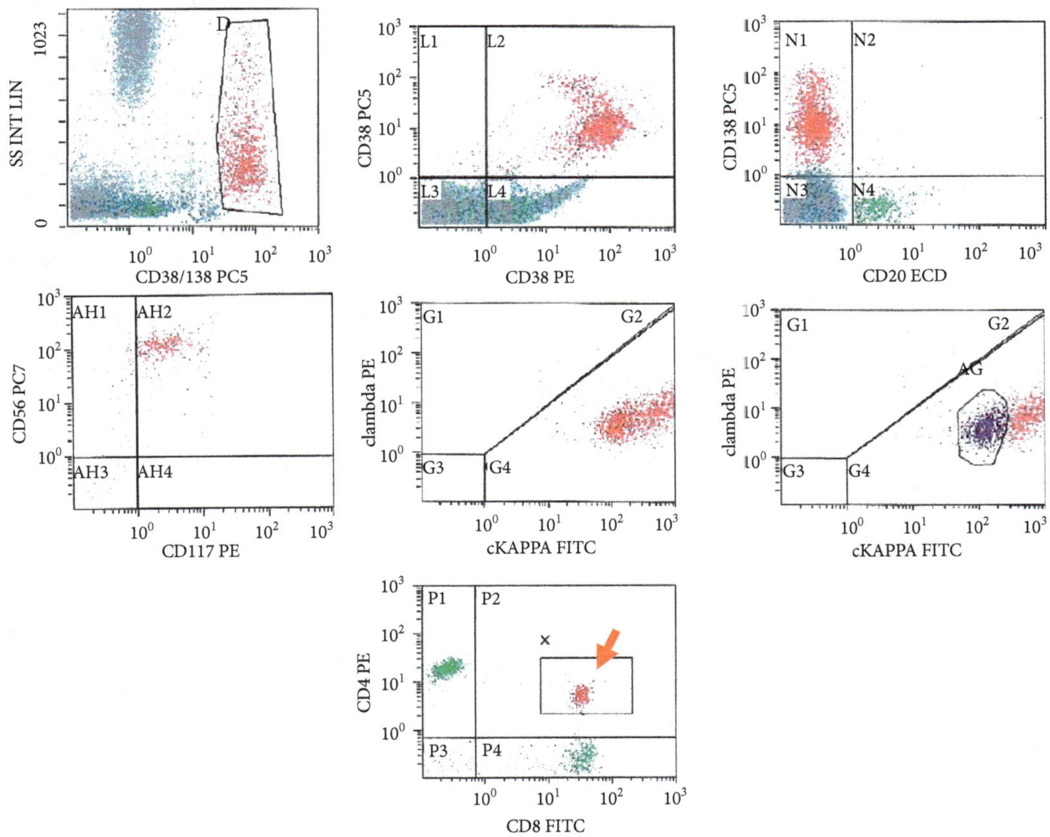

(b)

FIGURE 2: BM aspirate smear (Wright's stain, 100x) revealing ~18% myeloma plasma cells with a few atypical binucleated forms (a). FCM analysis on BM aspirate (b) showing a population of monotypic plasma cells ~5% expressing CD45, CD38, and CD138 with cytoplasmic kappa light chain restriction and aberrant expression of CD56 and CD117. The plasma cells show no significant expression of CD20. LGLs included the same population of CD4/CD8 double-positive cells (~2%) (red arrow) showing a dimmer expression of CD4 and CD7.

described [21–24]. It also seems that the expansion of clonal CD4/CD8 double-positive T-LGL, although fulfilling WHO diagnostic criteria for T-LGLL, has an even more indolent clinical course than the typical CD8+ T-LGL leukemia as our patient's case lacked the typical clinical features such as neutropenia and splenomegaly.

3. Conclusion

To our knowledge, this the first case report of T-LGLL with the extremely rare phenotype (CD4/CD8 double-positive) associated with multiple myeloma. This might suggest that there is either an underestimation of this rare phenotype in large granular lymphocytic leukemia or, indeed, a rare entity that requires further studies. Another distinguishing feature is that the diagnosis of LGL was made before establishing MM, and is again another unusual scenario, when compared with previous reports. Whether the relationship between the two hematologic neoplasms is a cause-and-effect relationship or simply a time to diagnose issue is yet to be investigated. Furthermore, uncontrolled expansion of clonal T cells (LGL) as one of the mechanisms of host immune response to multiple myeloma is also a possibility.

According to published data on patients who had a concomitant PCM and T-LGL, therapy directed towards the T-LGL component was needed in few patients, and the therapy consisted of cyclophosphamide and prednisone with good response and resolution of the cytopenias in most patients.

Consent

Consent was waived from the patients.

Authors' Contributions

First and second authors contributed equally. All coauthors contributed to this case report.

Acknowledgments

This case was encountered at Hamad Medical Corporation.

References

[1] M. V. Shah, C. C. Hook, T. G. Call, and R. S. Go, "A population-based study of large granular lymphocyte leukemia," *Blood Cancer Journal*, vol. 6, no. 8, p. e455, 2016.

[2] S. H. Swerdlow, E. Campo, N. L. Harris et al., "The 2016 revision of the World Health Organization classification of lymphoid neoplasms," *Blood*, vol. 127, no. 20, pp. 2375–2390, 2016.

[3] D. P. O'Malley, "T-cell large granular leukemia and related proliferations," *American Journal of Clinical Pathology* vol. 127, no. 6, pp. 850–859, 2007.

[4] T. Lamy and T. P. Loughran Jr., "How I treat LGL leukemia," *Blood*, vol. 117, no. 10, pp. 2764–2774, 2011.

[5] S. N. Steinway, F. LeBlanc, T. P. Loughran, and Loughran Jr., "The pathogenesis and treatment of large granular lymphocyte leukemia," *Blood Reviews*, vol. 28, no. 3, pp. 87–94, 2014.

[6] S. A. Greenberg, J. L. Pinkus, A. A. Amato, T. Kristensen, and D. M. Dorfman, "Association of inclusion body myositis with T cell large granular lymphocytic leukaemia," *Brain*, vol. 139, no. 5, pp. 1348–1360, 2016.

[7] R. N. Germain, "T-cell development and the CD4-CD8 lineage decision," *Nature Reviews Immunology*, vol. 2, no. 5, pp. 309–322, 2002.

[8] S. V. Rajkumar and R. A. Kyle, "Multiple myeloma: diagnosis and treatment," *Mayo Clinic Proceedings*, vol. 80, no. 10, pp. 1371–1382, 2005.

[9] N. A. Carreau, J. Y. Lee, B. Petersen, L. Silverman, and A. Chari, "Dual diagnosis of multiple myeloma and T-cell large granular lymphocytic leukemia: a case report and literature review," *Annals of Hematology & Oncology*, vol. 2, no. 9, p. 1062, 2015.

[10] J. Cheng, G. Talamo, J. Malysz et al., "Report of 6 cases of large granular lymphocytic leukemia and plasma cell dyscrasia," *Clinical Lymphoma Myeloma and Leukemia*, vol. 14, no. 5, pp. e169–e172, 2014.

[11] X. Xu, E. H. Broome, H. H. Rashidi, T. Sarah et al., "CD20dim-positive T-cell large granular lymphocytic leukemia in a patient with concurrent hairy cell leukemia and plasma cell myeloma," *International Journal of Clinical and Experimental Pathology*, vol. 3, no. 8, p. 798, 2010.

[12] M. H. Sidiqi, M. A. Aljama, D. S. Viswanatha, and D. Dingli, "T-cell large granular lymphocytic leukemia and plasma cell disorders," *Haematologica*, vol. 104, no. 3, pp. e108–e110, 2019.

[13] A. D. Viny, A. Lichtin, B. Pohlman, T. Loughran, and J. Maciejewski, "Chronic B-cell dyscrasias are an important clinical feature of T-LGL leukemia," *Leukemia & Lymphoma*, vol. 49, no. 5, pp. 932–938, 2008.

[14] M. Hashiguchi, T. Okamura, K. Nomura et al., "A case of refractory multiple myeloma with proliferation of large granular lymphocytes by lenalidomide treatment and its association with clinical efficacy," *Molecular and Clinical Oncology*, vol. 4, no. 4, pp. 574–578, 2016.

[15] A. C. Chan, P. Neeson, E. Leeansyah et al., "Natural killer T cell defects in multiple myeloma and the impact of lenalidomide therapy," *Clinical & Experimental Immunology*, vol. 175, no. 1, pp. 49–58, 2014.

[16] T. Goyal, B. Thakral, S. A. Wang et al., "T-cell large granular lymphocytic leukemia and coexisting B-cell lymphomas," *American Journal of Clinical Pathology*, vol. 149, no. 2, pp. 164–171, 2018.

[17] K. L. Wolniak, C. L. Goolsby, Y.-H. Chen et al., "Expansion of a clonal $CD8^{+}CD57^{+}$ large granular lymphocyte population after autologous stem cell transplant in multiple myeloma," *American Journal of Clinical Pathology*, vol. 139, no. 2, pp. 231–241, 2013.

[18] O. Benjamini, P. Jain, N Sergej et al., "$CD4^{-}/CD8^{-}$ variant of T-cell large granular lymphocytic leukemia or hepatosplenic T-cell lymphoma: a clinicopathologic dilemma," *Clinical Lymphoma, Myeloma and Leukemia*, vol. 13, no. 5, pp. 610–613, 2013.

[19] P. Garrido, F. Ruiz-Cabello, P. Bárcena et al., "Monoclonal TCR-$V\beta13.1^{+}/CD4^{+}/NKa^{+}/CD8^{-}/^{+}$dim T-LGL lymphocytosis: evidence for an antigen-driven chronic T-cell stimulation origin," *Blood*, vol. 109, no. 11, pp. 4890–4898, 2007.

[20] M. Mizuki, S. Tagawa, T. Machii et al., "Phenotypical heterogeneity of $CD4^{+}CD8^{+}$ double-positive chronic T lymphoid leukemia," *Leukemia*, vol. 12, no. 4, pp. 499–504, 1998.

[21] S. Raza, S. Naik, V. P. Kancharla, F. Tafera, and M. R. Kalavar, "Dual-positive ($CD4^{+}/CD8^{+}$) acute adult T-cell leukemia/ lymphoma associated with complex karyotype and refractory

hypercalcemia: case report and literature review," *Case Reports in Oncology*, vol. 3, no. 3, pp. 489–494, 2010.

[22] M. S. Pombo De Oliveira, P. Loureiro, A. Bittencourt et al., "Geographic diversity of adult *t*-cell leukemia/lymphoma in Brazil," *International Journal of Cancer*, vol. 83, no. 3, pp. 291–298, 1999.

[23] K. Tamura, T. Unoki, K. Sagawa et al., "Clinical features of $OKT4^+/OKT8^+$ adult T-cell leukemia," *Leukemia Research*, vol. 9, no. 11, pp. 1353–1359, 1985.

[24] S. Kamihira, H. Sohda, S. Atogami et al., "Phenotypic diversity and prognosis of adult T-cell leukemia," *Leukemia Research*, vol. 16, no. 5, pp. 435–441, 1992.

24

Extramedullary Solitary Plasmacytoma with Anaplastic Features of the Nasopharynx

Parikshit Padhi[1] **and Radwa El-Behery**[2]

[1]*Memorial Medical Cancer Center, 2530 S Telshor Blvd, Las Cruces, NM 88011, USA*
[2]*Integrated Oncology, 5005 S 40th St, Phoenix, AZ 85040, USA*

Correspondence should be addressed to Parikshit Padhi; parikshit.padhi@gmail.com

Academic Editor: Vincent Ribrag

Extramedullary plasmacytomas (ESPs) are rare forms of plasma cell dyscrasias and usually are seen in the upper aerodigestive tract. ESPs with anaplastic features are extremely rare, and no treatment guidelines exist. We present a 75-year-old gentleman presented with left nasal blockage, and on examination, a polypoid left nasal mass was seen. He was, then, referred to ENT after a CT scan revealed a mass in the left nasopharynx for a biopsy. The preliminary reports suggested a high-grade lymphoma; however, after further testing, it was revealed to be an anaplastic plasma cell neoplasm. PET scan, bone marrow biopsy, serum and urine protein electropheresis, serum immunofixation and light chains were all unremarkable for systemic disease. Differential diagnosis included plasmablastic lymphoma, NK/T cell lymphoma-nasal type, and squamous cell cancers of the head and neck. He was treated with radiation alone given his comorbidities. Given there are no treatment guidelines, we would like to highlight this rare case and discuss different potential management options such as radiation, chemotherapy, surgery, or a combination of different modalities.

1. Introduction

Extramedullary plasmacytomas (ESP) are rare forms of plasma cell dyscrasias with anaplastic variants mentioned in only a few case reports. There are no guidelines for the management of ESP; however, most are treated with radiation alone since they tend to be radiosensitive. It is unclear whether ESP with anaplastic features require more aggressive management with radiation and chemotherapy. This entity can resemble plasmablastic lymphoma, and it is paramount to rule out plasmablastic lymphoma since the management is different. We present a case of ESP with anaplastic features of the nasopharynx and will discuss the features and management of this rare entity.

2. Case Presentation

A 75-year-old gentleman with a history of Usher Syndrome with retinitis pigmentosa presented to his family doctor because of a sensation of left-sided nasal blockage especially on deep inspiration. He denied any nasal pain, nasal swelling, or epistaxis. He was legally blind in both eyes but had minimal vision in his left eye. On examination of his nose, a pink-colored polypoid mass was arising from the left nasal orifice. The extension could not be determined on physical examination. He has no history of hepatitis, HIV, or any chronic viral illnesses. He was a former smoker with a 60 pack year history, but no IV drug use or alcohol use. He had no family history of cancer.

A computed tomography (CT) scan of the sinuses revealed a $3.1 \times 4.4 \times 3.2$ cm mass arising from the left nasopharynx, causing rightward deviation of the nasal septum (Figure 1). He followed up with the ENT surgeon who performed a biopsy of this mass. Initially the frozen section revealed small round blue cells suggestive of an aggressive lymphoma, but it was sent for a second opinion. A CT scan of the chest, abdomen, and pelvis and, eventually, a PET scan showed no other sites of disease. Eventually, the biopsy from

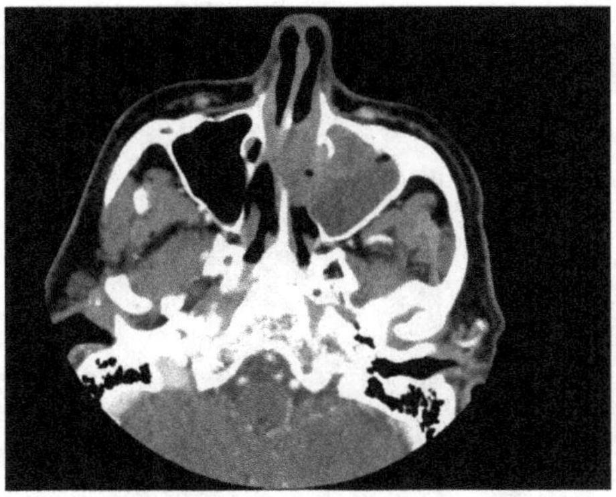

Figure 1: CT scan of the sinus showing an expansile mass in the left nasopharyngeal region leading to rightward nasal septum deviation and destruction of the etmoid cells.

the nasopharyngeal mass revealed a diffuse infiltrate of large atypical cells with variably eccentric nuclei, fairly abundant amphophilic cytoplasm, prominent nucleoli, and occasional binucleated forms. Few Dutcher bodies were seen. Mitosis was markedly increased, and atypical mitotic figures were identified. Apoptosis was also increased, and focal necrosis was present. Immunostains revealed the neoplastic cells to be positive for CD38 (strong), CD138, CD79a, MUM-1, kappa, IgA, BCL-2, and CD43 and negative for CD20, PAX-5, CD45, CD30, EMA, EBER by ISH, ALK-1, HHV8, lambda, IgG, IgM, IgD, CD56, CD5, CD10, BCL-6, BCL-1, CAM5.2/AE1, and CD117. Ki-67 was positive, variable 30–80% and overall 60% (Figure 2). He was diagnosed with an anaplastic plasma cell neoplasm. He, then, came to our cancer center for further management. Initial blood tests included complete blood counts (white blood count: 6.22×10^3/microlitre, hemoglobin: 15.9gm/dL, platelet count: 244×10^3/microlitre, and absolute neutrophil count: 3.42×10^3/microlitre), chemistries (sodium: 134 mmol/L, potassium: 4.3 mmol/L, chloride: 105 mmol/L, BUN: 17 mg/dL, creatinine: 0.86 mg/dL, and calcium: 10.2 mg/dL, and liver enzymes were within the normal range), and myeloma parameters (M protein: not observed, total protein: 7.2 gm/dL, albumin: 4 gm/dL, globulin 2.9 gm/gL, IgG 852 mg/dL, IgA 241 mg/dL, IgM 98 mg/dL, kappa light chains: 18.1 mg/L, lambda light chains: 13.7 mg/L, and kappa/lambda ratio: 1.34). A bone marrow biopsy revealed a normal cellular marrow for age (20–30%) with normal trilineage hematopoiesis, and no increased plasma cells were noted.

Our differentials included plasmablastic lymphoma, NK/T cell lymphoma, or a nasopharyngeal squamous cell carcinoma. We had to ensure that the patient did not have plasmablastic lymphoma as there is some overlap with the morphological and immunohistochemistry features with anaplastic plasma cell neoplasm. However, the absence of HIV history, the negative EBER by ISH, the presence of several Dutcher bodies, occasional binucleated forms, the Ki-67 that is well below 90%, the positive BCL-2, and negative EMA and CD30 are all in favor of a plasma cell neoplasm over a plasmablastic lymphoma. Histology analysis showed no evidence of a carcinoma or a, NK/T cell pathology.

We initially discussed with the patient that options include radiation to the nasophayngeal mass followed by either lenalidomide- or bortezomib-based therapy versus radiation alone. His case was discussed in our multidisciplinary tumor board, and based on his age, performance status, and comorbidities, it was decided to treat him with radiation alone (50 Gy/25 fractions) and reserve systemic treatment in the event of recurrence. He completed radiation treatment and, however, received 40 Gy due to the concern of complete blindness in his left eye. Postradiation PET scan and CT scan showed a complete response. Myeloma workup continued to show no evidence of systemic disease. He has remained in remission for 6 months, and we are monitoring him with imaging every 4–6 months and blood work (complete blood counts, chemistries, and myeloma parameters) every 3 months.

3. Discussion

Solitary plasmacytoma (SP) is a rare form of plasma cell dyscrasias in which neoplastic proliferation of monoclonal plasma cells are present in one location such as the bone or soft tissue without any evidence of bone marrow or systemic involvement. Solitary plasmacytomas only comprise of 2–5% of all plasma cell dyscrasias, and extramedullary solitary plasmacytomas (ESPs) are rarer making up only 3–4% of all SPs, while other reports mention that incidence of solitary bone plasmacytomas (SBPs) is 40% higher than that of ESPs [1, 2]. The incidence of ESPs with anaplastic features such as our case is unknown as they are very rare.

ESPs most commonly occur in the 6th to 8th decade of life, and compared to bone plasmacytomas, there is a higher male predominance for an ESP of 3–4:1 [3, 4]. ESPs most commonly occur in the head and neck or the upper aerodigestive tract region. [5] Other sites of ESPs (extramedullary plasmacytomas) that are reported are the retroperitoneum, muscle, lungs, and GI tract. [6–8] The symptoms of ESPs depend upon the location of the tumors; in the head and neck area, they can range from pain, airway obstruction, anosmia, change of speech, dysphagia, or localized bleeding. The workup for an ESP should include serum and urine electrophoresis, serum immunofixation, free light chain assay, bone marrow biopsy, and a metastatic bone survey, either via X-rays or a PET scan.

The differential diagnosis for an ESP with anaplastic features includes plasmablastic lymphoma, ALK-positive large B-cell lymphoma, and extracavitary primary effusion lymphoma. These four neoplasms share a high-grade morphology with variable plasmacytoid morphologic features, express plasma cell markers, including CD38, CD138, and MUM-1, lack pan-B-cell markers such as CD19, CD20, and PAX-5, and show variable expression of CD45, CD79a, CD30, EMA, CD56, and heavy and light chains. Plasmablastic lymphoma characteristically occurs not only in immunocompromised patients, most commonly in HIV-positive patients, but also in older individuals and in association with iatrogenic immunosuppression as in post-transplant patients and patients with autoimmune diseases. It typically shows high proliferation with a Ki-67 close to a

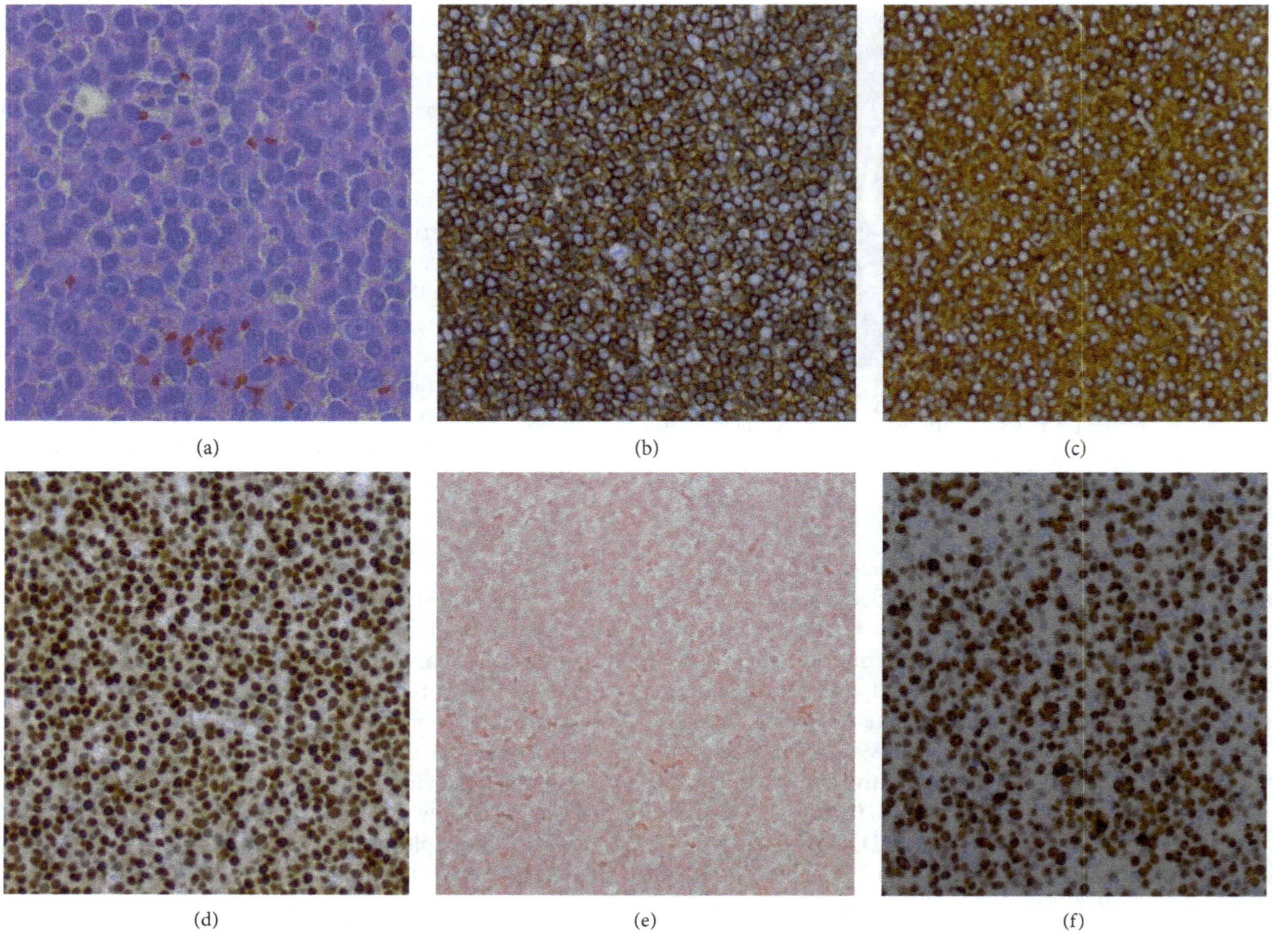

FIGURE 2: Nasopharyngeal mass biopsy reveals diffuse infiltrate of large atypical cells with variably eccentric neuclei, ampophilic cytoplasm, prominent nucleoli, and occasional uninucleated forms (a), that are CD138 positive (b), kappa restricted (c), MUM-1 positive (d), EBER negative (e), and a Ki-67 overall of 60% (f).

100% and with increased apoptosis, sometimes imparting a starry-sky appearance. The majority of cases (60–75%) are positive for EBER by ISH, while CD56 expression is detected in about 25% of cases. ALK-positive large B-cell lymphoma is characterized, as the name implies, by ALK-1 positivity (mostly granular cytoplasmic staining pattern with few cases showing a cytoplasmic, nuclear, and nucleolar staining pattern), while extracavitary primary effusion lymphoma is characterized by coexpression of HHV8 and EBER by ISH. A high-grade neoplasm with plasmacytoid features which lacks HHV8, EBER by ISH, and ALK-1 expression in an immunocompetent patient is most likely to represent a plasma cell neoplasm, especially if a monoclonal protein, bone marrow involvement, or lytic bone lesions are present. It is of note that some plasma cell neoplasms (plasmacytoma or plasma cell myeloma) can express EBV, so a positive EBER by ISH should not be used in isolation, to establish the diagnosis of plasmablastic lymphoma, and a correlation with all clinical, laboratory, radiologic, morphologic, and immunohistochemical findings is required for definitive diagnosis; however, in some cases with overlapping features, a descriptive diagnosis of "plasmablastic neoplasm consistent with plasmablastic lymphoma or anaplastic plasmacytoma" may be acceptable, according to the 2016 WHO classification of tumor of hematopoietic and lymphoid tissues [9]. It is also of note that tumors resembling plasmablastic lymphoma can develop in a patient with a documented prior history of a plasma cell neoplasm, and these cases are best classified as plasmablastic transformation of a plasma cell neoplasm as opposed to a primary plasmablastic lymphoma.

Whether management should be more aggressive for this entity is unknown. Some case reports have shown that radiation or surgery alone will suffice; however, there are reports of this entity not responding to chemotherapy or radiation [6, 10, 11]. The location of the plasmacytoma may affect its response to different modalities of treatment. ESP still has a lower rate of converting into multiple myeloma when compared to solitary bone plasmacytoma (SBP), and a myeloma-free survival at10 yr for ESP was 71.2% while SBP was 0% [12]. Progression to multiple myeloma for ESP with anaplastic features is unknown.

The management of head and neck ESP includes resection of the tumor, radiation (RT) alone, or surgery followed by radiation. Head and neck ESP are radiosensitive with one case series of 18 patients treated with RT alone having local recurrence in only 1 patient [13]. Bachar et al.

reviewed 68 cases and suggested that patients treated with radiation had an improved local free recurrence survival [2]. Sasaki et al. treated 67 patients with RT alone, and the 5-year and 10-year local control rates were 95% and 87%, respectively [14]. Another study revealed a 10-year local control of 88.9% with radiation alone [15]. The average dose of radiation should be at least 40–50 Gy given over 20–25 fractions. The role of chemotherapy in ESP is unknown. In the case report by Aluko et al., the patient had nasopharyngeal ESP similar to ours and was treated with 2 cycles of chemotherapy (cyclophosphamide, thalidomide, and dexamethasone) followed by radiation [1]. In the article by Bachar et al., 3 patients did receive concurrent chemoradiation as well with no difference in the outcomes when compared to RT alone [2]. Chemotherapy can be considered for high-grade tumors or large tumors as recurrence rates for higher grade ESP is high with RT alone. [16].

In our case, there was a strong consideration for adjuvant chemotherapy given the anaplastic features, but due to his comorbidities, we decided against it. We believe that RT alone should suffice for treatment of head and neck ESP; however, adjuvant chemotherapy should be considered in patients with anaplastic features. Surgery should only be performed for emergent issues or contraindications to RT.

4. Conclusions

Extramedullary plasmacytomas are very rare subtypes of plasma cell dyscrasias with anaplastic features being rarer. The head and neck, as well as the upper aerodigestive tract, are the most common sites of extramedullary plasmacytomas. Solitary bone plasmacytomas tend to have a higher rate of progressing to multiple myelomas when compared to extramedullary plasmacytomas. Extramedullary plasmacytomas of the head and neck region are radiosensitive, and in majority of the cases, radiation alone with a dose of approximately 40–50 Gy should be curative. However, ideal management is unknown. Extramedullary plasmacytomas with anaplastic features closely resemble plasmablastic lymphoma (PBL), and PBL needs to be ruled out because this tends to be more aggressive and usually requires systemic chemotherapy.

References

[1] A. A. A. Aluko, G. Hasheem, and A. Auwal, "Extramedullary plasmacytoma of the nasopharynx: a case report and review of literature," *Pyramid Journal of Medicine*, vol. 2, no. 1, 2019.

[2] G. Bachar, D. Goldstein, D. Brown et al., "Solitary extramedullary plasmacytoma of the head and neck-Long-term outcome analysis of 68 cases," *Head & Neck*, vol. 30, no. 8, pp. 1012–1019, 2008.

[3] P. Galieni, M. Cavo, A Pulsoni et al., "Clinical outcome of extramedullary plasmacytoma," *Haematologica*, vol. 85, no. 1, pp. 47–51, 2000.

[4] R. Soutar, H. Lucraft, G. Jackson et al., "Guidelines on the diagnosis and management of solitary plasmacytoma of bone and solitary extramedullary plasmacytoma," *British Journal of Haematology*, vol. 124, no. 6, pp. 717–726, 2004.

[5] S. Kilciksiz, O. Karakoyun-Celik, F. Y. Agaoglu, and A. Haydaroglu, "A review for solitary plasmacytoma of bone and extramedullary plasmacytoma," *Scientific World Journal*, vol. 2012, p. 895765, 2012.

[6] S. Madi, V. Senthil, M. Naik, and S. Vijayan, "Multiple solitary extramedullary anaplastic plasmacytomas," *Indian Journal of Medical and Paediatric Oncology*, vol. 37, no. 4, pp. 303-304, 2016.

[7] S. Nie, D. Peng, H. Gong, C. Ye, X. Nie, and H. Li, "Primary pulmonary plasmacytoma: a case report introduction," *World Journal of Surgical Oncology*, vol. 14, p. 205, 2016.

[8] I. Zihni, R. Dinc, S. Canpolat, F. Cengiz, and A. Uslu, "Extramedullary plasmacytoma of colon: a case report," *Turkish Journal of Surgery*, vol. 30, no. 4, pp. 231–233, 2014.

[9] S. H. Swerdlow, E. Campo, N. H Harris et al., *WHO Classification of Haematopoietic and Lymphoid Tissues*, International Agency for Reseach on Cancer, Lyon, France, 2017.

[10] M. J. Ashraf, N. Azarpira, and B. Khademi, "Anaplastic solitary plasmacytoma of the mandible, masquerading as sarcoma," *Pakistan Journal of Medical Sciences*, vol. 29, no. 3, pp. 872-873, 2013.

[11] W. Ding, W. Tan, Y Qian et al., "Primary plasmablastic plasmacytoma in the stomach of an immunocompetent adult," *Medicine(Baltimore)*, vol. 98, no. 4, Article ID e14235, 2019.

[12] Y.-G. Suh, C.-O. Suh, J. S. Kim, S.-J. Kim, H. O. Pyun, and J. Cho, "Radiotherapy for solitary plasmacytoma of bone and soft tissue," *Annals of Hematology*, vol. 91, no. 11, pp. 1785–1793, 2012.

[13] K. M. Creach, R. L. Foote, M. A. Neben-Wittich, and R. A. Kyle, "Radiotherapy for extramedullary plasmacytoma of the head and neck," *International Journal of Radiation Oncology Biology Physics*, vol. 73, no. 3, pp. 789–794, 2009.

[14] R. Sasaki, K. Yasuda, E. Abe et al., "Multi-institutional analysis of solitary extramedullary plasmacytoma of the head and neck treated with curative radiotherapy," *International Journal of Radiation Oncology Biology Physics*, vol. 82, no. 2, pp. 626–634, 2012.

[15] B. Khademi, Z. Zandifar, M Mohammadianpanah et al., "Head and neck solitary extramedullary plasmacytomas," *Journal of Oral Oncology*, vol. 2014, p. 5, 2014.

[16] S. Susnerwala, J. Shanks, S. Banerjee, J. Scarffe, W. Farrington, and N. Slevin, "Extramedullary plasmacytoma of the head and neck region: clinicopathological correlation in 25 cases," *British Journal of Cancer*, vol. 75, no. 6, pp. 921–927, 1997.

25

Cerebral Venous Thrombosis in the Setting of Malignancy: Case Report and Review of the Literature

Constantine N. Logothetis[1] **and Charles Pizanis**[2]

[1]*Department of Internal Medicine, University of South Florida Morsani College of Medicine, 17 Davis Blvd, Suite 308, Tampa, FL 33606, USA*
[2]*Division of Hospital Medicine Department of Internal Medicine, University of New Mexico School of Medicine, University of New Mexico, MSC10 5550, Albuquerque, NM 87131, USA*

Correspondence should be addressed to Charles Pizanis; cpizanis@salud.unm.edu

Academic Editor: Kostas Konstantopoulos

Cerebral venous thrombosis (CVT) is a rare condition that can be difficult to diagnose due to its vague and nonspecific symptoms. It is even more unusual to identify CVT in association with malignancy. Given the rarity of this disease, treatment and management of CVT in the setting of malignancy is not well defined. This case report and review of the literature addresses the epidemiology, pathophysiology, and medical treatment for malignancy-related CVT.

1. Introduction

Venous thromboembolism (VTE) is a common complication of cancer and cancer-related treatment. Among the possible VTEs that can occur are thromboses of the dural sinuses or cerebral veins. Cerebral venous thrombosis (CVT) is an uncommon clinical entity and is often difficult to identify due to its vague and nonspecific findings. Management of CVT can similarly pose a challenge for clinicians given the risk of bleeding complications with treatment. This case highlights a patient whose diagnosis of CVT was initially missed as was the underlying etiology of the disorder. This article reviews the epidemiology, pathophysiology, and medical management of CVT in patients with malignancy.

2. Case Presentation

A 60-year-old woman with a medical history of type 2 diabetes mellitus, papillary thyroid cancer status post resection, and hypertension presented to a referring hospital with worsening headaches and visual disturbances. For four months prior to her presentation, she had experienced intermittent unilateral, pulsating headaches as well as visual disturbances in the right eye. Upon arrival to the emergency department, she was febrile and noted to have meningismus. CBC revealed white blood cells at 9,800/L, hemoglobin at 12.9 g/dL, and platelets at 223,000/uL. Lumbar puncture was performed with a cerebrospinal fluid (CSF) profile demonstrating colorless fluid, total nucleated cells 43/mm^3, red blood cells 4/mm^3, glucose 134 mg/dL, total protein 50 mg/dL, and an opening pressure of 21 cm H20. CSF herpes simplex virus 1/2, West Nile virus, cytomegalovirus, enterovirus, varicella zoster virus PCRs, venereal disease research laboratory (VDRL), and coccidioides antibodies were negative or nonreactive, respectively. Serum HIV 1/2 antibodies, QuantiFERON-TB Gold, and autoimmune panel consisting of antinuclear antibody, rheumatoid factor, anti-mitochondrial antibody, and macrophage 2 antibodies were also nonrevealing. Magnetic resonance imaging (MRI) of the brain was obtained at the time which showed acute-to-subacute thrombosis of the right transverse sinuses (Figure 1). Given her constellation of symptoms and negative infectious and autoimmune workup, she was initially treated for aseptic meningitis and discharged home with warfarin anticoagulation for the thrombosis. Her symptoms did not fully resolve, however, and she was readmitted one week later to the hospital for further evaluation and workup.

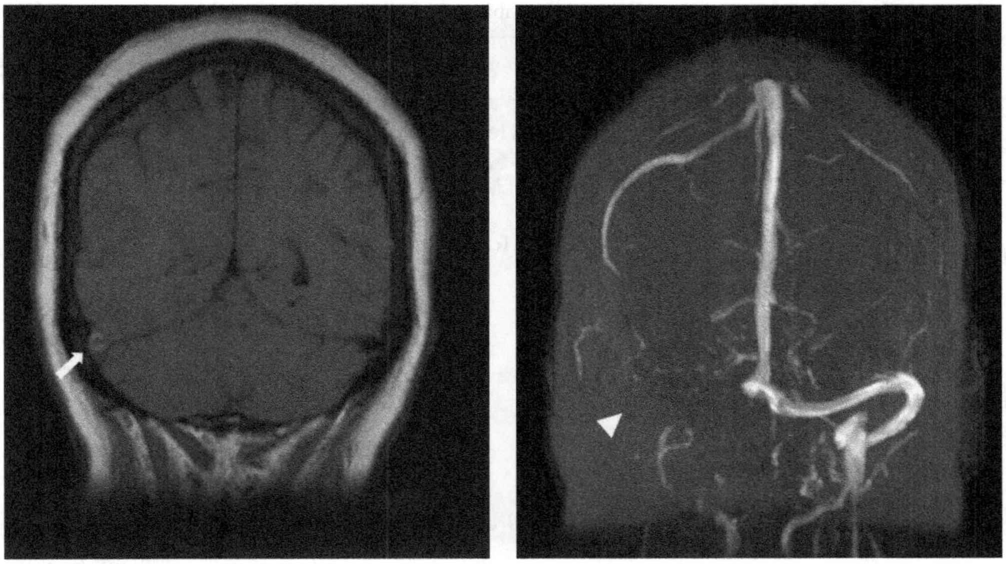

(a) (b)

FIGURE 1: Magnetic resonance imaging demonstrating flow void at right transverse sinus (arrow) and absence of contrast (arrowhead) along transverse sinus consistent with transverse sinus thrombus.

On readmission, her CBC demonstrated elevated white blood cells at 17,000/L (38% polymorphonuclear cells, 34% lymphocytes, and 23% variant lymphocytes). Due to the presence of variant lymphocytes noted at that time, a peripheral blood smear was obtained which revealed precursor B-cells and 30% circulating blasts consistent with B-cell acute lymphoblastic leukemia (ALL). A repeat lumbar puncture was performed with CSF profile demonstrating total nucleated cells 728/mm^3, red blood cells 0/mm^3, glucose 93 mg/dL, and total protein 42 mg/dL. CSF flow cytometry demonstrated 97% blasts expressing CD34, CD19, bright CD10, and dim CD33 consistent with CNS involvement. After consultation with hematology, the patient was started on the ALL202 protocol with cyclophosphamide, daunorubicin, vincristine, methotrexate, cytarabine, and imatinib (given Ph chromosome positivity) as well as intrathecal methotrexate. During her hospitalization, her dural sinus thrombosis was treated with therapeutic-dosing enoxaparin at 1.5 mg/kg/day (100 mg).

During the course of her ALL treatment, the patient experienced repeated episodes of thrombocytopenia with clinical concerns for subarachnoid hemorrhage. After a year and a half of anticoagulation with enoxaparin, a follow-up MRI was obtained which demonstrated stability in the thrombosis since initial diagnosis. Because of the chronicity of the thrombus and the ongoing bleeding concerns, enoxaparin was discontinued. The patient underwent subsequent brain imaging during the course of her ALL treatment which did not demonstrate any increase in size of the dural sinus thrombosis despite lack of anticoagulation.

3. Discussion

Due to the rare nature the disease, there is little literature on the epidemiology, pathophysiology, and management of malignancy-related CVT. The prevalence of CVT in patients with malignancy is believed to be approximately 0.3% [1, 2]. Malignancy-related thromboses of the dural sinus or cerebral veins are thought to represent roughly 7.4% of all CVT cases, with cancer increasing risk for CVT roughly 5-fold[3]. Hematologic malignancies appear to be implicated more so than solid organ malignancies; however, the underlying reasons for this are not completely understood [4]. CVT has also been described in the setting of antineoplastic therapy. Several agents have been reported in the development of this condition including bevacizumab and lenalidomide [1, 5].

3.1. Pathophysiology. The pathophysiology behind the development of CVT is complex and follows Virchow's triad. While more clearly described in the setting of infection wherein localized inflammatory processes related to septic emboli, thrombi formation, and localized infection are thought to drive thrombus formation, the pathogenesis of CVT in the setting of malignancy is not well defined [6]. Several potential mechanisms have been proposed including direct tumor compression, tumor invasion, and the hypercoagulable state of malignancy [2, 7, 8]. In the absence of tumor compression or invasion, malignancy-related prothrombotic states are thought to drive development of VTE via a variety of mechanisms including a tumor's ability to increase the expression of tissue factor (TF), cancer procoagulant, and inflammatory cytokines as well as to downregulate the expression of thrombomodulin and the protein C system [9].

3.2. Medical Management. The treatment strategy for patients with malignancy-related CVT can be challenging. Similar to other causes of CVT, malignancy-related CVT carries risks of hemorrhage and hematoma formation.

Table 1: Review of the literature describing sinus thromboses in malignancies.

Reference	Number of patients	Cancer	Anticoagulant	Duration of therapy	Outcome
Oda et al.[15]	1	Stage IV lung adenocarcinoma	Heparin, warfarin	4 weeks	Radiographic resolution at 4 weeks
Iqbal and Sharma [13]	1	Metastatic colorectal adenocarcinoma	LMWH, warfarin	5 months	Clinical improvement in symptoms at 5 months
Mutreja et al.[14]	1	JAK2V617F mutation-positive hematolymphoid malignancy	Heparin, warfarin, dabigatran	21 days	Death at 21 days
Tuncel et al. [16]	1	Advanced-stage small cell lung cancer	LMWH	N/A	Clinical improvement at 1 month
Marvin et al. [3]	1	Metastatic renal cell carcinoma (brain metastases)	Heparin	N/A	Radiographic resolution and death at 4 months (unknown cause)
Shimizu et al. [17]	1	Tongue cancer	Heparin	N/A	Clinical and radiographic improvement
Akai et al. [18]	1	Malignant melanoma with meningeal dissemination	Urokinase, heparin	24 hours	Recanalization of straight sinus
Ho et al. [19]	1	Acute lymphoblastic leukemia	Heparin, warfarin	N/A	Radiographic resolution at 20 days
Vargo et al. [1]	1	Anaplastic gemistocytic astrocytoma	Heparin, enoxaparin	N/A	Stabilization and interval improvement on MRI
Eudo et al. [5]	1	Multiple myeloma	LMWH	N/A	Clinical improvement in symptoms at 1 month
Li et al. [20]	1	Grade 2, stage IIIC serous ovarian cancer	Enoxaparin	5 weeks	Death at 5 weeks
Chang et al. [21]	1	Acute myeloid leukemia, M1	Enoxaparin, warfarin	N/A	Clinical improvement in vision
Wang et al. [22]	1	Acute lymphoblastic leukemia	Enoxaparin	7 months	Clinical and radiographic improvement at six months
Iurlaro et al. [23]	9	Breast cancer x2, gastric cancer, NHL x3, HL, kidney cancer and melanoma, and rhinopharyngeal cancer	Unfractionated , LMWH	N/A	Based off of modified Rankin scale (mRS): complete recovery in 4 patients (mRS 0), mild sequelae in 4 patients (mRS 1-2), and moderate sequelae in one patient (mRS 3)
Karam and Koussa [24]	2	Germ-cell carcinoma of the testis; poorly differentiated pericardial carcinoma	Unknown anticoagulation; heparin	20 days	Clinical and radiographic improvement at 1 month; unknown outcome
Ross et al. [25]	4	T-cell ALL; pre-B-cell ALL; ALL; pre-B-cell ALL	LMWH; unfractionated heparin, LMWH, warfarin; LMWH; LMWH	7 months; n/a; 3 months; 4 months	Radiographic partial recanalization; clinical improvement in symptoms; complete resolution on imaging at 1 month; resolution on imaging at 1 month
Song et al. [26]	1	Acute promyelocytic leukemia	LMWH, warfarin	N/A	Radiographic recanalization of straight sinus with continued occlusion of transverse and confluens sinuum at 1 month
Imamura et al. [27]	2	B-precursor ALL; T-cell type NHL	No anticoagulation; LMWH; ATIII concentrate supplementation	N/A; N/A	Death at 40 days; complete neurologic recovery
Lee et al. [28]	1	Acute lymphoblastic leukemia	Heparin, warfarin	N/A	Radiographic recanalization of the superior sagittal sinus
Ciccone et al. [29]	1	Acute promyelocytic leukemia	Unfractionated heparin, warfarin		Complete recovery from the coma and almost complete resolution of the sinuses thrombosis.

Table 1: Continued.

Reference	Number of patients	Cancer	Anticoagulant	Duration of therapy	Outcome
Motohashi et al. [30]	1	Acute myeloid leukemia	Heparin, warfarin	N/A	Recanalization of straight sinus but continued occlusion of the right transverse and sigmoid sinuses. No neurologic sequelae at 10 months
Corso et al. [31]	2	Ph + ALL; Ph + ALL	Heparin; heparin	N/A; N/A	Radiographic resolution of thrombus; progressive but slow resolution of symptoms

Moreover, patients with malignancy frequently experience thrombocytopenia and other coagulopathies as a result of the cancer and/or cancer therapies, making treatment decisions even more difficult. Lack of treatment, however, can lead to thrombus propagation, neurologic sequelae, and death [4]. As such, an individualized approach to treatment is recommended.

Much like other VTEs, the medical management of CVT primarily consists of systemic anticoagulation to reduce the risk of thrombosis growth and to facilitate vessel recanalization. Several agents have been described in the treatment of CVT including heparin, low-molecular weight heparins (LMWHs), vitamin-K antagonists (VKAs), and direct oral anticoagulants (DOACs). In 2011, the American Heart Association (AHA) and American Stroke Association (ASA) released a set of guidelines on the diagnosis and management of CVT. Contained within the recommendations were guidelines on acute as well as long-term treatments. Acute treatment options included heparins, LMWHs, and VKAs with VKAs being the primary recommendation for long-term treatment [4]. Additionally, the European Academy of Neurology (EAN) released similar recommendations in 2017 [10]. Notable differences include the recommendation of LMWHs over heparin in the acute treatment for CVT based in part on a more recent randomized controlled trial suggesting better recovery with LMWH [11]. Specific guidelines were limited, however, for malignancy-related CVT in both societal recommendations.

The existing literature on agent of choice for cancer-related CVT is primarily found in case reports. Several reports have been published demonstrating safety and positive outcomes of various anticoagulation regimens including heparin, LMWHs, and VKAs (Table 1) [1, 5, 12, 13–17, 18–31]. LMWHs have for several years been recommended over VKAs in malignancy-related VTE leading to the question of their superiority in malignancy-related CVT [32]. To date, however, no prospective trials evaluating LMWHs over VKAs have occurred. Despite these established recommendations for malignancy-related VTE elsewhere, specific recommendations for treatment of malignancy-related CVT were neither elaborated upon in the 2011 AHA/ASA nor the 2017 EAN CVT treatment guidelines [4, 10].

The emergence of the direct oral anticoagulants (DOACs) in the treatment of malignancy-related VTE is a new focus of great interest with multiple studies and societal recommendations supporting DOAC use to treat DVT and pulmonary embolism [33–36]. The role of DOACs in the treatment of CVT, however, is unclear [37]. In one randomized controlled trial examining the safety and efficacy of dabigatran versus dose-adjusted warfarin in patients with CVT, dabigatran was at least as safe, if not safer, than warfarin with regard to major bleeding risk. Neither group experienced recurrent VTE, and both had similar degrees of recanalization (60.0% in the dabigatran group and 67.3% in the warfarin group). Neither noninferiority nor superiority of either therapy could be demonstrated because of limited sample size [38].

Two case series exist describing the use of DOACs beyond the acute phase of treatment for CVT, one of which contained one patient with malignancy and CVT [39, 40]. In these series, DOACs appeared to be associated with favorable outcomes without significant bleeding concerns though absence of recanalization in the patient with malignancy was noted. Neither the Hokusai VTE Cancer Investigators nor the SELECT-D trials investigating DOAC treatment of malignancy-related VTE included patients with CVT. Given also the association of venous hemorrhage with CVT, use of DOACs may pose a clinical issue given limited (albeit growing) options for reversal agents [4]. In the 2017 European Academy of Neurology guidelines, DOAC therapy was not recommended for CVT based on low quality of evidence with a high risk for bias [10]. Further research is, therefore, needed into the efficacy and safety of DOACs for the management of malignancy-related CVT.

3.3. Duration of Therapy. The main goal of treatment beyond the acute therapy for CVT is prevention of thrombosis recurrence. New thrombosis following CVT has been reported as high 6.5% annually [41]. Optimal duration of long-term therapy to prevent recurrent CVT is often a question [42]. In the 2011 AHA/ASA and 2017 EAN CVT guidelines, a 3–12 month or indefinite anticoagulation duration was recommended depending on reversibility of the underlying etiology [4, 10]. Provoked CVT with a transient risk factor may be treated for 3–6 months, while unprovoked CVT may be treated for 6–12 months. Other authors have suggested ranges of weeks to several months or durations based on radiologic resolution of the thrombus. In the setting of malignancy, however, in which the provoking event may not be reversed prior to suggested end of therapy, an individualized decision should be made weighing risks of ongoing treatment as well as the risk for recurrence.

Currently, there are no consensus guidelines for the specific management of malignancy-related CVT with a majority of evidence for treatment found in case reports or extrapolated from guidelines focused on nonmalignant CVT. At this time, there is not a clearly superior anticoagulant for the management of malignancy-related CVT though it may be reasonable to consider LMWHs over VKAs given existing data on LMWH superiority in preventing VTE recurrence in patients with malignancy. DOAC therapy for malignancy-related CVT is not recommended at this time given lack of studies of efficacy and safety though they may emerge as future treatment options. Optimal treatment duration is similarly unclear though should be extended beyond acute treatment for CVT barring contraindications.

4. Conclusion

As described in this case, anticoagulation was administered upon the initial diagnosis of CVT. Given ongoing malignancy, the patient was treated with therapeutic-dosing enoxaparin for nearly two years which was eventually terminated after the complications of anticoagulation were thought to outweigh the risk of thrombus recurrence. While malignancy-related CVT is a rare phenomenon, further prospective study is warranted to establish firmer guidelines for anticoagulation. Until this occurs, treatment and duration should remain individualized. Data to date support the use of heparin, LMWH, and warfarin in the treatment of malignancy-related CVT. DOAC efficacy and safety are unclear at this time for the treatment of malignancy-related CVT though should be a focus of future investigation.

Acknowledgments

The authors would like to thank Allison Burnett, PharmD, PhC, CACP, for her review and support of this article.

References

[1] J. A. Vargo, B. M. Snelling, E. R. Ghareeb et al., "Dural venous sinus thrombosis in anaplastic astrocytoma following concurrent temozolomide and focal brain radiotherapy plus bevacizumab," *Journal of Neuro-Oncology*, vol. 104, no. 2, pp. 595–598, 2011.

[2] J. J. Raizer and L. M. DeAngelis, "Cerebral sinus thrombosis diagnosed by MRI and MR venography in cancer patients," *Neurology*, vol. 54, no. 6, pp. 1222–1226, 2000.

[3] S. M. Silvis, S. Hiltunen, E. Lindgren et al., "Cancer and risk of cerebral venous thrombosis: a case–control study," *Journal of Thrombosis and Haemostasis*, vol. 16, no. 1, pp. 90–95, 2018.

[4] G. Saposnik, F. Barinagarrementeria, R. D. Brown et al., "Diagnosis and management of cerebral venous thrombosis," *Stroke*, vol. 42, no. 4, pp. 1158–1192, 2011.

[5] C. Eudo, J.-P. Cottier, A. Petit et al., "Cerebral venous thrombosis in an individual with multiple myeloma treated with lenalidomide," *Journal of the American Geriatrics Society*, vol. 59, no. 12, pp. 2371-2372, 2011.

[6] J. R. Ebright, M. T. Pace, and A. F. Niazi, "Septic thrombosis of the cavernous sinuses," *Archives of Internal Medicine*, vol. 161, no. 22, pp. 2671–2676, 2001.

[7] A. W. Kim and J. D. Trobe, "Syndrome simulating pseudotumor cerebri caused by partial transverse venous sinus obstruction in metastatic prostate cancer," *American Journal of Ophthalmology*, vol. 129, no. 2, pp. 254–256, 2000.

[8] L. R. Rogers, "Cerebrovascular complications in patients with cancer," *Seminars in Neurology*, vol. 24, no. 4, pp. 453–460, 2004.

[9] G. J. Caine, P. S. Stonelake, G. Y. H. Lip, and S. T. Kehoe, "The hypercoagulable state of malignancy: pathogenesis and current debate," *Neoplasia*, vol. 4, no. 6, pp. 465–473, 2002.

[10] J. M. Ferro, M.-G. Bousser, P. Canhão et al., "European stroke organization guideline for the diagnosis and treatment of cerebral venous thrombosis-endorsed by the European Academy of Neurology," *European Journal of Neurology*, vol. 24, no. 10, pp. 1203–1213, 2017.

[11] U. K. Misra, J. Kalita, S. Chandra, B. Kumar, and V. Bansal, "Low molecular weight heparin versus unfractionated heparin in cerebral venous sinus thrombosis: a randomized controlled trial," *European Journal of Neurology*, vol. 19, no. 7, pp. 1030–1036, 2012.

[12] E. Marvin, J. Synkowski, and M. Benko, "Tumor cerebri: metastatic renal cell carcinoma with dural venous sinus compression leading to intracranial hypertension; a case report," *Surgical Neurology International*, vol. 8, no. 1, p. 175, 2017.

[13] N. Iqbal and A. Sharma, "Cerebral venous thrombosis: a mimic of brain metastases in colorectal cancer associated with a better prognosis," *Case Reports in Oncological Medicine*, vol. 2013, Article ID 109412, 3 pages, 2013.

[14] D. Mutreja, R. Saxena, T. S. V. G. Tilak, V. Tewari, N. Moorchung, and B. Nandi, "A 37-year-old male with extensive cerebral venous thrombosis: clinicopathological correlation of a rare case," *Indian Journal of Pathology and Microbiology*, vol. 61, no. 2, pp. 219–224, 2018.

[15] N. Oda, M. Sakugawa, A. Bessho et al., "Cerebral venous sinus thrombosis concomitant with leptomeningeal carcinomatosis, in a patient with epidermal growth factor receptor-mutated lung cancer," *Oncology Letters*, vol. 8, no. 6, pp. 2489–2492, 2014.

[16] T. Tuncel, A. Ozgun, L. Emirzeoğlu et al., "Broca's aphasia due to cerebral venous sinus thrombosis following chemotherapy for small cell lung cancer: a case report and review of literature," *Oncology Letters*, vol. 9, no. 2, pp. 937–939, 2015.

[17] T. Shimizu, A. Musha, Y. Takayama, and S. Yokoo, "A case of cerebral venous sinus thrombosis associated with chemoradiation therapy for oral cancer," *International Journal of Oral and Maxillofacial Surgery*, vol. 46, p. 293, 2017.

[18] T. Akai, N. Kuwayama, T. Ogiichi, M. Kurimoto, S. Endo, and A. Takaku, "Leptomeningeal melanoma associated with straight sinus thrombosis-case report," *Neurologia Medico-Chirurgica*, vol. 37, no. 10, pp. 757–761, 1997.

[19] C. L. Ho, Y. C. Chen, C. Y. Chen, and T. Y. Chao, "Cerebral dural sinus thrombosis in acute lymphoblastic leukemia with early diagnosis by fast fluid-attenuated inversion recovery (FLAIR) MR image: a case report and review of the literature," *Annals of Hematology*, vol. 79, no. 2, pp. 90–94, 2000.

[20] H. K. Li, V. Harding, R. Williamson, S. Blagden, H. Gabra, and R. Agarwal, "Cerebral sinus thrombosis and leptomeningeal

carcinomatosis in a patient with ovarian cancer," *Journal of Clinical Oncology*, vol. 30, no. 2, pp. e19–e20, 2012.

[21] H. Chang, T.-L. Lin, W.-J. Ho, and L.-A. Hsu, "Acute myeloid leukemia associated with acute myocardial infarction and dural sinus thrombosis: the possible role of leukemia-related hyperhomocysteinemia," *Journal of the Chinese Medical Association*, vol. 71, no. 8, pp. 416–420, 2008.

[22] T.-Y. Wang, H.-J. Yen, G.-Y. Hung, M.-Y. Hsieh, and R.-B. Tang, "A rare complication in a child undergoing chemotherapy for acute lymphoblastic leukemia: superior sagittal sinus thrombosis," *Journal of the Chinese Medical Association*, vol. 74, no. 4, pp. 183–187, 2011.

[23] S. Iurlaro, A. Silvani, M. Mauri et al., "Headache in cerebral venous thrombosis associated with extracranial tumors: a clinical series," *Neurological Sciences*, vol. 36, no. S1, pp. 149–151, 2015.

[24] C. Karam and S. Koussa, "Cerebral dural sinus thrombosis following cisplatin chemotherapy," *Journal of Clinical Neuroscience*, vol. 15, no. 11, pp. 1274-1275, 2008.

[25] C. S. Ross, T. M. Brown, S. Kotagal, and V. Rodriguez, "Cerebral venous sinus thrombosis in pediatric cancer patients," *Journal of Pediatric Hematology/Oncology*, vol. 35, no. 4, pp. 299–302, 2013.

[26] L.-x. Song, H.-y. Lu, C.-k. Chang, X. Li, and Z. Zhang, "Cerebral venous and sinus thrombosis in a patient with acute promyelocytic leukemia during all-trans retinoic acid induction treatment," *Blood Coagulation & Fibrinolysis*, vol. 25, no. 7, pp. 773–776, 2014.

[27] T. Imamura, A. Morimoto, R. Kato et al., "Cerebral thrombotic complications in adolescent leukemia/lymphoma patients treated with L-asparaginase-containing chemotherapy," *Leukemia & Lymphoma*, vol. 46, no. 5, pp. 729–735, 2005.

[28] J.-H. Lee, S.-W. Kim, and J. Sung Kim, "Sagittal sinus thrombosis associated with transient free protein S deficiency after L-asparaginase treatment: case report and review of the literature," *Clinical Neurology and Neurosurgery*, vol. 102, no. 1, pp. 33–36, 2000.

[29] M. Ciccone, G. M. Rigolin, G. M. Viglione, M. Borrelli, M. L. Serino, and A. Cuneo, "Thrombosis of the cerebral veins and sinuses in acute promyelocytic leukemia after all-trans retinoic acid treatment: a case report," *Blood Coagulation & Fibrinolysis*, vol. 19, no. 7, pp. 721–723, 2008.

[30] K. Motohashi, M. Hagihara, S. Ito et al., "Cerebral venous sinus thrombosis after allogeneic stem cell transplantation," *International Journal of Hematology*, vol. 91, no. 1, pp. 154–156, 2010.

[31] A. Corso, C. Castagnola, and C. Bernasconi, "Thrombotic events are not exclusive to the remission induction period in patients with acute lymphoblastic leukemia: a report of two cases of cerebral sinus thrombosis," *Annals of Hematology*, vol. 75, no. 3, pp. 117–119, 1997.

[32] C. Kearon, E. A. Akl, J. Ornelas et al., "Antithrombotic therapy for VTE disease," *Chest*, vol. 149, no. 2, pp. 315–352, 2016.

[33] G. E. Raskob, N. van Es, P. Verhamme et al., "Edoxaban for the treatment of cancer-associated venous thromboembolism," *New England Journal of Medicine*, vol. 378, no. 7, pp. 615–624, 2018.

[34] A. M. Young, A. Marshall, J. Thirlwall et al., "Comparison of an oral factor xa inhibitor with low molecular weight heparin in patients with cancer with venous thromboembolism: results of a randomized trial (SELECT-D)," *Journal of Clinical Oncology*, vol. 36, no. 20, pp. 2017–2023, 2018.

[35] E. Cosma and J. J. Prunty, "Direct oral anticoagulant in cancers patients," *U.S. Pharmacist*, vol. 43, no. 8, pp. 2–11, 2018.

[36] N. S. Key, K. Bohlke, and A. Falanga, "Venous thromboembolism prophylaxis and treatment in patients with cancer: ASCO clinical practice guideline update," *Journal of Oncology Practice*, vol. 15, no. 12, pp. 661–664, 2019.

[37] T. Duman, D. Uluduz, I. Midi et al., "A multicenter study of 1144 patients with cerebral venous thrombosis: the VENOST study," *Journal of Stroke and Cerebrovascular Diseases*, vol. 26, no. 8, pp. 1848–1857, 2017.

[38] J. M. Ferro, J. M. Coutinho, F. Dentali et al., "Safety and efficacy of dabigatran etexilate vs dose-adjusted warfarin in patients with cerebral venous thrombosis: a randomized clinical trial," *JAMA Neurology*, vol. 76, no. 12, p. 1457, 2019.

[39] C. Geisbüsch, D. Richter, C. Herweh, P. A. Ringleb, and S. Nagel, "Novel factor xa inhibitor for the treatment of cerebral venous and sinus thrombosis," *Stroke*, vol. 45, no. 8, pp. 2469–2471, 2014.

[40] M. D. Mendonça, R. Barbosa, V. Cruz-e-Silva, S. Calado, and M. Viana-Baptista, "Oral direct thrombin inhibitor as an alternative in the management of cerebral venous thrombosis: a series of 15 patients," *International Journal of Stroke*, vol. 10, no. 7, pp. 1115–1118, 2015.

[41] J. M. Ferro, P. Canhão, J. Stam, M.-G. Bousser, and F. Barinagarrementeria, "Prognosis of cerebral vein and dural sinus thrombosis," *Stroke*, vol. 35, no. 3, pp. 664–670, 2004.

[42] V. Desa and R. Green, "Cavernous sinus thrombosis: current therapy," *Journal of Oral and Maxillofacial Surgery*, vol. 70, no. 9, pp. 2085–2091, 2012.

26

An Incidental Finding of Gastric Mucosa-Associated Lymphoma (MALToma) in a Sleeve Gastrectomy with Literature Review

Brenda Mai, Michaelangelo Friscia, Pamela Younes, Jaiyeola Thomas-Ogunniyi, and Lei Chen

Department of Pathology and Laboratory Medicine, McGovern Medical School at the University of Texas Health Science Center, 6431 Fannin Street, Houston, TX, USA

Correspondence should be addressed to Lei Chen; lei.chen.1@uth.tmc.edu

Academic Editor: John Frater

Mucosal-associated lymphoid tissue (MALT) lymphoma can typically be identified as a mass lesion or nodularity endoscopically and macroscopically. We report an incidental finding of a *Helicobacter pylori* gastric mucosal-associated lymphoid tissue (MALT) lymphoma in a sleeve gastrectomy specimen with no gross examination findings.

1. Introduction

The macroscopic examination of specimens and the selection of representative sections for subsequent microscopic examination are crucial and fundamental to the accurate diagnoses in pathology. William Grossman claims that in over 90% of specimens, an accurate diagnosis can be made with just the gross examination only [1]. The decline of autopsies and the rise in reliance on pathologists' assistants (PAs) for handling and processing specimens have resulted in a decrease in exposure to gross findings for pathologists and residents in training [2]. However, the gross examination and description can greatly aid in diagnoses and reveal new incidental lesions that are important to patient outcomes. We report an incidental finding of a gastric mucosal-associated lymphoid tissue (MALT) lymphoma in a sleeve gastrectomy specimen.

2. Case Presentation

This case report describes a 54-year-old male who underwent a laparoscopic sleeve resection procedure for morbid obesity. Prior to the procedure, the patient had a weight of 115.9 kilograms and a body mass index (BMI) of 49.77 and had failed both diet and medical weight management. His other medical history included hypertension, dyslipidemia, and sigmoid diverticulosis. His surgical history comprised of a laparoscopic cholecystectomy and an open reduction internal fixation of fracture on his ankle. He has a family history of diabetes mellitus type 2 in both parents. The patient admitted to drinking alcohol weekly but denied tobacco and recreational drug use. Physical examination did not reveal lymphadenopathy or hepatosplenomegaly. Preoperative evaluation of the peripheral blood was within normal limits with no evidence of a hematological malignancy or lymphoproliferative process. In addition, the patient did not have any positive findings on review of systems or any symptoms. Preoperative gastroduodenoscopy did not reveal any lesions; however, two antral biopsies were taken which revealed mild chronic inactive gastritis. A "sleeve gastrectomy specimen" was received in the pathology department. On gross examination, the gastric mucosa was described as tan-pink, smooth, and glistening with a focal area of hemorrhage (Figure 1). There were no masses, no nodularities, no ulceration, or abnormal rugal folds. Representative sections of the hemorrhagic region were taken, along with several routine random areas of normal-appearing mucosa. Other than the focal area of hemorrhage,

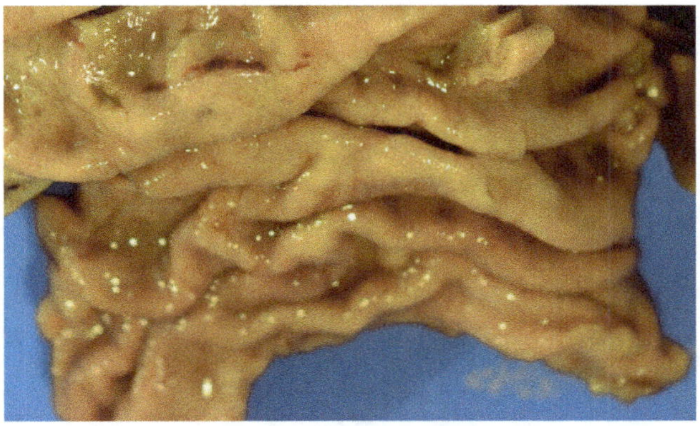

Figure 1: Sleeve gastrectomy specimen with focal area of petechial hemorrhage.

there was little evidence to indicate an underlying pathological process or malignancy, as small hemorrhagic areas are common findings in surgical specimens. On histological examination, sections taken from the hemorrhagic areas showed a diffuse atypical lymphoid infiltrate extending into the lamina propria and submucosa, with nodular pattern and focal germinal centers (Figure 2). Proliferation of plasma cells was also evident. In addition, there was an associated architectural distortion with gastric glandular atrophy (Figure 3). Immunohistochemical stains with the appropriate controls were obtained revealing diffuse sheets of lymphoma cells that were positive for CD20, CD43, and BCL-2. They were negative for CD3, CD5, CD23, CD138, BCL-6, and Cyclin D1. The plasma cells were monoclonal with kappa restriction. The proliferation index by Ki-67 was low, approximately 1–5%, except for the reactive germinal centers. *Helicobacter (H.) pylori* stain on three of the blocks was negative. With these histological findings, the patient was diagnosed with a MALToma. Positron emission tomography (PET) scan was performed which revealed a lesion in the sigmoid colon. Subsequently, the patient underwent another round of biopsies which showed mild chronic inactive gastritis within the stomach and benign lymphoid aggregates in the colon. The patient was placed on omeprazole, clairthromycin, and amoxicillin. And, six-month follow-up established endoscopic and histologic remission.

3. Discussion

This is not the first case report of an incidental MALT lymphoma in a sleeve gastrectomy, as several other investigators have identified a MALT lymphoma in other bariatric specimens [3–6]. A literature review found 4 other case reports with a MALToma diagnosed within a sleeve gastrectomy specimen (Table 1). There was no sex predilection as there were 3 males and 2 females. The average age at diagnosis was 47 years of age with an age range of 28 to 59. The BMIs averaged 49.1 with a range of 45 to 60. One of the cases did not comment on the gross examination of the sleeve gastrectomy specimen, whereas the remaining 3 cases reported a mass ranging in size from 1.2 to 18 cm. The

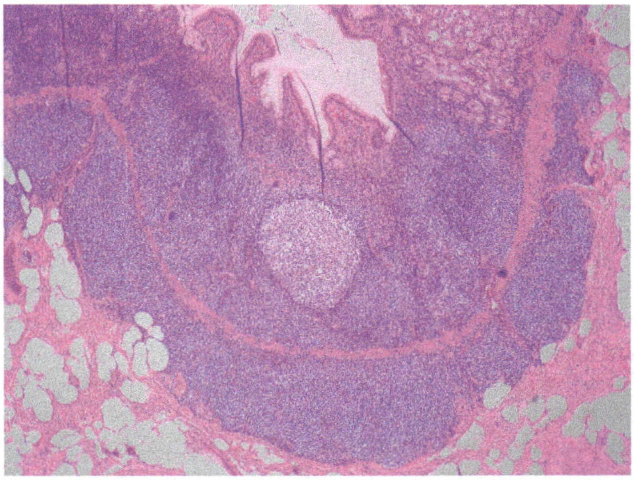

Figure 2: Atypical lymphoid aggregates expanding the lamina propria (hematoxylin and eosin; 40*x*).

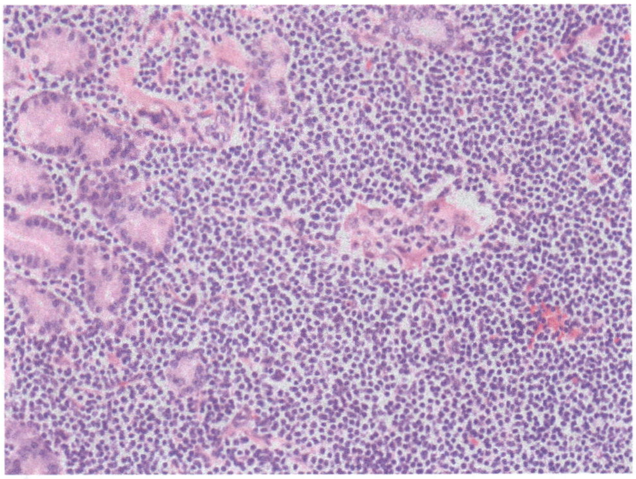

Figure 3: Glandular destruction secondary to the neoplastic lymphoid cells (hematoxylin and eosin; 200*x*).

Table 1: Incidental MALToma in sleeve gastrectomy samples.

	This case	De Silva et al.	Kopach et al.	Quesada et al.	Helman et al.
Age	54	59	39	53	28
Sex	M	F	M	M	F
BMI	49.77	45	44.8	60	46
Gross findings	Focal hemorrhage	18 × 3 cm mass	No information	8 cm mass	1.8 × 1.2 cm mass
H. pylori	Negative	Negative	Negative	No information	Negative

H. pylori status was available for all but 1 of the cases and they were negative.

Interestingly, this case report was the only case report that had no significant gross findings, whereas all the other cases reported identified a mass lesion in the specimen. A recent article by AbdullGaffar et al. challenges the need for routine microscopic evaluation of bariatric sleeve gastrectomy specimens [7]. Their prospective study identified 546 specimens and reported that there was no malignancy and less than five of the specimens had benign incidental findings. The researchers emphasize a thorough macroscopic evaluation only of these specimens to save time and cost, as incidental malignant findings are rare. A metanalysis study by Zullo et al. combined the data from 38 manuscripts with a total of over 2000 patients with MALTomas and concluded that MALTomas had the following endoscopic findings: 52.1% ulcerative pattern, 23.5% hypertrophic rugal folds, 12.7% normal or hyperemic mucosa, 9.7% exophytic mass, and 1% petechial hemorrhage. We would like to comment that although incidental findings are rare, they are still significant and greatly impact patient care and outcomes [8]. In addition, with the rising epidemic in obesity and bariatric procedures, we suggest that the practice of gross examination, proper sampling techniques, and microscopic examination be preserved for bariatric specimens.

In conclusion, our case emphasizes the importance of examining surgical specimens both macroscopically and microscopically for the identification of incidental malignant findings in asymptomatic patients. Although a large majority of MALTomas can be identified with gross lesions endoscopically and macroscopically on the specimen, a small percent of MALTomas have no gross findings. It is imperative to perform representative sampling on these specimens.

References

[1] I. W. Grossman, *A Primer of Gross Pathology*, Charles C Thomas Pub, Springfield, IL, USA, 1972.

[2] S. A. Geller and R. E. Horowitz, "Gross examination," in *Histopathology. Methods in Molecular Biology (Methods and Protocols)*, C. Day, Ed., vol. 1180, pp. 3–19, Humana Press, New York, NY, USA, 2014.

[3] R. Piyumal De Silva, S. Jaffar, and M. Devadas, "Laparoscopic sleeve gastrectomy—an unexpected finding: MALT lymphoma in a *H. pylori*-negative patient," *International Journal of Surgery Research and Practice*, vol. 4, p. 56, 2017.

[4] P. Kopach, E. M. Genega, S. N. Shah, J. J. Kim, and Y. Suarez, "The significance of histologic examination of gastrectomy specimens: a clinicopathologic study of 511 cases," *Surgery for Obesity and Related Diseases*, vol. 13, no. 3, pp. 463–467, 2017.

[5] B. M. Quesada, H. E. Roff, and L. T. Chiappetta Porras, "Intraoperative finding of a gastric lymphoma during gastric bypass surgery," *Obesity Surgery*, vol. 17, no. 6, pp. 847-848, 2007.

[6] R. Helman, P. P. Dos Santos Teixeira, C. J. L. Mendes, T. Szegö, and N. Hamershlak, "Gastric MALT lymphoma and grade II obesity: gastric bypass surgery as a therapeutic option," *Obesity Surgery*, vol. 21, no. 3, pp. 407–409, 2011.

[7] B. AbdullGaffar, L. Raman, A. Khamas, and F. AlBadri, "Should we abandon routine microscopic examination in bariatric sleeve gastrectomy specimens?" *Obesity Surgery*, vol. 26, no. 1, pp. 105–110, 2016.

[8] A. Zullo, C. Hassan, A. Andriani et al., "Primary low-grade and high grade gastric MALT lymphoma presentation," *Journal of Clinical Gastroenterology*, vol. 44, no. 5, pp. 340–344, 2010.

27

A Rare Case of Histiocytic Sarcoma Secondary to Gastrointestinal Stromal Tumor in the Stomach: Transdifferentiation or Synchronicity?

Jiankun Tong,[1] Jean Luo,[1] Pierre F. Saldinger,[2,3] and William H. Rodgers[1,3]

[1]*Department of Pathology, New York Presbyterian Queens, 56-45 Main Street, Flushing, NY 11355, USA*
[2]*Department of Surgery, New York Presbyterian Queens, 56-45 Main Street, Flushing, NY 11355, USA*
[3]*Weill Cornell Medical College, 525 East 68th Street, Box 130, New York, NY 10065, USA*

Correspondence should be addressed to Jiankun Tong; jtong90@hotmail.com

Academic Editor: Kostas Konstantopoulos

Histiocytic sarcoma is a rare malignant histiocytic neoplasm composed of cells with morphologic and immunophenotypic features of mature tissue histiocytes. It occurs anywhere in the body and behaves aggressively. However, its etiology is unknown. Here, we report a 68-year-old female who developed histiocytic sarcoma following chemotherapy with imatinib (Gleevec) for gastrointestinal stromal tumor. Possible mechanisms of transdifferentiation from gastrointestinal stromal tumor to histiocytic sarcoma are discussed based on the features of our case and other two similar cases in the literature.

1. Case Presentation

A 68-year-old female was suspected to have recurrent gastrointestinal stromal tumor (GIST) of stomach and was admitted to the hospital for an exploratory laparotomy with gastric wedge resection of greater curvature.

The patient had a history of GIST six years ago, being in remission after chemotherapy with imatinib (Gleevec) and partial gastrectomy. Four months ago, she had abdominal stress and chronic constipation. She denied fever, chills, nausea, vomiting, or abdominal pain. Laboratory analysis revealed mild anemia. An abdominal CT scan detected a gastric mass in the left upper quadrant, arising from the posterior aspect of the gastric body adjacent to the greater curvature and measuring $13.1 \times 11.4 \times 10.7$ cm (Figure 1(a)). Endosonography confirmed a round intramural lesion in the body of the stomach, which appeared to originate from the muscularis propria involving the submucosal layer. Fine needle biopsy of the gastric mass showed epithelioid and short spindle cells with nuclear hyperchromasia and mild pleomorphism (Figures 2(a) and 2(b)). The tumor cells were positive for CD34 (Figure 2(c)) and CD117 (Figure 2(d))—immunohistochemical features that are diagnostic of gastrointestinal stromal tumor (GIST).

After treatment with imatinib for 6 months, the patient was admitted for selective partial gastrectomy after a follow-up CT scan of the tumor only indicated a slight interval decrease in size (Figure 1(b)).

2. Diagnosis

The partial gastrectomy specimen was submitted for histopathologic examination. Grossly, a mass lesion (9.5 cm) was identified between muscularis propria and serosa. The lesion consisted of a central cavity (6.0 cm) that contained two small distinct nodules (1.0 cm and 0.6 cm) along its border. The lesion consisted of fibrotic stroma (80% of the entire mass) with postchemotherapy effects (Figure 3(a)). This cavity represented the previous GIST biopsy site. Microscopically, both small nodules consisted of large atypical epithelioid cells with abundant eosinophilic, finely granular cytoplasm, and round nuclei with prominent nucleoli (Figures 3(b) and 3(c)). Mitotic figures were markedly increased (approximately 7 per 10 high power field). Small

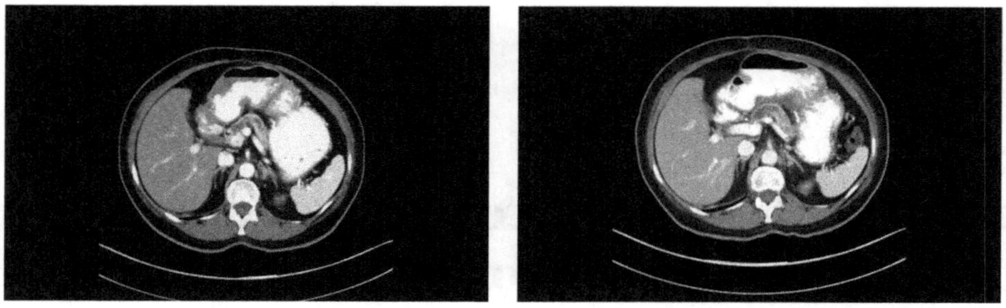

(a) (b)

FIGURE 1: CT scan of abdomen showing a 13.1 × 11.4 × 10.7 cm mass from the posterior aspect of the gastric body (a). Repeat CT scan of abdomen revealing the persistent presence of the mass after chemotherapy with imatinib for 6 months (b).

reactive lymphocytes were present in the background. Immunohistochemically, the large neoplastic cells were positive for CD4 (Figure 3(d)), CD10, CD31, CD45 (weak) (Figure 3(e)), CD68 (Figure 3(f)), CD163 (Figure 3(g)), HLA-DR, lysozyme, and vimentin, while they were negative for ALK-1, AE1/AE3, calretinin, CAM5.2, CD1a, CD3, CD15, CD20, CD21, CD30, CD34 (Figure 3(h)), CD35, CD43, CD117 (Figure 3(i)), CD123, chromogranin, desmin, DOG-1, EMA, HepPar-1, HMB-45, MART-1, MPO, S100, SMA, synaptophysin, TdT, and WT-1. The Ki-67 proliferative index was approximately 20–25%. The overall immunohistologic features were typical of histiocytic sarcoma (HS). Unexpectedly, there was no residual GIST despite histologic examination of the entire lesion. No BRAF mutation was detected by molecular analysis of both the original biopsy specimen of GIST and the current surgical specimen of HS.

3. Discussion

Histiocytic sarcoma (HS) is a rare malignancy that accounts for less than 1% of all hematolymphoid neoplasms [1, 2]. Lymph nodes are most commonly involved. The gastrointestinal tract is the most frequent extranodal site. Other less frequent extranodal sites are spleen, soft tissue, and skin [3, 4]. HS can be localized and disseminated. It affects the patients with a wide age range, from infancy to elderly; but it most commonly occurs in adults with the median age of 52 [3–6].

The rarity of HS makes it a difficult diagnosis, and it is often confused with other benign or malignant neoplasms. Its diagnosis is mainly based on morphology and immunohistochemistry, following exclusion of other hematopoietic and nonhematopoietic neoplasms. The former includes other histiocytic and dendritic cell neoplasms, myeloid sarcoma, anaplastic large cell lymphoma, and diffuse large B-cell lymphoma. The latter comprises malignant melanoma and undifferentiated or poorly differentiated carcinoma. Although each of the differential diagnoses shares morphologic and immunophenotypic features with HS, a correct diagnosis can be reached by careful examination and comprehensive immunohistochemical analysis.

The etiology of HS is unknown. Based on the 2017 World Health Organization (WHO) classification, HS is described as a malignant proliferation of cells showing morphological and immunophenotypic features of mature tissue histiocytes. Some cases report clonal IG and T-cell receptor gene rearrangements, most likely constituting examples of transdifferentiation [6]. Transdifferentiation, also known as lineage reprogramming, is the conversion of a cell type present in one tissue or organ into a cell type from another tissue or organ without going through a pluripotent cell intermediate. Previous publications report an association or concurrence of HS with a variety of malignancies, especially B-cell-associated hematopoietic neoplasms such as B-lymphoblast leukemia/lymphoma [7–10], chronic lymphocytic leukemia/small lymphocytic lymphoma [11], follicular lymphoma [12–15], hairy cell leukemia [16], MALT lymphoma [17], and mantle cell lymphoma [18]. It has been reported that HS occurred with myeloid neoplasms such as acute monocytic leukemia [19], chronic myeloid leukemia [20], chronic myelomonocytic leukemia [21], and idiopathic primary myelofibrosis [22]. These publications have provided direct and indirect evidence of the possibility of transdifferentiation between the two otherwise morphologically and immunohistochemically distinct neoplasms. A subset of HS cases occurs in patients with mediastinal germ cell tumors, most frequently malignant teratoma, with or without a yolk sac tumor component [23].

GIST is the most common mesenchymal tumor occurring in the gastrointestinal tract, especially in the stomach (56%), followed by the small intestine (32%), colorectum (6%), and esophagus (<1%) [24]. It rarely involves the omentum, mesentery, and peritoneum [24]. Interstitial cells of Cajal (ICCs) have been identified as the likely precursor cells of GIST. ICCs are located between the layers of the muscularis propria of the gastrointestinal tract in the regulation of gut peristalsis [25, 26]. They are thought to be pacemaker cells of the gastrointestinal tract. Immunohistochemically, they are usually positive for CD117 (KIT), CD34, and DOG-1. Some cases are focally or diffusely positive for SMA. Less than 5% of cases are weakly positive for Desmin and S100. Therefore, it is believed that these ICCs may have ultrastructural and immunophenotypic features of smooth muscle and neuronal differentiation.

In general, GISTs show a remarkable variability in their differentiation pathways, and GISTs can be roughly divided

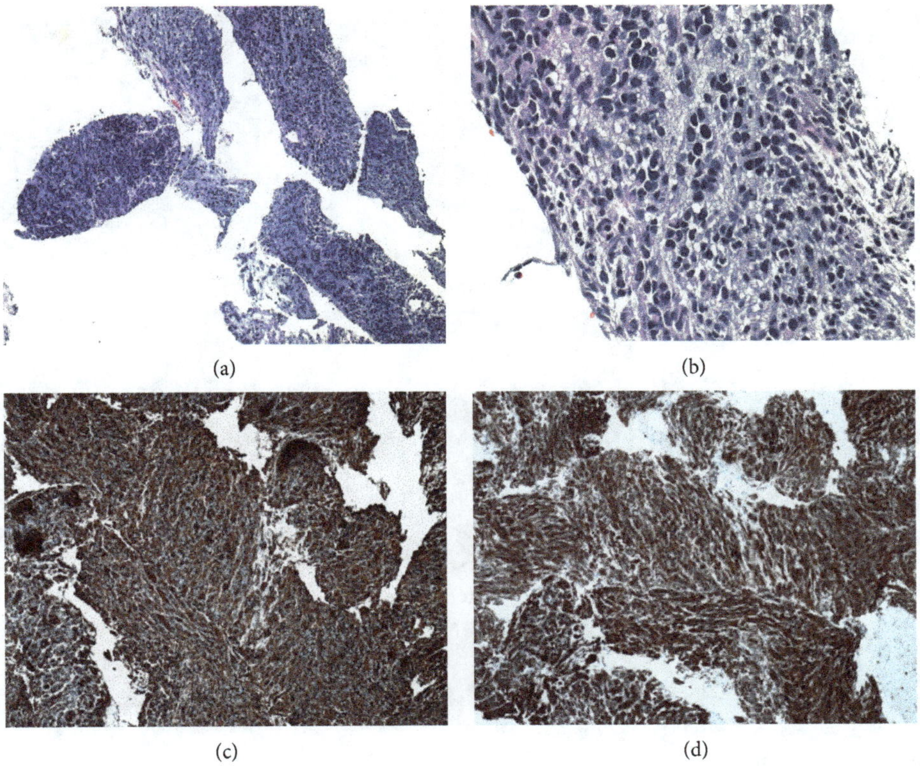

FIGURE 2: H&E sections showing atypical cellular proliferation of epithelioid cells and some spindle cells (×10) (a). The tumor cells showing round or oval nuclei with nuclear hyperchromasia (×40) (b) and expressing CD34 (c) and CD117 (d).

into four categories: tumors showing differentiation toward smooth muscle cells, neural-type elements, dual differentiation toward smooth muscle and neural-type elements, and those lacking differentiation toward either cell type [27]. Morphologically, GIST shows the spindle cell growth pattern, the epithelioid growth pattern, and the mixed growth pattern.

3.1. Is It Possible That HS in Our Case Is Transdifferentiated from GIST? Recently, there have been two case reports of HS together with GIST. One report of HS in the intestine occurred in a previously treated case of GIST in the stomach, following two years of treatment [28]. A second case report documented synchronous HS and GIST as a single gastric mass [29]. Now, we report a rare case of a 68-year-old female developing HS secondary to GIST in the stomach after chemotherapy with imatinib and partial gastrectomy.

In our case, we observed two very interesting phenomena. First, both the GIST and HS demonstrated a similar epithelioid morphology although the tumor cells exhibited different immunophenotypes and cellular sizes. The cell size of HS is much bigger than that of GIST. Secondly, the two nodules with HS are located in the inner surface of the mass cavity with stromal fibrosis, which represents the previous biopsy site of GIST. This may imply that the HS developed concurrently or subsequently from GIST after chemotherapy, suggesting that chemotherapy may be a triggering factor for the interstitial cells of Cajal (ICCs) or GIST to transdifferentiate to HS.

3.2. Can Treatment Cause a Transdifferentiation from GIST to HS? It has been observed that the interval between the occurrence of lymphoma and that of HS varies between 2 months and 17 years [5]. In our case, the patient received imatinib treatment initially seven years ago and then again one year after recurrence of the mass. Imatinib therapy has been successfully used for treating chronic myeloid leukemia (CML). Imatinib discontinuation trials typically follow two distinct outcomes: one group with relapse and the other group remaining disease-free throughout the duration of follow-up [30]. Tang et al. explained this mechanism in the imatinib-treated CML patients by suggesting that imatinib therapy leads to a rise of leukemic clones, which have different growth and differentiation properties compared to the predominant clone at the start of therapy [30].

Accordingly, transdifferentiation between cell types can occur naturally in response to tissue damage, and it can also be induced experimentally. It has been reported that blockade of KIT signaling induces transdifferentiation of interstitial cells of Cajal to a smooth muscle phenotype [31]. Perhaps transdifferentiation toward HS may be a product of the interaction of interstitial cells of Cajal with the effects of imatinib plus other intrinsic host factors, such as immune system and tumor microenvironment factors.

3.3. BRAF Mutation in Both GIST and HS. BRAF V600 E point mutation activates the preoncogene BRAF and has been reported in many hematopoietic and non-hematopoietic neoplasms. Although KIT and PDGFR are the

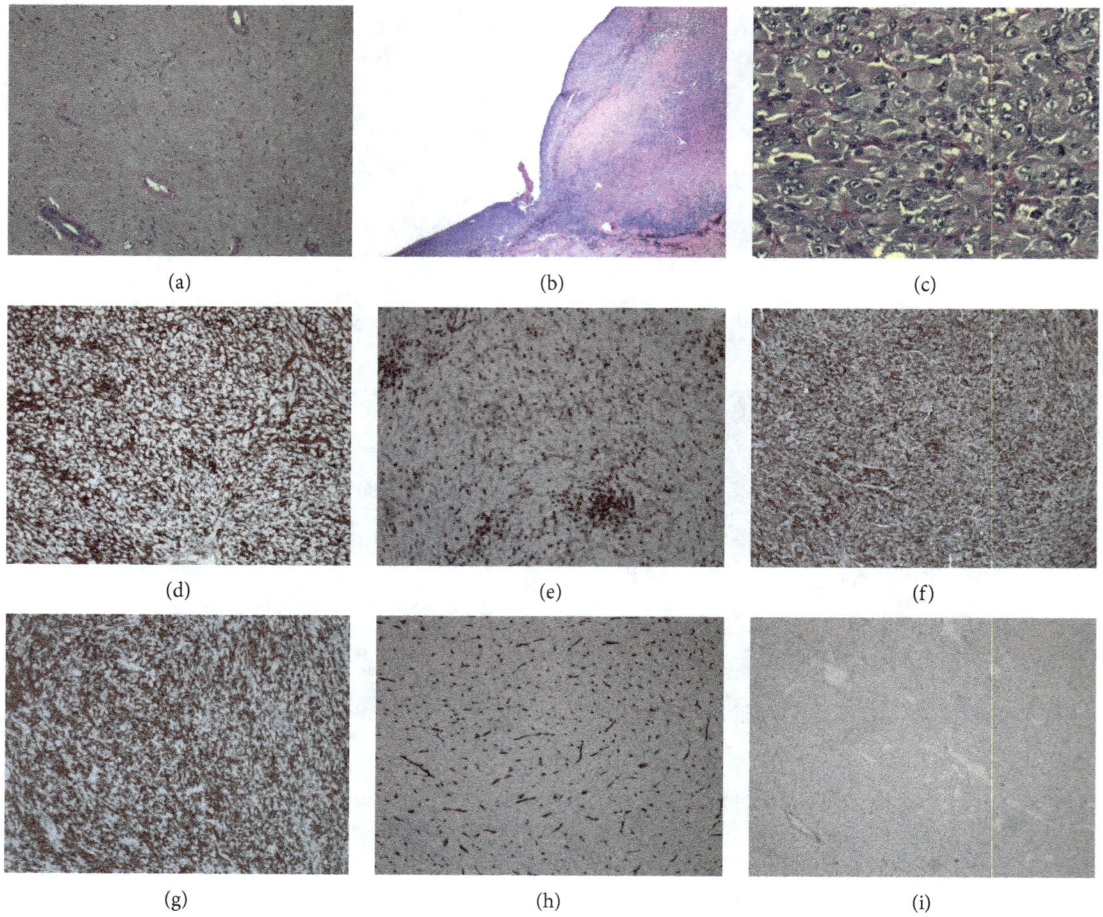

FIGURE 3: The 9.5 cm mass lesion consists predominantly of fibrotic stroma (80% of the mass) (×10) (a) with two distinct nodules measuring 1.0 cm and 0.6 cm (×2) (b). The two nodules are located in the inner surface of prior GIST cavity showing large atypical epithelioid cells with abundant eosinophilic cytoplasm and prominent nucleoli (×40) (c). The cells were positive for CD4 (d), CD45 (e), CD68 (f), and CD163 (g), while negative for CD34 (h) and CD117 (i).

two most common mutations in the GIST, BRAF V600 E mutation has been identified from 4% to 13% of the patients with KIT/PDGFRA wild-type GIST [32, 33]. BRAF V600 E mutation has also been found in some HS cases [16, 34, 35]. In one study, 5 of 8 HS cases were noted to have BRAF V600 E mutation [34]. To investigate whether BRAF V600 E mutation acts as a driver mutation favoring malignant transdifferentiation from GIST to HS, molecular studies for BRAF mutation were performed on previous and current specimens. No BRAF mutation was detected in either the GIST or HS tumors in our case.

3.4. RAS-MAPK Pathway Mutations. Just recently, Hornick's group has identified diverse and activating RAS-MAPK and PI3K-AKT-MTOR pathway mutations and CDKN2A tumor-suppressor gene alterations in the majority of histiocytic sarcomas by using a targeted next-generation sequencing approach [36]. Furthermore, a subset of cases harboring these mutations also show striking genetic similarities with B-cell lymphomas [36]. Whether these mutations concurrently exist in our GIST and HS cases is not clear. We believe that the targeted next-generation sequencing approach will provide a very useful tool to investigate these mutations and shed light on the future direction of demonstrating the possible mechanism of transdifferentiation from GIST to HS.

In conclusion, here, we reported a rare case of HS secondary to GIST in the stomach and discussed the possibility of transdifferentiation and synchronicity.

References

[1] C. A. Hanson, W. Jaszcz, J. H. Kersey et al., "True histiocytic lymphoma: histopathologic, immunophenotypic and genotypic analysis," *British Journal of Haematology*, vol. 73, no. 2, pp. 187–198, 1989.

[2] E. Ralfkiaer, G. Delsol, N. T. J. O'Connor et al., "Malignant lymphomas of true histiocytic origin. A clinical, histological, immunophenotypic and genotypic study," *The Journal of Pathology*, vol. 160, no. 1, pp. 9–17, 1990.

[3] J. L. Hornick, E. S. Jaffe, and C. D. M. Fletcher, "Extranodal histiocytic sarcoma," *American Journal of Surgical Pathology*, vol. 28, no. 9, pp. 1133–1144, 2004.

[4] E. Takahashi and S. Nakamura, "Histiocytic sarcoma: an updated literature review based on the 2008 WHO classification," *Journal of Clinical and Experimental Hematopathology*, vol. 53, no. 1, pp. 1–8, 2013.
[5] S. A. Pileri, T. M. Grogan, N. L. Harris et al., "Tumours of histiocytes and accessory dendritic cells: an immunohistochemical approach to classification from the International Lymphoma Study Group based on 61 cases," *Histopathology*, vol. 41, no. 1, pp. 1–29, 2002.
[6] S. H. Swerdlow, E. Campo, N. L. Harris et al., *WHO Classification of Tumor of Haematopoietic and Lymphoid Tissue*, pp. 468–470, WHO, Geneva, Switzerland, 2017.
[7] R. McClure, J. Khoury, A. Feldman, and R. Ketterling, "Clonal relationship between precursor B-cell acute lymphoblastic leukemia and histiocytic sarcoma: a case report and discussion in the context of similar cases," *Leukemia Research*, vol. 34, no. 2, pp. e71–e73, 2010.
[8] E. C. C. Castro, C. Blazquez, J. Boyd et al., "Clinicopathologic features of histiocytic lesions following ALL, with a review of the literature," *Pediatric and Developmental Pathology*, vol. 13, no. 3, pp. 225–237, 2010.
[9] R. Kumar, S. P. Khan, D.-D. Joshi, G. R. Shaw, R. P. Ketterling, and A. L. Feldman, "Pediatric histiocytic sarcoma clonally related to precursor B-cell acute lymphoblastic leukemia with homozygous deletion of CDKN2A encoding p16INK4A," *Pediatric Blood & Cancer*, vol. 56, no. 2, pp. 307–310, 2011.
[10] R. Bouabdallah, P. Abéna, B. Chetaille et al., "True histiocytic lymphoma following B-acute lymphoblastic leukaemia: case report with evidence for a common clonal origin in both neoplasms," *British Journal of Haematology*, vol. 113, no. 4, pp. 1047–1050, 2001.
[11] H. Shao, L. Xi, M. Raffeld et al., "Clonally related histiocytic/dendritic cell sarcoma and chronic lymphocytic leukemia/small lymphocytic lymphoma: a study of seven cases," *Modern Pathology*, vol. 24, no. 11, pp. 1421–1432, 2011.
[12] E. Wang, J. Papalas, C. B. Hutchinson et al., "Sequential development of histiocytic sarcoma and diffuse large B-cell lymphoma in a patient with a remote history of follicular lymphoma with genotypic evidence of a clonal relationship," *American Journal of Surgical Pathology*, vol. 35, no. 3, pp. 457–463, 2011.
[13] A. L. Feldman, D. A. Arber, S. Pittaluga et al., "Clonally related follicular lymphomas and histiocytic/dendritic cell sarcomas: evidence for transdifferentiation of the follicular lymphoma clone," *Blood*, vol. 111, no. 12, pp. 5433–5439, 2008.
[14] D. Zhang, J. McGuirk, S. Ganguly, and D. L. Persons, "Histiocytic/dendritic cell sarcoma arising from follicular lymphoma involving the bone: a case report and review of literature," *International Journal of Hematology*, vol. 89, no. 4, pp. 529–532, 2009.
[15] P. Brunner, A. Rufle, S. Dirnhofer et al., "Follicular lymphoma transformation into histiocytic sarcoma: indications for a common neoplastic progenitor," *Leukemia*, vol. 28, no. 9, pp. 1937–1940, 2014.
[16] D. Michonneau, S. Kaltenbach, C. Derrieux et al., "BRAFV600E mutation in a histiocytic sarcoma arising from hairy cell leukemia," *Journal of Clinical Oncology*, vol. 32, no. 35, pp. e117–e121, 2014.
[17] T. Álvaro, R. Bosch, M. T. Salvadó, and M. A. Piris, "True histiocytic lymphoma of the stomach associated with low-grade B-cell mucosa-associated lymphoid tissue (Malt)-type lymphoma," *The American Journal of Surgical Pathology*, vol. 20, no. 11, pp. 1406–1411, 1996.
[18] M. C. Hure, C. P. Elco, D. Ward et al., "Histiocytic sarcoma arising from clonally related mantle cell lymphoma," *Journal of Clinical Oncology*, vol. 30, no. 5, pp. e49–e53, 2012.
[19] J. Zhao, X. Niu, Z. Wang, H. Lu, X. Lin, and Q. Lu, "Histiocytic sarcoma combined with acute monocytic leukemia: a case report," *Diagn Pathol*, vol. 10, p. 110, 2015.
[20] J. Ansari, A. R. Naqash, R. Munker et al., "Histiocytic sarcoma as a secondary malignancy: pathobiology, diagnosis, and treatment," *European Journal of Haematology*, vol. 97, no. 1, pp. 9–16, 2016.
[21] M. Mori, A. Matsushita, Y. Takiuchi et al., "Histiocytic sarcoma and underlying chronic myelomonocytic leukemia: a proposal for the developmental classification of histiocytic sarcoma," *International Journal of Hematology*, vol. 92, no. 1, pp. 168–173, 2010.
[22] M. Fukunaga and H. Kato, "Histiocytic sarcoma associated with idiopathic myelofibrosis," *Archives of Pathology & Laboratory Medicine*, vol. 128, no. 10, pp. 1167–1170, 2004.
[23] S. H. deMent, "Association between mediastinal germ cell tumors and hematologic malignancies: an update," *Human Pathology*, vol. 21, no. 7, pp. 699–703, 1990.
[24] L. C. Harlan, J. Eisenstein, M. C. Russell, J. L. Stevens, and K. Cardona, "Gastrointestinal stromal tumors: treatment patterns of a population-based sample," *Journal of Surgical Oncology*, vol. 111, no. 6, pp. 702–707, 2015.
[25] L. G. Kindblom, H. E. Remotti, F. Aldenborg, and J. M. Meis-Kindblom, "Gastrointestinal pacemaker cell tumor (GIPACT): gastrointestinal stromal tumors show phenotypic characteristics of the interstitial cells of Cajal," *The American Journal of Pathology*, vol. 152, no. 5, pp. 1259–1269, 1998.
[26] K. Sircar, B. R. Hewlett, J. D. Huizinga, K. Chorneyko, I. Berezin, and R. H. Riddell, "Interstitial cells of Cajal as precursors of gastrointestinal stromal tumors," *The American Journal of Surgical Pathology*, vol. 23, no. 4, pp. 377–389, 1999.
[27] R. Juan, *Rosai and Ackmerman's surgical pathology*, Elsevier, vol. 2pp. P638–P644, Amsterdam, Netherlands, Tenth edition, 2018.
[28] A. Gangoli, K. Sharma, and K. Chaudhary, "A histiocytic twist in a tale of GIST," *Case Reports in Clinical Pathology*, vol. 3, no. 4, 2016.
[29] I. Obiorah, S. Han, and O. Metin, "Synchronous histiocytic sarcoma and gastrointestinal stromal tumor presenting as a gastric mass," *AJCP*, vol. 150, p. S32, 2018.
[30] M. Tang, J. Foo, M. Gönen, J. Guilhot, F.-X. Mahon, and F. Michor, "Selection pressure exerted by imatinib therapy leads to disparate outcomes of imatinib discontinuation trials," *Haematologica*, vol. 97, no. 10, pp. 1553–1561, 2012.
[31] S. Torihashi, K. Nishi, Y. Tokutomi, T. Nishi, S. Ward, and K. M. Sanders, "Blockade of kit signaling induces transdifferentiation of interstitial cells of cajal to a smooth muscle phenotype," *Gastroenterology*, vol. 117, no. 1, pp. 140–148, 1999.
[32] A. Kalfusova, Z. Linke, M. Kalinova et al., "Gastrointestinal stromal tumors - summary of mutational status of the primary/secondary KIT/PDGFRA mutations, BRAF mutations and SDH defects," *Pathology - Research and Practice*, vol. 215, no. 12, p. 152708, 2019.
[33] I. Hostein, N. Faur, C. Primois et al., "BRAFMutation status in gastrointestinal stromal tumors," *American Journal of Clinical Pathology*, vol. 133, no. 1, pp. 141–148, 2010.
[34] H. Go, "Frequent detection of BRAF (V600E) mutations in histiocytic and dendritic cell neoplasms," *Histopathology*, vol. 65, no. 2, pp. 261–272, 2014.

[35] J. L. Vaughn, C. E. Freitag, J. A. Hemminger, and J. A. Jones, "BRAF V600E expression in histiocytic sarcoma associated with splenic marginal zone lymphoma: a case report," *Journal of Medical Case Reports*, vol. 11, no. 1, p. 92, 2017.
[36] V. Shanmugam, G. K. Griffin, E. D. Jacobsen, C. D. M. Fletcher, L. M. Sholl, and J. L. Hornick, "Identification of diverse activating mutations of the RAS-MAPK pathway in histiocytic sarcoma," *Modern Pathology*, vol. 32, no. 6, pp. 830–843, 2019.

28

Dasatinib and FLAG-IDA is an Effective Therapy for Initial Myeloid Blast Crisis but Involves a High Risk of Opportunistic Infections

Jorge Labrador, Gerardo J. Hermida, Rodolfo Alvarez, Victor Anso, Pilar de Vicente, Mercedes Goñi, and Tomas Jose Gonzalez-Lopez

Department of Hematology, University Hospital of Burgos, Burgos, Spain

Correspondence should be addressed to Tomas Jose Gonzalez-Lopez; tjgonzalez@saludcastillayleon.es

Academic Editor: Håkon Reikvam

Blast crisis (BC) continues to be the major challenge in the treatment of chronic myeloid leukemia. Best results have been observed in a few patients who were successfully transplanted after returning to chronic phase. Recent studies focus on the combination of chemotherapy with imatinib, but results remain unsatisfactory. Since dasatinib induces deeper and faster responses, a reasonable strategy might be to combine it with chemotherapy, taking into account the alterations in T-cell response induced by dasatinib. However, there are no published studies or case reports supporting the use of dasatinib as first line treatment for initial myeloid BC, and very little is known about infectious complications associated with this drug. Based on this, we present the case of a patient diagnosed with an initial nonlymphoid phenotype BC, who achieved molecular response ($MR^{4.5}$) with dasatinib and FLAG-IDA, but he suffered a pulmonary aspergillosis, CMV infection, and a CMV reactivation, prior to an allogeneic hematopoietic stem cell transplantation (HSCT). In conclusion, dasatinib and FLAG-IDA is an effective therapy for initial BC. However, a warning call is needed owing to the high risk of opportunistic infections, such as CMV.

1. Introduction

The outcome of patients diagnosed with chronic myeloid leukemia (CML) has improved considerably since the introduction of tyrosine kinase inhibitors (TKIs) in clinical practice. However, the prognosis of patients who progress to blast crisis (BC) remains extremely poor [1]. In addition, 10–15% of patients initially present with blast crisis.

According to blast lineage, BC is classified into lymphoid (20–30%) and myeloid (70%), with different treatment approaches [2]. While lymphoid BC often responds to treatment used for Ph + acute lymphoblastic leukemia, myeloid BC does not respond well to standard induction regimens used for acute myeloid leukemia [3].

Imatinib alone induces hematological responses in 24–32% of patients with myeloid blast crisis, including 2–8% of complete cytogenetic responses [4–7]. But, unfortunately, duration of these responses is very short [1]. The median response duration in different studies varies between 3 and 10 months (range, 1–43 months) [4–7].

Dasatinib induces 23% of hematological responses in these patients with a higher rate of complete cytogenetic responses (14–21%) [8]. Moreover, it has a faster response (between 1 and 2 months) and has the advantage that it crosses the blood-brain barrier. However, approximately half of patients relapse within 4 months (95% CI: 3.0–6.2 months), and median overall survival is only 8 months [8].

The best results have been observed in a few patients who could receive an allogeneic hematopoietic stem cell transplantation (HSCT) after returning to chronic phase [1]. Therefore, the objective must be to obtain a complete response or a second chronic phase to proceed with an allogeneic HSCT as soon as possible [1].

A reasonable strategy might be to combine TKIs with acute leukemia-like chemotherapy prior to HSCT to improve the prognosis of these patients. Some studies have shown better results when using various chemotherapy agents in combination with imatinib 600 mg daily [9], but these results remain unsatisfactory. Since dasatinib induces more profound and faster responses, it could be an effective option in combination with chemotherapy prior to allogeneic HSCT. In fact, dasatinib and FLAG-IDA has shown to be an effective and safety bridge to HSCT in a small study including 4 patients with BC transformation after failure with imatinib treatment [10]. However, there are no published studies or case reports that support the use of dasatinib as first line treatment for initial myeloid BC, that is, for patients who did not previously receive imatinib.

In addition, in spite of alterations in T-cell response induced by dasatinib, little is known about infectious complications in these patients.

Based on all these, a case is presented of a patient diagnosed with an initial nonlymphoid phenotype BC who achieved a molecular response ($MR^{4.5}$) with dasatinib and FLAG-IDA but presented with high infectious toxicity including several opportunistic infections.

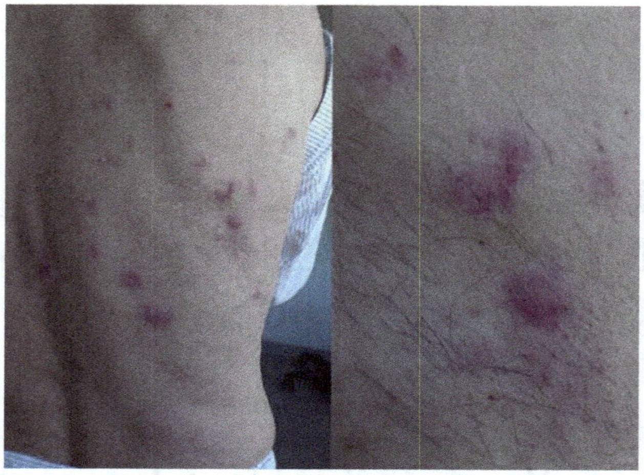

Figure 1: Erythematous, round, well-grouped plaques located at the rear right costal arch. A biopsy of the skin lesions was performed and reported as compatible with leukemia cutis.

2. Case Presentation

We present the case of a 67-year-old male patient, diagnosed with an initial nonlymphoid phenotype BC. At diagnosis, a physical examination revealed splenomegaly of 6 cm (splenomegaly was confirmed by abdominal ultrasound) and erythematous round well-defined grouped, not itchy, plaques located at the rear right costal arch (Figure 1). A biopsy of the skin lesions was performed and reported as compatible with leukemia cutis. Complete blood counts had values of hemoglobin 11.2 g/dL (13–17.5 g/dL), leukocytosis (WBC) 53.3×10^9/L (4.5–11×10^9/L) and platelets 48×10^9/L (140–450×10^9/L). A peripheral blood smear showed basophilia (3%), immature granulocytes (3% of bands forms, 2% of metamyelocytes, 10% of myelocytes), and 28% of blasts. Bone marrow aspirate showed granulocytic hyperplasia with 31% of myeloperoxidase negative blasts. Flow cytometry showed 33% blasts distributed in 3 populations (Figure 2): 1st, myeloid without differentiation (15%); 2nd, dendritic (13%); and 3rd, myeloid (5%).

Treatment was started with Hydrea until WBC $<50 \times 10^9$/L, and subsequently treatment began with fludarabine 30 mg/m^2 i.v. days 1 to 4, cytarabine 2 g/m^2 i.v. days 1 to 4, and idarubicin 10 mg/m^2 i.v. days 1 to 3 (FLA-IDA). G-CSF was omitted due to hyperleukocytosis.

After that, the karyotype showed Philadelphia chromosome t (9; 22) (q34; q11) in all metaphases, and BCR-ABL fusion gene was evidenced by FISH and RT-PCR analysis with a break in the minor breakpoint region. Thereafter, the patient was diagnosed with myeloid-phenotype initial BC, and dasatinib was added at a dose of 100 mg initially and 140 mg thereafter.

On day +21, with recovered neutrophils but only 20×10^9/L platelets, a bone marrow aspirate was performed to evaluate response, which showed 3% of blasts and negative minimal residual disease by flow cytometry (sensitivity 10–4). On day +41, due to hematological toxicity (grade 4 neutropenia and thrombocytopenia), a new bone marrow aspirate was performed which confirmed that the patient was still in complete response without platelets recovery, with negative minimal residual disease by flow cytometry, complete cytogenetic response, and major molecular response (detectable disease at a level of 0.024% by quantitative RT-PCR); moreover, both splenomegaly and cutaneous lesions disappeared. Therefore, dasatinib was temporally withdrawn for one week.

On day +47, neutrophil counts were recovered, but with platelets of 47×10^9/L, a second dasatinib and FLAG-IDA cycle was started (including G-CSF 300 μg/m^2 s.c. on days 1–5).

During the second cycle, the patient developed bacteremia with *S. epidermidis* from his peripherally inserted central catheter (PICC). A few days after discharge, he was admitted to the hospital again due to probable aspergillosis in the right superior lobule. The chest X-ray was compatible with this (Figure 3) and with a positive galactomannan in the bronchoalveolar lavage, he was treated with oral voriconazole 200 mg/12 h. Of note, the absolute neutrophil count was normal.

On day +45, approximately 10 days after the bronchoalveolar lavage, the patient sought urgent medical attention, presenting with fever. He was asymptomatic, with hemodynamic stability, good performance status, and normal physical examination. ANC was 2.2×10^9/L, so he was treated with empirical antibiotherapy, in accordance with the guidelines of our center, and continued with voriconazole. Both legionella and pneumococcal antigens were negative, as well as microbiological cultures. Since the patient remained febrile after 3 days of antibiotic treatment and had a questionable radiological worsening (on chest X-ray), it was decided to administer antifungal combination therapy consisting of voriconazole and liposomal amphotericin B at 5 mg/kg/d. On the seventh day, fever persisted despite empirical antibiotics and combined antifungal treatment, but the ophthalmogical investigation revealed no signs of fungal dissemination. In addition, galactomannan

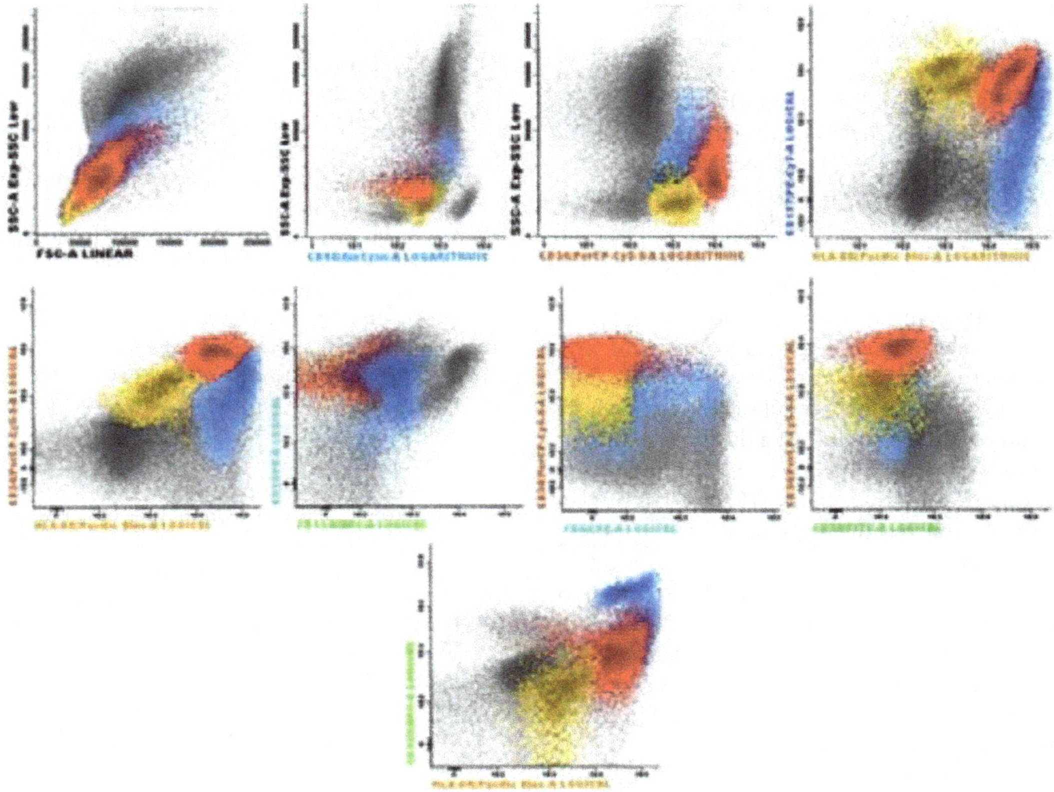

FIGURE 2: Flow cytometry at diagnosis showed 33% of blasts distributed in 3 populations. 1st population, myeloid without differentiation (15%), in red: CD34++, CD117 +, HLA-DR +, CD45 + d, CD13+, CD64 –, CD35–/+ d, CD36–, CD33 +, CD71–/ +, CD105 + d, CD7–/ +, CD15–/ +, CD22–, CD38 +, CD123 +, CD4+d, and cMPO–. 2nd population, dendritic (13%), in blue: CD34+d, CD117–/+, HLA-DR++, CD45+d, CD13 +, CD64–/ +, CD35–, CD36–/ +, CD33++, CD71–/+, CD105 + d, CD7–/+, CD15–/+, CD22–, CD38 +, CD123++, CD4 + d, and cMPO–/ +. 3rd population, myeloid (5%), in yellow: CD34 + d, CD117 + d, HLA-DR–/+, CD45 + d, CD13 +, CD64–, CD35–, CD36–, CD33–, CD71–, CD105–, CD7–, CD15–, CD22 +, CD38–, CD123–, CD4–/+d, and cMPO–. Blasts were negative for CD10, CD16, CD11b, CD14, IREM-2, nTdT, CD56, CD19, 7.1, CD42, CD61, CD203c, cCD79a, cCD3, and CD3.

antigen was negative; however, CMV antigen was positive (5 infected leukocytes per 2×10^5 leukocytes/mL). Therefore, it was concluded that the patient had a CMV infection, and the liposomal amphotericin B was discontinued. The CT scan was canceled and antiviral treatment was started with valganciclovir 900 mg every 12 hours, with good response.

It is noteworthy that, at 3 months of this CMV infection, the patient suffered a second CMV reactivation, which again responded to valganciclovir.

Besides infectious toxicity, the patient developed gastrointestinal toxicity (diarrhea), related to dasatinib, which required several admissions and temporary withdrawal of dasatinib with subsequent dose escalation to the maximum tolerated dose (100 mg/d).

The patient is currently in complete cytogenetic response, with molecular response ($MR^{4.5}$), and was admitted for an allogeneic HSCT from a matched unrelated donor with a reduced-intensity conditioning.

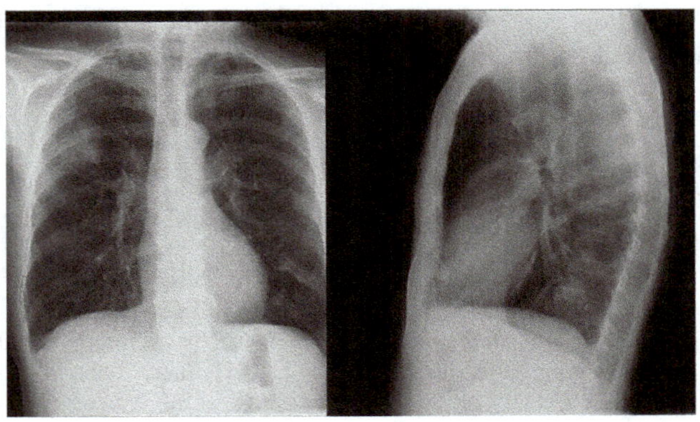

FIGURE 3: Chest X-ray showing a triangular consolidation in the right superior lobule.

3. Discussion

The efficacy of dasatinib and FLAG-IDA was demonstrated in our patient, who achieved a complete cytogenetic response after the first induction cycle and even subsequently improved (reaching $MR^{4.5}$), which allowed the subsequent performance of an allogeneic HSCT. However, although the response was excellent, the significant infection toxicity associated with this regimen must be taken into account.

Apart from grade 3-4 neutropenia induced by dasatinib in 79% of patients with CML in advanced stages, requiring discontinuation of treatment in 60% of patients [11], which in our case was aggravated by the administration of chemotherapy, there are few data on infectious complications associated with dasatinib. Some *in vitro* studies suggest disturbance in the T-cell response [12–14], which has been confirmed in *ex vivo* studies [15]. Also, during treatment with dasatinib, there is a decrease in the number of B lymphocytes, CD4+ T lymphocytes, cytotoxic T lymphocytes, and natural killer cells [15] and inhibition of T-cell activation [15], and all these are dose-dependent [12]. These alterations in T cell immune response would involve an increased risk for reactivation of herpes family viruses (CMV, HHV-6, etc.) or other opportunistic infections. In this regard, there are several published clinical cases of viral reactivation following treatment with dasatinib [16]. Furthermore, it is noteworthy that in a small retrospective study of 16 patients who received dasatinib at a dose of 140 mg, 12 out of 16 patients experienced an infectious complication, including three opportunistic infections [15]. But it is not yet clear whether these viral reactivations observed in the literature, as in our patient, were due solely to the effect of dasatinib on T-cell response, or it was a cumulative effect on cellular immunity due to prior treatment with imatinib, or in our case, due to combination with fludarabine. However, it seems reasonable what some authors propose, suggesting prospective studies to evaluate the effectiveness of CMV monitoring in those patients treated with dasatinib [17], especially if they have additional risk factors as in our case, even outside the usual context of allogeneic HSCT.

In conclusion, dasatinib and FLAG-IDA is an effective therapy for initial BC. However, the high risk of opportunistic infections, such as CMV, should taken into account.

Authors' Contributions

All authors contributed equally to this work and read and approved the final manuscript for submission.

References

[1] R. Hehlmann, "How I treat CML blast crisis," *Blood*, vol. 120, no. 4, pp. 737–747, 2012.

[2] S. H. Swerdlow, International Agency for Research on Cancer, and World Health Organization, *WHO Classification of Tumours of Haematopoietic and Lymphoid Tissues*, International Agency for Research on Cancer, Lyon, France, 2008.

[3] S. Sacchi, H. M. Kantarjian, S. O'Brien et al., "Chronic myelogenous leukemia in nonlymphoid blastic phase," *Cancer*, vol. 86, no. 12, pp. 2632–2641, 1999.

[4] B. J. Druker, C. L. Sawyers, H. Kantarjian et al., "Activity of a specific inhibitor of the BCR-ABL tyrosine kinase in the blast crisis of chronic myeloid leukemia and acute lymphoblastic leukemia with the Philadelphia chromosome," *New England Journal of Medicine*, vol. 344, no. 14, pp. 1038–1042, 2001.

[5] C. L. Sawyers, A. Hochhaus, E. Feldman et al., "Imatinib induces hematologic and cytogenetic responses in patients with chronic myelogenous leukemia in myeloid blast crisis: results of a phase II study," *Blood*, vol. 99, no. 10, pp. 3530–3539, 2002.

[6] H. M. Kantarjian, J. Cortes, S. O'Brien et al., "Imatinib mesylate (STI571) therapy for Philadelphia chromosome-positive chronic myelogenous leukemia in blast phase," *Blood*, vol. 99, no. 10, pp. 3547–3553, 2002.

[7] F. Palandri, F. Castagnetti, N. Testoni et al., "Chronic myeloid leukemia in blast crisis treated with imatinib 600 mg: outcome of the patients alive after a 6-year follow-up," *Haematologica*, vol. 93, no. 12, pp. 1792–1796, 2008.

[8] G. Saglio, A. Hochhaus, Y. T. Goh et al., "Dasatinib in imatinib-resistant or imatinib-intolerant chronic myeloid leukemia in blast phase after 2 years of follow-up in a phase 3 study," *Cancer*, vol. 116, no. 16, pp. 3852–3861, 2010.

[9] S. Fruehauf, J. Topaly, E. C. Buss et al., "Imatinib combined with mitoxantrone/etoposide and cytarabine is an effective induction therapy for patients with chronic myeloid leukemia in myeloid blast crisis," *Cancer*, vol. 109, no. 8, pp. 1543–1549, 2007.

[10] D. Milojkovic, A. Ibrahim, A. Reid, L. Foroni, J. Apperley, and D. Marin, "Efficacy of combining dasatinib and FLAG-IDA for patients with chronic myeloid leukemia in blastic transformation," *Haematologica*, vol. 97, no. 3, pp. 473-474, 2012.

[11] E. Jabbour, J. Cortes, and H. Kantarjian, "Dasatinib for the treatment of Philadelphia chromosome-positive leukaemias," *Expert Opinion on Investigational Drugs*, vol. 16, no. 5, pp. 679–687, 2007.

[12] R. Weichsel, C. Dix, L. Wooldridge et al., "Profound inhibition of antigen-specific T-cell effector functions by dasatinib," *Clinical Cancer Research*, vol. 14, no. 8, pp. 2484–2491, 2008.

[13] A. E. Schade, G. L. Schieven, R. Townsend et al., "Dasatinib, a small-molecule protein tyrosine kinase inhibitor, inhibits T-cell activation and proliferation," *Blood*, vol. 111, no. 3, pp. 1366–1377, 2008.

[14] F. Fei, Y. Yu, A. Schmitt et al., "Dasatinib inhibits the proliferation and function of CD4+CD25+regulatory T cells," *British Journal of Haematology*, vol. 144, no. 2, pp. 195–205, 2009.

[15] C. Sillaber, H. Herrmann, K. Bennett et al., "Immunosuppression and atypical infections in CML patients treated with dasatinib at 140 mg daily," *European Journal of Clinical Investigation*, vol. 39, no. 12, pp. 1098–1109, 2009.

[16] R. García-Muñoz, A. Galar, C. Moreno et al., "Parvovirus B19 acute infection and a reactivation of cytomegalovirus and herpesvirus 6 in a chronic myeloid leukemia patient during treatment with dasatinib (BMS-354825)," *Leukemia & Lymphoma*, vol. 48, no. 12, pp. 2461–2464, 2007.

[17] H. A. Torres and R. F. Chemaly, "Viral infection or reactivation in patients during treatment with dasatinib: a call for screening?" *Leukemia & Lymphoma*, vol. 48, no. 12, pp. 2308-2309, 2007.

29

Severe Aplastic Anemia as First Manifestation of Classical Hodgkin Lymphoma

Cláudia L. Pedrosa,[1] Patrícia Rosinha,[2] Patrícia Seabra,[1] Gisela Ferreira,[3] Cláudia Rosado,[2] Luísa Regadas,[1] Cláudia Casais,[1] and Jorge Coutinho[1]

[1]*Department of Clinical Hematology, Centro Hospitalar Universitário Do Porto, Porto, Portugal*
[2]*Department of Internal Medicine, Centro Hospitalar Do Baixo Vouga, Aveiro, Portugal*
[3]*Department of Clinical Hematology, Centro Hospitalar Do Baixo Vouga, Aveiro, Portugal*

Correspondence should be addressed to Cláudia L. Pedrosa; claudiamlpedrosa@gmail.com

Academic Editor: Tatsuharu Ohno

Autoimmune cytopenia, a known paraneoplastic complication of lymphoid neoplasms, may occur before, concurrently, at relapse, or even years after completion of lymphoma treatment. In the case of Hodgkin lymphoma (HL), it is thought that immune dysregulation, typical of this neoplasm, may be involved in the genesis of these manifestations. We report a 57-year-old male presenting with stage IIIA, International Prognostic Score (IPS) 4, nodular sclerosis HL, and severe AA (SAA) confirmed on the histologic exam of the bone marrow that showed severe marrow hypoplasia due to a decrease in the elements of the three cell linages with left shift of the myeloid maturation. Immunosuppression with steroids and cyclosporine A was started. Eltrombopag and G-CSF were also added. In spite of prompt initiation of immunosuppressive therapy, the patient presented an unfavorable outcome with progressive pancytopenia and severe acute cerebral hemorrhagic event. The patient died 59 days after admission. Although autoimmune disorders are described in HL, its concomitant diagnosis is extremely rare. Our case shows a rare instance of SAA as the first manifestation of HL.

1. Introduction

Hodgkin lymphoma (HL) accounts for approximately 10% of all malignant lymphomas, commonly affecting young adults. It usually presents with localized disease involving cervical, supraclavicular, and mediastinal regions. The classical form represents about 95% of the HL, nodular sclerosis being the most frequent subtype [1].

Autoimmune cytopenias are frequent paraneoplastic complications of non-Hodgkin lymphomas, but more rarely seen in HL. These may occur before, concurrently, at relapse, or even years after completion of lymphoma treatment [2].

The pathophysiology of this phenomenon is not completely understood. However, in HL, it is thought that immune deregulation, typical of this neoplasm, may be involved in the genesis of these manifestations.

Aplastic anemia (AA) is a hematopoietic stem cell disorder defined by reduced bone marrow cellularity and impaired peripheral blood cells production [3, 4]. It is classified according to the marrow cellularity and repercussion on the peripheral blood. Severe aplastic anemia (SAA) comprises bone marrow cellularity less than 25% and depression of at least two of the three hematopoietic lineages (absolute neutrophil count (ANC) $<0.5\times10^9$/L; platelets $<20\times10^9$/L; reticulocytes $<60\times10^9$/L). SAA designates patients who fulfill SAA criteria but present with an ANC $<0.2\times10^9$/L [5].

The underlying cause of AA seems to be an autoimmune process mediated by *T* cytotoxic cells that suppress hematopoiesis. Coincidentally, these cytotoxic T lymphocytes are abundantly present in HL, playing an important role in the pathogenesis of the disease and in tumor cells' survival and proliferation. This fact raises the possibility of a causal relationship between the two diseases.

Here, we report a rare case of a patient presenting SAA as the first manifestation of nodular sclerosis classical HL.

2. Case Report

A 57-year-old male, with no comorbidities, Eastern Cooperative Oncology Group (ECOG)-Performance Status 1, presented with asthenia, lower gastrointestinal and mucocutaneous bleeding, and right axillar adenomegaly, two months before admission.

Blood workup showed pancytopenia and reticulocytopenia with no morphologic atypia on the peripheral blood smear. Erythrocyte sedimentation rate was elevated. All tumor markers, including $\beta 2$-microglobulin and LDH, were negative. The patient had neither renal nor hepatic impairment. There was neither hemolysis pattern nor vitamin deficiencies. Microbiologic and autoimmune screening was also negative (Table 1).

A PET-CT scan was performed and documented hypermetabolic activity on supra- and infradiaphragmatic adenopathies and spleen. No bulky mass was identified.

The excisional biopsy of the axillar lymph node confirmed the diagnosis of nodular sclerosis classical HL (Figures 1(a)–1(d)).

A bone marrow biopsy was performed. The histologic exam revealed severe marrow hypoplasia due to a decrease in the elements of the three cell linages with left shift of the myeloid maturation. No blastic, dysplastic, or lymphoma cells were identified (Figures 2(a)–2(b)). Karyotype was normal (46, XY).

Next generation sequencing gene panel excluded mutations suggestive of inherited bone marrow failure syndrome or hypoplastic myelodysplastic syndrome/acute myeloid leukemia (Table 1). Immunophenotyping of the peripheral blood excluded paroxysmal nocturnal hemoglobinuria clone.

The concomitant diagnosis of advanced stage (Ann-Arbor IIIA) nodular sclerosis HL, IPS 4, and SAA was made.

Considering the myelotoxicity of standard HL's chemotherapy regimens, it was decided to start immunosuppressive therapy for SAA and postpone the introduction of chemotherapy. Prednisolone (1 mg/kg/day) was initiated. After one month on corticosteroids with no response, cyclosporine A was added. On day 15 of double immunosuppressive therapy, an agonist of thrombopoetin (eltrombopag 150 mg per day) was introduced.

After thirty days on immunosuppression, no improvement was documented on the blood counts (Hb <7 g/dL; neutrophils $<1\times10^9$/L; platelets $<10\times10^9$/L). G-CSF was started. During hospitalization, the patient was dependent on red blood cells and platelets transfusion.

Despite all the adopted measures, the patient's clinical status worsened and he was admitted to intensive care unit (ICU) for septic shock with multiorgan failure. Broad spectrum antibiotics and ventilatory and cardiovascular support were initiated. A multisensitive *Escherichia coli* was isolated on the peripheral blood cultures.

On the third day at the ICU, neurologic deterioration was noticed. A brain CT scan was performed showing "de novo" acute subdural hematoma and hydrocephaly.

Due to refractoriness to the immunosuppressive therapy and progressive deterioration of performance status of the patient in the context of septic shock and severe acute cerebral hemorrhagic event with hydrocephaly, it was decided to withdraw measures and begin palliative care.

The patient died 59 days after admission.

3. Discussion

Classical HL is characterized by the presence of B cells derived from germinal center, called Hodgkin or Reed–Sternberg cells (HRS). Although these cells derived from B lymphocytes, they do not express the majority of germinal center makers, do not produce immunoglobulins or undergo somatic hypermutation, under normal circumstances, a cell like this would be destined to apoptosis. However, in HL, the environment surrounding the HRS is the main element for tumor cell survival [6].

Autoimmune disorders are known complications of HL. Data suggest that HL's patients present a higher incidence of AA compared to the general population [7]. This may possibly be justified by the dysregulated immune response characterizing these neoplasms. In HL, an inflammatory background, constituted by *T* and B cells, macrophages, histiocytes, eosinophils, neutrophils, and plasma cells secreting cytokines, plays an important role in the survival of the HRS. In their turn, these cells also produce multiple cytokines and chemokines, such as tumor necrosis factor alpha (TNF-α), interleukin-4 (IL-4), IL-5, IL-6, chemokine ligand-5 (CCL-5), and fibroblast growth factor (FGF), which perpetuate this inflammatory activity [1].

The constitutive activation of the nuclear factor-kappa B and the Janus kinase-signal (JAK-STAT) signaling results in the upregulation of programmed death 1 ligand (PD1-ligand) and JAK2. This allows the interaction between the PD1-ligand on the surface of the HRS and PD1 on the T cell, downregulating the latest and compromising the function of cytotoxic T cells. Not only these cells but also *T* helper lymphocytes play a role in promoting tumor cell survival.

This immune dysregulation may represent a risk factor for AA [7].

Considering AA as a paraneoplastic manifestation of HL, the reasonable was to treat the underlying cause: the lymphoma. However, current chemotherapy regimens for HL are extremely myelotoxic and would not be feasible in a scenario of severe pancytopenia.

In recent studies, cases in which AA and HL arise simultaneously, the outcome of AA prevails over that of the lymphoma in the majority of the cases. The initiation of immunosuppressive treatment for AA plays a role in avoiding permanent and irreversible damage in the myelopoiesis [8]. The major challenges of these treatment regimens are severe complications, such as febrile neutropenia and infections by atypical or opportunistic agents, due to deep prolonged pancytopenia and extreme state of immunosuppression. In

Table 1: Patient's initial blood workup.

Laboratorial hematology	
Hemogram	
Hemoglobin	5.8 g/dL
Leucocytes	2.8×10^9/L
Neutrophils	1.36×10^9/L
Platelets	$<10 \times 10^9$/L
Reticulocytes	26×10^9/L
Erythrocyte sedimentation rate	92 mm/h
Biochemical profile	
Creatinine	65.43 μmol/L
Alanine/aspartate aminotransferase	28/32 U/L
Total bilirubin	15.56 μmol/L
Triglycerides	1.12 mmol/L
Ferritin	553 μg/L
LDH	221 U/L
β2-microglobulin	1.98 mg/L
Immunologic screening	
Antinuclear antibodies (ANA) (immunofluorescence)	<1/160 (1/160)
Antineutrophil cytoplasmic antibodies (c-ANCA) (immunofluorescence)	<1/20 (<1/10)
Antineutrophil cytoplasmic antibodies (p-ANCA) (immunofluorescence)	<1/20 (<1/10)
Serological/microbiological screening	
Interferon gamma release assay (IGRA) for *Mycobacterium tuberculosis* infection (*in vitro* stimulation)	<0.01 UI/mL
Human hepatitis virus B (HBs antigen)	<0.10 (<1.00)
Human hepatitis virus B (HBs antibody)	0.16 (<1.40)
Human hepatitis virus B (HBs antibody)	13.78 m UI/mL (<8.00)
Human Hepatitis virus C antibody	0.21 (<1.00)
Human immunodeficiency virus	0.10 (<0.90)
Epstein-Barr virus, viral capsid antigen (VCA) IgM antibody	0.40 RU/mL (<0.80)
Epstein-Barr virus, viral capsid antigen (VCA) IgG antibody	97.10 RU/mL (<16.00)
Cytomegalovirus, IgM antibody	0.15 UA/mL (<0.90)
Cytomegalovirus, IgG antibody	11.80 UA/mL (<0.90)
Parvovirus B19, IgM antibody (immunoassay)	Nonreactive
Parvovirus B19, IgG antibody (immunoassay)	3 UI/mL
Venereal Disease Research Laboratory (VDRL) test	Nonreactive
Treponema pallidum haemagglutination assay (TPHA)	Negative
Rubella virus, IgM antibody	0.00 UI/mL (<0.80)
Rubella virus, IgG antibody	16.50 UI/mL (<5.00)
Toxoplasma gondii, IgM antibody	0.20 UI/mL (<0.90)
Toxoplasma gondii, IgG antibody	5.20 UI/mL (<6.40)
Borrelia burgdorferi screening antibodies (enzyme-fluorescent assay)	Nonreactive
Bartonella henselae, IgM antibody (indirect immunofluorescence)	Nonreactive
Bartonella henselae, IgG antibody (indirect immunofluorescence)	<320
NGS panel (genes tested)	
ASXL1, CEBPA, NPM1, ETV6, FLT3, CSF3R, DNMT3A, EZH2, GATA1, IDH1-2, IKZF1, RUNX1, SFEB1, TET2, WT1, TP53	Unmutated

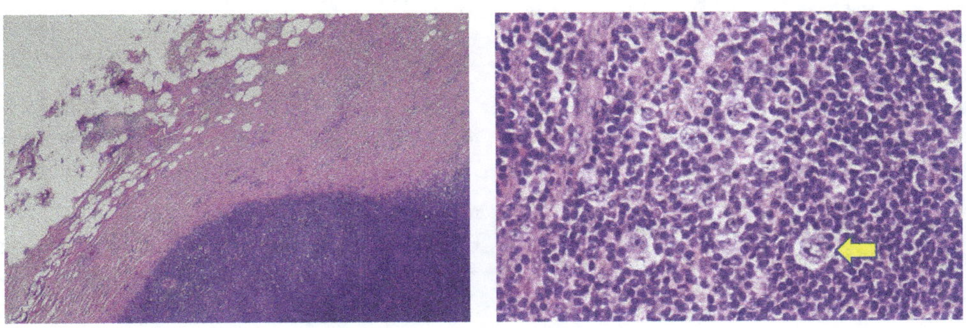

(a) (b)

Figure 1: Continued.

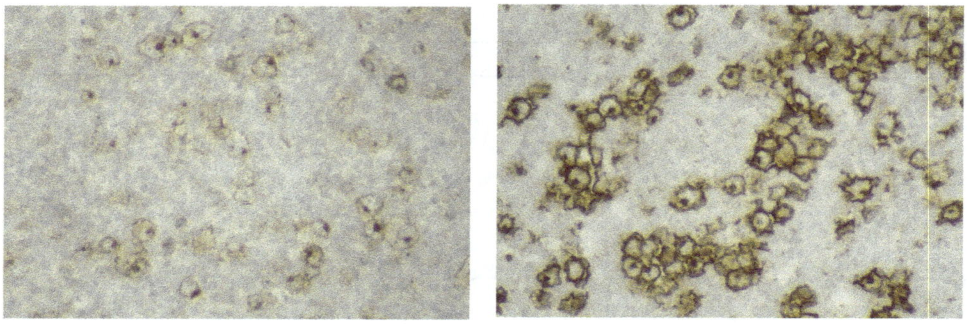

(c) (d)

Figure 1: Histology and immunochemistry of axillar lymph node. (a) Lymph node with enlarged capsule and disruptive morphologic structure (hematoxylin-eosin staining). (b) Reed–Sternberg cells (arrow) (hematoxylin-eosin staining). (c) Redd–Sternberg cells showing low affinity to CD30 antibody. (d) Redd–Sternberg cells showing high affinity to CD15 antibody.

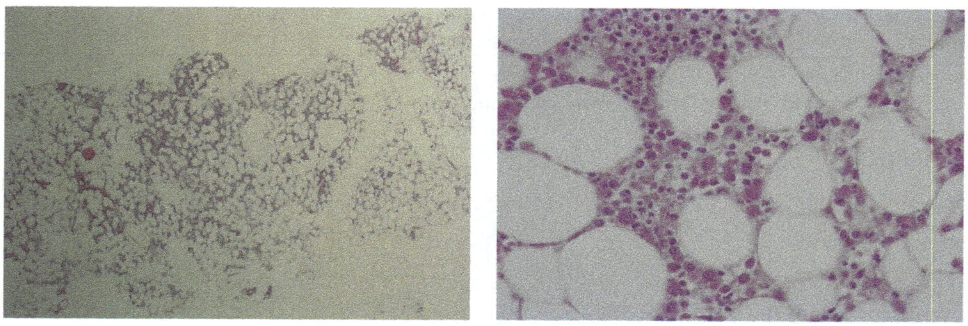

(a) (b)

Figure 2: Histology of bone marrow (hematoxylin-eosin staining). (a) Severe marrow hypoplasia (cellularity between 10% and 30%). (b) Histologic exam of bone marrow showing reduced presence of elements of the three cell lineages with left shift of the myeloid maturation. No blastic, dysplastic, or lymphoma cells were identified.

this case, we decided to start a mild-moderate immunosuppressive therapy in order to improve peripheral blood counts, allowing the patient to start chemotherapy. However, that was not possible due to sudden unfavorable progression of the patient's clinical situation. Nowadays, the advent of novel agents allows treating these patients with fewer side effects, mainly concerning myelotoxicity. Unfortunately, at the time of diagnosis, neither brentuximab nor checkpoint inhibitors were approved in Portugal.

To conclude, we consider the early recognition of the association between these two entities extremely important, since it allows a more accurate diagnosis and thus prompt initiation of effective immunosuppressive therapy. Despite being a malignant disease, HL shows high rates of complete remission and overall survival. On the other hand, AA is a benign disease with high rates of relapse/refractoriness to treatment and complications, certainly having an evident negative impact on the outcome of these patients.

Authors' Contributions

Cláudia L. Pedrosa and Patrícia Rosinha contributed equally to this work.

References

[1] B. Allen Pamela and M. Evens Andrew, *Hodgkin Lymphoma in: American Society of Hematology Self-Assessment Program*, American Society of Hematology, Washington, DC, USA, 7th edition, 2019.

[2] K. Lechner and Y.-A. Chen, "Paraneoplastic autoimmune cytopenias in Hodgkin lymphoma," *Leukemia & Lymphoma*, vol. 51, no. 3, pp. 469–474, 2010.

[3] A. Tzankov and M. Medinger, "Aplastic anemia: possible associations with lymphoproliferative neoplasms," *International Journal of Laboratory Hematology*, vol. 36, no. 3, pp. 382–387, 2014.

[4] T. Saitoh, T. Matsushima, A. Yamane et al., "Hodgkin lymphoma accompanied by aplastic anemia and polyclonal expansion of large granular lymphocytes," *Acta Haematologica*, vol. 117, no. 4, pp. 238–241, 2007.

[5] E. DeZern Amy and C. Smith, "Acquired marrow failure syndromes: aplastic anemia, paroxysmal nocturnal hemoglobinuria and myelodysplastic syndromes," *American Society of Hematology Self-Assessment Program*, American Society of Hematology, Washington, DC, USA, 7th edition, 2019.
[6] S. Poppema, "Immunobiology and pathophysiology of Hodgkin lymphomas," *Hematology*, vol. 2005, no. 1, pp. 231–238, 2005.
[7] T. Linabug, R. Davis Adam, V. Frey Noelle et al., "Classical Hodgkin lymphoma patients have an increased incidence of idiopathic acquired aplastic anemia," *Blood*, vol. 14, no. 4, Article ID e0215021, 2019.
[8] A. Rovó, A. Kulasekararaj, M. Medinger et al., "Association of aplastic anaemia and lymphoma: a report from the severe aplastic anaemia working party of the European Society of Blood and Bone Marrow Transplantation," *British Journal of Haematology*, vol. 184, pp. 279–310, 2019.

30

Clonally Related Plasmablastic Lymphoma Simultaneously Occurring with Diffuse Large B-Cell Lymphoma

Norisato Hashimoto,[1] Tomoki Ueda,[1] Shinichiro Hiraiwa,[2] Takuma Tajiri,[2] Naoya Nakamura,[3] and Kenji Yokoyama[1]

[1]*Department of Hematology/Oncology, Tokai University Hachioji Hospital, 1838 Ishikawa-machi, Hachioji 1920032, Japan*
[2]*Department of Pathology, Tokai University Hachioji Hospital, 1838 Ishikawa-machi, Hachioji 1920032, Japan*
[3]*Department of Pathology, Tokai University, School of Medicine, 143 Shimokasuya, Isehara 2591193, Japan*

Correspondence should be addressed to Kenji Yokoyama; yk092750@tsc.u-tokai.ac.jp

Academic Editor: Kostas Konstantopoulos

Plasmablastic lymphoma (PBL) is a rare aggressive lymphoma. Although it was first described in HIV- (human immunodeficiency virus-) infected patients, PBL has been diagnosed in patients with other immunodeficiencies as well as in immunocompetent patients. PBL immunohistochemically expresses plasmacytic markers and lacks pan B-cell markers. The cells of origin of PBL are considered to be plasmablasts. MYC gene rearrangement and MYC overexpression are frequently found in PBL, but the pathogenesis of PBL is yet to be elucidated. Here, we report a case of composite lymphoma of PBL and diffuse large B-cell lymphoma (DLBCL); that is, PBL in the urinary bladder and DLBCL in the nasal cavity occurred simultaneously. We extracted DNA from the two lymphomas for polymerase chain reaction and sequenced the amplified immunoglobulin heavy variable genes and the complementarity-determining region- (CDR-) 3. The sequence of the CDR3 region of both tumors matched. MYC rearrangement was found in the bladder tumor but not in the nasal tumor. The patient was treated with R-CHOP (rituximab, cyclophosphamide, vincristine, doxorubicin, and prednisone), and durable remission had been obtained. The results of the DNA analysis indicated that both PBL and DLBCL emerged from common postgerminal B cells. This case may help to elucidate the pathogenesis of PBL.

1. Introduction

Plasmablastic lymphoma (PBL) is a rare aggressive lymphoma that was first described in 1997 as a new clinical entity related to human immunodeficiency virus infection and is recognized as a variant of diffuse large B-cell lymphoma (DLBCL) [1]. PBL has the morphologic and immunophenotypic features of plasmablasts that lack activating B-cell markers such as CD20 and harbor plasma cell markers such as CD138. Although PBL was initially reported as a neoplasm arising in the oral cavity of HIV-positive patients, PBL has been diagnosed in patients with other causes of immunodeficiency (e.g., transplant recipients), in immunocompetent patients, and in various anatomic locations. In the latest World Health Organization classification, PBL is categorized as a distinct mature B-cell lymphoma with specific pathologic and immunohistochemical characteristics [2].

Plasmablasts are considered to be the cells of origin of PBL, but the mechanisms of tumor evolution remain unclear [3]. Here, we report a case of composite lymphoma of PBL and DLBCL. We demonstrated that the two lymphomas derived from a common postgerminal center B cell. These findings provide insight into the possible tumor evolution of PBL from DLBCL.

2. Case Report

A 37-year-old previously healthy man presented with swelling of the right nasal root and frequent urination. Otolaryngologic examination revealed thickened mucosa inside the right nasal cavity. Despite the use of both antibiotics and antihistamines, the symptoms deteriorated and the patient underwent diagnostic biopsy of the nasal mucosa. Hematoxylin and eosin (H&E) staining showed diffuse proliferation of atypical lymphoid cells with a prominent nucleolus and clear cytoplasm. Immunohistochemical staining revealed that the atypical cells were positive for CD20 and negative for CD138 (Figure 1). These cells were also positive for CD79a, PAX5, BCL2, BCL6, Mum-1, and CD45 and negative for CD56. A few cells were positive for in situ hybridization of Epstein–Barr virus- (EBV-) encoded RNA (data not shown). Based on these findings, the nasal tumor was diagnosed as nongerminal center B-cell (non-GCB) type DLBCL.

To evaluate the cause of frequent urination, ultrasonography of the urinary bladder was performed, and it revealed numerous irregular surfaced masses scattered on the wall of the urinary bladder. Biopsy specimens of one of the tumors showed the proliferation of atypical lymphoid cells with abundant basophilic cytoplasm and pleomorphic nucleoli. Immunohistochemical staining indicated that these atypical cells were negative for CD20 and positive for CD138 (Figure 2). These cells were also positive for CD56 and light chain kappa and negative for CD79a or PAX5 (data not shown). The serologic test for HIV was negative. According to these findings, the urinary bladder tumor was diagnosed as PBL. The patient did not complain of night sweats, weight loss, or fever. Blood laboratory tests indicated increased lactate dehydrogenase (334 U/ml), serum creatinine (1.67 mg/dl), and soluble interleukin-2 receptor (2650 U/ml) concentrations. Urinary tests revealed proteinuria and positivity for occult blood. Atypical cells were detected by urine cytology. A bone marrow trephine biopsy and cerebrospinal fluid cytology disclosed no lymphoma involvement. Fluorodeoxyglucose positron emission tomography/computed tomography (PET/CT) showed increased uptake at the lymph nodes on both the upper and lower sides of the diaphragm, and four extra nodal lesions in the right nasal mucosa, bilateral tonsils, prostate, and urinary bladder.

To identify the cell type of origin of the two lymphoma subtypes occurring simultaneously in one patient, we extracted DNA from frozen sections of each biopsy sample for polymerase chain reaction and sequenced the immunoglobulin heavy variable (IGHV) genes and the complementarity-determining region- (CDR-) 3, as previously described [4, 5] (see Supplementary Materials). The sequence of the CDR3 region of both tumors matched (Figure 3), indicating that both PBL and DLBCL emerged from a common clonal B cell. We also performed fluorescence in situ hybridization (FISH) in the biopsy specimens to detect MYC rearrangement. The split signal was detected in the bladder tumor, but not in the nasal tumor, indicating MYC rearrangement in the bladder PBL, but not in the nasal DLBCL (Figure 4).

This case was diagnosed as composite lymphoma of PBL and DLBCL and classified as stage 4A and IPI high/intermediate (elevated LDH, more than one extranodal lesion, and stage 4A). The patient underwent eight courses of R-CHOP (rituximab, cyclophosphamide, vincristine, doxorubicin, and prednisone) with four intrathecal infusions of methotrexate, cytarabine, and hydrocortisone to prevent central nervous system relapse, achieving a complete metabolic response based on PET/CT. Four years after completion of chemotherapy, he developed a soft tissue tumor on the cheek, and a biopsy specimen revealed recurrence of DLBCL.

3. Discussion

PBL is an aggressive lymphoma with the distinct morphologic features of large immunoblasts. The characteristic immunophenotype usually seen in PBL is the expression of plasmacytic markers, including CD138, CD38, and IRF4/MUM1, and the absence of pan B cell markers, including CD20 and PAX5. CD45 is weakly expressed or absent, and CD79a is often expressed in PBL [6]. The bladder tumor in our case was both morphologically and immunohistochemically compatible with PBL, and the nasal cavity tumor was morphologically and immunohistochemically compatible with non-GCB type DLBCL. Therefore, our case was diagnosed as composite lymphoma of PBL and DLBCL. Composite lymphoma is a rare manifestation of malignant lymphoma, which was first reported in 1954 [7], and there are several reports of non-Hodgkin lymphoma and Hodgkin lymphoma or two distinct subtypes of non-Hodgkin lymphoma. Most cases of composite lymphoma occur in the same organ, but some concurrently arise in different organs, such as in our case, the so-called discordant lymphoma [8].

The cells of origin of PBL are thought to be plasmablasts. Plasmablasts are precursor plasma cells derived from activated B cells. Several studies, including gene expression profiling studies, have investigated the pathogenesis of PBL, but it remains unclear. PBL was first reported in HIV patients, and EBV is detected in tumor cells of 74% of patients with HIV-associated PBL [9]. EBV, human herpes virus 8, MYC, p53, and BCL-6 gene aberrations may be involved in the development of AIDS-related lymphoma [10]. These mechanisms might also contribute to the pathogenesis of PBL, not only in HIV-infected patients but also in patients immunocompromised due to other causes as well as in immunocompetent individuals. Compared to HIV-associated PBL, approximately two-thirds of PBL cases in transplant recipients are EBV-positive and only half of the PBL cases in immunocompetent individuals are EBV-positive [11]. Chapman et al. [12] profiled the gene expression in 15 cases of PBL and compared them with the gene expression profiles of DLBCL and extramedullary (extraosseous) plasmacytoma. Overall, the gene expression profiles of PBLs were more similar to extramedullary (extraosseous) plasmacytoma than DLBCLs. They found that the transcriptional profile of PBL was distinct from that of DLBCL with regard to the activation of B-cell receptor signaling and the targets of MYC and MYB. They found that neither EBV positivity nor HIV status affected the gene expression profiles of PBL [12]. These findings suggest that the role of EBV or HIV in the pathogenesis of PBL may be limited.

MYC gene rearrangement is detected in up to 60% of PBL cases, and a common partner of the MYC gene is the

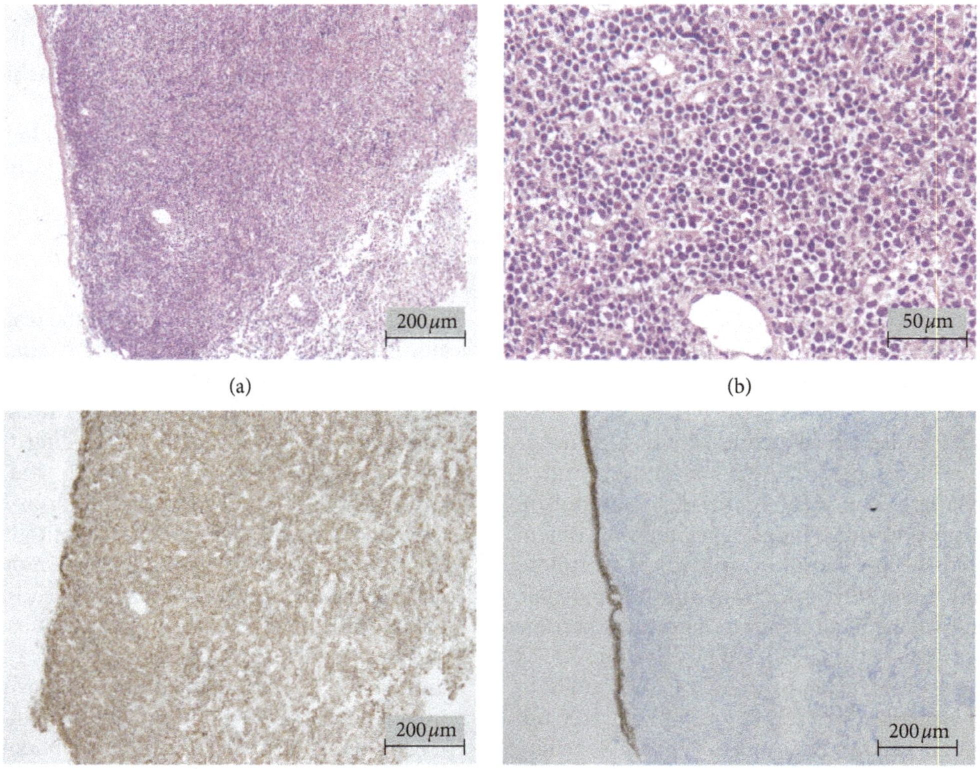

(a) (b) (c) (d)

Figure 1: Hematoxylin and eosin- (H&E-) stained section of nasal mucosa (a, b). Immunohistochemical staining of CD20 (c) and CD138 (d). H&E staining showed diffuse proliferation of atypical lymphoid cells with prominent nucleoli and clear cytoplasm (a, b). Immunohistochemical staining revealed that atypical cells were positive for CD20 (c) and negative for CD138 (d).

immunoglobulin gene [13, 14]. Gene expression profiles of PBL show the overexpression of MYC at the mRNA level, which is correlated with MYC protein overexpression [12]. Montes-Moreno et al. [15] profiled the gene expression in 36 PBL cases and demonstrated that MYC overexpression is not restricted to MYC-translocated or MYC-amplified cases. These findings suggest that MYC overexpression has an important role in the pathogenesis of PBL. They also found recurrent somatic mutations in PRDM1 in 50% of PBL cases [15]. PRDM1 encodes the protein Blimp1, which is considered to regulate plasma cell differentiation. MYC rearrangement was found only in the bladder PBL in our case, suggesting that MYC rearrangement might be critical in the pathogenesis of PBL.

DNA sequence analysis in our case revealed that PBL in the urinary bladder and DLBCL in the nasal cavity had matched sequences at the CDR3 region of IGHV. These results indicated that both PBL and DLBCL were derived from the same clone. The clonal relation between PBL and low-grade lymphoma has been demonstrated in a case series [16]. Marini et al. [17] reported a case with transformed PBL from previously diagnosed DLBCL, but they did not show a clonal relation between the two tumors. To the best of our knowledge, this is the first case that demonstrates the simultaneous occurrence of clonally related PBL with DLBCL. Although gene expression profiling was not performed in our case, this case may help to elucidate the pathogenesis of PBL. We speculate that a master regulator of plasma cell differentiation, like BLIMP1, is aberrantly expressed in DLBCL, leading to the development of PBL.

R-CHOP is a standard treatment for patients with DLBCL, and two-thirds of nonelderly patients with advanced-stage DLBCL can be cured with 6 to 8 cycles of R-CHOP. A standard treatment for PBL has not been established due to the rarity of the disease and its aggressive clinical course. Median survival time for PBL patients is estimated to be less than 1 year. A standard-dose CHOP-like regimen is considered inadequate because it provides the least possibility of cure [3]. The National Comprehensive Cancer Network recommends more intensive chemotherapy [18]. Bortezomib, a proteasome inhibitor that is a highly effective drug in multiple myeloma, is a promising agent for PBL because it targets plasma cells [19]. A recent study reported that the addition of bortezomib to dose-adjusted EPOCH (etoposide, prednisolone, vincristine, cyclophosphamide, hydroxydaunorubicin) led to a better response and survival in both HIV-positive and HIV-negative PBL patients, but the study was limited due to its retrospective design and small sample size [20]. Our case had composite lymphoma of PBL and DLBCL, and we selected R-CHOP as the first-line therapy. Our patient achieved a complete metabolic response after completing eight courses of R-CHOP, and durable remission for four years had been obtained. PBL does not usually express CD20, and therefore,

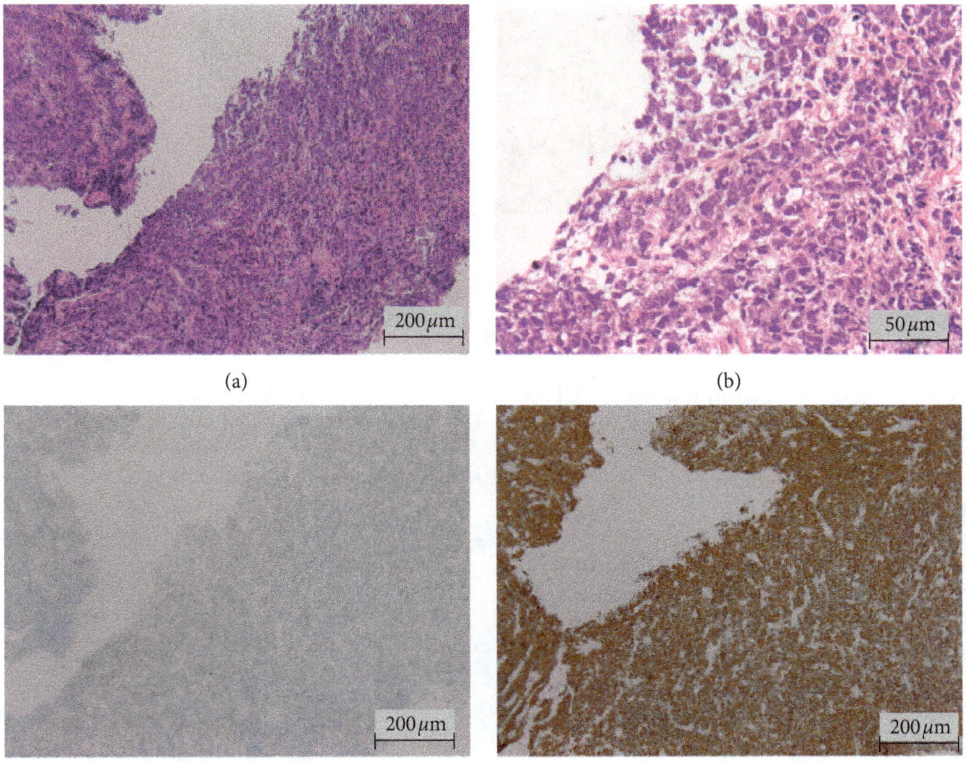

(c) (d)

Figure 2: H&E-stained section of bladder tumor (a, b). Immunohistochemical staining of CD20 (c) and CD138 (d). H&E staining showed the proliferation of atypical lymphoid cells with abundant basophilic cytoplasm and pleomorphic nucleoli (a, b). Immunohistochemical staining revealed that these atypical cells were negative for CD20 (c) and positive for CD138 (d).

```
                                 ----->  ____________CDR3-IMGT ______
H1503920_1C                      gtgtattactgtgcgagacgggagggatatagcagcagttggtacggcgtgagctggttc
AB019439 Homsap IGHV4-39*01 F     ----------a
M95116 Homsap IGHV4-39*05 F      ------------
X05715 Homsap IGHV4-39*02 F      ----------ga
```

(a)

```
                                 ----->  ____________CDR3-IMGT ______
H1504016_1C                      gtgtattactgtgcgagacgggagggtatagcagcagctggtacggctgagctggttc
X05715 Homsap IGHV4-39*02 F      ----------ga
AB019439 Homsap IGHV4-39*01 F    ----------a
M95116 Homsap IGHV4-39*05 F      --------
```

(b)

Figure 3: Sequences of the CDR3 region in the IGHV of the bladder tumor (a) and nasal tumor (b). The sequence of the CDR3 region in both tumors matched.

the addition of rituximab to the chemotherapy may not improve the response to chemotherapy. In the largest retrospective cohort study of PBL, CD20 was positive in 10% of patients, while 18% of patients received rituximab combined with or without chemotherapy [21]. When combined with chemotherapy, rituximab tended to improve the complete remission (CR) rate compared to chemotherapy alone, irrespective of CD20 or EBV positivity [21]. Considering our case and this cohort study, the addition of rituximab to the chemotherapy might be beneficial in selected cases of PBL. Our patient had been in CR for four years, but DLBCL relapsed as a soft tissue tumor. Serum soluble interleukin-2 receptor was markedly elevated at diagnosis, and increased serum soluble interleukin-2 receptor at diagnosis has been reported to be related to poor prognosis of DLBCL [22, 23]. Autologous stem cell transplantation (ASCT) in first CR has been shown to improve the outcomes of PBL patients [24]. Although the optimal treatment of composite lymphomas

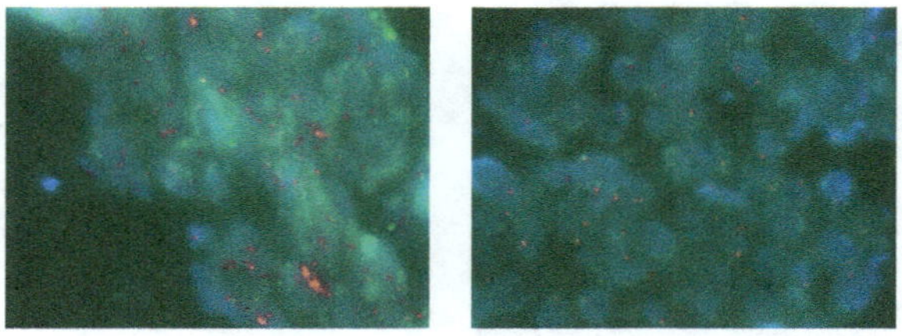

(a) (b)

FIGURE 4: FISH analysis of the MYC of the bladder tumor (a) and nasal tumor (b). The split signal was detected in the bladder tumor, whereas no split signal was detected in the nasal tumor.

has not been established, ASCT after completion of R-CHOP might reduce the risk of recurrence of lymphoma in our case.

Supplementary Materials

The primer sequences were used to amplify the immunoglobulin heavy chain gene by seminested polymerase chain reaction (PCR) as described previously [13, 14]. The PCR products were treated with EXO SAP IT (USB, Affymetrix Japan) according to the supplier's protocol and sequenced using the ABI PRISM 3100 Genetic Analyzer (Applied Biosystems Japan). Sequences were compared with the germline sequences using the IMGT site (*Supplementary Materials*)

References

[1] H. J. Delecluse, I. Anagnostopoulos, F. Dallenbach et al., "Plasmablastic lymphomas of the oral cavity: a new entity associated with the human immunodeficiency virus infection," *Blood*, vol. 89, no. 4, pp. 1413–1420, 1997.

[2] S. H. Swerdlow, E. Campo, S. A. Pileri et al., "The 2016 revision of the World Health Organization classification of lymphoid neoplasms," *Blood*, vol. 127, no. 20, pp. 2375–2390, 2016.

[3] J. J. Castillo, M. Bibas, and R. N. Miranda, "The biology and treatment of plasmablastic lymphoma," *Blood*, vol. 125, no. 15, pp. 2323–2330, 2015.

[4] N. Nakamura, T. Kuze, Y. Hashimoto et al., "Analysis of the immunoglobulin heavy chain gene of secondary diffuse large B-cell lymphoma that subsequently developed in four cases with B-cell chronic lymphocytic leukemia or lymphoplasmacytoid lymphoma (Richter syndrome)," *Pathology International*, vol. 50, no. 8, pp. 636–643, 2000.

[5] N. Nakamura, T. Kuze, Y. Hashimoto et al., "Analysis of the immunoglobulin heavy chain gene variable region of CD5-positive and-negative diffuse large B cell lymphoma," *Leukemia*, vol. 15, no. 3, pp. 452–457, 2001.

[6] F. Vega, C.-C. Chang, L. J. Medeiros et al., "Plasmablastic lymphomas and plasmablastic plasma cell myelomas have nearly identical immunophenotypic profiles," *Modern Pathology*, vol. 18, no. 6, pp. 806–815, 2005.

[7] R. Custer, "Pitfalls in the diagnosis of lymphoma and leukemia from pathologist's point of view," *Proceedings of Second National Conference*, pp. 554–557, American Cancer Society, Atlanta, GA, New York, 1954.

[8] R. Küppers, U. Dührsen, and M.-L. Hansmann, "Pathogenesis, diagnosis, and treatment of composite lymphomas," *The Lancet Oncology*, vol. 15, no. 10, pp. e435–e446, 2014.

[9] J. Castillo, L. Pantanowitz, and B. J. Dezube, "HIV-associated plasmablastic lymphoma: lessons learned from 112 published cases," *American Journal of Hematology*, vol. 83, no. 10, pp. 804–809, 2008.

[10] A. Carbone, "Emerging pathways in the development of AIDS-related lymphomas," *The Lancet Oncology*, vol. 4, no. 1, pp. 22–29, 2003.

[11] J. Morscio, D. Dierickx, J. Nijs et al., "Clinicopathologic comparison of plasmablastic lymphoma in HIV-positive, immunocompetent, and posttransplant patients," *The American Journal of Surgical Pathology*, vol. 38, no. 7, pp. 875–886, 2014.

[12] J. Chapman, A. J. Gentles, V. Sujoy et al., "Gene expression analysis of plasmablastic lymphoma identifies downregulation of B-cell receptor signaling and additional unique transcriptional programs," *Leukemia*, vol. 29, no. 11, pp. 2270–2273, 2015.

[13] A. Valera, O. Balagué, L. Colomo et al., "IG/MYC rearrangements are the main cytogenetic alteration in plasmablastic lymphomas," *The American Journal of Surgical Pathology*, vol. 34, no. 11, pp. 1686–1694, 2010.

[14] L. Taddesse-Heath, A. Meloni-Ehrig, J. Scheerle, J. C. Kelly, and E. S. Jaffe, "Plasmablastic lymphoma with MYC translocation: evidence for a common pathway in the generation of plasmablastic features," *Modern Pathology*, vol. 23, no. 7, pp. 991–999, 2010.

[15] S. Montes-Moreno, N. Martinez-Magunacelaya, T. Zecchini-Barrese et al., "Plasmablastic lymphoma phenotype is determined by genetic alterations in MYC and PRDM1," *Modern Pathology*, vol. 30, no. 1, pp. 85–94, 2017.

[16] D. Martinez, A. Valera, N. S. Perez et al., "Plasmablastic transformation of low-grade B-cell lymphomas," *The American Journal of Surgical Pathology*, vol. 37, no. 2, pp. 272–281, 2013.

[17] C. Marini, H. Baldaia, F. Trigo, and J. J. Castillo, "Transformation of a previously diagnosed diffuse large B-cell lymphoma to plasmablastic lymphoma," *American Journal of Hematology*, vol. 91, no. 8, p. E324, 2016.

[18] National Comprehensive Cancer Network, "NCCN clinical practice guidelines in oncology: b-cell lymphomas. AIDS-related b cell lymphomas," 2020, https://www.nccn.org/professionals/physician_gls/pdf/b-cell.pdf.

[19] T. A. Guerrero-Garcia, R. J. Mogollon, and J. J. Castillo, "Bortezomib in plasmablastic lymphoma: a glimpse of hope for a hard-to-treat disease," *Leukemia Research*, vol. 62, pp. 12–16, 2017.

[20] J. J. Castillo, J. L. Reagan, W. M. Sikov, and E. S. Winer, "Bortezomib in combination with infusional dose-adjusted EPOCH for the treatment of plasmablastic lymphoma," *British Journal of Haematology*, vol. 169, no. 3, pp. 352–355, 2015.

[21] E. Tchernonog, P. Faurie, P. Coppo et al., "Clinical characteristics and prognostic factors of plasmablastic lymphoma patients: analysis of 135 patients from the Lysa Group," *Annals of Oncology*, vol. 28, no. 4, pp. 843–848, 2017.

[22] T. Morito, M. Fujihara, H. Asaoku et al., "Serum soluble interleukin-2 receptor level and immunophenotype are prognostic factors for patients with diffuse large B-cell lymphoma," *Cancer Science*, vol. 100, no. 7, pp. 1255–1260, 2009.

[23] K. Umino, S.-I. Fujiwara, D. Minakata et al., "Prognostic impact of serum soluble interleukin-2 receptor level at diagnosis in elderly patients with diffuse large B-cell lymphoma treated with R-CHOP," *Leukemia & Lymphoma*, vol. 60, no. 3, pp. 734–741, 2019.

[24] M. M. Al-Malki, J. J. Castillo, J. M. Sloan, and A. Re, "Hematopoietic cell transplantation for plasmablastic lymphoma: a review," *Biology of Blood and Marrow Transplantation* vol. 20, no. 12, pp. 1877–1884, 2014.

31

Extensive Bone Marrow Necrosis: A Rare Presentation of Acute Lymphoblastic Leukaemia

I. Ranathunga,[1] **N. R. Muthumala**,[2] **H. W. C. K. Kulathilake**,[2] **S. Weerasinghe**,[3] **and N. L. A. Shyamali**[4]

[1]*Professorial Medical Unit, Colombo South Teaching Hospital, Colombo, Sri Lanka*
[2]*Department of Haematology, Faculty of Medicine, University of Sri Jayewardenepura, Colombo, Sri Lanka*
[3]*Cancer Institute, Maharagama, Colombo, Sri Lanka*
[4]*Department of Medicine, Faculty of Medicine, University of Sri Jayewardenepura, Colombo, Sri Lanka*

Correspondence should be addressed to I. Ranathunga; ish_75@yahoo.com

Academic Editor: Håkon Reikvam

Background. Bone marrow necrosis (BMN) is a rare entity which presents with bone pain, fever, and peripheral cytopenia. Acute lymphoblastic leukaemia (ALL) is characterized by malignant proliferation of immature lymphocytes, and patients usually present with fatigue and bleeding manifestations. Presentation with BMN is an extremely rare finding and only few cases had been reported in the literature. *Case Presentation.* A 22-year-old male presented with nocturnal lower back ache, pleuritic central chest pain, and fever for two weeks. He was extensively investigated for a cause. His investigations revealed pancytopenia with severe neutropenia. Initial bone marrow aspiration and biopsy did not provide a positive result due to extensive necrosis. However, immunohistochemical analysis of few immature lymphoid cells on repeated BM biopsy showed evidence of acute lymphoblastic leukaemia. *Conclusions.* ALL usually presents with fatigue and bleeding manifestations. Presentation with BMN is extremely rare. The diagnosis was extremely challenging as this patient had only occasional atypical cells in the peripheral blood film and the repeat bone marrow (BM) biopsy showed extensive necrosis.

1. Background

Bone marrow necrosis (BMN) is characterized by necrosis of the medullary stroma and myeloid tissues of the haematopoietic bone marrow (BM), leaving an amorphous eosinophilic background, necrotic cells, and preserved cortical bone [1]. It is a rare disorder with only few reported cases in the literature. The reported prevalence of the disease is variable between 0.3 and 37% with low prevalence among the living [2–5]. Severity is graded as severe, moderate, and mild according to the percentage of the diameter of the biopsy showing necrosis [1]. Trephine biopsy shows disruption of BM architecture with loss of fat spaces [6]. BMN is caused by a variety of medical conditions and drugs, of which haematological malignancies play a major role. Acute lymphoblastic leukaemia (ALL) is a haematological malignancy characterized by malignant proliferation of immature lymphocytes [7]. Depending on the extent of bone marrow involvement, the clinical manifestations may range from insidious onset nonspecific symptoms to acute onset, severe, life-threatening presentations [8, 9]. Only few cases of ALL have been reported as presenting with extensive bone marrow necrosis in the literature [1].

2. Case Presentation

A 22-year-old previously healthy male presented with nocturnal lower back ache, pleuritic central chest pain, and intermittent fever for two weeks. He did not have other constitutional symptoms or bleeding manifestations. Prior to admission, he had been treated with antibiotics and steroids by a general practitioner. His symptoms have subsided temporarily during this treatment. On admission, he was not pale and his vital parameters were stable. He had

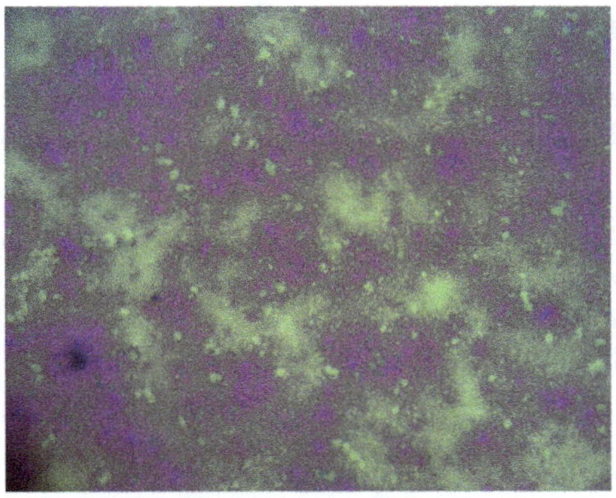

FIGURE 1: Bone marrow aspiration (Leishman stain) showing bone marrow necrosis.

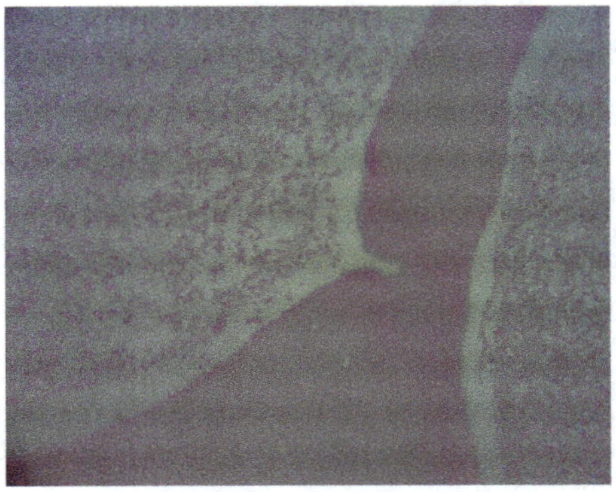

FIGURE 2: Bone marrow trephine biopsy (haematoxylin and eosin) showing extensive bone marrow necrosis.

bone tenderness over the sternum and lower lumbar spine. His cardiovascular, respiratory, abdominal, and neurological examination was normal.

On investigation, his white blood cell count (WBC) was $2.91 \times 10^3/\mu L$ with 51% neutrophils, heamoglobin was 13.6 g/dL, and platelet count was $28 \times 10^3/\mu L$. Blood picture revealed bicytopenia with leucoerythroblastic picture and occasional atypical cells. Reticulocyte count was 0.8%. Initial C-reactive protein was 520 mg/L, erythrocyte sediment rate was 110 mm/1st hour, and lactate dehydrogenase (LDH) was 4834 U/L. His alkaline phosphatase was 803 U/L (30–120 U/L), gamma glutamyl transferase was 171 U/L (<55 U/L), and total bilirubin was 67 μmol/L (5–21 μmol/L) with increased direct fraction. His renal function and coagulation profile were normal. During the hospital stay, his WBC dropped to $0.69 \times 10^3/\mu L$ with an absolute neutrophil count of $0.04 \times 10^3/\mu L$. Haemoglobin and platelets dropped to 7.4 g/dL and $6 \times 10^3/\mu L$, respectively. His viral studies including hepatitis A, hepatitis B, cytomegalovirus, Epstein-Barr, and human immunodeficiency were negative. Blood, urine, and sputum cultures were sterile. BM tuberculosis polymerase chain reaction and culture was negative.

BM aspiration and trephine biopsy revealed extensive necrosis with absence of cells. Repeated BM biopsy showed marrow spaces contained amorphous eosinophilic debris mixed with poorly demarcated cells (Figures 1 and 2). Nuclear details could not be appreciated. A clearly visible focus of immature lymphoid cells, which demonstrated nuclear terminal deoxynucleotidyl transferase (TdT) positivity on immunohistochemistry, was detected leading to the diagnosis of ALL. Immunophenotyping of peripheral blood by flow cytometry concluded 1-2% blasts of B lymphobast phenotype.

He was started on broad-spectrum antibiotics and high-dose steroids and required transfusion of several packed red cells and platelets before transfer to National Cancer Institute, Maharagama, for further management. ALL treatment protocol adapted from Hoelzer's (GMALL/BFM) 5/93 treatment regimen was started, and he has undergone the induction, consolidation 1, reinduction, and halfway of the consolidation 2 phase. He is responding well to treatment.

3. Discussion and Conclusions

Conditions that can cause BMN are haematological malignancies, sickle cell anaemia, infections, anorexia nervosa, haemolytic ureamic syndrome, antiphospholipid syndrome, hyperparathyroidism, and disseminated intravascular coagulation. Cytokines, antineoplastic drugs, and granulocyte colony-stimulating factors are some of the causative drugs [1]. The pathophysiology of BM necrosis can be due to several processes and mainly involves failure of the microcirculation [6]. Microcirculatory occlusion may occur as a result of fibrin thrombi formation, cytotoxic injury to vessels, tumor embolization, and tumor compression [10]. This process can be initiated by toxic effects of chemotherapy, irradiation, bacterial endotoxins, tumor cell infiltration, and cytokines [11].

Common manifestations of BMN are bone pain, fever, and peripheral cytopenia. All three cell lines may be affected while anaemia and thrombocytopenia are seen commonly [1]. Leucoerythroblastic blood picture, high LDH, and uric acid levels can be seen [1]. Our patient presented with bicytopenia and a leucoerythroblastic blood picture which can be a common presentation of hematological malignancies. The diagnosis of BMN is pathognomically made on the basis of bone marrow aspiration and biopsy findings. Due to extensive necrosis, BM aspiration is generally unsuccessful and multiple aspirations are necessary to arrive at a diagnosis [12]. Aspirated samples are opaque, whitish or reddish purple fluid. Stained smear shows amorphous pink stained material with faint outline of necrotic cells with nuclei appearing as dark stain smudges. Trephine biopsies are more informative with early stages showing pyknotic nuclei, granular cytoplasm, and indistinct cell margins. Later, nuclear karyorrhexis and complete loss of cell outlines result in amorphous eosinophilic debris with considerable loss of fat spaces [6]. Immunohistochemistry may be misleading if used to investigate neoplastic cells in necrotic areas due to loss of antigens and tendency of antibodies to adhere in a nonspecific way to necrotic tissue [6]. Though the radiological investigations may play a limited role in evaluation, MRI demonstrates a characteristic geographic pattern of signal abnormalities with diffuse and extensive involvement [13]. Characteristically, the marrow demonstrates a central region of varying signal intensity which is surrounded by a low signal intensity peripheral band [13]. Favorable prognosis depends on the underling diagnosis, especially when mild degree of bone marrow necrosis is present. BMN usually has an unfavorable outcome [9, 14]. Prolonged BMN can lead to secondary bone marrow fibrosis [1]. Median survival ranges from weeks to months [1].

ALL usually presents with fatigue and bleeding manifestations [6]. Presentation with BMN is extremely rare [1, 9]. The diagnosis was extremely challenging as this patient had only occasional atypical cells in the peripheral blood film, and the BM biopsy showed extensive necrosis. This case highlights the rare presentation of ALL and importance of repeated bone marrow examination and usage of complimentary tools in haematopathology.

Abbreviations

BMN: Bone marrow necrosis
ALL: Acute lymphoblastic leukaemia
BM: Bone marrow
WBC: White blood cell count
LDH: Lactate dehydrogenase
MRI: Magnetic resonance imaging.

Consent

The patient's consent was taken to report his clinical details anonymously. The authors have taken informed written consent from the patient to report and publish about his illness anonymously.

Authors' Contributions

N. L. A. Shyamali and I. Ranathunga involved in the history taking, examination, diagnosing, and management of the patient's condition and prepared the manuscript for publication. N. R. Muthumala and H. W. C. K. Kulathilake performed and reported the blood pictures, bone marrow aspirations, and biopsies and were actively involved in the diagnosis of the patient's condition and provided images for publication. S. Weerasinghe was involved in the management of the patient's condition after he was transferred to the National Cancer Institute of Sri Lanka and provided details of management. All authors read and approved the final manuscript.

Acknowledgments

The authors acknowledge the support from staff of ward 1 in Colombo South Teaching Hospital, Haematology Team, and staff of National Cancer Institute in the management of this patient's condition.

References

[1] S. Paydas, M. Ergin, F. Baslamisli et al., "Bone marrow necrosis: clinicopathologic analysis of 20 cases and review of the literature," *American Journal of Hematology*, vol. 70, no. 4, pp. 300–305, 2002.

[2] J. F. Kiraly and M. S. Wheby, "Bone marrow necrosis," *The American Journal of Medicine*, vol. 60, no. 3, pp. 361–368, 1976.

[3] M. J. Norgard, J. T. Carpenter, and M. E. Conrad, "Bone marrow necrosis and degeneration," *Archives of Internal Medicine*, vol. 139, no. 8, pp. 905–911, 1979.

[4] A. M. Jassens, F. C. Offner, and W. Z. Van Hove, "Bone marrow necrosis," *Cancer*, vol. 88, pp. 1769–1780, 2000.

[5] B. A. Nies, D. W. Kundel, L. B. Thomas, and E. J. Freireich, "Leukopenia, bone pain, and bone necrosis in patients with acute leukemia," *Annals of Internal Medicine*, vol. 62, no. 4, pp. 698–705, 1965.

[6] B. J. Bain, D. M. Clark, and B. S. Wilkins, *Bone Marrow Pathology*, John Wiley and Sons Ltd Publication, London, UK, 4th edition, 2010.

[7] R. A. Larson and J. Anastasi, *Acute Lymphoblastic Leukemia: Clinical Presentation, Diagnosis, and Classification*, Springer, Berlin, Germany, 2008.

[8] O. Frankfurt, L. A. Petersen, S. Martin, and Tallman, *Acute Lymphocytic Leukemia—Clinical Features and Making the Diagnosis*, Humana Press, Totowa, NJ, USA, 2010.

[9] T. Badar, A. Shetty, C. Bueso-Ramos et al., "Bone marrow necrosis in acute leukemia: clinical characteristic and outcome," *American Journal of Hematology*, vol. 90, no. 9, pp. 769–773, 2015.

[10] D. Maisel, J. Y. Lim, W. J. Pollock, and P. I. Liu, "Bone marrow necrosis: an entity often overlooked," *Annals of Clinical & Laboratory Science*, vol. 18, pp. 109–115, 1998.

[11] P. Ricci, G. Bandini, M. Baccarani, F. Bazzocchi, G. Martinelli, and S. Tura, "Bone marrow necrosis by diffuse metastatic intravascular obstruction," *Haematologica*, vol. 67, no. 5, pp. 754–759, 1982.

[12] C. Knupp, P. H. Pekala, and P. Cornelius, "Extensive bone marrow necrosis in patients with cancer and tumor necrosis factor activity in plasma," *American Journal of Hematology*, vol. 29, no. 4, pp. 215–221, 1988.

[13] Y. M. Tang, S. Jeavons, S. Stuckey, H. Middleton, and D. Gill, "MRI features of bone marrow necrosis," *American Journal of Roentgenology*, vol. 188, no. 2, pp. 509–514, 2007.

[14] L. A. Al-Gwaiz, "Bone marrow necrosis," *Annals of Saudi Medicine*, vol. 17, no. 3, pp. 374–376, 1997.

32

CNS Involvement in a Patient with Chronic Myeloid Leukemia

Marcus A. Healey,[1] **Daniel J. Allendorf**,[2] **Uma Borate**,[3] **and Ankit Madan**[4]

[1]*Edward Via College of Osteopathic Medicine, Blacksburg, VA, USA*
[2]*Alabama Oncology, Alabaster, AL, USA*
[3]*School of Medicine, Oregon Health & Science University, Portland, OR, USA*
[4]*SOVAH Cancer Center, Danville, VA, USA*

Correspondence should be addressed to Ankit Madan; ankmadan@gmail.com

Academic Editor: Massimo Breccia

Inspite of medication compliance, some chronic myeloid leukemia (CML) patients will relapse/progress into an accelerated phase or blast crisis. Central nervous system (CNS) involvement is a rare manifestation of such a relapse. Here, we report a case of 23-year-old female who was diagnosed with CML in the accelerated phase and subsequently treated with imatinib. She developed early relapse in her CNS, and her treatment was switched to dasatinib and intrathecal chemotherapy with cytarabine and methotrexate. Her CNS disease went into remission, and she underwent matched unrelated donor (MUD) hematopoietic stem cell transplant (HSCT). We discuss various mechanisms of treatment failure, importance of vigilance for symptoms and signs of treatment failure/relapse, indications for use of different tyrosine kinase inhibitors (TKIs), and management of blast crises in CML.

1. Introduction

CML is a clonal proliferation of progenitor stem cells, resulting from a reciprocal translocation between chromosomes 9 and 22 forming the Philadelphia chromosome t (9; 22) (q34; q11). The chimeric BCR-ABL fusion gene resulting from this translocation subsequently codes for constitutively active tyrosine kinase that activates several intracellular proteins which leads to clonal proliferation. CML represents a success for targeted therapies known as tyrosine kinase inhibitors (TKIs). These agents are small molecule antagonists used in treatment of several cancers. In the case of CML, they are directed against the constitutively activated BCR-ABL protein. Approximately 90% of patients with CML are diagnosed in the chronic phase (CP). A fraction of patient's experience relapse or progress to an accelerated phase or blast crisis in the form of acute leukemia, either myeloid (AML) or lymphoid (ALL), respectively. Treatment with first generation TKI, imatinib, leads to complete hematologic, cytogenetic, and molecular remissions in approximately 90%, 70%, and 30% of patients, respectively [1]. The second generation TKIs, dasatinib and nilotinib, enjoy higher rates of cytogenetic and molecular remissions, roughly 90% and 70%, respectively, and these generally occur more rapidly than observed after treatment with imatinib [2, 3]. Patients require monitoring of complete blood count with differential every 2 weeks until patients attain a complete hematological response. Molecular response is measured by ratio of BCR-ABL1 transcripts to ABL1 transcript according to the international scale. This is performed by peripheral blood quantitative polymerase chain reaction (PCR). Cytogenetics should be performed in marrow cell metaphases at diagnosis through chromosome banding analysis or interphase fluorescence in situ hybridization (FISH), and in patients with atypical translocations, and when PCR is unable to measure atypical or rare BCR-ABL1 transcripts [4, 5]. These responses are measured against a set of temporal benchmarks that prompt changes in management if they are not met. It is reported that response rates for those patients presenting in the accelerated phase or blast crisis are decreased regardless of the TKI used but are still improved by the use of second generation TKIs [6].

Some patients fail to respond to treatment or relapse despite treatment. There are numerous mechanisms of treatment failures which include nonadherence, resistance, particularly in the form of ATP-binding pocket mutations within the BCR/ABL fusion protein, expression of transporter proteins, and epigenetic modifications of the fusion transcript, among others [7, 8]. Despite the achievement of therapeutic milestones including hematologic, cytogenetic, and molecular remissions, treatment failures as a consequence of above mechanisms can occur. Clinicians should always remain vigilant for evidence of treatment failures despite these milestones and change management appropriately. We report a patient undergoing treatment for CML with TKIs who had a very unusual presentation of relapsed disease, presenting with CNS involvement, despite adherence to therapy. We will discuss potential mechanisms of disease resistance or progression and briefly discuss the management of CML in blast crisis.

2. Case Presentation

Our patient is a 23-year-old female who presented with two weeks of fatigue, symmetric lower extremity edema, and easy bruising. Her white blood cell count (WBC) was 385,000 cells/μL with basophilia and 15% blasts, platelet count (PC) of 1×10^6 cells/μL, and hemoglobin of 8.2 g/dL. Bone marrow aspiration and biopsy (BMBx) showed a hypercellular marrow (>95% cellularity) with 14% blasts, having an immature myeloid immunophenotype. Karyotype and FISH from the bone marrow aspirate were positive for t (9; 22) (q34; q11). She was diagnosed with CML in the accelerated phase defined by the WHO criterion of 15% circulating blasts [9] Treatment began with imatinib 400 mg twice daily. Within two weeks, her WBC count had normalized. After 10 weeks, she achieved a complete hematological response (CHR) with normal blood counts. At this time, she developed headache. She reported adherence to imatinib therapy. Her neurological exam revealed normal cranial nerve examination, normal deep tendon reflexes, and intact motor and sensory exam. She was evaluated and empirically treated with nonsteroidal anti-inflammatory drugs (NSAIDS) but found no relief. One week later, she underwent a gadolinium-contrasted MRI brain revealing enhancement in the left posterior frontal lobe involving the subarachnoid space. A lumbar puncture revealed an elevated opening pressure and increased cerebrospinal fluid (CSF) cell count of 468 cells/μL with 51% blasts with the same immature myeloid immunophenotype. FISH from the CSF revealed evidence of t (9; 22) (q34; q11) in 200/200 cells analyzed. At the writing of this report, mutational status of CSF sample and CD 93 was not available. At this time, her CBC was normal, and she continued to be in complete hematological remission. BMBx showed no evidence of CML, suggesting an isolated CNS relapse of CML in blast crisis as per the WHO criterion of extramedullary infiltration of blasts [10]. Based on data suggesting superior CNS penetration by dasatinib, imatinib was discontinued, and dasatinib 100 mg daily was started [11–13]. In addition, she received one dose each of intrathecal cytarabine and intrathecal methotrexate on consecutive days. Thereafter, she received weekly intrathecal cytarabine for two additional weeks at which time the myeloid blast population was not detectable in the CSF. She continued to have no evidence of recurrent myeloid blasts in the CNS for six months after her relapse. Her CBC remained normal. BMBx performed four months after the relapse demonstrated no evidence of t (9; 22) (q34; q11) by karyotype or FISH, and quantitative reverse transcriptase PCR (QT-PCR) from the peripheral blood revealed no copies of the BCR/ABL transcript. Given her young age, outstanding performance status, the good support system, and the aggressive nature of her CML, she underwent a matched unrelated donor (MUD) hematopoietic stem cell transplant (HSCT) in the absence of a suitable sibling donor.

3. Discussion

Isolated CNS symptoms are rare in CML; however, there have been case reports that show a pattern of demographic data. Typically, but not seen in our case, males are more affected than females at a ratio of 4.5 : 1. The median age at diagnosis is 40 years old, and patients who had isolated CNS relapse were on imatinib therapy for a median of 2.4 years. Importantly, headache and vomiting are the most common presenting symptoms in isolated CNS relapse, and their presentation should prompt clinical suspicion of CML relapse. Papilledema remains the most common finding on fundoscopy, and leptomeningeal enhancement is the most common finding on imaging [14].

Durable remissions in patients with CML can be achieved with TKIs. A fraction of patients, though, will fail to respond or will have disease progression to the accelerated phase or blast crisis. At present, there are multiple sets of criteria in use to define the accelerated phase or blast crisis. In terms of prognosis, the most important factor appears to be blast count with the poorest prognosis found at a peripheral blood count of >30% blasts [15]. Myeloid immunophenotype and the use of TKI therapy prior to blast crisis from either the chronic phase or accelerated phase portends a worse prognosis [16]. There are multiple observed and hypothesized mechanisms of TKI failure including, but not limited to, nonadherence, resistance, particularly in the form of ATP-binding pocket mutations within the BCR/ABL fusion protein, expression of transporter proteins, and epigenetic modifications of the BCR/ABL fusion transcript [6, 7]. In the event of treatment failure, relapse, or progression to blast crisis, the management depends on the immunophenotype of the blasts.

Nonadherence defined by the Basel Assessment of Adherence Scale with immunosuppressive medication has been demonstrated in up to one-third of patients taking imatinib, and correlation studies have demonstrated an inverse relationship between nonadherence and the probability of achieving a complete cytogenetic response [17–19]. Mutations in the BCR/ABL protein are found in more than 50% of patients' refractory to imatinib [20]. Indications for mutation analysis include failure to achieve a hematologic response by three months, minimal cytogenetic response by six months, relapse (including increases in BCR/ABL transcript by QT-PCR), and presentation in or progression to the accelerated phase or blast crisis [7, 19]. Many of these mutations occur in the adenosine triphosphate- (ATP-) binding pocket of the protein, and one of these, the T315I mutation accounting for up to 15% of mutations, confers resistance to imatinib, dasatinib, and nilotinib [6]. Mutation status can be detected by RT-PCR with sequence analysis, and the sensitivity of various BCR/ABL mutants to available TKIs has been assessed in vitro to help guide treatment [21]. Newer generation TKIs are being designed to overcome this current limitation [22]. For instance, ponatinib is a 3rd generation TKI that is FDA approved for all CML patients harboring the T3151 mutation. Ponatinib should be considered in CML patients who have failed first and second-line therapies either through relapse or inability to tolerate side effects. The European Leukemia Network also recommends using ponatinib in patients who are resistant to second generation TKI and do not have a specific mutation [4]. One recent study showed that the identification of CD93 on CML cells may be important in identifying a population of tumor cells that are resistant to TKI therapy [23]. Thus, other therapies may need to be considered in patients expressing this marker. Transporter proteins and drug efflux pumps contribute to the resistance of tumors to many conventional and targeted therapies. Treatment of CML with TKIs is no exception. The P-glycoprotein efflux pump and ATP-binding cassette (ABC) transporter have been identified on primary CML isolates and have been shown to expel TKIs [24]. Indeed, it has been shown that imatinib concentration in the CNS is decreased by the P-glycoprotein pump at the blood-brain barrier [25]. Epigenetic regulation of BCR/ABL and other genes relevant to the survival of CML tumor cells is also described. There is a recent description of epigenetic silencing through hypermethylation of microRNA-203 whose targets include ABL1. Restoration of microRNA-203 expression through transfection with a vector containing microRNA-203 was shown to decrease the expression of the BCR/ABL transcript in a CML cell line. Epigenetic silencing also occurs through polycomb group (PcG) proteins, which are thought to play an important role in stem cell differentiation and hematopoiesis [26]. Last, sirtuin 1 is a histone deacetylase that is upregulated in CML cells positive for CD34. In studies of patients with CML treated with imatinib, SIRT1 expression was diminished but not entirely absent. Thus, direct sirtuin 1 inhibition may prove to be a potential novel therapy for CML patients [27].

Any treatment decision regarding management of CML in blast crisis should include consideration of allogeneic HSCT. The immunophenotype of the blasts should be assessed to determine if the cells are myeloid or lymphoid. Treatment should include a TKI with the specific choice dependent on prior therapy and mutation analysis (Table 1) [20]. Treatment with TKI only may be a sufficient bridge to allogeneic HSCT or it can be combined with conventional AML or ALL induction regimens for myeloid and lymphoid blast crises, respectively. Ponatinib has shown promise as potential additional therapy with allogeneic HSCT in patients with extramedullary blast crisis harboring the T315I mutation [28]. In the case of our presented patient, she only had evidence of myeloid blasts in the CNS, which is an uncommon presentation. Her treatment plan was influenced by evidence that imatinib has low CNS penetration, whereas dasatinib, in animal models, had improved CNS penetration [12]. In addition, dasatinib has been shown to decrease microglial and astrocytic neuro-inflammatory responses, which may have important implications for therapy in isolated CNS blast crises [29]. Local control in the CNS was achieved further by using cytarabine, a drug with activity against myeloid blasts [10, 30].

Table 1: European Leukemia Network' summary of the most appropriate alternative therapeutic options based on BCR-ABL KD mutation status [4].

Mutation	Therapeutic options
T315I	Ponatinib
F317L/V/I/C, T315A	Nilotinib, bosutinib[#], or ponatinib
V299L	Nilotinib or ponatinib
Y253H, E255V/K, F359V/I/C	Dasatinib, bosutinib[#], or ponatinib

[#]Limited in vivo data suggest resistance to bosutinib in vivo in patients with E255K and, to a reduced extent, the E255V mutation.

In summary, significant therapeutic advances in the treatment of CML have been made in the past fifteen years, most notably, by the development of TKIs. Despite these advances, a fraction of patients fail to respond optimally to treatment while others will relapse while receiving therapy. The mechanisms driving these clinical challenges include nonadherence, acquired mutations in the BCR/ABL fusion protein, the expression of TKI efflux systems by tumor cells, and failure of epigenetic silencing of the BCR/ABL transcript. Treatment decisions in these situations need to be highly individualized. In addition to the development of newer TKIs (such as radotinib in South Korea) and next generation TKIs (such as ponatinib), emphasis should be placed on the development of novel strategies to combat other mechanisms of treatment failure [4]. Clinicians must also remain vigilant for evidence of therapeutic failure or progressive/relapsed disease and be aware of unusual patterns of treatment failure as illustrated by our case.

Authors' Contributions

All authors contributed to the acquisition of data and drafting, writing, and editing the manuscript. DA and UB were involved in clinical management of the patient.

References

[1] S. G. O'Brien, F. Guilhot, R. A. Larson et al., "Imatinib compared with interferon and low-dose cytarabine for newly diagnosed chronic-phase chronic myeloid leukemia," *New England Journal of Medicine*, vol. 348, no. 11, pp. 994–1004, 2003.

[2] H. Kantarjian, N. P. Shah, A. Hochhaus et al., "Dasatinib versus imatinib in newly diagnosed chronic-phase chronic

myeloid leukemia," *New England Journal of Medicine*, vol. 362, no. 24, pp. 2260–2270, 2010.

[3] H. M. Kantarjian, A. Hochhaus, G. Saglio et al., "Nilotinib versus imatinib for the treatment of patients with newly diagnosed chronic phase, Philadelphia chromosome-positive, chronic myeloid leukaemia: 24-month minimum follow-up of the phase 3 randomised ENESTnd trial," *The Lancet Oncology*, vol. 12, no. 9, pp. 841–851, 2011.

[4] A. Hochhaus, M. Baccarani, R. T. Silver et al., "European LeukemiaNet 2020 recommendations for treating chronic myeloid leukemia," *Leukemia*, vol. 34, no. 4, pp. 966–984, 2020.

[5] M. Baccarani, S. Pileri, J.-L. Steegmann, M. Muller, S. Soverini, and M. Dreyling, "Chronic myeloid leukemia: ESMO clinical practice guidelines for diagnosis, treatment and follow-up," *Annals of Oncology*, vol. 23, no. 7, pp. vii72–vii77, 2012.

[6] K. Porkka, S. Mustjoki, and B. Simonsson, "Suboptimal responses in chronic myeloid leukemia: milestones and mechanisms," *Expert Review of Hematology*, vol. 2, no. 1, pp. 81–91, 2009.

[7] M. Deininger, "Resistance and relapse with imatinib in CML: causes and consequences," *Journal of the National Comprehensive Cancer Network*, vol. 6, no. 2, pp. S11–S21, 2008.

[8] P. La Rosée and M. W. Deininger, "Resistance to imatinib: mutations and beyond," *Seminars in Hematology*, vol. 47, no. 4, pp. 335–343, 2010.

[9] D. A. Arber, A. Orazi, R. Hasserjian et al., "The 2016 revision to the World Health Organization classification of myeloid neoplasms and acute leukemia," *Blood*, vol. 127, no. 20, pp. 2391–2405, 2016.

[10] S. Swerdlow, E. Campo, N. Harris et al., *WHO Classification of Tumours of Haematopoietic and Lymphoid Tissues*, WHO Press, Geneva, Switzerland, 4th edition, 2008.

[11] K. J. Aichberger, S. Herndlhofer, H. Agis et al., "Liposomal cytarabine for treatment of myeloid central nervous system relapse in chronic myeloid leukaemia occurring during imatinib therapy," *European Journal of Clinical Investigation*, vol. 37, no. 10, pp. 808–813, 2007.

[12] S. Bujassoum, J. Rifkind, and J. H. Lipton, "Isolated central nervous system relapse in lymphoid blast crisis chronic myeloid leukemia and acute lymphoblastic leukemia in patients on imatinib therapy," *Leukemia & Lymphoma*, vol. 45, no. 2, pp. 401–403, 2004.

[13] K. Porkka, P. Koskenvesa, T. Lundan et al., "Dasatinib crosses the blood-brain barrier and is an efficient therapy for central nervous system Philadelphia chromosome-positive leukemia," *Blood*, vol. 112, no. 4, pp. 1005–1012, 2008.

[14] A. Jain and N. Gupta, "Isolated CNS blast crises in chronic myeloid leukemia presenting as hypertrophic pachymeningitis and bilateral optic neuritis: a case report," *Journal of Clinical and Diagnostic Research: JCDR*, vol. 10, no. 1, Article ID OE01-5, 2016.

[15] M. K. Lauseker, A. Turkina, E. Faber et al., "Prognosis of patients with chronic myeloid leukemia presenting in advanced phase is defined mainly by blast count, but also by age, chromosomal aberrations and hemoglobin," *American Journal of Hematology*, vol. 94, no. 11, pp. 1236–1243, 2019.

[16] P. Bachl, H. M. Kantarjian, A. Ghorab et al., "Prognostic factors and survival outcomes in patients with chronic myeloid leukemia in blast phase in the tyrosine kinase inhibitor era: cohort study of 477 patients," *Cancer*, vol. 123, no. 22, pp. 4391–4402, 2017.

[17] P. Kantarjian, T. G. Sagar, B. Dubashi et al., "Nonadherence to imatinib adversely affects event free survival in chronic phase chronic myeloid leukemia," *American Journal of Hematology*, vol. 86, no. 6, pp. 471–474, 2011.

[18] D. Marin, A. Bazeos, F. X. Mahon et al., "Adherence is the critical factor for achieving molecular responses in patients with chronic myeloid leukemia who achieve complete cytogenetic responses on imatinib," *Journal of Clinical Oncology*, vol. 28, no. 14, pp. 2381–2388, 2010.

[19] L. Noens, M. A. van Lierde, R. De Bock et al., "Prevalence, determinants, and outcomes of nonadherence to imatinib therapy in patients with chronic myeloid leukemia: the ADAGIO study," *Blood*, vol. 113, no. 22, pp. 5401–5411, 2009.

[20] S. Branford and T. P. Hughes, "Mutational analysis in chronic myeloid leukemia: when and what to do?" *Current Opinion in Hematology*, vol. 18, no. 2, pp. 111–116, 2011.

[21] S. Soverini, A. Hochhaus, F. E. Nicolini et al., "BCR-ABL kinase domain mutation analysis in chronic myeloid leukemia patients treated with tyrosine kinase inhibitors: recommendations from an expert panel on behalf of European LeukemiaNet," *Blood*, vol. 118, no. 5, pp. 1208–1215, 2011.

[22] T. O'Hare, M. W. N. Deininger, C. A. Eide, T. Clackson, and B. J. Druker, "Targeting the BCR-ABL signaling pathway in therapy-resistant Philadelphia chromosome-positive leukemia," *Clinical Cancer Research*, vol. 17, no. 2, pp. 212–221, 2011.

[23] R. Kinstrie, G. A. Horne, H. Morrison et al., "CD93 is expressed on chronic myeloid leukemia stem cells and identifies a quiescent population which persists after tyrosine kinase inhibitor therapy," *Leukemia*, vol. 34, no. 6, pp. 1613–1625, 2020.

[24] S. Shukla, A. P. Skoumbourdis, M. J. Walsh et al., "Synthesis and characterization of a BODIPY conjugate of the BCR-ABL kinase inhibitor tasigna (nilotinib): evidence for transport of Tasigna and its fluorescent derivative by ABC drug transporters," *Molecular Pharmaceutics*, vol. 8, no. 4, pp. 1292–1302, 2011.

[25] H. Dai, P. Marbach, M. Lemaire, M. Hayes, and W. F. Elmquist, "Distribution of STI-571 to the brain is limited by P-glycoprotein-mediated efflux," *Journal of Pharmacology and Experimental Therapeutics*, vol. 304, no. 3, pp. 1085–1092, 2003.

[26] J. Bugler, R. Kinstrie, M. T. Scott, and D. Vetrie, "Epigenetic reprogramming and emerging epigenetic therapies in CML," *Frontiers in Cell and Developmental Biology*, vol. 7, Article ID 136, 2019.

[27] H. Z. Yuan, L. Li, H. Zhang et al., "Activation of stress response gene SIRT1 by BCR-ABL promotes leukemogenesis," *Blood*, vol. 119, no. 8, pp. 1904–1914, 2012.

[28] J. Zhang, X. Zhang, Y. Lu, J. Jiao, Y. Chen, and D. Lin, "Extramedullary blast crisis in a patient with T315I BCR-ABL mutated chronic myeloid leukemia," *Clinical Laboratory*, vol. 64, no. 1, pp. 193–196, 2018.

[29] K.-Y. Ryu, H.-J. Lee, H. Woo et al., "Dasatinib regulates LPS-induced microglial and astrocytic neuroinflammatory responses by inhibiting AKT/STAT3 signaling," *Journal of Neuroinflammation*, vol. 16, no. 1, Article ID 190, 2019.

[30] E. Morra, M. Lazzarino, E. Brusamolino et al., "The role of systemic high-dose cytarabine in the treatment of central nervous system leukemia clinical results in 46 patients," *Cancer*, vol. 72, no. 2, pp. 439–445, 1993.

33

A Rare Case of Coexisting Breast Cancer and Refractory Acute Myeloid Leukemia

L. Ballotta,[1] S. M. Trisolini,[1] A. P. Iori,[1] U. La Rocca,[1] A. Micozzi,[1] G. Gentile,[1] T. De Giacomo,[2] A. Guarini,[1] R. Foà,[1] and S. Capria[1]

[1]*Hematology, Department of Translational and Precision Medicine, Sapienza University of Rome, Rome, Italy*
[2]*Department of Cardiovascular and Thoracic Surgery "Paride Stefanini", Sapienza University, Policlinico Umberto I, Rome, Italy*

Correspondence should be addressed to L. Ballotta; ballotta@bce.uniroma1.it

Academic Editor: Yusuke Shiozawa

The occurrence of acute myeloid leukemia (AML) within six months from a diagnosis of breast cancer (BC) is rarely reported in the literature, and it is associated with a poor prognosis. We report herein the case of a 40-year-old woman referred to our centre affected by BC and simultaneous AML. The patient proved refractory to first line therapy and achieved complete remission (CR) with a clofarabine-based regimen followed by allogeneic stem cell transplantation (ASCT). Both during salvage chemotherapy and after ASCT, the patient presented severe infectious complications (acute cholecistytis and *Nocardia* pneumonia, respectively) treated with surgery, and currently she is alive in CR for both diseases after 29 months of follow-up. The case highlights the importance of a diagnostic assessment of any unexplained cytopenia in association with solid neoplasia under treatment, underlining the feasibility and priority of a timely treatment of the haematological neoplasm in order to achieve long-term survival.

1. Introduction

The prognosis of early-stage breast cancer (BC) in women has radically improved after the introduction of neoadjuvant chemotherapy regimens including anthracyclines and alkylating agents [1]. However, the association between cytotoxic agents and secondary acute myeloid leukemia (AML) has been frequently reported in the literature, and it is included in the 2016 edition of WHO classification as "therapy-related myeloid neoplasms." While this association is a late complication of chemotherapy and depends on the cumulative dose administered, the synchronous occurrence (within 6 months) of two neoplasms is rarely observed [2]. We hereby report a rare case of coexisting BC and refractory AML focusing on the importance of an early diagnosis of both diseases, and of a shared approach between the hematologist and the oncologist to tailor both the treatment choices and the timing of intervention.

2. Case Report

In October 2016, a 40-year-old woman was admitted to another hospital for a diagnosis of BC. One month prior to admission, a routinary mammography had shown the presence of a mass of 15 mm in diameter confirmed by a subsequent MRI scan. She was treated with right quadrantectomy and axillary dissection, and the histopathology provided a diagnosis of grade III invasive poorly differentiated ductal carcinoma. Immunohistochemistry was positive for estrogen and progesterone receptors (75%), with a high Ki67 proliferation index (30%) and mild expression of HER-2 (+1). However, fluorescent in situ hybridization for the HER2 gene was negative (staging pT1N2M0). In November, she started adjuvant chemotherapy regimen with doxorubicin 60 mg/m^2/day and cyclophosphamide 600 mg/m^2/day for 4 cycles, followed by maintenance with paclitaxel 80 mg/m^2 since April 2017 and endocrine therapy with tamoxifen. Peripheral blood cell count at the start of chemotherapy showed leukopenia (white blood cells count

1.0×10^9/L), not further investigated, with mild anemia (hemoglobin 11.6 g/dl) and normal platelets count (168×10^9/L). In June 2017, during breast adjuvant radiotherapy, the patient was persistently pancytopenic (hemoglobin 9.6 g/dl, white blood cells 0.9×10^9/L, and platelets 101×10^9/L). Bone marrow was cellular (+3) and showed 82% of CD34/CD117/CD13+ and CD33/CD7/CD11b/CD14/cMPO blasts of small-medium size, round nucleus, and basophilic cytoplasm with rare granules, consistent with a diagnosis of AML. Cytogenetic analysis showed a normal karyotype (46, XX), and the gene mutation status was wild type for FLT3/ITD and TKD, AML1/ETO, Cbf/MYH11, NPM1, PML-RARα, BCR-ABL1, and MLL. The patient was treated with ICE induction chemotherapy, consisting of a combination of idarubicin 10 mg/m^2 days 1, 3, and 5, cytarabine 100 mg/m^2 days 1–7, and etoposide 100 mg/m^2 days 1–5, but proved refractory. In September 2017, the patient was referred to our centre and underwent a salvage chemotherapy with the G-CLAC schedule: clofarabine 30 mg/m^2 days 1–5, cytarabine 2000 mg/m^2 days 1–5, and granulocyte colony stimulating factor (G-CSF) until hemopoietic recovery. On day +13 from chemotherapy, the patient was pancytopenic (hemoglobin 8.5 g/dl, white blood cells 0.750×10^9/L, neutrophils 0.2×10^9/L, and platelets 20×10^9/L) and presented a septic shock, associated with acute abdominal pain with positive Murphy sign and positive blood cultures for *Escherichia coli, Staphylococcus haemolyticus,* and *Candida glabrata.* She received antibiotic and antifungal treatment (meropenem, tigecycline, and caspofungin) and supportive care with fluids and inotropic agents. An abdominal ultrasound and an MRI allowed to make a diagnosis of acute cholecistytis and in October 2017 (on day +30 from chemotherapy), after a full hematologic recovery, she underwent a laparoscopic cholecystectomy. The microbiologic examination of pericholecistic liquid revealed a multidrug-resistant *Pseudomonas aeruginosa.* In the same period, she became a KPC-*Klebsiella pneumoniae* rectal carrier. On day +35, the bone marrow aspiration showed a complete remission (CR). For this reason, in November 2017, on day +56 from chemotherapy, she underwent an allogeneic hematopoietic stem cell transplantation (HSCT) from the haploidentical brother after a preparative regimen with TBF (thiotepa 5 mg/kg days −7, −6; fludarabine 50 mg/m^2 days −5, −4, −3; busulfan 3.2 mg/kg days −5, −4, −3). No major toxicity was observed during the aplastic phase, and the engraftment was obtained on day +17 for PMN and on day +25 for platelets. On day +20, the bone marrow aspirate confirmed a CR with complete donor chimerism, and on day +30, the patient was discharged.

Two months after discharge, she was readmitted to the hospital due to an acute left chest pain, fever, and neutropenia (hemoglobin 8.9 g/dl, white blood cells 0.62×10^9/L, neutrophils 0.34×10^9/L, and platelets 21×10^9/L); chest computed tomographic scan showed a basal bilateral pneumonia associated with diffuse pulmonary nodules and bronchial obliteration. A microbiological examination of bronchoalveolar lavage proved the presence of a *Nocardia* spp. Despite targeted antibiotic therapy with high-dose sulfametoxazole-trimethoprim in association with broad-spectrum and specific antibiotics in different timing (amikacin, ceftadizime-avibactam, levoxacin, ceftolozane-tazobactam, tigecycline, imipenem, and linezolid), pulmonary nocardial lesions persisted (and progressed toward) with the formation of a pulmonary organized abscess (Figure 1). Due to the persistence of fever and worsening of clinical conditions, the patient was submitted to a lower pulmonary lobectomy by left lateral thoracotomy; histological examination confirmed the presence of a *Nocardia* spp. She had a good postoperative course with disappearance of fever and complete resolution of the pneumonia.

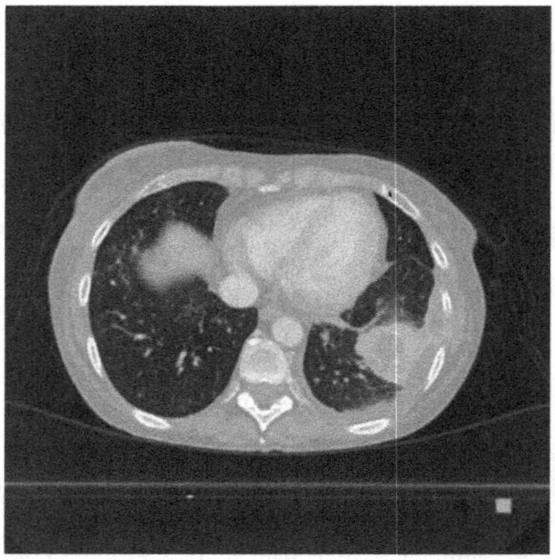

Figure 1: Pulmonary TC scan showing nocardial organized abscess in the left inferior lobe.

Currently, the patient is alive in continuous CR for AML and BC, with a follow-up from diagnosis of 29 months and 37 months, respectively. She is in good general conditions with an excellent quality of life.

3. Discussion

Herein we describe the case of a young woman presenting with unexplained and persistent cytopenia before and during chemotherapy for BC, due to the coexistence of BC and AML.

The onset of AML within 6 months from a diagnosis of BC is associated with a very poor prognosis with refractoriness to standard therapies and a limited chance to receive an allogeneic HSCT; only 7 cases of a synchronous occurrence of BC and AML have been so far described in the literature (Table 1), and only 3 of them reached a CR for AML. No patient, except the present case, could undergo an allogeneic HSCT and achieved a CR for both diseases. Our patient had a refractory disease for which an allogeneic HSCT currently represents the only recommended therapeutic approach aimed at achieving a long-term disease-free survival [7]. The timing of the different interventions was crucial to bridge this patient to allogeneic HSCT; despite the infectious complications, first of all the acute cholecistytis, she was subjected to laparoscopic cholecystectomy on day +30 from salvage chemotherapy, immediately after a complete hematologic recovery, and to allogeneic HSCT on day +56, after the demonstration of a CR for AML.

In the past years, the use of clofarabine-based regimens as a bridge to transplant has provided encouraging results [8]. Clofarabine is a second-generation purine nucleoside

Table 1: Cases of synchronous occurrence of BC and AML in the literature.

Case	Latency	Morphology	Phenotype	Karyotype	Genetics	Outcome
Jacobs and Carey [3]	Simultaneous	NA	NA	NA	NA	NA
Carey [3]	Simultaneous	NA	NA	NA	NA	Died during induction (no autopsy).
Rosner et al. (case 18) [4]	3 months	NA	NA	NA	NA	Died in CR of AML for diabetic coma and gastrointestinal hemorrhage.
Ershler (case 6 and 8) [5]	6 months	NA	NA	45, banding not possible	NA	**RD**. Died in 3 months.
	Simultaneous	M4	NA	NA	NA	Died during induction in 9 days.
Mishra et al. [2]	<1 month	M1	CD13+, CD33+, HLA–DR+, CD7+	46, XX	p53 mutation in both AML and BC	Died from septicemia, DIC, and intracerebral bleeding after reaching a **CR**.
Hu et al. [6]	Simultaneous	M4	HLA-DR+, CD117+, CD34+, CD33+, CD64+, CD11c+, CD13+, CD38+	47, XX, +11	NPM1 and CEBPA mutations	**RD**. Alive in **CR** after 3 lines of chemotherapy. stable BC.
Present case	6 months	—	CD34+, CD117+, CD133+, HLA-DR+, CD4+, CD7+, CD13+, TdT+, CD33+/–	46, XX	Negative	**RD**. Alive in **CR** of AML after allogeneic HSCT. CR of BC.
Our case, data not published	Simultaneous	M2	CD34+/–, CD117+, HLA–DR+, CD13+, CD33+, CD7+	46, XX	MLL self-fusion	**RD**. Died of AML in 13 months.

AML: acute myeloid leukemia; RD: refractory disease; CR: complete remission; NA: not available; BC: breast cancer.

analogue with strong antileukemia activity and an acceptable toxicity profile [9], but its high immunosuppressive effect is well known. It is conceivable that the deep immunosuppression related to clofarabine, associated with posttransplant cyclosporine treatment may have had a role in the occurrence of the *Nocardia* infection, whose incidence in transplanted patients is reported to be about 0.3%, with pulmonary nocardiosis as most frequent manifestation [10]. In the literature, the few cases of *Nocardia* infection described in HSCT patients were treated with antibiotic therapy; no one, with the exception of the hereby reported case, underwent a pulmonary lobectomy. The difficult decision to submit an allogeneic transplanted patient to thoracic surgery was guided by the absence of other therapeutic options.

In conclusion, the occurrence of unexplained cytopenia concomitant to a diagnosis of BC must be closely investigated, and collaboration between the oncologist and hematologist is essential both to reduce the diagnostic delay and to choose the appropriate therapeutic strategy. To our knowledge, our case is the only one described in the literature that is long surviving in complete remission of the two malignancies, characterized by an extremely severe prognosis if it arose simultaneously.

In the molecular era, the coexistence of BC and AML in a young woman could be explained by common pathogenetic mechanisms, and the mutation status of p53 seems to be the most involved: 20–40% of BC patients and 10–20% of AML patients show an acquired mutation of p53 at diagnosis [6]. The presence of p53 mutation is associated with a poor prognosis. In our patient, p53 was not mutated.

Alternative mechanisms involving p53 are described in AML with t(8;21) where the fusion gene AML1-ETO enables the cell to bypass the regulatory effect of p53 [6]. Also abnormalities of chromosome 11 may be involved in AML; chromosome 11 is frequently amplificated in the 11q23 region where the MLL proto-oncogene (myeloid/lymphoid leukemia or mixed-lineage leukemia) is located. In BC, nonrandom abnormalities of chromosome 11 are frequently reported, with involvement of 11p15, 11q13, and 11q23 [6].

In addition, the BRCA1 protein is important for the regulation of cell proliferation, DNA repair, and induction of apoptosis in damaged cells; BRCA1 expression is reduced in about 11–31% of BC, and recent evidences in t-AML have shown a low expression of BRCA1 in AML blasts which could contribute to secondary leukemogenesis, though further studies are necessary [11].

We expect that, in the near future, the new molecular diagnostic techniques as well as the modern biologic therapeutic tools will allow to better understand the molecular pathways possibly involved in the pathogenesis of both diseases, thus opening the way to a combined therapeutic approach.

Authors' Contributions

BL wrote the manuscript, TSM followed the clinical course of the patient during chemotherapy, IAP and LRU performed the stem cell transplant, MA and GG managed the infective complications, DGT performed the surgical intervention, GA performed the molecular analysis, and FR and CS reviewed the final manuscript and made therapeutic decisions about the patient.

References

[1] C. G. Valentini, L. Fianchi, M. T. Voso, M. Caira, G. Leone, and L. Pagano, "Incidence of acute myeloid leukemia after breast cancer," *Mediterranean Journal of Hematology and Infectious Diseases*, vol. 3, no. 1, Article ID e2011069, 2011.

[2] P. P. Mishra, M. Mahapatra, and V. P. Choudhry, "Synchronous occurrence of breast carcinoma and acute myeloid leukemia: case report and review of the literature," *Annals of Hematology*, vol. 83, pp. 541–543, 2004.

[3] R. W. Carey, J. F. Holland, P. R. Sheehe, and S. Graham, "Association of cancer of the breast and acute myelocytic leukemia," *Cancer*, vol. 20, no. 7, pp. 1080–1088, 1967.

[4] F. Rosner, R. W. Carey, and M. H. Zarrabi, "Breast cancer and acute leukemia: report of 24 cases and review of the literature," *American Journal of Hematology*, vol. 4, no. 2, pp. 151–172, 1978.

[5] W. B. Ershler, H. L. Davis, H. I. Robins et al., "Emergence of acute non-lymphocytic leukemia in breast cancer patients," *The American Journal of the Medical Sciences*, vol. 284, no. 2, pp. 23–31, 1982.

[6] G. Hu, D. K. Mallik, W. Yang et al., "Appropriate clinical strategies for breast cancer coexisting with acute myeloid leukemia in the genomic-molecular era: a case report," *Breast Care*, vol. 11, no. 2, pp. 145–147, 2016.

[7] M. R. Litzow, "The therapy of relapsed acute leukaemia in adults," *Blood Reviews*, vol. 18, no. 1, pp. 39–63, 2004.

[8] J. M. Middeke, R. Herbst, R. Herbst et al., "Clofarabine salvage therapy before allogeneic hematopoietic stem cell transplantation in patients with relapsed or refractory AML: results of the BRIDGE trial," *Leukemia*, vol. 30, no. 2, pp. 261–267, 2015.

[9] S. Faderl, M. Wetzler, D. Rizzieri et al., "Clofarabine plus cytarabine compared with cytarabine alone in older patients with relapsed or refractory acute myelogenous leukemia: results from the CLASSIC I Trial," *Journal of Clinical Oncology*, vol. 30, no. 20, pp. 2492–2499, 2012.

[10] U. Ibrahim, A. Saqib, F. Mohammad, and T. Terjanian, "An Unusual Presentation of Nocardiosis in an Allogeneic Transplant Recipient," *Cureus*, vol. 8, no. 10, p. e834, 2016.

[11] A. Scardocci, F. Guidi, F. D'Alo' et al., "Reduced BRCA1 expression due to promoter hypermethylation in therapy-related acute myeloid leukaemia," *British Journal of Cancer*, vol. 95, no. 8, pp. 1108–1113, 2006.

34

Combination of Dabrafenib and Trametinib for the Treatment of Relapsed and Refractory Multiple Myeloma Harboring BRAF V600E Mutation

Rūta Čepulytė,[1] Andrius Žučenka,[1] and Valdas Pečeliūnas[1,2]

[1]Vilnius University Hospital Santaros Klinikos, Center of Hematology, Oncology and Transfusion Medicine, Santariškių 2, Vilnius 08661, Lithuania
[2]Vilnius University Faculty of Medicine, Institute of Clinical Medicine, Clinic of Internal Diseases, Family Medicine and Oncology, Santariškių 2, Vilnius 08661, Lithuania

Correspondence should be addressed to Rūta Čepulytė; rcepulyte@yahoo.com

Academic Editor: Håkon Reikvam

Multiple myeloma (MM) is an incurable plasma cell neoplasia characterized by relapsed and/or refractory (R/R) disease course, which poses a major therapeutic challenge. New therapies, including BRAF V600E mutation targeting, may become a new treatment option for R/R MM. In combination with mitogen-activated protein kinase inhibitors (MEKi), BRAF inhibitors (BRAFi) could provide better tailored clinical management, although experience in this field is lacking. To this date, there is only one case describing R/R MM treatment with BRAFi vemurafenib and MEKi cobimetinib. This is the first case presenting a R/R MM patient treated with BRAFi dabrafenib and MEKi trametinib.

1. Introduction

Multiple myeloma (MM) is an incurable malignancy of mature lymphoid plasma cells located primarily in the bone marrow. Typically, its clinical course is characterized by a pattern of recurrent remissions and relapses, with patients becoming increasingly refractory to treatment [1]. Despite advances in therapy over the last two decades, overcoming drug resistance and salvaging patients with relapsed and/or refractory (R/R) MM are an unmet medical need [2]. Driver mutations in the BRAF gene, a key player in the RAS-RAF-MAPK-ERK pathway, are described in multiple tumor types, including subsets of melanoma, nonsmall cell lung cancer, and anaplastic thyroid cancer, making BRAF a desirable target for inhibition [3]. BRAF V600E, the most common BRAF mutation, has been identified in 2.4% to 5.3% multiple myeloma patients in the Western countries [4–8].

Despite experience in BRAF V600E targeted therapy in melanoma, nonsmall cell lung cancers, and anaplastic thyroid cancer [9], information on efficacy of such MM treatment is very limited. Available data present short-lived responses when treating with BRAF inhibitor (BRAFi) vemurafenib alone [7, 10–12]; thus, inhibition of mitogen-activated protein kinase (MEK) has emerged as a viable strategy to treat patients with BRAF mutated cancers [2, 13]. The rationale behind adding another RAS-RAF-MAPK-ERK pathway inhibitor to the treatment strategy is based on pathway reactivation [14–18]. When given alone, BRAFi can induce the pathway to become activated evading the blockade. By adding an inhibitor of a downstream effector (MEK), two nodes of the pathway are targeted, thus increasing its suppression [14].

The combination of BRAF and MEK inhibition has shown to improve response rates as well as progression-free survival (PFS) and overall survival (OS) compared to treatment with BRAF inhibition alone in melanoma [19, 20]. Only very few data are available regarding clinical activity of BRAF and MEK inhibitor combination in R/R MM [21]. To the best of our knowledge, no further case reports of BRAF and MEK kinases inhibitor combination in R/R MM were published. Therefore, we present the first report on BRAF kinase inhibitor dabrafenib and MEK1/MEK2 inhibitor (MEKi) trametinib in the posttransplant and conventional-therapy-resistant BRAF V600E positive MM patient.

2. Case Presentation

A 52-year-old male was first diagnosed with immunoglobulin G (IgG) kappa light chain (LC) symptomatic MM, Salmon and Durie stage II, in October 2002. Firstly, he presented with pathological fracture due to left femur plasmacytoma and multiple osteolytic lesions. Subsequent examination revealed 21% plasmocytic infiltration in the bone marrow. Risk profiling revealed an International Staging System score of II.

In seven years, he received four lines of MM treatment, alkylators, proteasome inhibitor bortezomib, and two autologous stem cell transplants in May 2009 and February 2016. Progression occurred nine months after the second transplantation, followed by VTD (bortezomib, thalidomide, and dexamethasone) therapy, which was discontinued after one cycle due to refractory disease and infectious complications.

Then, the patient received five lines of treatment, including proteasome inhibitor bortezomib, immunomodulators (thalidomide and lenalidomide), bendamustine, and maintenance with alkylators. At that time, daratumumab or carfilzomib was not available. Rapid extramedullary (plasmacytomas of the scull and vertebrae) and systematic progression of the disease followed. The durable response was not achieved in five years (Figure 1).

After 10th line treatment, bone marrow aspiration was performed, and the sample was submitted to genomic profiling in search of possible targeted therapy options. 14q32 (IGH) break-apart was negative, but PCR result of the bone marrow sample was BRAF gene V600E mutation positive. Single nucleotide polymorphism test revealed no clinically significant structural cytogenetic aberrations.

Having informed the patient of the experimental character of a targeted treatment approach in the absence of other available standard options and written informed consent, off-label use of dabrafenib 150 mg BID in combination with trametinib 2 mg QD was started on 12th August 2019. The treatment was approved by the local ethics committee. Dabrafenib and trametinib were kindly provided by Novartis on compassionate grounds.

Significant reduction of plasmacytomas was observed after just one week of therapy. After 46 days of treatment, *M* component decreased from 30,8 to 13,4 g/l, serum kappa light chain concentration declined from 1720,07 to 577 mg/l, skull plasmacytomas fully regressed. After four lines of sequential therapy, the first partial remission was achieved.

On 27th September, the patient was hospitalized due to febrile fever and diarrhea up to 3 times a day. *Clostridium difficile* colitis was confirmed. During colitis treatment, dabrafenib and trametinib were discontinued due to concerns of possible adverse effect of experimental therapy. After one week of *Clostridium difficile* eradication therapy with metronidazole and negative *Clostridium difficile* PGR test, diarrhea continued with decreasing intensity; therefore, it was considered that BRAFi and MEKi related toxicity. Diarrhea regressed after 3 weeks since discontinuation of the targeted therapy.

Having discontinued MM treatment for 24 days, new left upper arm 10 × 8 cm tumor (Figure 2) and former skull plasmacytomas (Figure 3) occurred while the *M* component remained stable. BRAFi and MEKi were resumed in reduced dosage to 75 mg BID and 1 mg QD, respectively. After diarrhea regression, dabrafenib and trametinib were continued in standard doses. The patient succumbed to death eleven days after BRAFi and MEKi reinitiation due to MM progression-related complications; therefore, the possibility to regain durable response to this kind of targeted therapy remains unknown.

3. Discussion

BRAF mutation is well-known for its activation of the Ras-Raf-MEK–ERK signaling pathway, thereby stimulating cellular growth, differentiation, and survival [21, 22]. This mutation has been observed in melanoma, nonsmall cell lung cancer, colorectal carcinoma, and a wide variety of other malignancies, but only some of these diseases have been studied for response to BRAF V600E-specific inhibitors [9, 12].

To date, the published experience in MM is mostly limited to case reports and case series [23]. Majority of them present vemurafenib monotherapy [7, 10–12] or its combination with bortezomib [24]. Upon initiation of vemurafenib, patients rapidly experienced decreased paraprotein levels, extramedullary disease reduction, and improvement of clinical performance status, although duration of response was limited to months since acquired resistance began to develop [11, 12, 24].

The reasons of delayed-onset treatment failure may be associated with spatial genomic heterogeneity in MM [2, 25] and paradoxical activation of the MAPK pathway by BRAF inhibition [26, 27]. Regarding that, a retrospective study conducted in 2016 by Heuck et al. reported 58 R/R MM patients with oncogenic mutations of NRAS, KRAS, or BRAF or GEP pathway activation [13]. All patients received treatment with MEKi trametinib monotherapy with overall response (ORR) of 40%.

The drawbacks of monotherapy encouraged to search for effective treatment combinations. To the best of our knowledge, there is only one case report published that presents combination of BRAFi vemurafenib and MEKi cobimetinib for highly resistant MM patients [21]. After 3 months of treatment, the best response was a very good partial remission (VGPR).

Several prospective studies are now underway and should provide a more comprehensive analysis of efficacy [23]. In the NCI-MATCH study (ClinicalTrials.gov identifier: NCT02465060), R/R MM patients with BRAF V600E/R/K/D mutation in a Phase 2 setting received dabrafenib and trametinib, whereas patients with BRAF fusion or BRAF

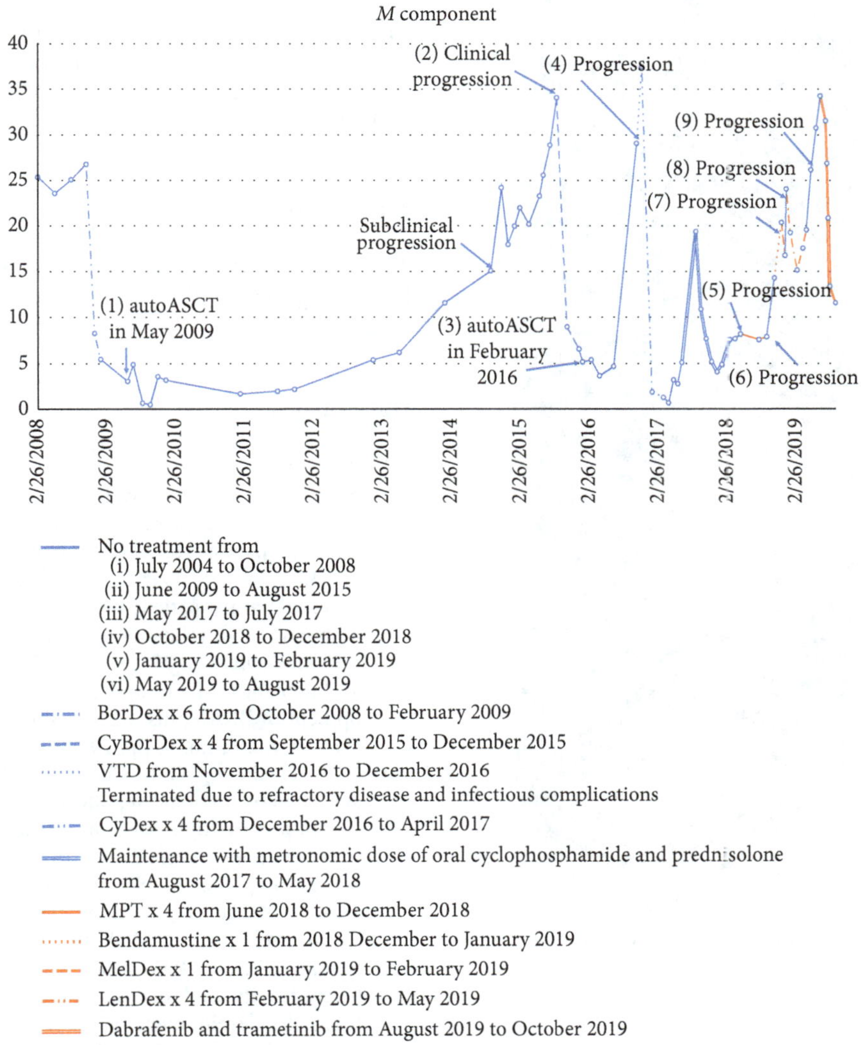

FIGURE 1: Treatment lines. Data on the *M* component are available from 2009. From 2002 to 2008, the *M* component could not be assessed due to laboratory limitations: (1) consolidation with autologous blood stem cell transplant (autoASCT) in May 2009 included stem cell mobilization and harvesting followed by conditioning with high-dose melphalan (Mel200 mg/m2). (2)In September 2015, the clinical progression manifested with pain in the chest and spine. (3) Consolidation with autologous blood stem cell transplant in February 2016. Conditioning with high-dose melphalan (Mel200 mg/m2), cryopreserved stem cells from 2009 harvest. (4) Nine months after second autoASCT, the fourth clinical progression was diagnosed based on the *M* component rising to 29.1 g/l, kappa LC 1250 mg/l. (5) During maintenance treatment, the new plasmacytoma in lumbar vertebrae occurred. This resulted in left leg paresis and spinal decompression was performed. (6) Worsening of bone pain and *M* component increase. (7) New skull plasmacytoma and *M* gradient increase. (8) New multiple skull plasmacytomas and worsening of bone pain and polyneuropathy, which led to significant decline in functional status. (9) Skull plasmacytomas regressed, but the disease response was minimal due to the stabile *M* component. During the first cycle, the patient experienced proximal left humerus fracture due to a trauma. Osteosynthesis was performed. Two months later, the patient was repeatedly operated due to left upper arm deformation and potential metal construction cutaneous perforation. Biopsy was taken from the left humerus fraction site. During the fourth LenDex cycle, the biopsy revealed plasmocytic infiltration.

non-V600 mutation received trametinib and patients with NRAS mutation in codon 12, 13, or 61 received binimetinib. Likewise, dabrafenib in combination with trametinib, dabrafenib alone, or trametinib alone are being evaluated in patients with R/R MM and BRAF/NRAS/KRAS mutations (ClinicalTrials.gov identifier: NCT03091257). In the GMMG-BIRMA Phase 2 study (ClinicalTrials.gov identifier: NCT02834364), R/R MM patients harboring the BRAF V600E/K mutation are being treated with the kinase inhibitor encorafenib (LGX818; RAF kinase inhibitor) in combination with the MEK inhibitor binimetinib (MEK162) [2].

Our report presents a patient with systemic, highly resistant, and rapidly progressing BRAFV600E mutated MM with extramedullary involvement. The disease was refractory to a variety of antimyeloma drugs including melphalan, cyclophosphamide, bortezomib, thalidomide, bendamustine, and lenalidomide. With BRAFV600E and MEK1/2

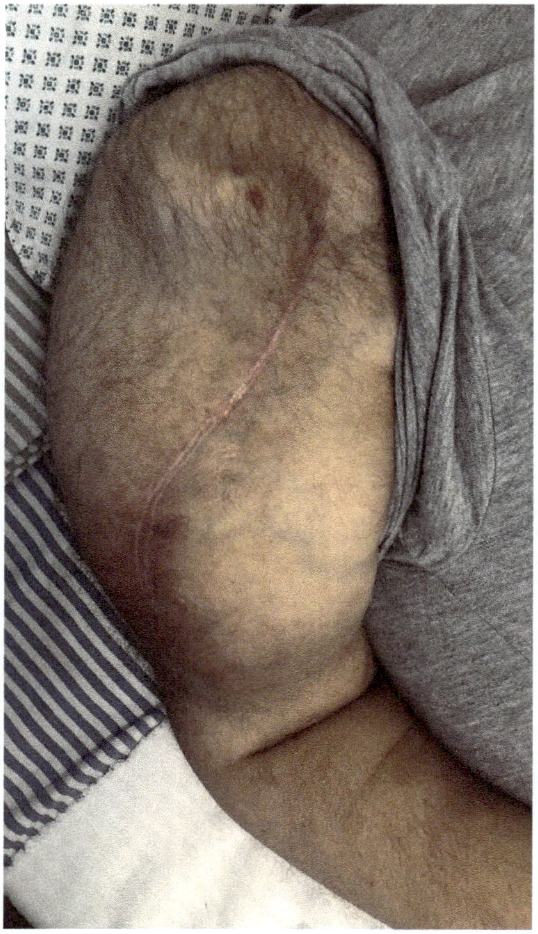

Figure 2: Left upper arm tumor.

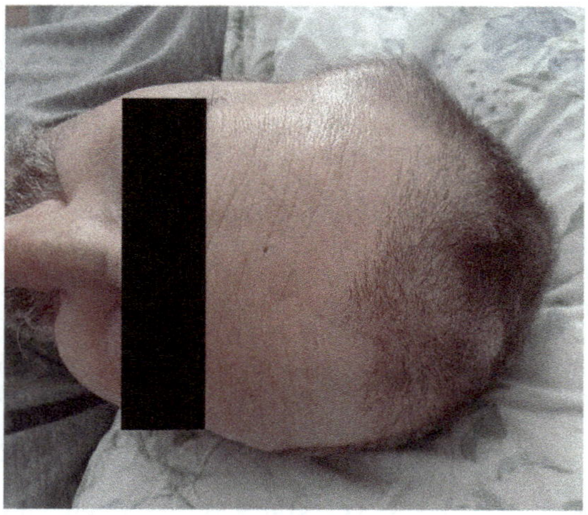

Figure 3: Skull plasmacytomas.

inhibition approaches, a rapid response was achieved but unsustained due to possible dabrafenib and trametinib toxicity-related discontinuation.

This report illustrates the significance of BRAF/MEK inhibition for patients with R/R MM. However, the duration of response may be limited, and the profile of side effects should be considered in heavily pretreated MM patients. Therefore, it encourages further investigation of therapeutic regimens targeting the BRAF and MEK pathway in patients with R/R MM within clinical trials.

Disclosure

This case report did not receive any specific grant from funding agencies in the public, commercial, or not-for-profit sectors.

References

[1] A. Laganà, I. Beno, D. Melnekoff et al., "Precision medicine for relapsed multiple myeloma on the basis of an integrative multiomics approach," *JCO Precision Oncology*, vol. 2018, no. 2, 17 pages, Article ID 18.00019, 2018.

[2] F. M. Uckun, S. Qazi, T. Demirer, and R. E. Champlin, "Contemporary patient-tailored treatment strategies against high risk and relapsed or refractory multiple myeloma," *EBioMedicine*, vol. 39, pp. 612–620, 2019.

[3] V. Subbiah, C. Baik, and J. M. Kirkwood, "Clinical development of BRAF plus MEK inhibitor combinations," *Trends Cancer*, vol. 6, no. 9, pp. 797–810, 2020.

[4] C. H. Y. Cheung, C. K. Cheng, K.-M. Lau et al., "Prevalence and clinicopathologic significance of BRAF V600E mutation in Chinese multiple myeloma patients," *Clinical Lymphoma Myeloma and Leukemia*, vol. 18, no. 7, pp. e315–e325, 2018.

[5] M. A. Chapman, M. S. Lawrence, J. J. Keats et al., "Initial genome sequencing and analysis of multiple myeloma," *Nature*, vol. 471, no. 7339, pp. 467–472, 2011.

[6] B. A. Walker, C. P. Wardell, L. Melchor et al., "Intraclonal heterogeneity and distinct molecular mechanisms characterize the development of t (4;14) and t (11;14) myeloma," *Blood*, vol. 120, no. 5, pp. 1077–1086, 2012.

[7] M. Andrulis, N. Lehners, D. Capper et al., "Targeting the BRAF V600E mutation in multiple myeloma," *Cancer Discovery*, vol. 3, no. 8, pp. 862–869, 2013.

[8] E. H. Rustad, H. Y. Dai, H. Hov et al., "BRAF V600E mutation in early-stage multiple myeloma: good response to broad acting drugs and no relation to prognosis," *Blood Cancer Journal*, vol. 5, no. 3, Article ID e299, 2015.

[9] A. Zaman, W. Wu, and T. G. Bivona, "Targeting oncogenic BRAF: past, present, and future," *Cancers*, vol. 11, no. 8, 2019.

[10] N. Raje, I. Chau, D. M. Hyman et al., "Vemurafenib in patients with relapsed refractory multiple myeloma harboring BRAFV600 mutations: a cohort of the histology-independent VE-BASKET study," *JCO Precision Oncology*, vol. 2, no. 9, 2018.

[11] O. L. Bohn, K. Hsu, D. M. Hyman, D. S. Pignataro, S. Giralt, and J. Teruya-Feldstein, "BRAF V600E mutation and clonal evolution in a patient with relapsed refractory myeloma with plasmablastic differentiation," *Clinical Lymphoma Myeloma and Leukemia*, vol. 14, no. 2, pp. e65–e68, 2014.

[12] J. P. Sharman, J. Chmielecki, D. Morosini et al., "Vemurafenib response in 2 patients with posttransplant refractory BRAF V600E-mutated multiple myeloma," *Clinical Lymphoma Myeloma and Leukemia*, vol. 14, no. 5, pp. e161–e163, 2014.

[13] C. J. Heuck, Y. Jethava, R. Khan et al., "Inhibiting MEK in MAPK pathway-activated myeloma," *Leukemia*, no. 4, pp. 976–980, 2016.

[14] J. N. Sanchez, T. Wang, and M. S. Cohen, "BRAF and MEK inhibitors: use and resistance in BRAF-mutated cancers," *Drugs*, vol. 78, no. 5, pp. 549–566, 2018.
[15] C. Zhang, W. Spevak, Y. Zhang et al., "RAF inhibitors that evade paradoxical MAPK pathway activation," *Nature*, vol. 526, no. 7574, pp. 583–586, 2015.
[16] S. J. Heidorn, C. Milagre, S. Whittaker et al., "Kinase-dead BRAF and oncogenic RAS cooperate to drive tumor progression through CRAF," *Cell*, vol. 140, no. 2, pp. 209–221, 2010.
[17] G. Hatzivassiliou, K. Song, I. Yen et al., "RAF inhibitors prime wild-type RAF to activate the MAPK pathway and enhance growth," *Nature*, vol. 464, no. 7287, pp. 431–435, 2010.
[18] M. Holderfield, H. Merritt, J. Chan et al., "RAF inhibitors activate the MAPK pathway by relieving inhibitory autophosphorylation," *Cancer Cell*, vol. 23, no. 5, pp. 594–602, 2013.
[19] K. B. Kim, R. Kefford, A. C. Pavlick et al., "Phase II study of the MEK1/MEK2 inhibitor Trametinib in patients with metastatic BRAF-mutant cutaneous melanoma previously treated with or without a BRAF inhibitor," *Journal of Clinical Oncology*, vol. 31, no. 4, pp. 482–489, 2013.
[20] K. T. Flaherty, J. R. Infante, A. Daud et al., "Combined BRAF and MEK inhibition in melanoma with BRAF V600 mutations," *New England Journal of Medicine*, vol. 367, no. 18, pp. 1694–1703, 2012.
[21] U. J. M. Mey, C. Renner, and R. von Moos, "Vemurafenib in combination with cobimetinib in relapsed and refractory extramedullary multiple myeloma harboring the BRAF V600E mutation," *Hematological Oncology*, vol. 35, no. 4, pp. 890–893, 2017.
[22] J. A. McCubrey, L. S. Steelman, W. H. Chappell et al., "Roles of the Raf/MEK/ERK pathway in cell growth, malignant transformation and drug resistance," *Biochimica et Biophysica Acta (BBA)-Molecular Cell Research*, vol. 1773, no. 8, pp. 1263–1284, 2007.
[23] C. Pawlyn and F. E. Davies, "Toward personalized treatment in multiple myeloma based on molecular characteristics," *Blood*, vol. 133, no. 7, pp. 660–675, 2019.
[24] M. S. Raab, N. Lehners, J. Xu et al., "Spatially divergent clonal evolution in multiple myeloma: overcoming resistance to BRAF inhibition," *Blood*, vol. 127, no. 17, pp. 2155–2157, 2016.
[25] L. Rasche, S. S. Chavan, O. W. Stephens et al., "Spatial genomic heterogeneity in multiple myeloma revealed by multi-region sequencing," *Nature Communications*, vol. 8, no. 1, p. 268, 2017.
[26] M. J. Garnett, S. Rana, H. Paterson, D. Barford, and R. Marais, "Wild-type and mutant B-RAF activate C-RAF through distinct mechanisms involving heterodimerization," *Molecular Cell*, vol. 20, no. 6, pp. 963–969, 2005.
[27] C. Zhang, W. Spevak, Y. Zhang et al., "RAF inhibitors that evade paradoxical MAPK pathway activation," *Nature*, vol. 526, no. 7574, pp. 583–586, 2015.

35

Concurrent Central Diabetes Insipidus and Acute Myeloid Leukemia

Stephanie L. Pritzl, Daniel R. Matson, Mark B. Juckett, and David J. Ciske

University of Wisconsin School of Medicine and Public Health, Madison, Wisconsin, USA

Correspondence should be addressed to David J. Ciske; dciske@dshealthcare.com

Academic Editor: Håkon Reikvam

Central diabetes insipidus (CDI) is a rare reported complication of acute myeloid leukemia (AML). The onset of AML-associated CDI often precedes the diagnosis of AML by weeks or months and is considered an adverse prognostic indicator in this setting. The mechanism of AML-associated CDI is not known; however, it is often reported in the setting of cytogenetic events resulting in MDS1 and EVI1 complex locus protein (MECOM) gene overexpression. Here, we describe a case of new onset CDI which preceded a diagnosis of AML by 1 month. We detail the clinical and laboratory evaluation of the patient's CDI, and we describe the pathological and laboratory workup of their AML, which ultimately yielded a diagnosis of AML with myelodysplasia-related changes. Additional cytogenetic findings included the identification of the t (2;3)(p23;q27), which leads to MECOM gene overexpression and which to our knowledge has not previously been reported in the setting of AML-associated CDI. The patient received induction chemotherapy followed by allogeneic hematopoietic stem cell transplantation but experienced disease relapse and passed away nine months after initial diagnosis. We emphasize that new onset CDI can occur as a rare complication of AML where it portends a poor prognosis and may be related to AML subtypes displaying MECOM gene dysregulation.

1. Introduction

Central diabetes insipidus (CDI) as a complication of acute myeloid leukemia (AML) is rare, and the underlying mechanism(s) of AML-associated CDI remains incompletely understood. When it occurs, the onset of CDI typically precedes the diagnosis of AML by 1-2 months [1]. However, CDI may also occur at the time of AML diagnosis or as the initial manifestation of AML relapse [1, 2]. AML-associated CDI is hypothesized to represent an adverse prognostic indicator of AML, even when CDI symptoms are ameliorated by administration of desmopressin (DDAVP) [1–3]. Here, we present a case of CDI preceding an initial diagnosis of AML.

2. Case Presentation

A previously healthy 71-year-old man presented to his primary care physician with abrupt onset of polyuria and polydipsia. Physical exam was notable for intact visual fields and no evidence of hypovolemia. His medications included only aspirin (81 mg daily) and simvastatin (40 mg daily). Laboratory testing revealed leukopenia and macrocytic anemia (Table 1), in the setting of a previously normal complete blood count (CBC) one year prior. Comprehensive metabolic panel, hemoglobin A1c, and urinalysis were unremarkable. However, urine osmolality was inappropriately low in conjunction with an elevated serum osmolality (Table 1). Polyuria was confirmed with a 24-hour urine collection. An 8-hour water deprivation test was completed and demonstrated worsening hypernatremia with a suboptimal response in urinary concentration (Table 1). A subsequent desmopressin challenge was notable for decreased urine output and increased urine osmolality (Table 1). Levels of plasma vasopressin and copeptin, which comprises a portion of the vasopressin precursor molecule, were not measured. Other hormones dependent on pituitary function including serum prolactin, free T4, cortisol (AM),

Table 1: Laboratory data.

Laboratory testing at diagnosis			
Assay	Result		Normal values
WBC	2.3 K/μL		3.8–10.5 K/μL
Hb	13.5 g/dL		13.6–17.2 g/dL
MCV	101 fL		80–97 fL
24-hour urine collection	12.5 L urine output		0.8–2.0 L
Prolactin	8.9 ng/mL		3.5–19.4 ng/mL
Cortisol (AM)	18.6 μg/dL		10–20 μg/dL
Free T4	0.81 ng/L		0.70–1.48 ng/L
Total testosterone	338 ng/dL		300–720 ng/dL
8-hour water deprivation test			
Assay	0 hours	8 hours	Normal values
Serum sodium	144 mmol/L	149 mmol/L	136–145 mmol/L
Serum osmolality	302 mOsm/kg	308 mOsm/kg	278–298 mOsm/kg
Urine osmolality	123 mOsm/kg	235 mOsm/kg	50–1200 mOsm/kg
Desmopressin challenge			
Time	Urine output (mL)		Urine osmolality (mOsm/kg)
12-1 PM	725		87
1 PM		2 mcg DDAVP SubQ	
1-2 PM	160		341
2-3 PM	80		467

and free testosterone were all within normal limits. MRI head demonstrated lack of the normal posterior pituitary bright spot. The laboratory and imaging findings were consistent with CDI, and the, patient began treatment with DDAVP nasal spray which led to rapid improvement in his symptoms.

During this 21-day period, serial CBCs revealed a persistent leukopenia (WBC 3.4 K/μL), worsening macrocytic anemia (Hb 11.7 g/Dl and MCV 107 fL), and a progressive thrombocytosis (PLT 500 K/μL and normal 160–370 K/μL). A manual differential performed on peripheral blood revealed 17% circulating blasts, and bone marrow biopsy demonstrated a hypercellular marrow virtually effaced by leukemic blasts (Figure 1(a)). Flow cytometry revealed a myeloid immunophenotype confirming a diagnosis of AML, without features worrisome for acute promyelocytic leukemia. Routine ancillary testing for newly diagnosed AML includes (minimally) the following studies performed on the leukemic blast population: karyotyping by classical cytogenetics, evaluation for core binding factor rearrangements by either fluorescence in situ hybridization (FISH) or classical cytogenetics, and mutational analysis of the fms-like tyrosine kinase 3 (FLT3) gene [4].

In this case, cytogenetic analyses revealed the t (2;3)(p23; q27), which is a chromosomal translocation often associated with MDS1 and EVI1 complex locus (MECOM) gene overexpression, as well as the del (5) q31;q33) (Figure 1(b)). FISH was negative for core binding factor rearrangements, and molecular analyses revealed no mutation in FLT3. Based on the presence of the del (5)(q31;q33), a final diagnosis of AML with myelodysplasia-related changes (AML-MRC) was rendered. AML-MRCs are a subtype of AML that are associated with a poor prognosis. They are diagnosed when AML patients have a known history of myelodysplastic syndrome, display significant morphologic dysplasia in the bone marrow at leukemic presentation, or when their AML harbors characteristic cytogenetic findings that are associated with myelodysplasia [5]. These characteristic cytogenetic findings include deletions in chromosome 5, as seen in our patient.

The patient received induction chemotherapy with liposomal daunorubicin and cytarabine which failed to reduce his bone marrow blast count. This was followed by two cycles of azacytidine and lenalidomide and reinduction with fludarabine, cytarabine, and granulocyte colony-stimulating factor. Three weeks following his second induction, the bone marrow blast count percentage was 95%. He then received an allogeneic stem cell transplantation (alloSCT) following pretreatment with an experimental radiolabeled anti-CD45 monoclonal antibody (IOMAB-01). Unfortunately, he experienced disease relapse 1 month after transplant and ultimately passed away 9 months after his initial diagnosis. Interestingly, prior to transplant, he required 40 mcg/day of DDAVP 0.01% nasal spray (20 mcg twice daily) to control his CDI symptoms, but following his transplant, he was able to space out the dosing of his DDAVP to every 4-5 days.

3. Discussion

AML-associated CDI is a rare but increasingly recognized complication of AML. In perhaps the largest study of AML-associated CDI to date, Ladigan et al. analyzed 51 reports of adults with myeloid malignancies and associated CDI [1]. They found a median age of diagnosis of 48 years, which is younger than the median age of 65 years reported across all new AML diagnoses [6]. At least 9 cases have also been reported in the pediatric population [7–13]. In addition,

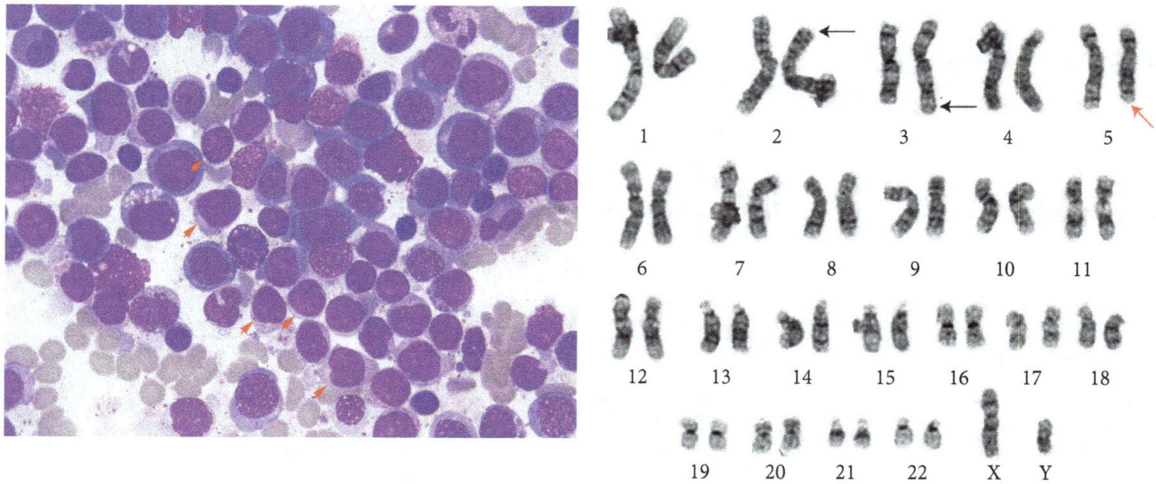

(a) (b)

Figure 1: Bone marrow aspirate and AML cytogenetic karyotype: (a) wright-stained bone marrow aspirate showing increased blasts (examples highlighted by red arrowhead; 1000x original magnification); (b) AML karyotype demonstrating the t (2;3)(p23;q27) (black arrows) and del (5q)(q31;q33) (red arrow).

patients with AML-associated CDI show a female predominance (59% female), compared to a mild male predominance across all AMLs. The majority (45/51) of these cases occur in the setting of *de novo* AMLs, wherein the patient has no known prior diagnosis of a primary bone marrow neoplasm. The remaining cases are comprised of either myelodysplastic syndrome (MDS), which is a common precursor to AML, or AML transformed from aplastic anemia, MDS, or chronic myelomonocytic leukemia (CMML).

The diagnosis of AML-associated CDI is essentially identical to the diagnosis of CDI in any other setting [14, 15]. Most patients (75%) will be diagnosed with CDI concurrently with their AML diagnosis, with most remaining cases presenting no more than 2 months prior to or following their AML diagnosis [1]. While the majority of patients with AML-associated CDI (61%) will have no associated brain imaging abnormalities, some may have pathologic findings including loss of the posterior pituitary bright spot or nodular thickening/attenuation of the pituitary stalk [1]. MRI of our patient revealed absence of the posterior pituitary bright spot which can be indicative of hypothalamic pituitary dysfunction. The normal pituitary bright spot seen on T1-weighted MRI is thought to result from the T1-shortening effect of stored vasopressin in the posterior pituitary [16].

The pathogenesis of AML-associated CDI remains unclear although there are hints that dysmegakaryopoiesis and resulting platelet dysfunction could lie at the heart of this disorder. Previously, clinicians hypothesized that CDI occurred secondary to pituitary damage as a consequence of tumor-mediated destruction or infection. Early cohort studies of deceased patients with leukemia-associated CDI noted two types of lesions that could be routinely identified at autopsy in the supraopticohypophyseal system: (1) leukemic infiltrates and/or (2) thrombosis of small vessels [16]. However, it should be noted that leukemic infiltrates are not uncommonly seen at autopsy in AML patients who never developed CDI [2, 17, 18]. More recently, multiple case series have revealed a strong association between AML-associated CDI and cytogenetic abnormalities in the concurrent AML, chiefly inversions involving chromosome 3 (inv (3)) and monosomies involving chromosome 7 (monosomy 7) [1, 3, 19, 20]. Interestingly, at least a subset of cases with inv (3) harbor fusion events leading to MECOM gene overexpression, which has been shown to drive both leukemogenesis and dysmegakaryopoiesis [3, 21, 22]. It is theorized that the resulting abnormal platelets could adversely impact circulating vasopressin function, as 90% of peripheral vasopressin is platelet-bound [1–3]. Cytogenetic studies in our patient revealed the t (2;3)(p23;q27), a translocation that also typically results in MECOM overexpression and which to our knowledge has not been previously reported in the setting of AML-associated CDI [23]. Interestingly, our patient also showed a progressive thrombocytosis, an uncommon event in AML that has nonetheless been reported in the setting of the t (2;3) and MECOM overexpression [24]. Finally, our patient showed a greatly decreased requirement for DDAVP following alloSCT, after which his circulating platelets would have been derived from donor marrow. This decreased requirement for DDAVP and even complete resolution of CDI following AML treatment has been previously reported [1] and argues against pituitary destruction as the cause of AML-associated CDI in these cases.

Clinicians treating a patient with AML-associated CDI must correct the patient's CDI while also identifying an optimal treatment strategy for their AML. 90% of reported AML-associated CDI cases have a documented response to a vasopressin analog (mainly DDAVP), with the majority of patients demonstrating a marked improvement in CDI symptoms upon treatment [1]. Our patient's CDI symptoms are rapidly improved with DDAVP nasal spray. In comparison, treatment of the underlying AML depends on a number of factors, including the presence or absence of prognostically important cytogenetic and molecular findings and the patient's ability to tolerate therapy. In this respect, it is important to note that both monosomy 7 and inv (3) constitute unfavorable-risk cytogenetic findings in AML and are independently associated with worse rates of complete remission and overall survival [25–27]. Thus, independent of CDI, most AML-associated CDI patients would already be expected to have a 5-year AML-related survival of only 5-10%, compared to a 5-year survival of 29% across all AMLs [6]. In general, there is also a paucity of data regarding optimal induction regimens for AML patients with associated CDI. In 39 patients who received treatment with either standard-dose cytarabine and daunorubicin (often referred to as 7 + 3) or high-dose cytarabine, the rate of complete remission (CR) was only 15% [28–33]. Sufficient reports of other treatment regimens are not readily available. Perhaps not surprisingly given these data, AMLs in patients with AML-associated CDI confer a dismal prognosis, with an overall 1-year survival as low as 20% and a median overall survival time of only 6 months [1, 3]. However, CDI-associated AML patients who underwent alloSCT showed markedly better outcomes, with 40% surviving to 12 months. This is consistent with the survival benefit seen with alloSCT following first CR in AML patients with unfavorable risk cytogenetics [34]. Thus, the best available evidence suggests that patients with AML-associated CDI typically have unfavorable-risk cytogenetics and stand to benefit from intensive induction chemotherapy regimens followed (when possible) by an alloSCT in the first CR. Unfortunately, our patient never achieved a CR despite receiving multiple induction regimens, and although he underwent an alloSCT facilitated by pretreatment with an experimental therapy, he rapidly relapsed.

We reiterate that CDI is a rare but recognized complication of AML which is associated with a poor prognosis. We support future studies examining the consequences of MECOM gene dysregulation in AML and vasopressin function in both the pituitary and peripheral circulation.

Disclosure

This case report was prepared as part of the employment of the authors at the University of Wisconsin Hospitals and Clinics.

Acknowledgments

The authors would like to acknowledge the Wisconsin State Lab of Hygiene for providing images of the cytogenetic findings in this case. DRM is further supported by Grant number T32-HL007899 from the NHLBI.

References

[1] S. Ladigan, T. Mika, A. Figge et al., "Acute myeloid leukemia with central diabetes insipidus," *Blood Cells, Molecules, and Diseases*, vol. 76, pp. 45–52, 2019.

[2] P. Dy, P. Chua, J. Kelly, and S. Liebman, "Central diabetes insipidus in the setting of acute myelogenous leukemia," *American Journal of Kidney Diseases*, vol. 60, no. 6, pp. 998–1001, 2012.

[3] E. H. Cull, J. M. Watts, M. S. Tallman et al., "Acute myeloid leukemia presenting with panhypopituitarism or diabetes insipidus: a case series with molecular genetic analysis and review of the literature," *Leukemia & Lymphoma*, vol. 55, no. 9, pp. 2125–2129, 2014.

[4] D. A. Arber, M. J. Borowitz, M. Cessna et al., "Initial diagnostic workup of acute leukemia: guideline from the college of American pathologists and the American society of hematology," *Archives of Pathology & Laboratory Medicine* vol. 141, no. 10, pp. 1342–1393, 2017.

[5] D. A. Arber and H. P. Erba, "Diagnosis and treatment of patients with acute myeloid leukemia with myelodysplasia-related changes (AML-MRC)," *American Journal of Clinical Pathology*, vol. 154, no. 6, pp. 731–741, 2020.

[6] NIH, *Acute Myeloid Leukemia-Cancer Stat Facts*, NIH, Bethesda, MD, USA, 2018, https://seer.cancer.gov/statfacts/html/amyl.html.

[7] M. C. Joseph and S. E. Levin, "Leukaemia and diabetes insipidus," *BMJ*, vol. 1, no. 4979, pp. 1328–1322, 1956.

[8] G. E. Bergman, H. J. Baluarte, and J. L. Naiman, "Diabetes insipidus as a presenting manifestation of acute myelogenous leukemia," *The Journal of Pediatrics*, vol. 88, no. 2, p. 355, 1976.

[9] D. J. Kanabar, D. R. Betts, B. Gibbons, J. E. Kingston, and O. B. Eden, "Monosomy 7, diabetes insipidus and acute myeloid leukemia in childhood," *Pediatric Hematology and Oncology*, vol. 11, no. 1, pp. 111–114, 1994.

[10] S. Roy and W. W. Johnson, "Diabetes insipidus in a child with erythromyelocytic leukemia," *Archives of Pediatrics & Adolescent Medicine*, vol. 119, no. 1, pp. 82–85, 1970.

[11] U. Betkerur, A. Shende, and P. Lanzkowsky, "Acute myeloblastic leukemia presenting with diabetes insipidus," *The American Journal of the Medical Sciences*, vol. 273, no. 3, pp. 325–328, 1977.

[12] H. A. Frangoul, D. W. W. Shaw, D. Hawkins, and J. Park, "Diabetes insipidus as a presenting symptom of acute myelogenous leukemia," *Journal of Pediatric Hematology/Oncology*, vol. 22, no. 5, pp. 457–459, 2000.

[13] W. Wössmann, A. Borkhardt, R. Gossen, F.-J. Göbel, and A. Reiter, "Acute myeloid leukemia presenting with diabetes insipidus," *European Journal of Pediatrics*, vol. 161, no. 3, pp. 161-162, 2002.

[14] A. Garrahy, C. Moran, and C. J. Thompson, "Diagnosis and management of central diabetes insipidus in adults," *Clinical Endocrinology*, vol. 90, no. 1, pp. 23–30, 2019.

[15] W. Fenske and B. Allolio, "Current state and future perspectives in the diagnosis of diabetes insipidus: a clinical review," *The Journal of Clinical Endocrinology & Metabolism* vol. 97, no. 10, pp. 3426–3437, 2012.

[16] V. I. Miller and W. G. Campbell, "Diabetes insipidus as a complication of leukemia: a case report with a literature review," *Cancer*, vol. 28, no. 3, pp. 666–673, 1971.

[17] K. Yamagami and K. Yoshioka, "Central diabetes insipidus presenting as an early sign of acute myeloid leukemia," *Clinical Advances in Hematology & Oncology: H&O*, vol. 10, no. 6, pp. 400-401, 2012.
[18] K. Loukidis, E. Papadakis, N. Anagnostou et al., "Polyuria due to central diabetes insipidus presenting as an early manifestation of acute myeloid leukemia," *Clinical Advances in Hematology & Oncology: H&O*, vol. 10, no. 6, pp. 399-400, 2012.
[19] C. Castagnola, M. Morra, B. Bemasconi, C. Astori, S. Santagostino, and C. Bemasconi, "Acute myeloid leukemia and diabetes insipidus: results in 5 patients," *Acta Haematologica*, vol. 93, no. 1, pp. 1–4, 1995.
[20] A. De La Chapelle and R. Lahtinen, "Monosomy 7 predisposes to diabetes insipidus in leukaemia and myelodysplastic syndrome," *European Journal of Haematology*, vol. 39, no. 5, pp. 404–411, 1987.
[21] M. Sonmez, N. Erkut, T. S. Tat, F. Celep, U. Cobanoglu, and H. O. Ersoz, "Can a high platelet count be responsible for diabetes insipidus in acute myelogenous leukemia with monosomy 7 and inversion 3 (q21q26)?" *International Journal of Hematology*, vol. 90, no. 2, pp. 273-274, 2009.
[22] K. Morishita, E. Parganas, C. L. William et al., "Activation of EVI1 gene expression in human acute myelogenous leukemias by translocations spanning 300-400 kilobases on chromosome band 3q26," *Proceedings of the National Academy of Sciences*, vol. 89, no. 9, pp. 3937–3941, 1992.
[23] J. L. Huret, M. Ahmad, M Arsaban et al., "Atlas of genetics and cytogenetics in oncology and haematology in 2013," *Nucleic Acids Research*, vol. 41, no. Database issue, pp. D920–D924, 2013.
[24] K. Yamamoto, A. Okamura, Y. Sanada, K. Yakushijin, H. Matsuoka, and H. Minami, "Marked thrombocytosis and dysmegakaryopoiesis in acute myeloid leukemia with t (2;3) (p22; q26.2) and EVI1 rearrangement," *Annals of Hematology*, vol. 92, no. 12, pp. 1713–1715, 2013.
[25] D. Grimwade, H. Walker, F. Oliver et al., "The importance of diagnostic cytogenetics on outcome in AML: analysis of 1,612 patients entered into the MRC AML 10 trial," *Blood*, vol. 92, no. 7, pp. 2322–2333, 1998.
[26] M. L. Slovak, K. J. Kopecky, P. A. Cassileth et al., "Karyotypic analysis predicts outcome of preremission and postremission therapy in adult acute myeloid leukemia: a Southwest oncology group/eastern cooperative oncology group study," *Blood*, vol. 96, no. 13, pp. 4075–4083, 2000.
[27] J. C. Byrd, K. Mrózek, R. K. Dodge et al., "Pretreatment cytogenetic abnormalities are predictive of induction success, cumulative incidence of relapse, and overall survival in adult patients with de novo acute myeloid leukemia: results from cancer and leukemia group B (CALGB 8461)," *Blood*, vol. 100, no. 13, pp. 4325–4336, 2002.
[28] F. Nakamura, Y. Kishimoto, T. Handa, Y. Arai, and K. Mitani, "Myelodysplastic syndrome with central diabetes insipidus manifesting hypodipsic hypernatremia and dehydration," *American Journal of Hematology*, vol. 75, no. 4, pp. 213–216, 2004.
[29] R. P. Mozersky, V. K. Bahl, D. Meisner, and H. Patel, "Diabetes insipidus, acute myelogenous leukemia, and monosomy 7," *The Journal of the American Osteopathic Association*, vol. 96, no. 2, pp. 116–118, 1996.
[30] P. Nieboer, E. Vellenga, R. Adriaanse, and A. A. van de Loosdrecht, "Central diabetes insipidus preceding acute myeloid leukemia with t (3;12) (q26;p12)," *The Netherlands Journal of Medicine*, vol. 56, no. 2, pp. 45–47, 2000.
[31] L. Pagano, M. T. Voso, S. Sica, and G. Leone, "Recovery from diabetes insipidus associated with AML after a BMT conditioning regimen including busulfan," *Bone Marrow Transplantation*, vol. 11, no. 2, pp. 175-176, 1993.
[32] C. C. Yen, C. H. Tzeng, J. H. Liu et al., "Acute myelomonocytic leukemia preceded by secondary amenorrhea and presenting with central diabetes insipidus: a case report," *Zhonghua Yi Xue Za Zhi*, vol. 60, no. 4, pp. 213–218, 1997.
[33] A. Lawrie, D. A. J. Stevenson, T. N. Doig, M. A. Vickers, and D. J. Culligan, "Acute myeloid leukemia presenting in a mother and daughter pair with the identical acquired karyotypic abnormality consisting of inversion 3q21q26 and monosomy 7: a review of possible mechanisms," *Cancer Genetics*, vol. 205, no. 11, pp. 599–602, 2012.
[34] W.-J. Hong and B. C. Medeiros, "Unfavorable-risk cytogenetics in acute myeloid leukemia," *Expert Review of Hematology*, vol. 4, no. 2, pp. 173–184, 2011.

36

Hemophagocytic Syndrome-Associated Variant of Methotrexate-Associated Intravascular Large B-Cell Lymphoma in a Rheumatoid Arthritis Patient

Yukiko Komeno,[1] Minako Akiyama,[2] Yasumi Okochi,[3] Hitoshi Tokuda,[3] Keiko Abe,[4] Kuniko Iihara,[4] and Tomiko Ryu[1]

[1]*Department of Hematology, Japan Community Healthcare Organization (JCHO) Tokyo Yamate Medical Center, Hyakunin-cho, Shinjuku, Tokyo 169-0073, Japan*
[2]*Department of Nephrology, JCHO Tokyo Yamate Medical Center, Hyakunin-cho, Shinjuku, Tokyo 169-0073, Japan*
[3]*Department of Respiratory Medicine, JCHO Tokyo Yamate Medical Center, Hyakunin-cho, Shinjuku, Tokyo 169-0073, Japan*
[4]*Department of Pathology, JCHO Tokyo Yamate Medical Center, Hyakunin-cho, Shinjuku, Tokyo 169-0073, Japan*

Correspondence should be addressed to Yukiko Komeno; ykomeno-tky@umin.ac.jp

Academic Editor: Salah Aref

A 59-year-old man was treated for rheumatoid arthritis (RA) for 12 years with methotrexate (MTX) and prednisolone. After MTX-associated interstitial pneumonia developed, he was treated with cyclophosphamide and prednisolone for 7 months. Arthritis worsened, and tacrolimus was added to the treatment regimen. One month later, he had fever, loss of appetite, and dyspnea on exertion. Blood tests showed pancytopenia with large, atypical lymphocytes. Computed tomography showed mild splenomegaly. Bone marrow examination demonstrated CD20-positive, EBER-positive atypical lymphocytes, and hemophagocytosis. Random skin biopsy led to the diagnosis of intravascular large B-cell lymphoma (IVLBCL). The final diagnosis was a hemophagocytic syndrome-associated variant of IVLBCL. Complete remission was achieved after seven courses of R-CHOP. However, within a month, he complained of dizziness. Magnetic resonance imaging revealed focal infarctions in the cerebellum and around the left lateral ventricle. Central nervous system relapse was suspected. Although salvage chemotherapy (CHASER), whole brain irradiation, and intrathecal injection of cytarabine and prednisolone were temporarily effective, he died. Autopsy revealed infiltration of lymphoma cells in the brain and adrenal glands. To the best of our knowledge, this is the sixth case of IVLBCL and the first case of the hemophagocytic syndrome-associated variant of IVLBCL in RA patients in the literature.

1. Introduction

According to WHO classification, intravascular large B-cell lymphoma (IVLBCL) is a rare type of extranodal large B-cell lymphoma characterized by the selective growth of lymphoma cells within the lumina of vessels, in particular capillaries, with the exception of larger arteries and veins [1, 2]. It comprises three major subtypes: a classic variant, a hemophagocytic syndrome-associated variant, and a cutaneous variant. The former variants were originally known as Western and Asian variants, respectively, based on geographical distributions. Murase et al. proposed diagnostic criteria of the hemophagocytic syndrome-associated (Asian) variant [3]. IVLBCL disseminates to almost all organs, while lymphadenopathy is absent in most cases. The prognosis of IVLBCL is very poor, partly because disease presentation can be varied and nonspecific, which makes early diagnosis difficult. CNS relapse occurs in up to 25% of IVLBCL cases, and its outcome is dismal. Unlike the other two variants, the cutaneous variant is restricted to the skin and is associated with a better prognosis.

Lymphoid proliferations or lymphomas arising in patients treated with immunosuppressive drugs for autoimmune diseases, excluding transplantation recipients, are classified as "other iatrogenic immunodeficiency-associated lymphoproliferative disorders (OIIA-LPD)" according to WHO classification [2]. Rheumatoid arthritis (RA) is the most representative underlying disorder, typically treated with methotrexate (MTX). The most dominant histopathology of MTX-associated LPD is diffuse large B-cell lymphoma (DLBCL) and Hodgkin lymphoma [2]. As for IVLBCL arising in RA patients, only five cases have been reported in the literature [4–8].

Here, we present the first case of the hemophagocytic syndrome-associated variant of IVLBCL that developed during the follow-up of rheumatoid arthritis treated with MTX.

2. Case Presentation

A 43-year-old Japanese man was diagnosed with RA in 1995. In 1998, treatment with methotrexate (MTX) and prednisolone (PSL) was started. In November 2010, he was diagnosed with MTX-induced interstitial pneumonia, and MTX was discontinued. He was treated with pulse steroid therapy, followed by a tapering dose of prednisolone. In January 2011, cyclophosphamide (CPA) was added to treat dyspnea due to interstitial pneumonia. In July 2011, tacrolimus was added for the treatment of arthralgia. In the following months, hemoglobin and platelet levels gradually decreased, and lactate dehydrogenase (LDH) levels increased. Tacrolimus side effects were suspected, and tacrolimus was discontinued. Two weeks later (August 2011, at the age of 59), he visited the hospital for fever, appetite loss, dyspnea on exertion, and skin rash. Blood testing revealed anemia, thrombocytopenia, and elevated levels of LDH and CRP. He was hospitalized for further examination.

On admission, he was administered PSL 10 mg/day daily and CPA 50 mg/day every other day. Skin eruptions were observed on his back and lateral regions. Blood testing revealed pancytopenia with large atypical lymphocytes and elevated C-reactive protein levels (Table 1). Soluble interleukin-2 receptor (sIL-2R) was elevated to 12,600 U/mL. Blood culture was negative. Computed tomography (CT) showed inactive interstitial shadows in the subpleural region and mild splenomegaly but no lymphadenopathy. Bone marrow aspiration demonstrated atypical lymphocytes (3.0% of all nucleated cells) (Figure 1(a)) and hemophagocytosis by macrophages, suggesting lymphoma-associated hemophagocytic syndrome (Figure 1(b)). Bone marrow biopsy revealed hypercellular marrow with diffuse infiltration of large atypical lymphocytes, which were CD20(+), CD79a(+), Bcl-2(−), CD10(−), Epstein–Barr virus-encoded RNA (EBER) in situ hybridization (+), and high Ki-67 index level (100%) (Figures 1(c) and 1(d)). One of the four samples of random skin biopsy was angiolipoma containing relatively large atypical lymphocytes within the lumina of vessels (CD20(+), CD79a(+), CD10(−), Bcl-6(−), MUM-1(+), and Ki-67(+)) (Figure 2). These findings fulfilled the diagnostic criteria of the hemophagocytic-syndrome associated (or Asian) variant of IVLBCL (International Prognostic Index (IPI) high intermediate) [3].

Table 1: Summary of the patient's initial laboratory data.

White blood cells	3750/μL
Monocyte	15.5%
Lymphocyte	10.0%
Basophil	0.0%
Eosinophil	0.0%
Segmented	51.0%
Band	20.0%
Metamyelocyte	0.5%
Myelocyte	0.5%
Atypical lymphocyte	2.5%
Red blood cells	$299 \times 10^4/\mu$L
Hemoglobin	9.4 g/dL
MCV	90.6 fL
Reticulocytes	$6.94 \times 10^4/\mu$L
Platelets	$5.0 \times 10^4/\mu$L
TP	5.1 g/dL
Albumin	2.6 g/dL
LDH	1336 IU/L
AST	83 IU/L
ALT	23 IU/L
ALP	385 IU/L
γ-GTP	80 IU/L
TB	1.3 mg/dL
DB	0.3 mg/dL
BUN	22 mg/dL
Creatinine	0.8 mg/dL
CRP	8.2 mg/dL
Fe	101 μg/dL
Ferritin	5854.7 ng/mL
sIL-2R	12600 U/mL
PT	84%
PT-INR	1.09
aPTT	33.2 sec
D-dimer	2.8 μg/mL

Segmented, segmented neutrophil. Band, band neutrophil. MCV, mean corpuscular volume. TP, total protein. LDH, lactate dehydrogenase. AST, aspartate transaminase. ALT, alanine aminotransferase. ALP, alkaline phosphatase. γ-GTP, γ-glutamyltransferase. TB, total bilirubin. DB, direct bilirubin. BUN, blood urea nitrogen. CRP, C-reactive protein. Fe, iron. sIL-2R, soluble interleukin-2 receptor. PT, prothrombin time. PT-INR, the international normalized ratio of prothrombin time. aPTT, activated partial thromboplastin time.

Pulse steroid therapy (methylprednisolone 500 mg/day for 3 days) was started on day 2 after admission, which relieved dyspnea. After the diagnosis of IVLBCL, one course of CHOP (cyclophosphamide, doxorubicin, vincristine, and prednisone) and six courses of R-CHOP (rituximab plus CHOP) were administered. Splenomegaly was resolved, and blood cell counts returned to the normal levels. Normal hematopoiesis was confirmed by bone marrow biopsy. However, at the final (sixth) R-CHOP therapy (January 2012) as an outpatient, he complained of staggering gait, which started one month earlier. He was afebrile. Magnetic resonance imaging (MRI) performed in February 2012 revealed a fresh infarction in the white matter around the left lateral ventricle, which was possibly caused by IVLBCL. He was hospitalized. Laboratory findings were as follows: WBC 2,040/μL, neutrophil 1,300/μL, hemoglobin 14.0 g/dL, platelet $10.0 \times 10^4/\mu$L, LDH 241 IU/L, ferritin 141.4 ng/mL, and sIL-2R 319 U/mL. The finger-to-nose test was positive

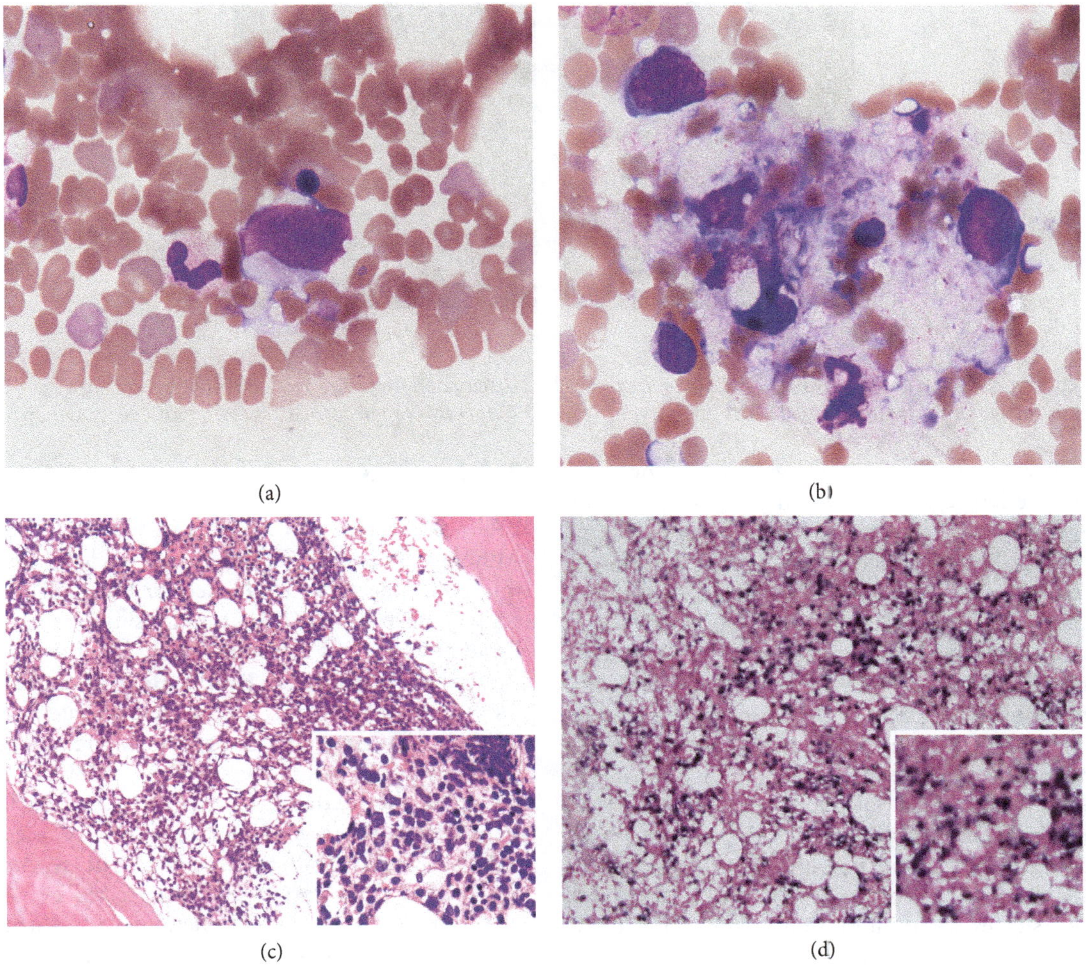

FIGURE 1: Bone marrow aspiration/biopsy findings. (a, b) Bone marrow aspirate. Wright-Giemsa staining. (a) A large, atypical lymphocyte (×1,000). (b) Hemophagocytosis (×1,000). (c, d) Bone marrow biopsy showing hypercellular marrow. (c) Hematoxylin and eosin staining. Low-magnification image (×40). Inset: high-magnification image (×200). (d) Epstein–Barr virus-encoded RNA (EBER) in situ hybridization. Large atypical lymphocytes are positive. Low-magnification image (×40). Inset: high-magnification image (×200).

on the right side. Cytology of cerebrospinal fluid (CSF) was class II. Bone marrow aspiration/biopsy revealed no evidence of lymphoma or hemophagocytosis. As he had a past history of MTX-induced interstitial pneumonia, cyclophosphamide, cytosine arabinoside, dexamethasone, etoposide, and rituximab (CHASER) instead of high-dose MTX was administered as salvage therapy.

In March 2012, he was hospitalized for the second course of chemotherapy. On admission, MRI revealed a new 2.3-cm mass in the infarction lesion in the white matter around the left lateral ventricle (Figures 3(a) and 3(b)). It had low intensity in the T1-weighted image, higher intensity than cerebral parenchyma in the T2-weighted image (T2WI) and fluid-attenuated inversion recovery (FLAIR) (Figure 3(a)), and high intensity in the diffusion weighted image, and its apparent diffusion coefficient value was low. It was evenly enhanced in contrast-enhanced MRI (Figure 3(b)). These results suggested infiltration of lymphoma. Cytology of CSF was class II. The second course of CHASER was administered, followed by whole brain irradiation, and MRI revealed shrinkage of the mass.

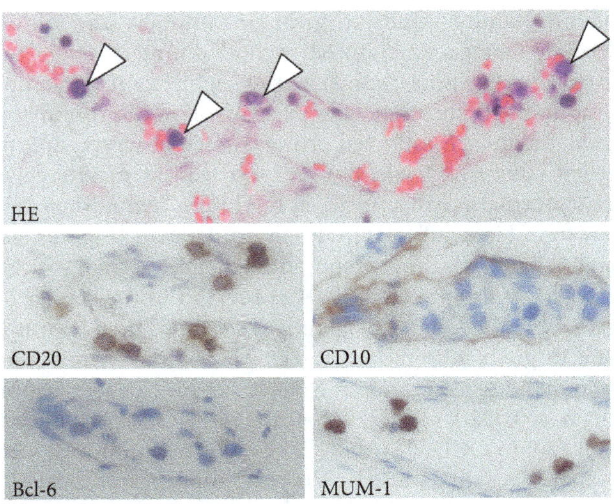

FIGURE 2: Histopathology of the angiolipoma. Large atypical lymphocytes in the lumina of the capillaries. Lymphoma cells are indicated by arrowheads. They are CD20(+), CD10(−), Bcl-6(−), and MUM-1(+). Magnification: ×400. HE, hematoxylin and eosin stain.

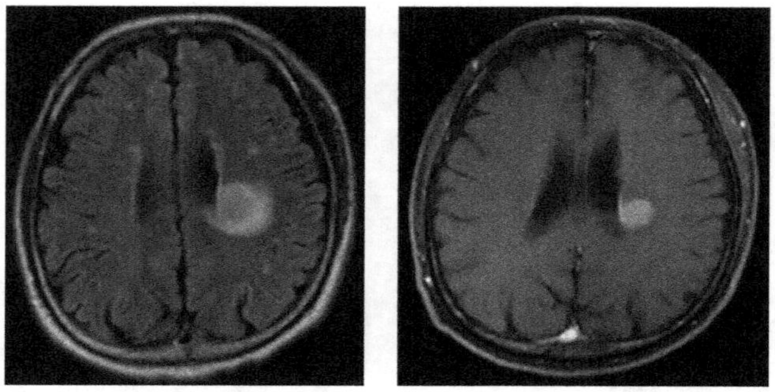

(a) (b)

Figure 3: Magnetic resonance imaging (MRI) for CNS relapse. (a) Fluid-attenuated inversion recovery image showing a 2.3-cm mass in the infarction lesion in the white matter near the left lateral ventricle. (b) Contrast-enhanced MRI showing an evenly enhanced mass.

In May 2012, he had staggering gait, headache, and dysesthesia in the left leg. MRI showed that the mass was smaller than it was before treatment, but it still had high intensity in T2WI/FLAIR and diffusion enhanced images, while no enhancement was noted in contrast-enhanced images. Cytology of CSF was class V. CNS relapse of IVLBCL was suggested. High-dose cytarabine and prednisolone therapy was administered for 3 days, and repeated intrathecal injections of cytarabine and prednisolone were administered. On MRI, the low-density area remained the same size and showed no enhancement on contrast-enhanced images. Continuous injection of oxycodone was administered for headache. In June 2012, dizziness, nausea, paresis of the right oculomotor nerve, and left leg paralysis manifested. Abdominal CT showed swelling of the bilateral adrenal glands, suggestive of infiltration of lymphoma cells, but neither lymphadenopathy nor hepatosplenomegaly was detected. Within the next two weeks, he had high fever and developed shock. Chest radiography revealed bilateral diffuse pneumonia. Despite antibiotic therapy and intrathecal injections of cytarabine and prednisolone, he died in August 2012, one year after diagnosis.

Autopsy was performed with written consent from the patient's family. Multiple focal pneumonias and diffuse alveolar damage were noted in both lungs. Massive purulent sputum was found in the right main bronchus. Lymphoma infiltration was prominent in the brain and adrenal glands. Spotty red changes were observed around the left lateral ventricle, but no infarction, hemorrhage, or tumor formation was noted in the brain. Lymphoma cells were found in capillaries in the choroid plexus (Figures 4(a) and 4(b)) and pituitary gland. Bilateral adrenal glands were enlarged. Lymphoma cells were observed in the capillaries of the bilateral adrenal glands and fatty tissue around them (Figures 4(c) and 4(d)), ectopic adrenal cortex tissue around the spleen, and transverse colon. The lymphoma cells were CD20(+), CD79a(+), CD10(−), Bcl-6(−), MUM-1(+), CD5(−), CD3(−), and CD56(−). These findings were compatible with IVLBCL. No lymphoma infiltration was observed in the thyroid gland, liver, spleen, heart, skin, or bone marrow. No lymphadenopathy was detected. These results suggested that the cause of death was diffuse infiltration of IVLBCL in the brain and respiratory failure due to bilateral pan-lobular pneumonia.

3. Discussion

RA is associated with an increased risk of lymphoma [9]. Although its pathogenesis remains unclear, the increase in this risk appears to be related to the high inflammatory activity observed in RA, immunosuppressive agents, and Epstein–Barr virus infection. DLBCL is the most common subtype of lymphoma in RA [9]. Here, we reported a case of the hemophagocytic syndrome-associated variant of IVLBCL following immunosuppressive treatment for RA. To our knowledge, this is the sixth case of IVLBCL in RA reported in the literature [4–8]. Four cases, including ours, were from Japan [4–6]. However, of the six cases, ours is the only one involving the hemophagocytic syndrome-associated variant. This variant is characterized by bone marrow involvement, fever, hepatosplenomegaly, thrombocytopenia, and hemophagocytic syndrome [1–3].

Prior treatments for IVLBCL in RA patients have varied. Since most RA patients with OIIA-LPD have a history of treatment with MTX, the term "MTX-associated LPD" is commonly used. However, in most cases, several immunosuppressive agents were concomitantly used (such as PSL, etanercept, tumor necrosis factor inhibitor, and adalimumab) [4, 5, 7]. Our patient had MTX-associated interstitial pneumonia, and the prolonged use of PSL and CPA, and the use of tacrolimus for a month, was necessary after MTX cessation. In fact, MTX has not been proven to have a direct causative effect for lymphoma in RA patients [9]. Thus, the significance of the diagnosis of "MTX-associated LPD" needs further validation. In contrast, Willemze et al. reported on an RA patient who had been treated with only PSL 10 mg for 9 years and later developed IVLBCL [8]. The latency of IVLBCL in RA patients has ranged from 2 months [6] to 13 years (our case) after starting MTX treatment [4–6].

Approximately 40% of MTX-associated LPD cases show at least partial regression after drug withdrawal [2]. However, all the previously reported IVLBCL (classic variant) cases in RA patients were treated with chemotherapy. The outcomes were favorable, although the observation periods were relatively short. The clinical course of our case lasted for only one year, and massive infiltration of lymphoma cells into the CNS was noted during the autopsy; this is consistent with the fact that the hemophagocytic syndrome-associated variant shows a poor prognosis [3].

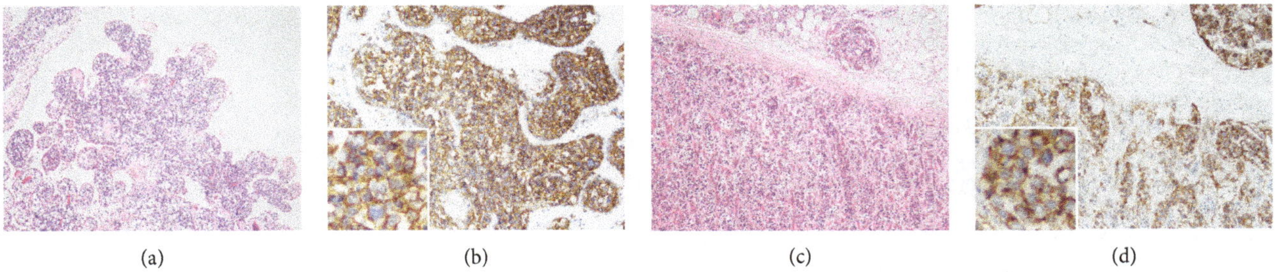

FIGURE 4: Autopsy findings. (a, b) Choroid plexus. (a) Hematoxylin and eosin staining. Magnification, ×100. (b) CD20 staining. Magnification, ×200. (c, d) Adrenal gland. (c) Hematoxylin and eosin staining. Magnification, ×100. (c) CD20 staining. Magnification, ×200.

As IVLBCL cells proliferate in blood vessels, R-CHOP is the standard therapy [1]. However, CNS invasion/relapse is one reason for the poor prognosis of IVLBCL [1, 2]. CNS invasion/relapse was reported in three previous RA-associated IVLBCL cases as well as in ours. Kikuchi et al. administered 8 courses of R-CHOP and 4 rounds of intrathecal (IT) injections (PSL, MTX, and cytarabine) [5]. Hagihara et al. administered six courses of R-THPCOP, three rounds of IT injections of MTX plus dexamethasone, and one course of high-dose MTX [4]. Kida et al. administered R-Hyper-CVAD/R-MA (rituximab plus cyclophosphamide, vincristine, doxorubicin, and dexamethasone, alternating with rituximab plus high-dose MTX and cytarabine) [6]. Our patient, who was initially treated with R-CHOP, experienced CNS relapse during the last course of R-CHOP. As our patient had a past history of MTX-associated interstitial pneumonia, high-dose MTX was not administered. After relapse, he received two courses of CHASER, whole brain irradiation, and repeated IT injections of cytarabine and PSL. The best way of CNS prophylaxis of IVLBCL is not clear [1]. According to the ESMO guideline on the management of "ultra-high-risk" lymphoma patients, IPI parameters (age > 60 years, high LDH levels, poor performance status, advanced disease stage, and more than one extranodal site) are risk factors for early CNS relapse following first-line treatment of DLBCL including IVLBCL [10]. In addition, the involvement of the testes, kidneys, adrenals, breast, bone marrow, and bone increases the risk of CNS disease [10]. Thus, our patient, with a high LDH level and bone marrow invasion at diagnosis, should have benefitted from CNS prophylaxis. Intrathecal injections of MTX, cytarabine, and prednisolone have been the traditional method of CNS prophylaxis. However, significance of IT chemotherapy is controversial, because it does not reach measurable concentrations of brain parenchyma [10]. Instead, intravenous prophylaxis, such as systemic high-dose MTX, is an alternative strategy of CNS prophylaxis [1, 10].

In our case, random skin biopsy resulted in the diagnosis of IVLBCL. Among the four biopsies, the only sample showing positive results contained angiolipoma. There are two previous reports of IVLBCL diagnosed by angiolipoma biopsies [11, 12]. Biopsies of the lung and kidney can also be used for the diagnosis of IVLBCL [3]. Moreover, we previously reported a case of IVLBCL diagnosed by colon biopsy [13].

In conclusion, here, we reported a rare case of the hemophagocytic syndrome-associated variant of IVLBCL that developed during RA treatment. IVLBCL should be considered as a differential diagnosis of pancytopenia during RA treatment or immunosuppressive therapy.

References

[1] M. Ponzoni, E. Campo, and S. Nakamura, "Intravascular large B-cell lymphoma: a chameleon with multiple faces and many masks," *Blood*, vol. 132, no. 15, pp. 1561–1567, 2018.

[2] S. Swerdlow, E. Campo, N. Harris et al., *WHO Classification of Tumours of Haematopoietic and Lymphoid Tissues*, IARC, Lyon, France, 2017.

[3] T. Murase, S. Nakamura, K. Kawauchi et al., "An Asian variant of intravascular large B-cell lymphoma: clinical, pathological and cytogenetic approaches to diffuse large B-cell lymphoma associated with haemophagocytic syndrome," *British Journal of Haematology*, vol. 111, no. 3, pp. 826–834, 2000.

[4] M. Hagihara, T. Mese, S. Ohara, J. Hua, S. Ide, and M. Inoue, "Methotrexate-associated intravascular large B-cell lymphoma in a patient with rheumatoid arthritis: a very rare case," *Internal Medicine*, vol. 57, no. 20, pp. 3001–3005, 2018.

[5] J. Kikuchi, Y. Kaneko, H. Kasahara et al., "Methotrexate-associated intravascular large B-cell lymphoma in a patient with rheumatoid arthritis," *Internal Medicine*, vol. 55, no. 12, pp. 1661–1665, 2016.

[6] T. Kida, M. Kohno, Y. Chinen et al., "Intravascular lymphoma in a rheumatoid arthritis patient following short-term methotrexate treatment," *Rheumatology*, vol. 56, no. 2, pp. 318–320, 2017.

[7] V. Bogomolski-Yahalom, I. S. Lossos, E. Okun, Y. Sherman, A. Lossos, and A. Polliack, "Intravascular lymphomatosis-an indolent or aggressive entity?," *Leuk Lymphoma*, vol. 29, no. 5-6, pp. 585–593, 1998.

[8] R. Willemze, M. R. J. Kruyswijk, C. D. D. Bruin, C. J. L. M. Meijer, and W. V. Berkel, "Angiotropic (intravascular) large cell lymphoma of the skin previously classified as malignant angioendotheliomatosis," *British Journal of Dermatology*, vol. 116, no. 3, pp. 393–399, 1987.

[9] A. Klein, A. Polliack, and A. Gafter-Gvili, "Rheumatoid arthritis and lymphoma: incidence, pathogenesis, biology, and outcome," *Hematological Oncology*, vol. 36, no. 5, pp. 733–739, 2018.

[10] M. Hutchings, M. Ladetto, C. Buske et al., "ESMO Consensus Conference on malignant lymphoma: management of "ultra-high-risk" patients," *Annals of Oncology*, vol. 29, no. 8, pp. 1687–1700, 2018.

[11] T. Saito, T. Matsuya, C. Takahashi et al., "Cutaneous variant of intravascular large B-cell lymphoma in a Japanese patient: an occult lesion localized in a solitary angiolipoma," *The Journal of Dermatology*, vol. 44, no. 3, pp. e28–e29, 2017.

[12] M. E. Smith, M. D. Stamatakos, and T. S. Neuhauser, "Intravascular lymphomatosis presenting within angiolipomas," *Annals of Diagnostic Pathology*, vol. 5, no. 2, pp. 103–106, 2001.

[13] D. Kaneyuki, Y. Komeno, H. Yoshimoto, N. Yoshimura, K. Iihara, and T. Ryu, "Intestinal intravascular large B-cell lymphoma mimicking ulcerative colitis with secondary membranoproliferative glomerulonephritis," *Internal Medicine*, vol. 55, no. 17, pp. 2475–2481, 2016.

37

Two Different Extranodal Lymphomas in an HIV$^+$ Patient: A Case Report and Review of the Literature

Clara Bertuzzi,[1] Elena Sabattini,[1] Francesco Bacci,[1] Claudio Agostinelli,[1] and Gian Gaetano Ferri[2]

[1]*Hematopathology Unit, Sant'Orsola University Hospital, Bologna, Italy*
[2]*ENT and Audiology Unit, Department of Experimental, Diagnostic and Specialty Medicine, Sant' Orsola Hospital, University of Bologna, Bologna, Italy*

Correspondence should be addressed to Clara Bertuzzi; clarabertuzzi@gmail.com

Academic Editor: Yusuke Shiozawa

Human immune deficiency virus- (HIV-) infected individuals present a higher risk of developing malignancies. Herein, we are presenting an unusual case of an untreated HIV$^+$ patient, who developed two distinct lymphoproliferative disorders in a period of 4 years: a primary cutaneous T-cell lymphoma (PCTCL) and a diffuse large B-cell lymphoma (DLBCL) not otherwise specified (NOS), the latter developed while commencing combined antiretroviral therapy (cART). The two lymphomas also showed peculiar features: PCTCL are rarely described in HIV$^+$ setting and particularly at such a low clinical stage, and the DLBCL showed uncommon cytology, non-GCB phenotype, EBER negativity, and absence of c-MYC translocation, all atypical features in this clinical context. This report not only confirms the increased risk of lymphoma for HIV$^+$ patients and HIV infection being one of the major risk factors for lymphoid disorders but draws the attention on the possible occurrence of unusual features, suggesting that HIV serology should always be investigated in the clinical suspicion of lymphoma.

1. Introduction

Human immune deficiency virus- (HIV-) infected individuals present a higher risk of developing malignancies. Among these latter, lymphomas are the most frequent neoplasms in USA and Europe within seropositive patients [1, 2]. Furthermore, aggressive B-cell lymphomas together with Kaposi's sarcoma and invasive cervical cancer are considered to be acquired immune deficiency syndrome (AIDS)-defining cancers [3]. Here, we are presenting an unusual case of an HIV$^+$ patient who developed two separate extranodal lymphomas and reviewing the literature focusing on lymphoproliferative disorders in the setting of HIV infection.

2. Case Presentation

In March 2010, a 43-year-old man underwent surgery to remove a subcutaneous nodule from the inguinal region. The patient had a known hepatitis B virus (HBV) and HIV infection since 1986; he had never been treated with a combined antiretroviral therapy (cART) and had never developed opportunistic infections. The histological examination of the removed lesion showed a proliferation of medium/large sized lymphoid cells infiltrating dermis and subcutaneous tissue, without epidermotropism or ulceration and absence of inflammatory background (Figure 1(a)). Immunohistochemical investigations of these cells showed a T-lymphoid phenotype: CD3$^+$, CD2$^+$ with partial expression of CD5, CD7, and TIA1. CD4, CD8, and granzyme B were negative. The tumoral population was highly proliferating (90% Ki67$^+$ cells). A strong and diffuse CD30 positivity was observed (Figure 1(b)), while B-cell markers were negative as well as EMA, Perforin, Alkc, HHV8, and CD56. Staging procedures failed to demonstrate other sites of involvement. The uniqueness and persistence of the lesion, the absence of ulceration, and the strong diffuse positivity for CD30 prompted a diagnosis of primary cutaneous CD30$^+$ T-cell

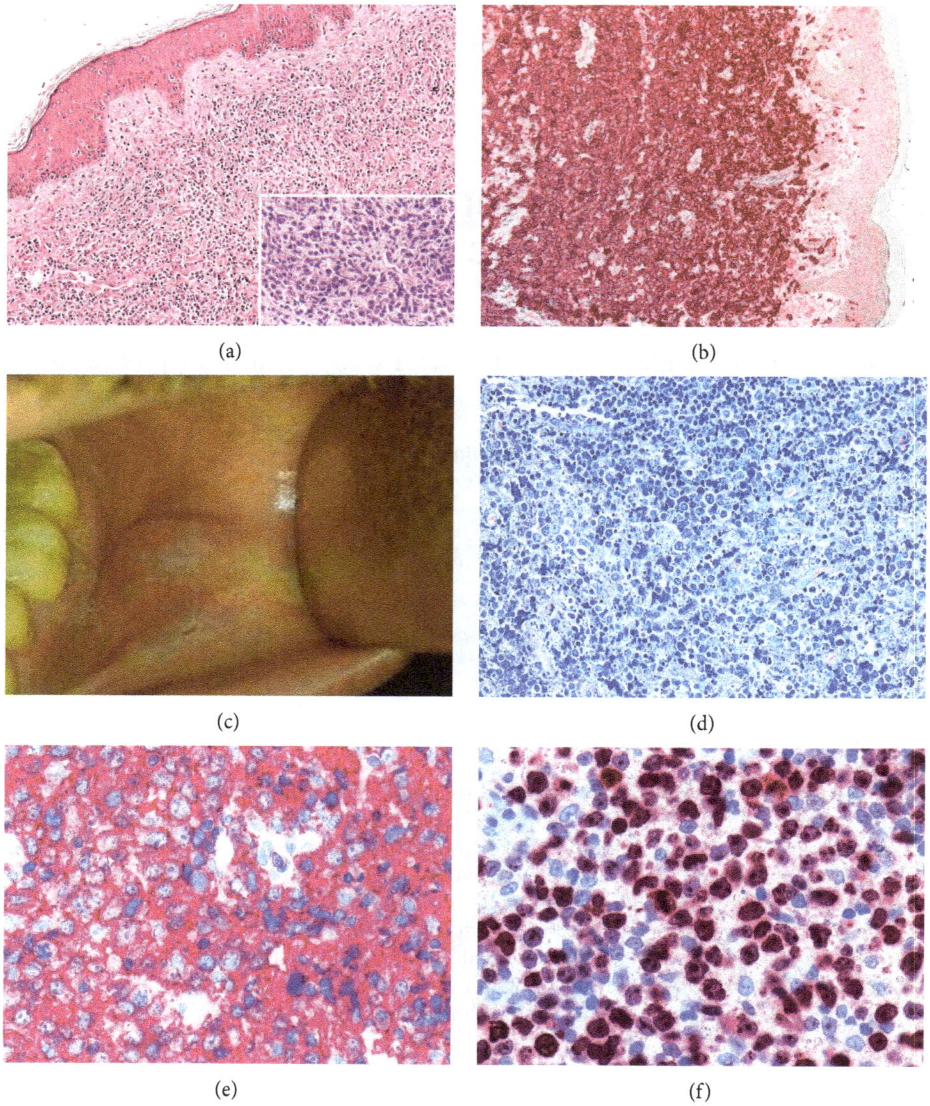

Figure 1: (a) Morphological features (haematoxylin and eosin ×100; insert ×400) and (b) CD30 expression (×100) of the skin lesion; (c) intraoperatory picture of gingival neoformation and (d) its morphologic features (Giemsa stain, ×200); immunohistochemical expression of (e) CD20 (×400) and (f) Ki67 (×400) in DLBCL.

lymphoproliferative disorders with the features of anaplastic large cell lymphoma. A targeted radiotherapy treatment was suggested.

In November 2013, the patient started cART and almost simultaneously he developed a hard, nonpainful, nonulcerated gingival lesion sited on the left anteroinferior genus mucosa. Few months later, this lesion had reached 3 cm in diameter (Figure 1(c)) and an incisional surgical biopsy was performed (February 2014). The gingival tissue was diffusely infiltrated by large lymphoid cells with a prevalent immunoblastic morphology (Figure 1(d)), expressing CD20 (Figure 1(e)), BCL6, and IRF4 while CD10, CD3, and CD30 were negative. The proliferation index was high (90% $Ki67^+$ cells) (Figure 1(f)). BCL2 resulted diffusely positive while cMYC protein was detected in 25% of the 57 cells and was thus considered negative, being the established cutoff positivity ≥40%. In situ hybridization analysis for Epstein–Barr virus (EBV) small encoded RNAs did not reveal EBV presence. The investigation for cMYC rearrangements by fluorescence in in situ hybridization was negative. Based on the molecular and morphophenotypic findings, a diagnosis of diffuse large B-cell lymphoma (DLBCL) not otherwise specified (NOS) with non-GCB phenotype was made, according to Hans' algorithm [4]. The staging positron emission tomography showed areas of hypercaptation in the left pleura and in the right obturatory site, indicating a multifocal disease. The patient refused the proposed treatment and was lost at follow-up.

3. Discussion

Lymphomas are one of the most common cancers among patients with HIV/AIDS [5, 6]. Before the introduction in 1996 of cART, the estimated risk to develop a non-Hodgkin lymphoma was 60–200 times higher in the HIV^+ individuals than in the general population [7]. Since the advent of cART, the mortality caused by infections has decreased and HIV-patients' life expectancy is now close to normal. However, despite the overall reduced incidence of lymphomas, these neoplasms are still the most important cause of cancer-related death, and HIV infection is so far the strongest risk factor for the onset of non-Hodgkin B-cell lymphoma (B-NHL) [5, 6].

The most frequent HIV-associated lymphomas are DLBCL (often involving the primary central nervous system) and Burkitt lymphoma (BL), both AIDS-defining illnesses, and accounts for 50% and 40% of NHLs, respectively [8, 9]; among non-AIDS-defining malignancies, Hodgkin's lymphoma (HL) is one of the most common [8]. The World Health Organization has grouped the HIV-associated lymphomas into three categories: [8] (a) lymphomas also occurring in immunocompetent patients such as BL, DLBCL, HL, plasmablastic lymphoma (PL), and other rarer subtypes (mycosis fungoides, anaplastic large cell lymphoma, NK/T-cell lymphoma, marginal zone lymphoma, and lymphoplasmacytic and lymphoblastic lymphoma); (b) lymphomas occurring more specifically in HIV-infected patients such as primary effusion lymphoma (PEL), PL, and human herpes virus-8 (HHV8) positive DLBCL; (c) lymphomas occurring in other immunodeficiency states, in which 84 include lymphoid proliferations resembling posttransplant lymphoproliferative disorders. Interestingly, the latter are far less common in the HIV setting than in transplanted patients, where they represent less than 5% of lymphomas [8].

The high prevalence of NHL also in cART era hints that additional mechanisms are involved in HIV lymphomagenesis beyond impaired immune surveillance. The chronic B-cell activation favoured by the HIV-mediated immune dysfunction, which is responsible for hypergammaglobulinemia, defective humoral immunity, and florid germinal centre hyperplasia (all characterizing early HIV-infection), was demonstrated to be critical for the development of lymphomas. This persistent polyclonal proliferation of B cells increases the risk of mistakes involving oncogenic genetic alterations during the germinal centre reaction. Chronic B-cell stimulation might be linked to: (a) HIV itself and various HIV-encoded proteins, (b) the Tat-induced abnormal production of interleukin 6 (IL-6) and IL-10, (c) the antigenic stimulation of opportunistic viral infections (i.e., Epstein–Barr virus (EBV), HHV8), and (d) the incorporation of host-derived CD40 L into virions and the ability of these latter to bind B lymphocytes mimicking the endogenous CD40-CD40 L interaction [10–15]. Furthermore, HIV preferentially infects T-follicular helper (TFH) cells altering B-cell development and function and the control of chronic viral infection [16, 17]. It was recently shown that expanded TFH-cell populations in HIV$^+$ patients are associated with an increase in germinal centre B-cells and plasma cells and a decrease of memory B-cells and immunoglobulin hypersecretion [18, 19]. HIV may also act as a local lymphomagenic factor through the effects of the virus encoded and secreted proteins. Tat functionally interacts with and enters into B lymphocytes, leading to deregulation of the pRb2/p130 oncosuppressor protein [20]. Variants of the HIV-1 matrix protein p17 (vp17s) recently detected in the NHL samples of HIV$^+$ patients, besides its impact on angiogenesis, displays also B-cell growth-promoting activity, due to activation of the Akt signaling pathway, suggesting its possible role in oncogenic transformation [21]. These vp17s are more frequently detected in HIV$^+$ patients with NHL than in patients without NHL. Moreover mice transgenic over-expressing the HIV proteins p17, gp120, and nef, develop B-cell lymphomas [22], and induction of RAG1 gene expression in costimulated human B-cells, treated with p17, has been recently observed. In this specific setting of costimulation, the activation of RAG genes could lead to genomic instability and transformation [23].

We report an unusual case of an HIV$^+$ patient who developed two distinct lymphoproliferative disorders in a period of 4 years after 25 years of HIV untreated and uncomplicated infection: a primary cutaneous T-cell lymphoma disorder and, three years later, an oral DLBCL, at the time he started cART.

In the HIV$^+$ population, DLBCL presents more frequently with disseminated disease (stages III and IV) and extranodal presentation than in HIV$^-$ people [8], the most common sites being the gastrointestinal tract, liver, bone marrow, and central nervous system (CNS). In particular, the risk of developing a primary CNS lymphoma (PCNSL) was 1000 times higher in the HIV$^+$ patients than in controls before cART although PCNSL still accounts for 20% of HIV-associated lymphomas and generally occurs in patients with very low CD4 cell counts (<100 cells/μl). HIV-related DLBCL usually consists of large cells characterized by centroblastic or immunoblastic cytology and displays a complete B-cell phenotype (CD20$^+$/CD19$^+$/CD79a$^+$/PAX5$^+$) [8], with a more frequent germinal centre B-cell (GCB) phenotype, although the prognostic impact of the cell of origin is not clear in the HIV setting [8]. Up to 80% of the cases are EBV$^+$, and this association reaches 100% in PCNSL [8]. The EBV-infected blasts carry a latency type II with expression of latent membrane protein 1 (LMP1). LMP1 and the mutation/deletion of TNFAIP3 gene, commonly observed in HIV$^+$ DLBCL, may contribute to lymphoma genesis activating the nuclear factor kB (NF-kB) pathway and consequently promoting cell proliferation and survival [8]. Additionally, cMYC and BCL6 gene rearrangements are frequently detected as well as aberrant somatic hypermutations involving PAX5, Rho/TTF, and PIM1 genes [8].

Our patient developed an extranodal DLBCL at the beginning of cART, when CD4 count was 437 cells/μl, and the PET scan revealed a disseminated disease. The finding of a rapidly growing neoformation in the oral cavity of an HIV$^+$ individual generally suggests an EBV$^+$ PL, which is the most common lymphoma arising at this site and setting. However, one should keep in mind that LBCL other than EBV + PL localizes in oral cavity, particularly in HIV-infected subjects, and therefore any oral LBCL should per se prompt clinical investigations for HIV infection. The described DLBCL showed peculiar features: in fact, it presented with immunoblastic (IB) cytology and a non-GCB phenotype, which are biologic features commonly associated to EBV positivity, which was however negative in our case by means of in situ hybridization analysis for EBV small encoded RNAs, although Mundo and colleagues [24] reported possible false negative results. We did not perform RNA scope or miRNAs qPCR and can not thus exclude the possibility of a previous EBV infection followed by the virus loss (so called "hit and run" event). Nonetheless, we considered our observations consistent, also considering the patient's CD4+ lymphocyte blood count which was still relatively high for an untreated long-lasting HIV infection, which had never been complicated by opportunistic infections. The cMYC rearrangement that is reported in about 20% of HIV-related IB-DLBCL was not revealed by FISH analysis in our case.

Interestingly, a primary cutaneous peripheral T-cell lymphoma (PC-PTCL) was diagnosed three years before the onset of gingival DLBCL. Although relative risk of developing NHL is increased among HIV^+ population, PTCL are rarely described; most data referred to small retrospective series and suggest a significantly lower incidence than the B-cell ones [25–27]. The PTCL frequency is estimated between 2% and 7% of all HIV-associated lymphoma, and it seems to be similar in pre- and post-cART era [25–27], with not otherwise specified and ALK-anaplastic large cell lymphoma types being mostly prevalent, and angioimmunoblastic T-cell lymphoma (AITL) sporadically found. Patients affected by systemic PTCL usually have advanced stage disease, multiple extranodal involvement, B-symptoms, poor performance status, and a haemophagocytic syndrome sometimes complicating the clinical course. [25–28]. Cutaneous T-cell lymphomas rarely occurs in HIV-infected patients: mycosis fungoides (MF) is definitely unusual, whereas primary cutaneous $CD30^+$ T-cell lymphoma ALCL type (PC-ALCL) seems to be more frequent [29–31]. The latter more frequently arises in severely immunocompromised patients with very low CD4 count and presents with a single deep skin, rapidly growing nodule. These HIV^+ cases share the same morphologic and phenotypic features as in HIV^- patients, although they more often express T-cell antigens (i.e., CD2, CD3, and CD4) [28–30]. Occasionally EBV positivity was reported, while HHV8 is regularly negative [30, 31]. Isolated lesions are treated with surgical excision or radiation therapy or both, while multifocal skin lesions may require multiagent chemotherapy [29–31]. Survival was correlated to the immune-suppression status and is good in patients without opportunistic infections. Occasional spontaneous and/or complete regression after immune recovery secondary to cART was also reported. In the presented case, the skin lesion consisted of large atypical cells diffusely and intensively expressing CD30. The T-cell origin was demonstrated by the expression of CD2, CD3, CD5, and CD7; however, the neoplasm turned out to be negative for both CD4 and CD8. This phenotypic profile suggested a diagnosis of CD30 + PTCL, which might be referred to as ALCL, despite negativity for EMA and cytotoxic markers. The primary cutaneous origin was ascertained by the clinical staging and the bone marrow biopsy which excluded any systemic involvement, and a targeted radiotherapy was suggested.

In conclusion, we presented an extremely unusual case of an HIV^+ patient who developed both a B-cell and T-cell neoplasms in a relatively short period of time, with one of them (PC-ALCL) being an unusual variant in the setting of HIV infection especially with still good clinical conditions and relatively high CD4 count. This case provides confirmation of higher exposure of HIV^+ patients to the lymphoma development, sometimes presenting with unusual biologic features, and of HIV being by itself one of the major risk factors for lymphoid disorders, indicating that the HIV status should always be investigated in the clinical suspicion of lymphoma.

References

[1] R. U. Hernández-Ramírez, M. S. Shiels, R. Dubrow, and E. A. Engels, "Cancer risk in HIVinfected people in the USA from 1996 to 2012: a population-based, registry-linkage study," *Lancet HIV*, vol. 4, pp. e495–e504, 2017.

[2] E. A. Engels, R. J. Biggar, H. I. Hall et al., "Cancer risk in people infected with human immunodeficiency virus in the United States," *International Journal of Cancer*, vol. 123, pp. 187–194, 2008.

[3] K. G. Castro, J. W. Ward, L. Slutsker, J. W. Buehler, H. W. Jaffe, and R. L. Berkelman, "1993 Revised classification system for HIV infection and expanded surveillance case definition for AIDS among adolescents and adults," *MMWR Recommendations and Reports*, vol. 41, pp. 1–19, 1992.

[4] C. P. Hans, D. D. Weisenburger, T. C. Greiner et al., "Confirmation of the molecular classification of diffuse large B-cell lymphoma by immunohistochemistry using a tissue microarray," *Blood*, vol. 103, pp. 275–282, 2004.

[5] E. P. Simard, R. M. Pfeiffer, and E. A. Engels, "Cumulative incidence of cancer among individuals with acquired immunodeficiency syndrome in the United States," *Cancer*, vol. 117, no. 5, pp. 1089–1096, 2011.

[6] F. Bonnet, C. Lewden, T. May et al., "Malignancy-related causes of death in human immunodeficiency virus-infected patients in the era of highly active antiretroviral therapy," *Cancer*, vol. 101, pp. 317–324, 2004.

[7] V. Beral, T. Peterman, R. Berkelman, and H. Jaffe, "AIDS-associated non-Hodgkin lymphoma," *The Lancet*, vol. 337, pp. 805–809, 1991.

[8] J. Said, E. Casarman, A. Rosenwald, and N. L. Harris, "Lymphoma associated with HIV infection," in *WHO Classification of Tumours of Haematopoietic and Lymphoid Tissues*, S. H. Swerdlow, E. Campo, N. L. Harris et al., Eds., IARC, Lyon, France, 2017.

[9] R. J. Biggar, "AIDS-related cancers in the era of highly active antiretroviral therapy," *Oncology (Williston Park)*, vol. 15, pp. 439–448, 2001.

[10] R. Dolcetti, A. Gloghini, A. Caruso, and A. Carbone, "A lymphomagenic role for HIV beyond immune suppression?," *Blood*, vol. 127, pp. 1403–1409, 2016.

[11] E. Vendrame, S. K. Hussain, E. C. Breen et al., "Serum levels of cytokines and biomarkers for inflammation and immune activation, and HIV-associated non-Hodgkin B-cell lymphoma risk," *Cancer Epidemiology, Biomarkers & Prevention*, vol. 23, pp. 343–349, 2014.

[12] G. Martin, J. Roy, C. Barat, M. Ouellet, C. Gilbert, and M. J. Tremblay, "Human immunodeficiency virus type 1-

associated CD40 ligand transactivates B lymphocytes and promotes infection of CD4+ T-cells," *Journal of Virology*, vol. 81, pp. 5872–5881, 2007.

[13] M. Imbeault, M. Ouellet, K. Giguère et al., "Acquisition of host-derived CD40L by HIV-1 in vivo and its functional consequences in the B-cell compartment," *Journal of Virology*, vol. 85, pp. 2189–2200, 2011.

[14] G. Scala, M. R. Ruocco, C. Ambrosino et al., "The expression of the interleukin 6 gene is induced by the human immunodeficiency virus 1 TAT protein," *Journal of Experimental Medicine*, vol. 179, pp. 961–971, 1994.

[15] V. Blazevic, M. Heino, A. Lagerstedt, A. Ranki, and K. J. Krohn, "Interleukin-10 gene expression induced by HIV-1 Tat and Rev in the cells of HIV-1 infected individuals," *Journal of Acquired Immune Deficiency Syndromes and Human Retrovirology*, vol. 13, pp. 208–214, 1996.

[16] S. L. Kohler, M. N. Pham, J. M. Folkvord et al., "Germinal center T follicular helper cells are highly permissive to HIV-1 and alter their phenotype during virus replication," *Journal of Immunology*, vol. 196, pp. 2711–2722, 2016.

[17] R. A. Cubas, J. C. Mudd, A. L. Savoye et al., "Inadequate T follicular cell help impairs B-cell immunity during HIV infection," *Nature Medicine*, vol. 19, pp. 494–499, 2013.

[18] O. Martínez-Maza and E. C. Breen, "B-cell activation and lymphoma in patients with HIV," *Current Opinion in Oncology*, vol. 14, pp. 528–532, 2002.

[19] A. De Milito, A. Nilsson, K. Titanji et al., "Mechanisms of hypergammaglobulinemia and impaired antigen-specific humoral immunity in HIV-1 infection," *Blood*, vol. 103, pp. 2180–2186, 2004.

[20] S. Lazzi, C. Bellan, G. De Falco et al., "Expression of RB2/p130 tumor-suppressor gene in AIDS-related non-Hodgkin's lymphomas: implications for disease pathogenesis," *Human Pathology*, vol. 33, pp. 723–731, 2002.

[21] R. Dolcetti, C. Giagulli, W. He et al., "Role of HIV-1 matrix protein p17 variants in lymphoma pathogenesis," *Proceedings of the National Academy of Sciences of the United States of America*, vol. 112, no. 46, pp. 14331–14336, 2015.

[22] S. Curreli, S. Krishnan, M. Reitz et al., "B-cell lymphoma in HIV transgenic mice," *Retrovirology*, vol. 10, p. 92, 2013.

[23] V. A. Carroll, M. K. Lafferty, L. Marchionni, J. L. Bryant, R. C. Gallo, and A. Garzino-Demo, "Expression of HIV-1 matrix protein p17 and association with B-cell lymphoma in HIV-1 transgenic mice," *Proceedings of the National Academy of Sciences of the United States of America*, vol. 113, no. 46, pp. 13168–13173, 2016.

[24] L. Mundo, M. R. Ambrosio, M. Picciolini et al., "Unveiling another missing piece in EBV-driven lymphomagenesis: EBV-encoded microRNAs expression in EBER-negative burkitt lymphoma cases," *Frontiers in Microbiology*, vol. 8, p. 229, 2017.

[25] R. J. Biggar, E. A. Engels, M. Frisch, J. J. Goedert, and AIDS Cancer Match Registry Study Group, "Risk of T-cell lymphomas in persons with AIDS," *Journal of Acquired Immune Deficiency Syndromes*, vol. 26, pp. 371–376, 2001.

[26] L. Gilardin, C. Copie-Bergman, L. Galicier et al., "Peripheral T-cell lymphoma in HIV-infected patients: a study of 17 cases in the combination antiretroviral therapy era," *British Journal of Haematology*, vol. 161, pp. 843–851, 2013.

[27] K. K. Arzoo, X. Bu, B. M. Espina, L. Seneviratne, B. Nathwani, and A. M. Levine, "T-cell lymphoma in HIV-infected patients," *Journal of Acquired Immune Deficiency Syndromes*, vol. 36, no. 5, pp. 1020–1027, 2004.

[28] J. J. Castillo, B. E. Beltran, M. Bibas et al., "Prognostic factors in patients with HIV-associated peripheral T-cell lymphoma: a multicenter study," *American Journal of Hematology*, vol. 86, no. 3, pp. 256–261, 2011.

[29] M. Beylot-Barry, B. Vergier, B. Masquelier et al., "The spectrum of cutaneous lymphomas in HIV infection," *The American Journal of Surgical Pathology*, vol. 23, no. 10, pp. 1208–1216, 1999.

[30] K. Wilkins, R. Turner, J. C. Dolev, P. E. LeBoit, T. G. Berger, and T. A. Maurer, "Cutaneous malignancy and human immunodeficiency virus disease," *Journal of the American Academy of Dermatology*, vol. 54, no. 2, pp. 189–206, 2006.

[31] A. Saggini, L. Anemona, S. Chimenti et al., "HIV-associated primary cutaneous anaplastic large cell lymphoma: a clinicopathological subset with more aggressive behavior? Case report and review of the literature," *Journal of Cutaneous Pathology*, vol. 39, no. 12, pp. 1100–1109, 2012.

38

Myelodysplastic Syndrome with Transfusion Dependence Treated with Venetoclax

Waqas Jehangir,[1] **Alexander Karabachev**,[2] **Taimoor Jahangir**,[3] **and Elvira Umyarova**[1]

[1]*University of Vermont Medical Center, Hematology and Medical Oncology, 89 Beaumont Ave., Burlington, VT 05405-0068, USA*
[2]*University of Vermont College of Medicine, Larner College of Medicine. 89 Beaumont Ave., Burlington, VT 05405-0068, USA*
[3]*University Hospitals of Leicester NHS Trust, Groby Rd., Leicester LE3 9QP, UK*

Correspondence should be addressed to Waqas Jehangir; wjehangir@hotmail.com

Academic Editor: Stephen E. Langabeer

Myelodysplastic syndromes are characterized by ineffective hematopoiesis in one or more lineages of the bone marrow. They are a group of heterogeneous clonal stem cell malignancies with a high risk to progress to acute myeloid leukemia. Currently, there are no curative FDA-approved medications for myelodysplastic syndromes. Hematopoietic cell transplantation is potentially the only curative option; however, treatment is often unavailable due to age and comorbidities. Hypomethylating agents, azacitidine and decitabine, and the immunomodulatory agent, lenalidomide, are the only FDA approved medications for the treatment of MDS, all of which are noncurative. Venetoclax, an inhibitor of the antiapoptotic protein BCL-2 used to treat chronic lymphocytic leukemia, is currently being evaluated in clinical trials as a monotherapy in high-risk myelodysplastic syndromes/acute myeloid leukemia. We present a patient with transfusion-dependent myelodysplastic syndromes refractory to the current standard of care treatment not a candidate for hematopoietic cell transplantation who responded well to monotherapy treatment with venetoclax and has since remained transfusion-independent.

1. Introduction

Myelodysplastic syndromes (MDS) are characterized by ineffective hematopoiesis in one or more lineages of the bone marrow. They are a group of heterogeneous clonal stem cell malignancies with a high risk to progress to acute myeloid leukemia (AML). Majority of adult MDS cases arise *de novo*; however, some are due to genotoxic damage from ionizing radiation or chemotherapy treatments [1]. In the United States, the incidence of MDS is 3-4 cases per 100,000 population per year and increases with age with 30 cases per 100,000 population per year among individuals of 70 years of age and older [2]. The prevalence of MDS is growing in part due to an ageing population and an increased awareness of these syndromes [3]. Prognosis of MDS is highly variable based on risk stratification ranging from several years in low-risk patients to several months in patients with high-risk disease [4].

Currently, there are no curative FDA-approved medications for MDS. Hematopoietic cell transplantation (HCT) is potentially the only curative option; however, treatment with HCT is often unavailable due to age and comorbidities or is not tolerated due to potential side effects. Hypomethylating agents (HMA), Azacitidine and Decitabine, and the immunomodulatory agent Lenalidomide are the only three FDA-approved drugs for the treatment of MDS, all of which are noncurative [5–7].

Venetoclax, a small molecule inhibitor of the antiapoptotic protein BCL-2, has demonstrated promising results as a monotherapy in high-risk MDS/AML in *in vitro* studies [8, 9] and is currently being evaluated in clinical trials as a single-agent and in combination with Azacitidine for relapsed/refractory MDS. In this case, we describe a patient with transfusion-dependent myelodysplastic syndrome refractory to the current standard of care treatments and not a candidate for hematopoietic cell transplantation who responded well to monotherapy treatment with Venetoclax and has since remained transfusion-independent.

2. Case Presentation

A 53-year-old male with past medical history of hypertension, hyperlipidemia, peptic ulcer disease, gout, coronary artery disease, and sleep apnea underwent a CABG procedure in December 2011. Following CABG, the patient's blood counts remained low, and in March of 2012, he was referred to Hematology at the VA for further evaluation. His CBC at that time demonstrated pancytopenia with a white count of 2100×10^6/L, hemoglobin of 9.7×10^9/L, and platelet count of 123,000 per microliter. He had 3% circulating blasts. The bone marrow demonstrated a hypercellular marrow with multilineage dysplasia. Cytogenetics were significant for translocation between chromosome 2 and 11 t(2; 11)(p21; q23). At that time, he was diagnosed with MDS (refractory anemia with excess blasts, intermediate 1) and was found to have a revised IPSS (International Prognostic Scoring System) score of 3. The initial bone marrow blast count was 4%, and the cytogenics was 46, XY, t(2; 11). A repeat bone marrow showed a blast count of 3%, and the cytgenics was 46, XY, t(2; 11).

The patient was started on Azacitidine in September of 2012. This was complicated by elevated liver function tests as well as prolonged neutropenia. The bilirubin peaked at approximately 5-6 mg/dL. In November 2012, he received a 20% dose reduction of Azacitidine which was again complicated by acute hepatitis and renal failure with a creatinine of approximately 6 mg/dL, a total bilirubin peaked at 10 mg/dL and AST and ALT of 401 and 414 units per liter. His CBC demonstrated pancytopenia, however, was stable and he had not required any further blood transfusions. The licensed indication for the use of Azacitidine in Europe is IPSS Int-2 and high; therefore, its use was off-label. He had a response to Azacitidine for almost 10 months. In May 2013, CBC showed a white blood cell count of $4,100 \times 10^6$/L with a hemoglobin of 13.9 g/dL and a platelet count of 161,000 per microliter. His differential indicates 56% segs and 37% lymphocytes. There was no evidence of circulating blasts. His repeat bone marrow biopsy revealed normocellular with persistent myelodysplasia, Grade 1 myelofibrosis, and cytogenetics 46, XY t(2; 11) in 100%. The diagnostic bone marrow analysis showed Grade 2 myelofibrosis.

Given acute hepatitis, acute renal failure, and prolonged cytopenias, he was not felt to be good candidate for continuation of Azacitidine. Given his worsening cytopenias, low dose lenalidomide 5 mg PO every other day was initiated in Dec 2013 and then stopped for prolonged cytopenia. Its use was off-label, given the patient did not have del (5q). In Feb 2014, repeat bone marrow biopsy for declining counts was performed (WBC 2.7×10^9/L, hemoglobin 12.3 g/dL and platelets 117,000 per microliter) which showed no change when compared to October 2012. He was evaluated at Dartmouth Hitchcock Medical Center for allogenic stem cell transplantation (alloHSCT) and had a 10/10 donor (sister) and, however, considered ineligible due to comorbidities of coronary artery disease and unstable angina. He remained on active surveillance until August 2018 when he became transfusion-dependent. He was on almost twice weekly transfusions through the VA. Bone marrow biopsy in August 2018 showed myelodysplastic syndrome: refractory cytopenia with multilineage dysplasia. On Novemeber 28, 2018, the patient was started on single-agent Venetoclax 100 mg daily. The use of Venetoclax was off-label and obtained through the compassionate use program through the VA.

After approximately one month of 100 mg Venetoclax monotherapy, he experienced no side effects and, however, remained neutropenic and required two packed red blood cell transfusions secondary to anemia. The dose of Venetoclax was increased to 200 mg daily. The twice weekly transfusions through the VA were stopped in January 2019 and the patient is monitored via Complete Blood Count (CBC) with differential and Basic Metabolic Panel (BMP). According to his most recent appointment with Hematology on January 15, 2020, he has been transfusion-independent for twelve months. The maximum cell counts since transfusion independence was achieved as follows: white blood cell count of 3.07×10^9/L, red blood cell count of 4.53, hemoglobin of 16 g/dL, and platelet count of 215,000 per microliter (Figures 1–3) His red blood cell count, hemoglobin and platelet counts are stable. No bone marrow analysis was performed after treatment with Venetoclax as the counts were improved. The patient continues to feel very well with no side effects from therapy. He remains intermittently neutropenic and, however, has not had any problems with infection.

3. Discussion

Hypomethylating agents are the standard treatment for myelodysplastic syndrome in the United States; however, in Europe and many countries outside the US, they are only standard of care for high-risk MDS. HMAs have been shown to prolong survival, but responses are usually transient and only 40–50% of patients respond to therapy [10]. Overall survival for patients that have lost response to HMAs is very poor at 4.3 months for high-risk MDS and 14 months for low-risk MDS [10]. MDS patients that relapse or become refractory to HMA have poor outcomes. AlloSCT is the only treatment with curative potential and, however, is associated with significant mortality, toxicity, and higher risk of relapse in patients with MDS in the context of HMA failure [11]. Currently, there are no approved standard of care options for patients with MDS that have failed initial HMAs and have contraindications to alloHSCT.

Venetoclax, a potent highly selective BCL-2 inhibitor, has been studied as a monotherapy or in combination with HMAs in MDS and AML patients. Venetoclax as a monotherapy for relapsed or refractory AML has demonstrated 19% overall response rate in heavily pretreated patients [12]. Recently, due to a phase Ib study (ClinicalTrials.gov identifier: NCT02203773), the FDA approved Venetoclax with HMAs for elderly patients (>65 years) with treatment naïve AML ineligible for chemotherapy. As a treatment for MDS,

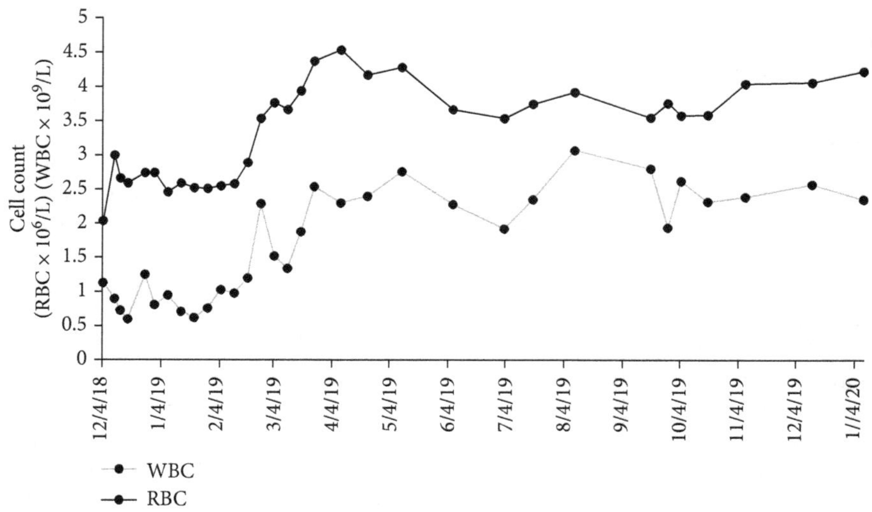

Figure 1: Red blood cell and white blood cell count recorded during Venetoclax monotherapy treatment from December 2018 to January 2020. The treatment initially began on November 28, 2018 at 100 mg and after one month was increased to 200 mg.

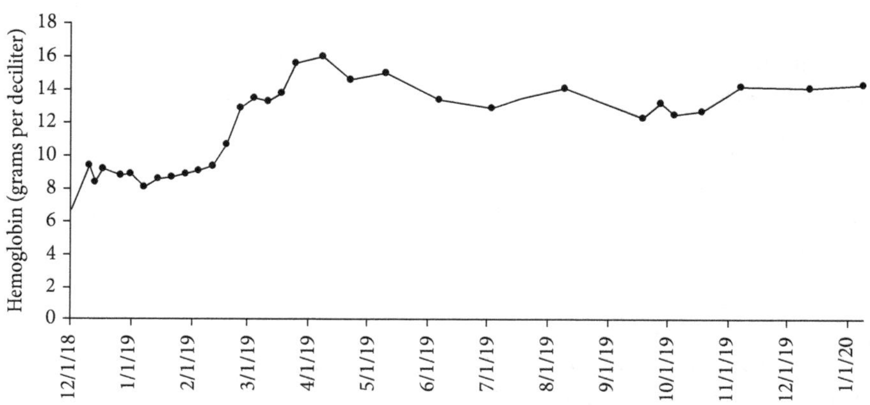

Figure 2: Hemoglobin recorded during Venetoclax monotherapy treatment from December 2018 to January 2020. The treatment initially began on November 28, 2018 at 100 mg and after one month was increased to 200 mg.

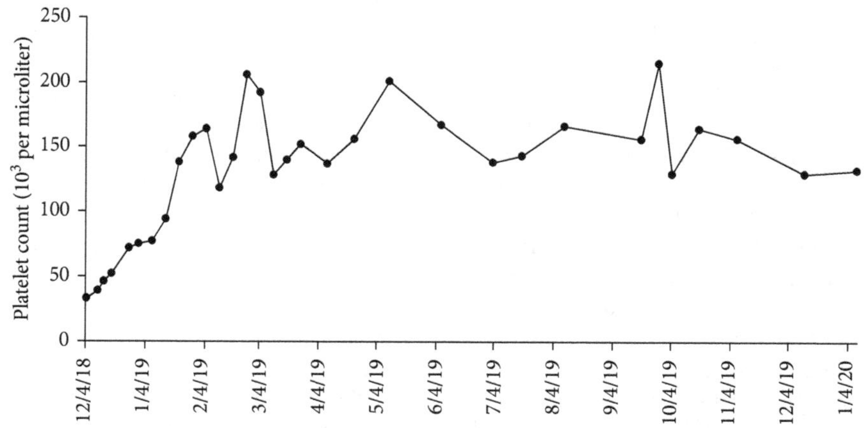

Figure 3: Platelet count recorded during Venetoclax monotherapy treatment from December 2018 to January 2020. The treatment initially began on November 28, 2018 at 100 mg and after one month was increased to 200 mg.

there is currently an ongoing Phase 1b, open-label, multi-center study evaluating the safety and pharmacokinetics as a monotherapy or in combination with hypomethylating agents for the treatment of relapsed/refractory myelodysplastic syndrome with an estimated completion date of August 2020 (ClinicalTrials.gov identifier: NCT02966782).

A recently accepted abstract to the American Society of Hematology (ASH) 2019 Annual meeting presented preliminary results demonstrating that venetoclax in combination with HMAs led to high rates of marrow remission (55%) and hematologic improvement (38%) in a very high-risk and heavily treated MDS population after performing a retrospective review [13].

In this case, a patient with myelodysplastic syndrome refractory to current standard of care treatments with contraindications to alloSCT was treated with Venetoclax as the sole agent. After three months of treatment, the patient became transfusion independent. As of June 2019, he has not required further transfusions, however, remains mildly neutropenic. The development of new therapeutic strategies for MDS refractory to HMAs is an important avenue of research and is being extensively studied in clinical trials. Our case aims to demonstrate the feasibility of Venetoclax monotherapy for refractory MDS in hopes that in conjunction with the results of current and future clinical trials will become a standard of care option for these patients.

Disclosure

This case was presented at the Northern New England Clinical Oncology Society Annual Meeting on October 19, 2019, in Rockport, Maine.

References

[1] N. Gangat, M. M. Patnaik, and A. Tefferi, "Myelodysplastic syndromes: contemporary review and how to treat," *American Journal of Hematology*, vol. 91, no. 1, pp. 76–89, 2016.

[2] M. A. Sekeres, "The epidemiology of myelodysplastic syndromes," *Hematology/Oncology Clinics of North America*, vol. 24, no. 2, pp. 287–294, 2010.

[3] S. J. Corey, M. D. Minden, D. L. Barber, H. Kantarjian, J. C. Y. Wang, and A. D. Schimmer, "Myelodysplastic syndromes: the complexity of stem-cell diseases," *Nature Reviews Cancer*, vol. 7, no. 2, pp. 118–129, 2007.

[4] P. L. Greenberg, H. Tuechler, J. Schanz et al., "Revised international prognostic scoring system for myelodysplastic syndromes," *Blood*, vol. 120, no. 12, pp. 2454–2465, 2012.

[5] P. Fenaux, G. J. Mufti, E. Hellstrom-Lindberg et al., "Efficacy of azacitidine compared with that of conventional care regimens in the treatment of higher-risk myelodysplastic syndromes: a randomised, open-label, phase III study," *The Lancet Oncology*, vol. 10, no. 3, pp. 223–232, 2009.

[6] H. Kantarjian, J.-P. J. Issa, C. S. Rosenfeld et al., "Decitabine improves patient outcomes in myelodysplastic syndromes: results of a phase III randomized study," *Cancer*, vol. 106, no. 8, pp. 1794–1803, 2006.

[7] A. List, S. Kurtin, D. J. Roe et al., "Efficacy of lenalidomide in myelodysplastic syndromes," *New England Journal of Medicine*, vol. 352, no. 6, pp. 549–557, 2005.

[8] S. Jilg, V. Reidel, C. Müller-Thomas et al., "Blockade of BCL-2 proteins efficiently induces apoptosis in progenitor cells of high-risk myelodysplastic syndromes patients," *Leukemia*, vol. 30, no. 1, pp. 112–123, 2016.

[9] V. Reidel, J. Kauschinger, R. T. Hauch et al., "Selective inhibition of BCL-2 is a promising target in patients with high-risk myelodysplastic syndromes and adverse mutational profle," *Oncotarget*, vol. 9, no. 25, pp. 17270–17281, 2018.

[10] E. Jabbour, G. Garcia-Manero, N. Batty et al., "Outcome of patients with myelodysplastic syndrome after failure of decitabine therapy," *Cancer*, vol. 116, no. 16, pp. 3830–3834, 2010.

[11] M. Festuccia, K. Baker, T. A. Gooley, B. M. Sandmaier, H. J. Deeg, and B. L. Scott, "Hematopoietic cell transplantation in myelodysplastic syndromes after treatment with hypomethylating agents," *Biology of Blood and Marrow Transplantation*, vol. 23, no. 9, pp. 1509–1514, 2017.

[12] M. Konopleva, D. A. Pollyea, J. Potluri et al., "Efficacy and biological correlates of response in a phase II study of venetoclax monotherapy in patients with acute myelogenous leukemia," *Cancer Discovery*, vol. 6, no. 10, pp. 1106–1117, 2016.

[13] B. Ball, C. Famulare, E. M. Stein et al., "4241 combined venetoclax and hypomethylating agent (HMA) therapy induces high response rates in patients with myelodysplastic syndrome including patients previously failing HMA," in *Proceedings of the American Society of Hematology 2019 Annual Meeting*, Orlando, FL, USA, December 2019.

Multiple Severe Toxicities of L-Asparaginase and their Innovative Management during Induction Therapy of Acute Lymphoblastic Leukemia in an Adult Patient

Guillaume Beziat ,[1] Suzanne Tavitian,[1] Muriel Picard,[2] Stanislas Faguer,[3] Christian Recher,[1] and Françoise Huguet[1]

[1]*Service d'Hématologie Clinique, Institut Universitaire du Cancer Oncopole, Toulouse, France*
[2]*Réanimation et Soins Intensifs, Institut Universitaire du Cancer Oncopole, Toulouse, France*
[3]*Secteur de Réanimation de l'Unité de Transplantation d'Organes, CHU Rangueil, Toulouse, France*

Correspondence should be addressed to Guillaume Beziat; guillaume.beziat@hotmail.fr

Academic Editor: Sergio Storti

L-asparaginase is a key chemotherapeutic agent in acute lymphoblastic leukemia (ALL). It is also known for multiple and severe specific toxicities, without consensual management. We report the case of a 51-year-old man treated with L-asparaginase for recently diagnosed T-cell ALL. During the treatment, he developed a coma due to multifactorial diffuse cerebral edema, by hepatic encephalopathy, cerebral venous thrombosis, and hyperammonemia, all linked to toxicity of L-asparaginase. Specific and innovative treatments were employed to manage these toxicities: supplementation with L-carnitine, thiamine, and pyridoxine for hepatic toxicity, perfusion of sodium benzoate to decrease ammonemia, and extrahepatic albumin-based dialysis sessions, along with anticoagulation. The patient improved within two weeks and is currently alive 13 months later, in first complete remission, without sequelae, on an alleviated chemotherapy regimen.

1. Introduction

L-asparaginase is known to play a key role in the treatment of childhood and adult acute lymphoblastic leukemia (ALL), particularly during the induction phase [1]. This drug can lead to various and frequent adverse events, resulting in delay or cessation of chemotherapy and in morbimortality. There are no clear recommendations for their management. Age is a major risk factor for L-asparaginase toxicity, and hepatic injury is more common in adults than in children. Here, we illustrate a successful strategy overcoming multiple severe toxicities of L-asparaginase during the induction phase in a T-cell ALL (T-ALL) adult patient.

2. Case Presentation

T-ALL was diagnosed in a 51-year-old man, with no medical history but obesity (BMI = 30.9 kg/m^2). He had mediastinal, pleural, pericardial, bone and pancreatic dissemination, no central nervous system involvement, normal karyotype, and high-risk NRAS mutation associated to FBXW7 and NOTCH1 mutations.

The patient was included in the GRAALL-2014 study (ClinicalTrials.gov Identifier: NCT02617004). After a seven-day prophase of steroids, the induction phase was composed of five drugs and prophylaxis of the central nervous system (CNS) involvement by repeated intrathecal injections (Figure 1). Native L-asparaginase is administered at the dose of 6000 UI/m2 on days 8, 10, 12, 20, 22, and 24. Of note, age-adapted doses of steroids, daunorubicin, and L-asparaginase are delivered to patients aged 46 to 60 years, as compared with patients aged 18 to 45 years, as a result of a high treatment-related mortality rate in the oldest patients in previous trials [2, 3].

According to the protocol, the patient received anticoagulant prophylaxis by unfractionated heparin from day 8 and was supplemented with antithrombin III if below 60%.

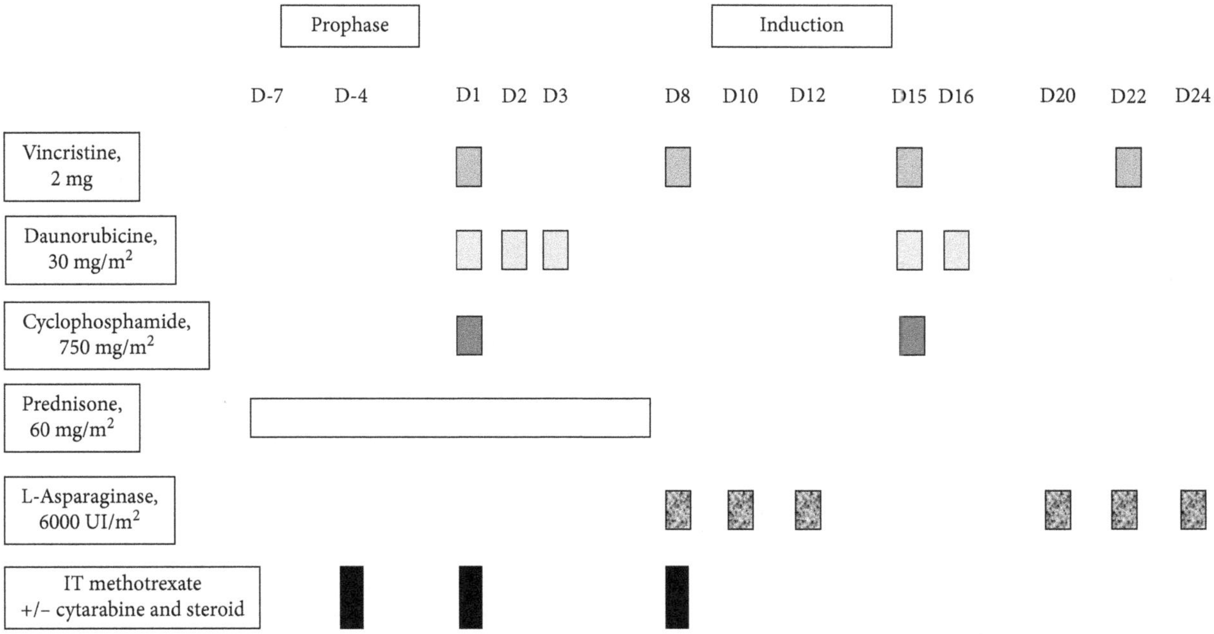

FIGURE 1: Prophase and induction phase of the GRAALL-2014 protocol for patients aged >45 years.

From day 24, cholestasis and conjugated hyperbilirubinemia appeared. Doppler ultrasonography of the liver showed previously unknown steatosis, no focal parenchymal lesion, no vascular lesion, particularly no portal thrombosis, and a discrete dilatation of intrahepatic bile ducts without any visible obstacle.

Autoimmune (antinuclear, ANCA, antimitochondria, anti-LKM1, antismooth muscle, and antiliver cytosol type 1 antibodies) and viral (detection of viremia by polymerase chain reaction of HBV, HCV, CMV, EBV, HSV 1&2, VZV, and HHV8) screenings were negative.

Transcutaneous liver biopsy was performed a few days later, showing marked steatosis and cholestasis, suggestive of drug toxicity attributable to L-asparaginase. It has to be noted that there was no concomittant medication with common potential hepatic toxicity, except for other chemotherapies such as daunorubicine and cyclophosphamide.

L-asparaginase was omitted on day 24, and the patient received supplementations in L-carnitine (4.8 g twice a day), thiamine (100 mg per day), and pyridoxine (250 mg per day) from this date to day 30. Evolution of hepatic parameters between D11 and D30 of the induction phase is described in Figure 2.

From day 28, headaches and nausea appeared, and vigilance progressively decreased.

On day 30, the patient was in a febrile coma, with no sign of focalization. Laboratory results revealed normal white blood cells and platelet counts. Bilirubinemia reached 7 folds, ammonemia reached 2 folds above normal value, prothrombin time was 68%, factor V 86%, and antithrombin III 46%.

Cerebral CT-scan showed cerebral venous thrombosis of the medial longitudinal sinus and diffuse cerebral edema.

This multifactorial diffuse cerebral edema was due to hepatic encephalopathy, hyperammoniemic encephalopathy, and cerebral venous thrombosis, all mechanisms that can be linked to specific toxicities of L-asparaginase.

The patient was admitted to intensive care unit on day 30.

After initiation of usual measures of neurological protection, deep sedation and intubation, curative anticoagulation by unfractionated heparin, and empirical piperacilline-tazobactam for probable aspiration pneumonia, two specific treatments were begun in order to manage hepatic and neurological deficiencies: intravenous sodium benzoate at the dose of 12 g per day was given for five days, and the patient followed daily albumin-based liver dialysis sessions of Molecular Adsorbents Recirculating System (Mars) type for 6 days.

Hepatic biologic parameters stabilized and ammonemia progressively decreased and finally normalized. Evolution of hepatic parameters between D30 and D43 of the induction phase is described in Figure 3; variation of bile acids and ammonemia from D30 to D43 is depicted in Figure 4. Deep sedation was stopped at day 41, and consciousness improved. However, the patient's condition deteriorated at day 42 because of acute subdural hematoma. Surgery was performed, and anticoagulants were stopped. A few days later, colloid epidural patches were performed to treat intracranial hypotension syndrome, related to lumbar punctures for CNS prophylaxis.

Meanwhile, complete remission (CR) was assessed on Day 26.

Currently, the patient is in continuous remission at 13 months, with negative minimum residual disease and normal neurological and hepatic functions. He still follows the GRAALL-2014 protocol and consolidation and delayed intensification phases, with decreased dosage and frequency of chemotherapy administration. Inclusion in the ATRIALL phase 2 substudy of nelarabine-containing

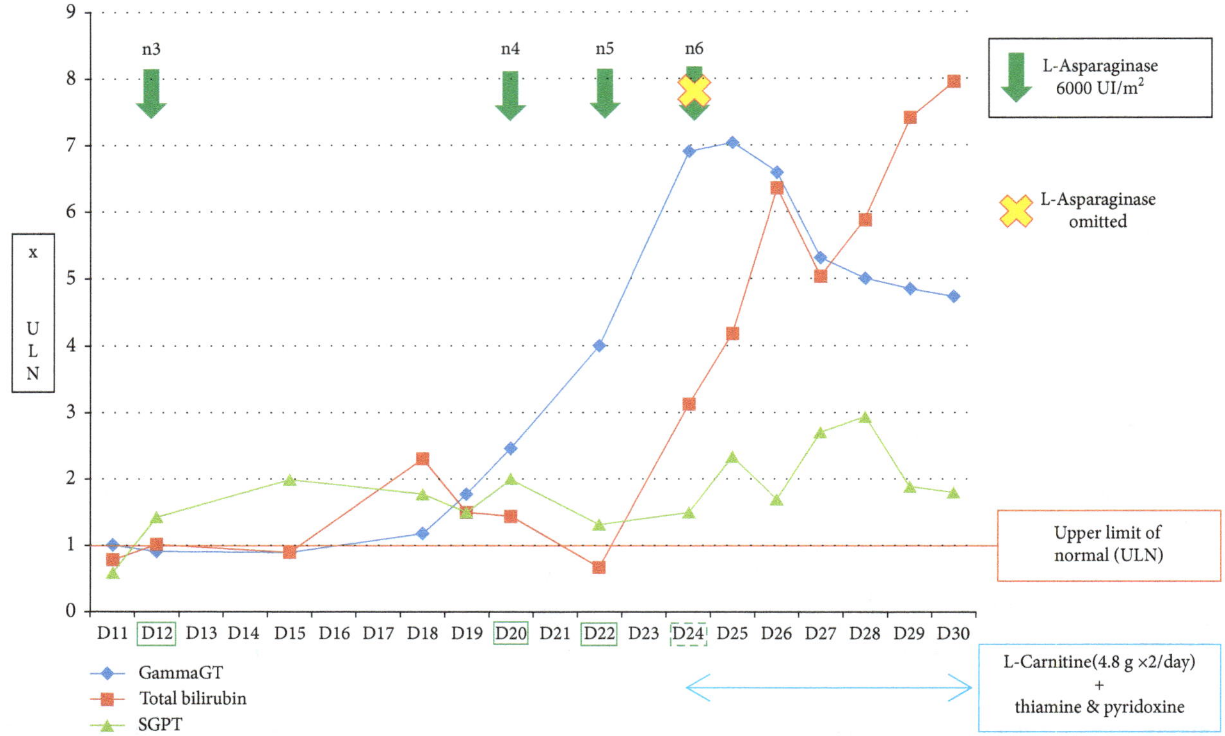

Figure 2: Variation of liver biologic parameters from D11 to D30 of the induction phase.

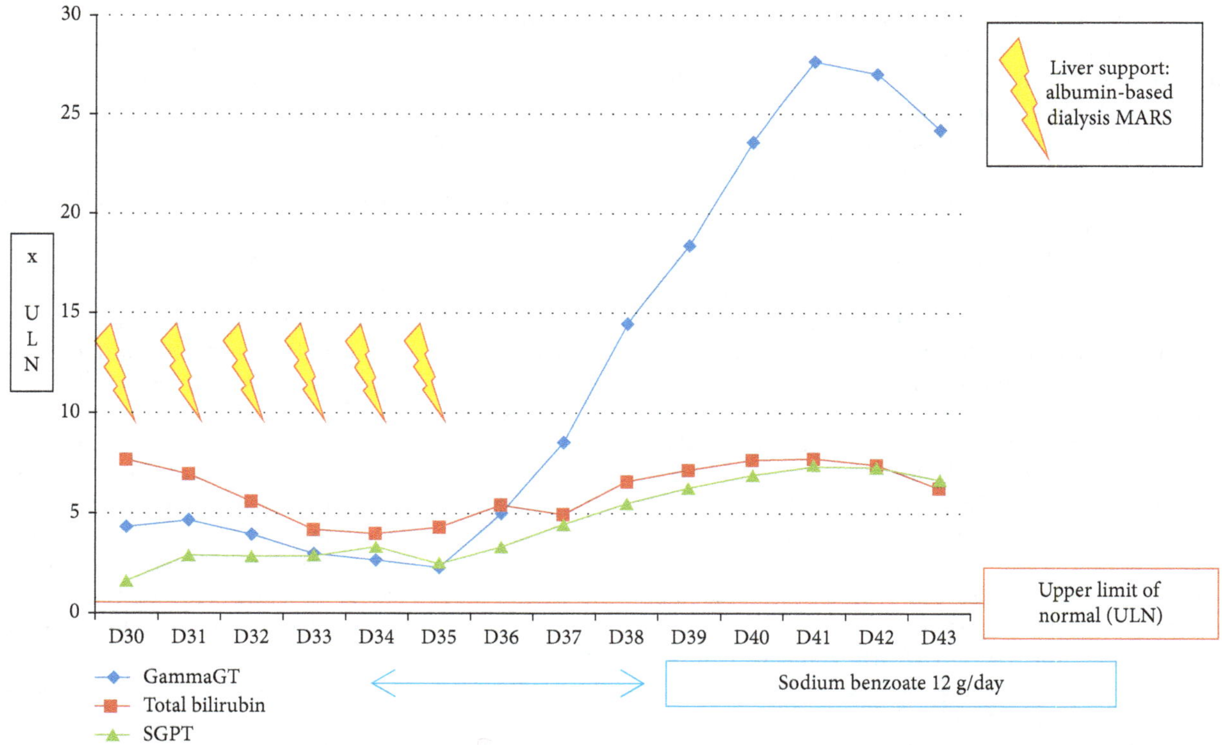

Figure 3: Variation of liver biologic parameters from D30 to D43 of the induction phase.

consolidation [4] in patients with an adverse oncogenetic profile was declined, due to the potential neurotoxicity of the drug. L-asparaginase and intrathecal injections were contraindicated for the rest of the treatment. Indeed, severe intracranial hypotension syndrome was directly linked to intrathecal injections performed during the induction phase, and it had to be treated with colloid epidural patches. Encephalic irradiation treatment has been

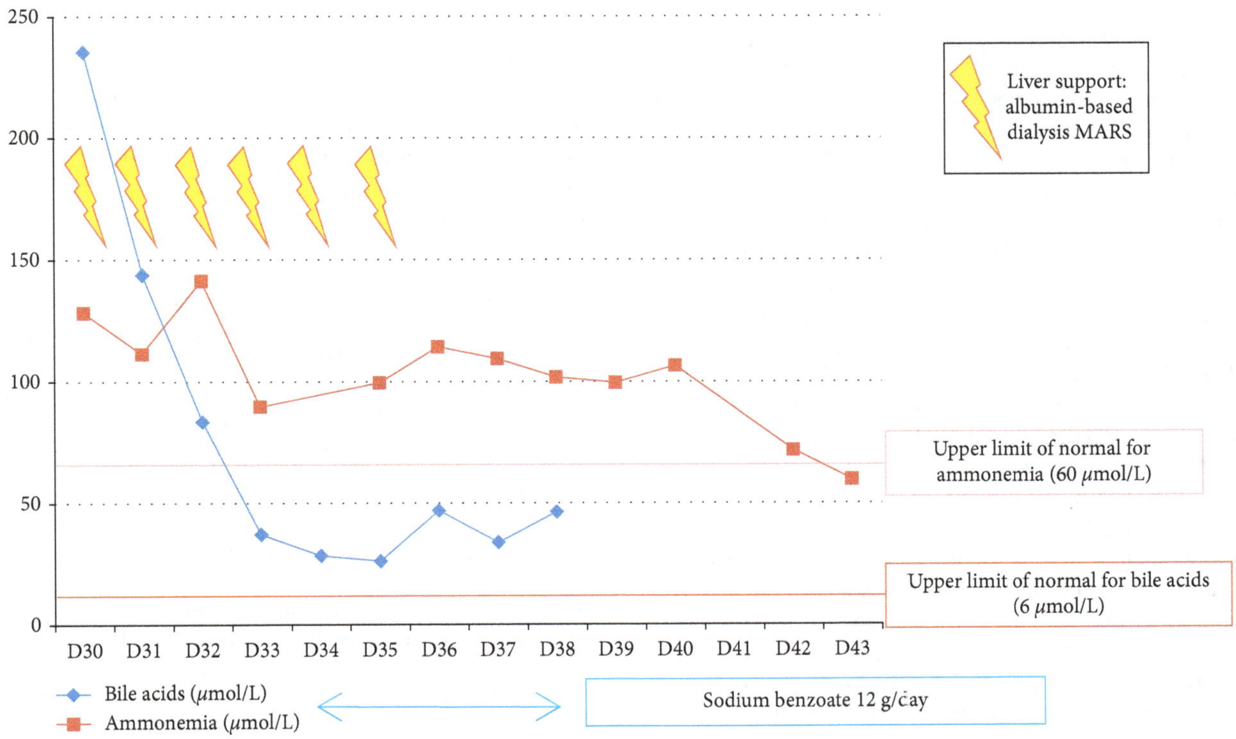

FIGURE 4: Variation of bile acids and ammonemia from D30 to D43 of the induction phase.

performed to ensure CNS prophylaxis. After achievement of negative minimal residual disease at the end of induction and at midconsolidation, allogeneic bone marrow transplantation was not indicated.

3. Discussion

Through this case, multiple severe and specific toxicities of L-asparaginase during induction therapy of ALL are illustrated. They led to neurologic failure linked to diffuse cerebral edema.

L-asparaginase hydrolyses asparagine into L-aspartic acid and ammonia, depriving leukemic cells of this key amino acid they cannot produce by themselves. L-asparaginase has also a weak glutaminase activity. Therefore, by its own mode of action, L-asparaginase produces three neurotoxic agents: ammonia, L-aspartic acid, and glutamic acid. These two amino acids can induce cell death in CNS neurons by excessive stimulation through NMDA (*N*-methyl-D-aspartate) receptor, leading to a major intracellular calcium influx and apoptosis. In our patient, glutamic acid at the onset of coma was normal and probably did not play a key role in the neurologic deficiency. On the contrary, ammonemia was high, due to probably in part to overproduction and in part to L-asparaginase-induced hepatic failure [5]. Sodium benzoate has been given with the aim of lowering ammonemia. Indeed, sodium benzoate may bypass the purification cycle of nitrogen toward alternative metabolic pathways which do not produce ammonia. In our case, ammonemia first stabilized, before normalizing five days after the end of sodium benzoate administration.

The patient presented a grade 3 cholestasis and a grade 3 cytolysis. Hepatic toxicity of L-asparaginase is common, and increased levels of bilirubin have been reported in 30 to 60% of patients receiving it. In most cases, liver toxicity and hyperbilirubinemia are not life-threatening and resolve several weeks after drug discontinuation [6]. As recently described [7], L-asparaginase induces liver injury with short latency and a marked steatosis, probably due to direct inhibition of hepatic protein synthesis caused by asparagine depletion. In our case, cholestasis was prominent, but other abnormalities can occur, such as cytolysis, sinusoidal obstruction syndrome, or fulminant acute hepatitis for example. This toxicity is more frequent and severe in obese patients [8], like our patient. It may be linked to more frequent hepatic steatosis in obese patients at the beginning of the treatment. Obesity may also impair efficacy of L-asparaginase because of the potency of adipocytes to release glutamine, which inhibits cell cytotoxicity induced by the drug [9]. Other risk factors for grade 3-4 hyperbilirubinemia include older age and previous hyperbilirubinemia.

Facing this situation, two therapeutic approaches were proposed. The first one was supplementation in L-carnitine (along with thiamine and pyridoxine). L-carnitine is a derivate of lysine, an amino acid involved in production of energy through fatty acid oxidation. It has shown efficacy in liver protection in case of nonalcoholic steatosis, and preclinical studies in murine models concerning hepatic toxicity of chemotherapy (including L-asparaginase) have shown promising results in reducing hepatic lesions [10]. Different mechanisms of hepatic protection by L-carnitine are known or proposed: reduction of oxygen consumption in steatotic livers and reduction of vascular resistance in the portal system. L-asparaginase induces mitochondrial dysfunction caused by amino acid depletion, resulting in accumulation of unoxidized fatty acids which are directly responsible for hepatic damages. L-carnitine, through its roles in fatty acids metabolism, helps to maintain normal mitochondrial function and cell viability under these abnormal cellular conditions [11]. Few clinical experiments of L-carnitine in management of hepatic toxicity of L-asparaginase exist, showing some cases of improvement of the liver enzyme counts [12], but there is no prospective or comparative study to affirm the efficacy of L-carnitine in this situation. Our second therapy for liver failure was dialysis with molecular adsorbent recirculating system (Mars). This treatment is currently indicated in severe hepatic failure with encephalopathy and often represents a "bridge-to-liver transplantation" in cirrhotic patients in intensive care units [13]. It replaces liver functions of purification of bilirubin, bile acid, ammonia, and several cytokines (nitric oxide, IL6, TNFα etc). In our patient, daily sessions for six days have been performed. Bile acid level decreased rapidly, ammonia more slowly. To our knowledge, it is the first report of the use of Mars to manage hepatic toxicity of chemotherapy. Although the role of each component of this integrative strategy is difficult to assess, sodium benzoate and Mars dialysis seem to have significantly contributed to the favorable biological and clinical outcome, with complete neurological recovery and ultimately successful treatment of ALL.

In this case, the native form of L-asparaginase was used. Other forms of L-asparaginase exist in the induction therapy of ALL, such as pegylated asparaginase. Compared with native L-asparaginase, pegylated form shares the same toxicity profile and does not seem less toxic in adult patients [14, 15]. Indeed, more than a third of the patients face grade 3 to 5 hepatic toxicity with pegylated asparaginase.

Daunorubicin was the main concomitant medication with a common hepatotoxicity. It may have played a role in the liver dysfunction in our patient since this drug is known to have a direct hepatic toxicity. The hepatic injury due to daunorubicin varies in severity from mild, transient, and asymptomatic liver enzyme elevations to acute liver failure due to sinusoidal obstruction syndrome. Nevertheless, the timing, type, and severity of the liver dysfunction indicated that it was more attributable to L-asparaginase.

4. Conclusion

Neurological deficiency under L-asparaginase chemotherapy for ALL may result from intricated toxicities. Albumin-based dialysis (Mars) and supplementation in L-carnitine, thiamine, and pyridoxine should be discussed in case of hepatic encephalopathy, along with sodium benzoate to limit hyperammonemia. We think that this innovative approach is warranted in front of life-threatening L-Asparaginase toxicities.

Acknowledgments

The authors thank Dr. Pierre Broue (Pediatric Hepatology Department) and Dr. Leonardo Astudillo (Internal Medicine Department), Toulouse University Hospital, for their expertise in constitutional metabolic abnormalities and their contribution to the treatment design.

References

[1] T. J. McElwain and R. M. Hardisty, "Remission induction with cytosine arabinoside and L-Asparaginase in acute lymphoblastic leukaemia," *BMJ*, vol. 4, no. 5683, pp. 596–598, 1969.

[2] F. Huguet, T. Leguay, E. Raffoux et al., "Pediatric-inspired therapy in adults with Philadelphia chromosome-negative acute lymphoblastic leukemia: the GRAALL-2003 study," *Journal of Clinical Oncology*, vol. 27, no. 6, pp. 911–918, 2009.

[3] F. Huguet, S. Chevret, T. Leguay et al., "Intensified therapy of acute lymphoblastic leukemia in adults: report of the randomized GRAALL-2005 clinical trial," *Journal of Clinical Oncology*, vol. 36, no. 24, pp. 2514–2523, 2018.

[4] Y. Abaza, H. M. Kantarjian, S. Faderl et al., "Hyper-CVAD plus nelarabine in newly diagnosed adult T-cell acute lymphoblastic leukemia and T-lymphoblastic lymphoma," *American Journal of Hematology*, vol. 93, no. 1, pp. 91–99, 2018.

[5] N. Strickler, S. Balabanov, K. Casauro, U. Schanz, M. G. Manz, and B. Gerber, "Acute central nervous system complications and ammonium levels in adult patients with acute lymphoblastic leukemia receiving l-asparaginase," *Leukemia and Lymphoma*, vol. 59, no. 4, pp. 855–862, 2018.

[6] V. Thu Huynh and S. Bergeron, "Asparaginase toxicities: identification and management in patients with acute lymphoblastic leukemia," *Clinical Journal of Oncology Nursing*, vol. 21, no. 5, pp. E248–E259, 2017.

[7] N. Kamal, for the Drug-Induced Liver Injury Network, C. Koh, N. Samala, R. J. Fontana, A. Stolz et al., "Asparaginase-induced hepatotoxicity: rapid development of cholestasis and hepatic steatosis," *Hepatology International*, vol. 13, no. 5, pp. 641–648, 2019.

[8] I. A. Nikonorova, R. J. T. Al-Baghdadi, E. T. Mirek et al., "Obesity challenges the hepatoprotective function of the integrated stress response to asparaginase exposure in mice," *Journal of Biological Chemistry*, vol. 292, no. 16, pp. 6786–6798, 2017.

[9] E. A. Ehsanipour, X. Sheng, J. W. Behan et al., "Adipocytes cause leukemia cell resistance to L-asparaginase via release of glutamine," *Cancer Research*, vol. 73, no. 10, pp. 2998–3006, 2013.

[10] A. Roesmann, M. Afify, J. Panse, A. Eisert, J. Steitz, and R. H. Tolba, "L-carnitine ameliorates L-asparaginase-induced acute liver toxicity in steatotic rat livers," *Chemotherapy*, vol. 59, no. 3, pp. 167–175, 2013.

[11] R. R. Schulte, M. V. Madiwale, A. Flower et al., "Levocarnitine for asparaginase-induced hepatic injury: a multi-institutional case series and review of the literature," *Leukemia and Lymphoma*, vol. 59, no. 10, pp. 2360–2368, 2018.

[12] R. Alshiekh-Nasany and D. Douer, "L-carnitine for treatment of pegasparaginase-induced hepatotoxicity," *Acta Haematologica*, vol. 135, no. 4, pp. 208–210, 2016.

[13] C. Sponholz, K. Matthes, D. Rupp et al., "Molecular adsorbent recirculating system and single-pass albumin dialysis in liver failure—a prospective, randomised crossover study," *Critical Care*, vol. 20, no. 1, 2015.

[14] M. Hunault-Berger, T. Leguay, F. Huguet et al., "A Phase 2 study of L-asparaginase encapsulated in erythrocytes in elderly patients with Philadelphia chromosome negative acute lymphoblastic leukemia: the GRASPALL/GRAALL-SA2-2008 study," *American Journal of Hematology*, vol. 90, no. 9, pp. 811–818, 2015.

[15] B. Patel, A. A. Kirkwood, A. Dey et al., "Pegylated-asparaginase during induction therapy for adult acute lymphoblastic leukaemia: toxicity data from the UKALL14 trial," *Leukemia*, vol. 31, no. 1, pp. 58–64, 2017.

40

Hodgkin Lymphoma Mimicking Inflammatory Breast Carcinoma: A Rare Case with Diagnostic Challenge and Novel Treatment

Eleni Thodou,[1] **Maria Befani**,[2] **George Triantafyllidis**,[3] **Theodosia Choreftaki**,[4] **George Kanellis**,[5] **and Nikolaos Giannakoulas**[6]

[1]*Department of Pathology, Medical School, University of Thessaly, Viopolis, 41500 Larisa, Greece*
[2]*Hematology, Private Practice, 61 Koumoundourou Str., 38221 Volos, Greece*
[3]*Radiology, Private Practice, 29 Glavani Str., 38221 Volos, Greece*
[4]*Department of Pathology, "G. Genimmatas", Athens General Hospital, 154 Mesogeion Ave., 11527 Athens, Greece*
[5]*Department of Hematopathology, "Evangelismos", General Hospital, 45 Ypsilantou Str., 10676 Athens, Greece*
[6]*Department of Hematology, Medical School, University of Thessaly, Viopolis, 41500 Larisa, Greece*

Correspondence should be addressed to Eleni Thodou; eleni.thodou@gmail.com

Academic Editor: Sylvain Choquet

Extranodal Hodgkin lymphoma involving the breast is infrequent. Most cases reported in the literature were diagnosed by histology after lumpectomy. We present a Hodgkin lymphoma mimicking inflammatory breast carcinoma in a 57-year-old woman. The diagnosis was performed by fine-needle aspiration (FNA) of the breast lesion and the axillary lymph nodes with rapid on-site evaluation followed by immunocytochemistry, and it was confirmed by histology. The patient after first-line chemotherapy developed relapse/refractory disease. Salvage chemotherapy regimens were applied with poor results and severe toxicity. Total remission was achieved with monotherapy of brentuximab vedotin, a novel anti-CD30-targeted antibody drug conjugate. This is a unique case of breast HL with misleading clinical presentation initially diagnosed by cytology. FNA as a minimally invasive diagnostic tool was crucial in avoiding unnecessary breast surgery and further delay of chemotherapy. It is also the first report highlighting the importance of this novel immunotherapy in the management of refractory Hodgkin lymphoma with breast involvement.

1. Introduction

Breast lymphomas account for less than 0.5% of all malignant breast tumors [1]. Particularly, in a large multicenter study, the prevalence of breast lymphoma has been defined at 1.6% among all cases with non-Hodgkin Lymphoma (NHL). Furthermore, primary breast lymphoma represents a small proportion of extranodal lymphomas ranging from 0.85% to 2.2% [2]. Primary breast lymphomas are usually NHL, in specific diffuse B large cell, Burkitt lymphoma, T anaplastic cell lymphoma, and mucosa-associated lymphoid tissue lymphoma [3].

Breast is an uncommon site of extranodal Hodgkin lymphoma (HL). Given that only sporadic cases of breast HL have been reported in the literature, the exact prevalence, either as a primary tumor or in the process of disseminated or recurrent disease, cannot be defined [4, 5].

The diagnosis of lymphomas is traditionally established by histology on a surgical biopsy material with an appropriate panel of immunostains. However, in the last decade, FNA has reached an important and definite role in the diagnosis of lymphomas and reactive lesions in both lymph nodes and extranodal sites with the use of ancillary techniques such as flow cytometry and immunocytochemistry. FNA assisted by flow cytometry can further contribute significantly in the subclassification of NHL [6]. Similarly, in lymphoid breast lesions, the combination of FNA cytology with these techniques can provide specific diagnoses, distinguishing reactive from neoplastic processes, with a sensitivity of 90% and specificity of 100%. Therefore, it simplifies patients' management preventing unnecessary biopsies [7]. Furthermore, the correct management of breast seroma cytological samples is critical for the diagnosis of implant-associated anaplastic large-cell lymphoma [8].

We report a unique case of HL, clinically presenting as inflammatory breast carcinoma diagnosed by FNA with rapid on-site evaluation (ROSE) and immunocytochemistry. This diagnostic procedure proved to be crucial for the patient's management for it prevented an unnecessary breast surgery and further delay of chemotherapy. It is also the first case of Hodgkin lymphoma with breast involvement and refractory disease, with an otherwise poor prognosis, successfully treated with monotherapy of brentuximab vedotin, the novel CD30-targeted immunotherapy.

2. Case Presentation

A 57-year-old woman presented with signs of inflammation, hardness, and lymphedema, with orange peel appearance of the skin of the right breast. A palpable mass of the right axilla preceded the breast lesion. It was gradually enlarging during a three-month period and did not respond to treatment with antibiotics. A mammography, performed when the axillary mass, was first observed, and it did not detect any abnormality in the breast, except of an enlarged lymph node in the axilla (Figure 1). Her medical history included hysterectomy for a mucinous borderline tumor of the right ovary four years ago.

Initially, a clinical diagnosis of inflammatory breast carcinoma was made and an FNA of the axillary lymph nodes was first attempted elsewhere. The cytology reported bloody material with few lymphoid cells and scant atypical epithelial cells, suspicious for malignancy. Immunocytochemistry was not performed. Following blind core biopsies of the breast did not reveal malignancy. The patient refused further investigation. A month later, she complained for further enlargement of the axillary mass and mild fever. At that time, clinical examination also showed palpable ipsilateral supraclavicular lymph nodes in the right region. A subsequent computed tomography (CT) scan confirmed the enlargement of axillary and supraclavicular lymph nodes. In addition, CT revealed a lesion with ill-defined border in the right breast considered suspicious for primary malignancy, skin thickening, and lymphedema (Figure 2). Her biochemical and full blood tests were within normal limits but showed an elevated red blood cell precipitation of 107 mm/h. The patient refused surgical biopsy of the axillary lymph node block; thus, she was referred to us for repeated FNA.

By ultrasound (US), we observed in the right breast a hypoechoic, partially ill-defined lesion with mild posterior acoustic enhancement, measuring 8 mm in its maximal diameter. It was classified as BIRADS 4 (Figure 3).

US-guided FNA targeted the breast lesion and the axillary lymph node block consecutively. FNA was performed with rapid on-site evaluation (ROSE) of the specimens using Hemacolor rapid staining (Merck, Darmstadt, Germany). The remaining slides were evaluated after Papanicolaou stain. The cytomorphology of the breast and axillary lesions was identical. Scattered large neoplastic lymphoid cells were observed among a reactive population of small lymphocytes and eosinophils. The neoplastic cells showed abundant faint basophilic cytoplasm and large nuclei with prominent nucleolus. A substantial number of them were binucleated with typical features of Reed–Sternberg cells and few were multinucleated. Immunostains were performed on some of the Hemacolor-stained slides. The neoplastic cells were immunopositive for CD30 and CD15 and negative for LCA. The latter was immunoreactive only in the small lymphocytes. Pan-keratin was negative. A nonepithelial neoplasm, consistent with HL, was reported. Following the unexpected cytological diagnosis, surgical biopsy of the axillary lymph node block was performed. A tissue specimen of aprox. 1.1 cm was forwarded for histology. Classical HL of nodular sclerosis subtype was reported, confirming the cytological diagnosis. The Hodgkin/Reed–Sternberg cells, in addition to CD30 and CD15 immunoreactivity, were positive for MUM1 and CD4 (approx. 50%). PAX5, CD20, CD3, and CD79a were negative. The small lymphocytes consisted of a mixed T (CD3 positive) and B (CD20 positive) population. Small CD4 positive lymphocytes focally formed rosettes around Hodgkin cells (Figure 4).

The disease stage was IV B with extranodal right breast involvement. The patient received ABVD regimen (doxorubicin, bleomycin, vinblastine, and dacarbazine). After two full cycles, she showed a satisfactory (more than 50%) reduction of the lymph nodes mass on CT. One month before completion of all ABVD cycles, the axillary mass was palpable again. She was restaged with CT, which showed a remarkable increase of the lymph nodes block, and a PET-CT showed increased fluorodeoxyglucose (FDG) uptake in the right axillary and breast region. The patient was considered primary refractory HL, and salvage chemotherapy with DHAP regimen (dexamethasone, cisplatin, and cytarabine) was given. After one cycle of DHAP with mild toxicity (grade II no febrile neutropenia), a new CT was performed to check for chemosensitivity in order to proceed to autologous transplantation consolidation. The CT scan showed no improvement, and a cycle of DICE (dexamethasone, ifosfamide, cisplatin, and etoposide) in combination with brentuximab vedotin (BV), a newly introduced anti-CD30 antibody-drug conjugate, was decided. Grade IV hematological toxicity was observed, and the patient was hospitalized due to febrile neutropenia, anemia, and pyelonephritis. After hospitalization for a week with fluid and antibiotics intake, granulocyte colony stimulating factor (GCSF) administration, and red blood cell and platelet transfusions, she gradually improved and was discharged from the hospital. The patient denied any further aggressive chemotherapy. The treatment continued with BV monotherapy at a dose of 1.8 mg/kg every three weeks. After four infusions, a CT scan showed total remission of lymphadenopathy, the breast lesion disappeared, and lymphedema diminished substantially. The above findings were also confirmed with a negative PET CT scan. The patient continued receiving nine more cycles of BV every three weeks. Therapy was completed after thirteen infusions in total. Repeated annual restaging with CT scan revealed no signs of

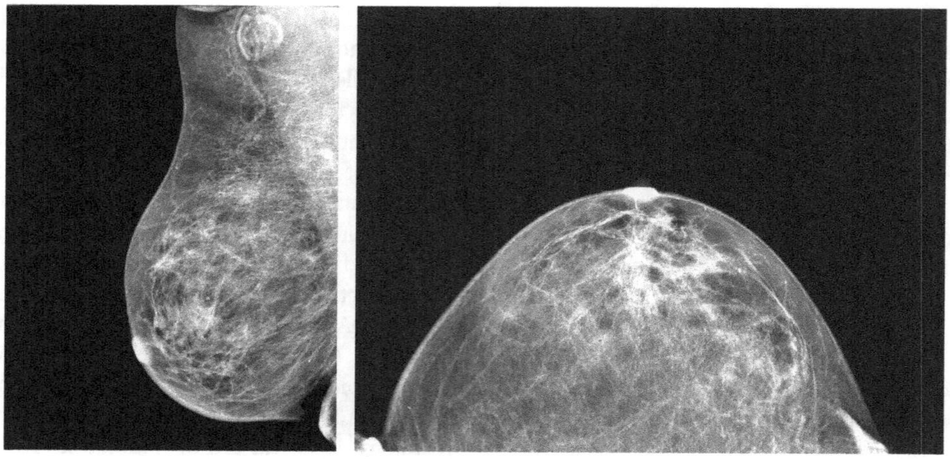

FIGURE 1: Mammography showing enlarged lymph node in the right axilla. No specific abnormalities were detected in the breast.

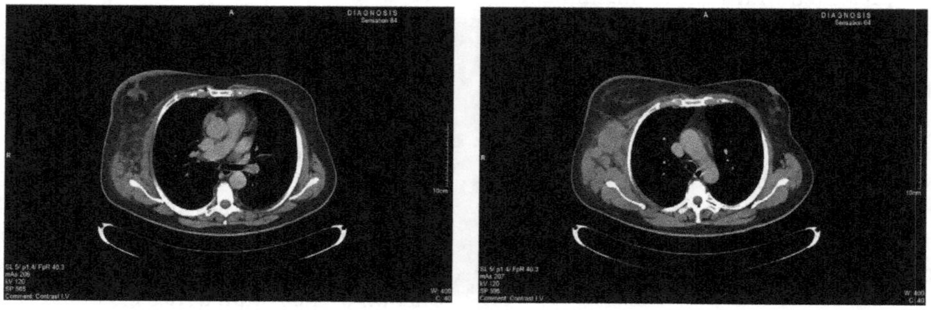

(a) (b)

FIGURE 2: CT revealing breast lesion with partially ill defined borders, thickening of the breast skin, and lymphedema (a) and enlarged axillary lymph nodes (b).

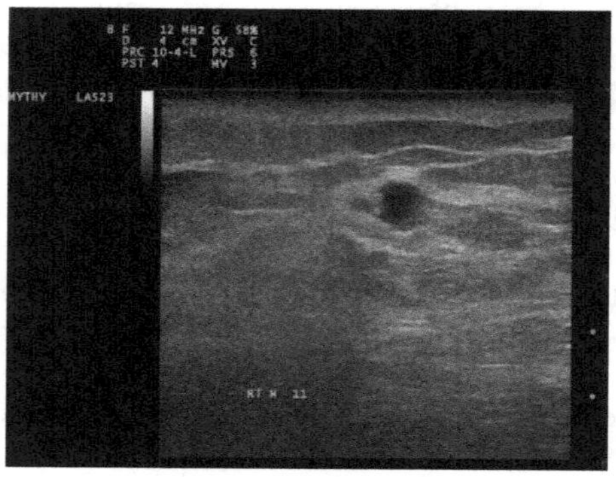

FIGURE 3: US revealing a small hypoechoic breast lesion with partially ill-defined borders and mild posterior acoustic enhancement.

relapse. After two and a half years of follow-up, the patient is free of disease, in good health, and the breast has turned to normal.

3. Discussion

Classic HL is a monoclonal neoplasm composed of Hodgkin/Reed–Sternberg cells admixed with a heterogeneous population of nonneoplastic immune cells usually arising in the lymph nodes [9]. Extranodal manifestation of Hodgkin lymphoma is less frequent than non-Hodgkin lymphoma. It can involve several organs mimicking other neoplasms or infectious processes [10]. Breast is an uncommon site affected by HL. According to a recent review, 19 cases of primary HL of the breast have been reported since the first description by Kueckens in 1928 [4, 11]. However, after a better search of the literature, we retrieved 5 additional cases [12–16]. Breast involvement in the process of disseminated or recurrent Hodgkin lymphoma has also been reported [5, 17].

Breast lymphoma presents as a palpable tumor with or without axillary lymph node involvement. Mammographic findings are not pathognomonic. In the majority

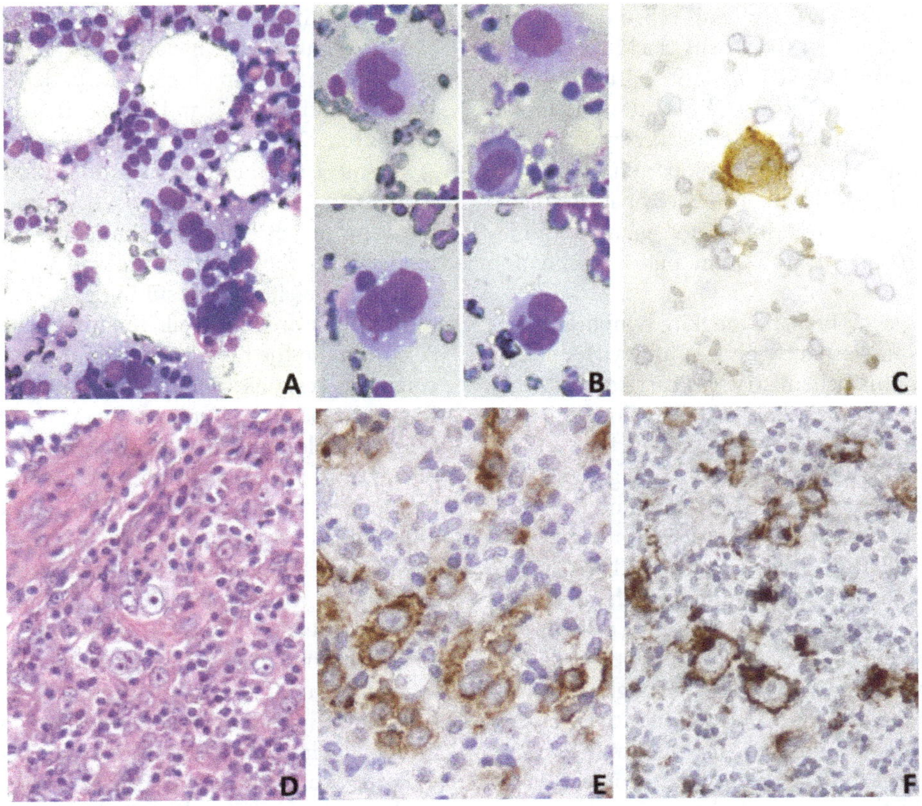

FIGURE 4: Cytology: (a) breast FNA showing scattered Reed–Sternberg and Hodgkin cells admixed with lymphocytes and eosinophils (Hemacolor stain, 20X); (b) Reed–Sternberg and Hodgkin cell variants (Hemacolor stain, 40X); (c) CD30 immunoreactive Hodgkin cell in cytology smear (ABC, 40X). Histology: (d) lymph node specimen showing Reed–Sternberg and Hodgkin cells in a classic milieu (H & E stain, 25X); (e) CD30 immunoreactive Reed–Sternberg and Hodgkin cells; typical Golgi pattern of chromogen distribution (25X); (f) Reed–Sternberg and Hodgkin cells with Golgi pattern immunopositive for CD15 (25X).

of cases, breast lymphomas appear as round or irregular masses with well- or ill-defined margins, showing no calcifications or sclerosis. In a smaller proportion, they can appear as architectural distortion or as a combination of a mass with architectural distortion pattern. Rarely, mammography shows no abnormalities [2, 18]. In the present case, mammography did not show any specific findings in the breast except of the enlarged axillary lymph node.

US in breast lymphomas demonstrates mostly oval or round lesions with distinct or microlobular margins, hypoechoic or with a mixed echo pattern, and posterior acoustic enhancement. Some cases, significantly hypoechoic or anechoic lesions closely, mimick cysts [2]. However, in a recent multicentre study of a large number of hematopoetic malignancies involving the breast, most lesions show irregular shape, complex echo pattern, indistinct margins, and various posterior acoustic phenomena [18]. In general agreement, US has a higher sensitivity in detecting hematological malignancy of the breast compared to mammography [2, 18]. In our case, the US features are in agreement with the literature [2].

On CT, the findings are not specific overlapping with other entities as cysts, fibroadenomas, and malignant tumors [2]. In the present case, the identified breast lesion, although not specific, it was considered suspicious for primary malignancy.

Although imaging studies in cases of breast lymphoma can suggest malignancy, they are not helpful in differentiating lymphoma from carcinoma. Therefore, accurate diagnosis is based on biopsy [19].

Breast lymphoma can rarely present with extended lymphedema, stimulating inflammatory breast carcinoma. To the best of our knowledge, three cases of HL with breast inflammatory presentation have been reported so far [14, 15, 20]. Our case shows similarities with the previous reports regarding the clinical appearance. However, it is unique, because unlike these cases which were diagnosed by histology, the initial diagnosis was achieved by FNA further confirmed by histology.

The role of cytology in the diagnosis of breast NHL is well established [7, 21]. HL can also be diagnosed reliably by cytology and immunocytochemistry performed on cytospin or cell block material [6]. However, most of the breast Hodgkin lymphoma cases reported in the literature have been diagnosed by histology of the surgical specimen after lumpectomy or on core needle biopsy material.

This fact is related to the rarity of the entity and to the limited use of FNA as a diagnostic approach of breast lesions in routine practice lately. A recent review states that breast HL cannot be diagnosed by FNA. This can be attributed mainly to inadequate or inconclusive material, particularly in cases of nodular sclerosis with abundant collagenous stroma [4]. In another case, cytology was reported as suspicious for malignancy [17]. Hodgkin cells may simulate carcinoma, in paucicellular specimens lacking the full spectrum of the lymphoid cell population. That was the reason for misdiagnosis in the first FNA attempt in our patient, in which no immunostains for keratin or other markers were performed. Even in core biopsy, in the absence of typical Reed–Sternberg cells, the presence of accumulated epithelioid histiocytes and multinucleated giant cells may lead to erroneous report of granulomatous inflammation [20].

In only two cases of breast Hodgkin lymphoma, the initial diagnosis was suggested by FNA cytology [13, 22]. In one of them, immunohistochemistry was carried out on the cell block. In both, the final diagnosis was confirmed by histology [22]. In our case, ROSE procedure during the FNA proved to be a valuable diagnostic tool. Using ROSE, we were able to ascertain the specimen sufficiency and recognize the lymphomatous nature of the breast lesion, leading to direct FNA of the axillary lymph node mass. Therefore, we obtained adequate material for immunocytochemistry. In our case, the presence of typical Reed–Sternberg cells was the diagnostic clue. This is in concordance with the two previous reports [13, 22]. Immunopositivity of the Hodgkin cells for CD30 and CD15 in conjunction with LCA negativity further sustained the diagnosis. In addition, negative immunostain for pankeratin excluded the diagnosis of carcinoma. Keratin markers are useful in the differential diagnosis between HL and metastatic carcinoma in lymph node FNA. Furthermore, keratin positivity in a breast FNA showing large malignant cells among abundant lymphoid population can confirm the diagnosis of medullary carcinoma, which may pause diagnostic difficulties. Histological study, which followed, confirmed the unexpected cytological diagnosis, reporting a classical HL of nodular sclerosis subtype, commonly observed involving the breast [4, 5, 12, 14, 15, 17, 20, 22].

Our case represents a successful example of cytological diagnosis of Hodgkin lymphoma in breast, despite the misleading clinical presentation. This minimally invasive diagnostic approach proved crucial for avoiding an unnecessary major breast surgery, which would further delay chemotherapy. Instead, the patient underwent minor lymph node biopsy for histology.

The therapeutic management of our patient was also challenging because she developed relapsed/refractory disease, not responding to salvage chemotherapy regimens, and she experienced severe side effects. BV is a novel therapeutic agent for CD30-positive lymphomas, the first immunotherapy that was approved by the United States Food and Drug Administration (US FDA) for the treatment of Hodgkin lymphoma. The drug consists of a tubulin toxin (monomethyl auristatin E) conjugated on anti-CD30 monoclonal antibody, which binds to the CD30-expressing neoplastic cells. The conjugate inhibits microtubule formation prohibiting mitosis, leading to cell cycle arrest and apoptosis [23, 24]. BV is being investigated in the management of relapse/refractory Hodgkin lymphoma as monotherapy or in combination with chemotherapy regimens with promising results [25]. In addition, it has recently been incorporated in the treatment of newly diagnosed HL patients with encouraging results, at least in some patients [26]. Previous studies have also proved the importance of BV as maintenance in high-risk patients after autologous transplantation [27] and as a bridge to allogenic transplantation [28].

In our case, the administration of DICE in combination with BV was discontinued, because of severe toxicity resulting in patient's unwillingness to receive any further intensive chemotherapy. Eventually, monotherapy with BV proved to be effective, resulting in total remission and long-term disease-free survival. The treatment was well tolerated. According to the literature, monotherapy with BV results in complete response in 35% of patients with relapsed/refractory Hodgkin lymphoma, causing minimal side effects [25]. The role of BV has already been established in different settings in the management of patients with HL and is regarded a valuable tool in the treatment of the disease. Therefore, the role of immunohistochemical markers such as CD30, also applied in cytologic material, is of paramount importance for therapy.

In conclusion, Hodgkin lymphoma, although very rare, should be included in the differential diagnosis of breast lesions with inflammatory presentation. FNA assisted by ROSE and immunocytochemistry may serve as a primary minimally invasive procedure for a prompt diagnosis in order to avoid unnecessary surgical management and delay of chemotherapy. In addition, it is the first case in the literature of Hodgkin lymphoma, with breast involvement and refractory disease, with an otherwise poor prognosis, cured with monotherapy of the novel CD30-targeted antibody drug conjugate. This report highlights the key role of the pathologist, not only in the diagnosis but also in the decision for therapy in the new era of precision medicine.

Acknowledgments

This work was supported by funds from the Medical School, University of Thessaly, Larissa, Greece.

References

[1] C. Wiseman and K. T. Liao, "Primary lymphoma of the breast," *Cancer*, vol. 29, no. 6, pp. 1705–1712, 1972.

[2] A. Surov, H. J. Holzhausen, A. Wienke et al., "Primary and secondary breast lymphoma: prevalence, clinical signs and radiological features," *The British Journal of Radiology*, vol. 85, no. 1014, pp. 195–205, 2012.

[3] S. R. Lakhani, I. O. Ellis, S. J. Schnitt et al., *WHO Classification of Tumours of the Breast*, International Agency for Research on Cancer, Lyon, France, 4th edition, 2012.

[4] M. Faenza, A. Ronchi, A. Santoriello et al., "What's new on primary Hodgkin's lymphoma of the breast? A case report and review of the literature," *International Journal of Surgery Case Reports*, vol. 38, pp. 149–153, 2017.

[5] J. M. Meis, J. J. Butler, and B. M. Osborne, "Hodgkin's disease involving the breast and chest wall," *Cancer*, vol. 57, no. 9, pp. 1859–1865, 1986.

[6] P. Zeppa, E. Vigliar, I. Cozzolino et al., "Fine needle aspiration cytology and flow cytometry immunophenotyping of non-Hodgkin lymphoma: can we do better?," *Cytopathology*, vol. 21, no. 5, pp. 300–310, 2010.

[7] E. Vigliar, I. Cozzolino, L. V. S. Fernandez et al., "Fine-needle cytology and flow cytometry assessment of reactive and lymphoproliferative processes of the breast," *Acta Cytologica*, vol. 56, no. 2, pp. 130–138, 2012.

[8] A. Ronchi, M. Montella, V. Argenzio et al., "Diagnosis of anaplastic large cell lymphoma on late peri-implant breast seroma: management of cytological sample by an integrated approach," *Cytopathology*, vol. 29, no. 3, pp. 294–299, 2018.

[9] S. H. Swerdlow, E. Campo, N. L. Harris et al., *WHO Classification of Tumours of Haematopoietic and Lymphoid tissues*, vol. 2, International Agency for Research on Cancer, Lyon, France, 4th edition, 2017.

[10] A. Guermazi, P. Brice, E. de Kerviler et al., "Extranodal Hodgkin disease: spectrum of disease," *Radiographics*, vol. 21, no. 1, pp. 161–179, 2001.

[11] H. Kueckens, "Ein locales lymphogranulom der brustin furm eines mammatumors," *Beiträge zur Pathologie*, vol. 80, pp. 135–137, 1928.

[12] G. C. Raju, N. Jankey, and K. Delpech, "Localized primary extranodal Hodgkin's disease (Hodgkin's lymphoma) of the Breast," *Journal of the Royal Society of Medicine*, vol. 80, no. 4, pp. 247–249, 1987.

[13] P. Karamanakos, J. Ziounas, J. Griniatsos, D. Trafalis, A. Mela, and E. Bastounis, "Primary Hodgkin's disease of the breast," *The Breast*, vol. 10, no. 6, pp. 546–549, 2001.

[14] E. A. Pillemer and N. L. Harris, "Case records of the Massachusetts General Hospital. Weekly clinicopathological exercises. Case16-2000. A 53-year-old woman with swelling of the right breast and bilateral lymphadenopathy," *New England Journal of Medicine*, vol. 342, no. 21, pp. 1590–1597, 2000.

[15] C. Hoimes, M. Selbst, N. Shafi et al., "Hodgkin's lymphoma of the breast," *Journal of Clinical Oncology*, vol. 28, no. 2, pp. 11–13, 2010.

[16] C. Osuji, G. Ahaneku, E. Onwubuya et al., "Hodgkin's lymphoma of the breast," *Journal of Cancer Research and Therapeutics*, vol. 9, no. 3, pp. 526–528, 2013.

[17] H. Shaaban, T. Layne, G. Guron, Y. Modi, and D. Thomas, "Nodular sclerosing Hodgkin's lymphoma with breast involvement: case report and review of the literature," *Journal of Natural Science, Biology and Medicine*, vol. 5, no. 2, pp. 467–469, 2014.

[18] S. Wienbeck, H. J. Meyer, J. Uhlig et al., "Radiological imaging characteristics of intramammary hematological malignancies: results from a German multicenter study," *Scientific Reports*, vol. 7, no. 1, p. 7435, 2017.

[19] S. D. Raj, M. Shurafa, Z. Shah, K. M. Raj, M. D. C. Fishman, and V. M. Dialani, "Primary and Secondary Breast Lymphoma: Clinical, Pathologic, and Multimodality Imaging Review," *Radiographics*, vol. 39, no. 3, pp. 610–625, 2019.

[20] N. O. Zarneascu, A. Ilesiu, A. Procop et al., "A challenging case of primary breast Hodgkin's lymphoma," *Maedica (Buchar)*, vol. 10, no. 1, pp. 44–47, 2015.

[21] S. K. Arora, N. Gupta, R. Srinivasan et al., "Non-Hodgkin's lymphoma presenting as breast masses: a series of 10 cases diagnosed on FNAC," *Diagnostic Cytopathology*, vol. 41, no. 1, pp. 53–59, 2013.

[22] J. Park, M. Rizzo, S. Jackson, S. R. Bates, V. Green, and G. Oprea-Ilies, "Reed-sternberg cells in breast FNA of a patient with left breast mass," *Diagnostic Cytopathology*, vol. 38, no. 9, pp. 663–668, 2010.

[23] C. J. Hoimes, "Antimicrotubule agents in cancer," in *Principles & Practice of Oncology*, V. T. DeVita JR, T. S. Lawrence, and S. A. Rosenberg, Eds., Wolters Kluwer, South Holland, Netherlands, 11th edition, 2019.

[24] A. Alperovich and A. Younes, "Targeting CD30 using brentuximab vedotin in the treatment of Hodgkin lymphoma," *The Cancer Journal*, vol. 22, no. 1, pp. 23–26, 2016.

[25] A. Kallam and J. M. Vose, "Hope after salvage therapy fails: novel agents for relapsed/refractory Hodgkin lymphoma," *Oncology (Williston Park)*, vol. 33, no. 5, pp. 192–198, 2019.

[26] J. M. Connors, W. Jurczak, D. J. Straus et al., "Brentuximab vedotin with chemotherapy for stage III or IV Hodgkin's Lymphoma," *New England Journal of Medicine*, vol. 378, no. 4, pp. 331–344, 2018.

[27] C. H. Moskowitz, A. Nademanee, T. Masszi et al., "Brentuximab vedotin as consolidation therapy after autologous stem-cell transplantation in patients with Hodgkin's lymphoma at risk of relapse or progression (AETHERA): a randomised, double-blind, placebo-controlled, phase 3 trial," *The Lancet*, vol. 385, no. 9980, pp. 1853–1862, 2015.

[28] S. Garciaz, D. Coso, F. Peyrade et al., "Brentuximab vedotin followed by allogeneic transplantation as salvage regimen in patients with relapsed and/or refractory Hodgkin's lymphoma," *Hematological Oncology*, vol. 32, no. 4, pp. 187–191, 2014.

41

Patient-Initiated Discontinuation of Tyrosine Kinase Inhibitor for Chronic Myeloid Leukemia

Stephen E. Langabeer,[1] **Rehman Faryal**,[2] **Michael O'Dwyer**,[2,3] **and Sorcha Ní Loingsigh**[2]

[1]*Cancer Molecular Diagnostics, St. James's Hospital, Dublin D08 W9RT, Ireland*
[2]*Department of Haematology, University Hospital Galway, Galway H91 YR71, Ireland*
[3]*National University of Ireland, Galway H91 TK33, Ireland*

Correspondence should be addressed to Stephen E. Langabeer; slangabeer@stjames.ie

Academic Editor: Tomás J. González-López

The introduction of tyrosine kinase inhibitors (TKI) has revolutionised the management of patients with chronic myeloid leukemia (CML) over the last twenty years, but despite significant improvements in survival, patients exhibit long-term side effects that impact on quality of life. A major advance in CML management has been the ability to discontinue TKI therapy achieving a treatment-free remission (TFR), yet this option is only available to eligible patients who present with low-risk disease and who subsequently attain deep and sustained molecular responses. A case is described of a patient with CML who self-initiated stopping of TKI therapy when in a less than optimal molecular remission. Despite this action, the patient continues to experience a TFR with prospective close molecular monitoring performed. It is emphasized that this approach may lead to ineffective treatment discontinuation, molecular relapse, and increased patient anxiety. As TFR for patients with CML moves from clinical trials into routine clinical practice, emphasis is placed on adherence to (evolving) guidelines critical to ensure optimal counselling, selection, monitoring, and continued management of patients whether TFR is successful or not.

1. Introduction

Chronic myeloid leukemia (CML) patients with optimal responses to tyrosine kinase inhibitors (TKI) have achieved long-term survival with life expectancy in younger CML patients approaching near normal [1]. Despite this improved outcome, long-term use of TKIs is associated with adverse events that may severely affect patient quality of life and impact on morbidity and mortality [2]. In the last decade, the remarkable phenomenon of treatment-free remission (TFR) has been witnessed: in a pivotal study, approximately 40% of CML patients on imatinib therapy for more than two years and in a deep molecular response remained in sustained clinical and molecular remission upon antileukemic TKI discontinuation [3]. TFR rates of 40–60% in eligible patients have been corroborated by numerous, subsequent, randomised clinical trials (in which the eligibility criteria of TKI, time on TKI, and length and depth of molecular response have varied) and have been recently reviewed [4, 5]. Outside of clinical trials, similar TFR rates are also achievable in the "real-world" setting [6–8]. Importantly, in all these studies where patients relapse after discontinuation (nearly always within the first six months of stopping), reintroduction of a TKI results in attainment of a favourable molecular response in the vast majority of patients [9]. The persistence of quiescent CML stem cells in those patients in successful TFR suggests some form of immunological interaction is partly responsible for control of the residual leukaemic clone, the mechanisms of which remain poorly defined [10, 11]. Of note is the recurrent adverse event in 20–30% of those CML patients attempting TFR of a transient TKI withdrawal syndrome manifesting as musculoskeletal pain [12].

With the increased acceptance and uptake of attempting TFR in routine clinical practice, recommendations for the minimal requirements for treatment discontinuation have been proposed by both European and North American experts groups [13, 14]. Similarities exist between these two sets of criteria although there remains limited consensus on the requirements for TKI treatment duration or depth and stability of the molecular remission prior to attempting TFR [15]. Both sets of guidelines concur on the importance of instigating frequent molecular monitoring so that molecular relapse can be rapidly captured prompting reintroduction of TKI.

Improving quality of life may alone provide sufficient rationale for TFR consideration. Younger patients may have a desire to lessen the potential of future adverse events or by personal/family goals, whereas older patients may seek to mitigate the adverse effects they currently experience on TKI therapy [16]. Given that nonadherence is not an uncommon pattern in patients on long-term TKI therapy [17] and an increased awareness of TFR, CML patients may be independently motivated to stop therapy.

2. Case Report

A 55-year-old man presented in November 2008 with fatigue, headache, left upper quadrant abdominal discomfort, and palpable splenomegaly. He had a hemoglobin of 11.6 g/dL, a white cell count of 53.7×10^9/L, and platelets of 165×10^9/L. Bone marrow aspirate revealed moderate hypercellularity with less than 2% myeloblasts, and cytogenetics demonstrated a karyotype of 46,XY,t(9;22)(q34;q11.2). Molecular analysis revealed high levels of e14a2 *BCR-ABL1* transcripts, all consistent with a diagnosis of chronic phase CML with a low-risk Sokal score of 0.75.

The patient was enrolled on an open label, single stage, multicentre, nonrandomized, phase II clinical trial to assess the efficacy of upfront nilotinib 300 mg twice daily [18]. Prospective molecular *BCR-ABL1* monitoring was performed in a European Treatment and Outcome Study (EUTOS)-certified laboratory according to standardized procedures with results reported in line with standardized definitions of response [19, 20]. The patient achieved a major molecular response (MMR; *BCR-ABL1/ABL1* IS $\leq$ 0.1% on the International Scale) at 16 months that was maintained for seven years (Figure 1). Thereafter, a deeper molecular response (MR4; *BCR-ABL1/ABL1* IS $\leq$ 0.01% on the International Scale) was transiently noted.

During his treatment he continued to have mild fatigue and headaches. Transient grade-II increase in serum lipase was also noted which normalised on temporary interruption of nilotinib. Later in the treatment, he reported having frequent nightmares, sleep disturbances, poor concentration, and in general, poor quality of life. Overall, his treatment was continuous with three short (<7 days) interruptions due to impairment in baseline renal functions and transient increase in serum lipase at one instance but was not considered a candidate for attempting TFR at any time due to the lack of a prolonged, deep molecular response. However, at a follow-up appointment, the patient stated that he had stopped taking his TKI in March 2018 and reported feeling much better having stopped nilotinib and did not wish to restart. He had not noticed any symptoms

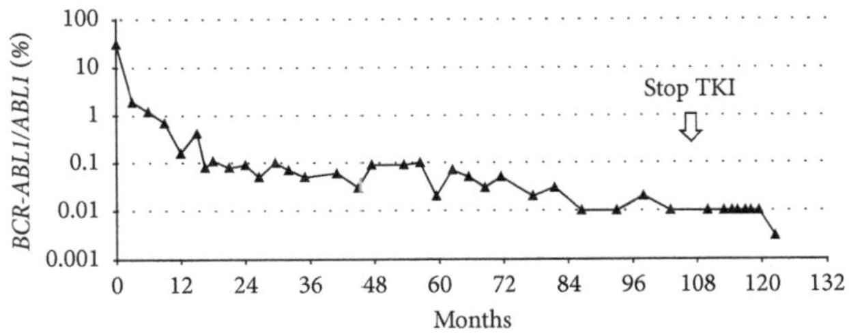

FIGURE 1: Patient *BCR-ABL1* levels throughout disease course.

suggestive of a TKI withdrawal syndrome. Counselled that his response could be lost and being offered treatment with an alternative TKI, he preferred to pursue a trial of treatment cessation, prompting immediate monthly *BCR-ABL1* monitoring to detect any loss of molecular response as per European guidelines [13]. The patient is now 18 months after TKI discontinuation maintaining a stable *BCR-ABL1* level of 0.01% (Figure 1) and remains clinically well. Given the less than optimal *BCR-ABL1* history, molecular monitoring continues at six weekly intervals.

3. Discussion

For many CML patients who have achieved stable and deep molecular responses with TKI therapy, evidence from both clinical trials and real-world settings has demonstrated the feasibility of TFR with current guidelines outlining minimal criteria for eligibility [13, 14]. While these guidelines concur that CML patients attempting TFR must be under the care of CML specialist physicians, have low-risk, chronic phase disease, and have been on continuous TKI therapy for a specified number of years, several aspects of these evolving guidelines remain equivocal (Table 1).

Initial TKI choice appears to have little impact on attaining TFR which has been achieved at a similar frequency of CML patients treated with first-line with imatinib, dasatinib, or nilotinib. The use of more potent inhibitors first-line may increase the number of patients eligible for TFR consideration and reduce overall TKI exposure [21]. Furthermore, in those patients who have switched TKI due to intolerance, TFR rates are comparable to those patients who received only a single agent, provided criteria regarding molecular response and other features are met and are superior to those patients previously experiencing resistance to their first-line TKI [16]. A further intriguing development is the de-escalation of TKI prior to cessation, recently demonstrated to improve the success of TFR protocols though the mechanism of this benefit is not yet clear [22].

Interest has focussed on the influence of the *BCR-ABL1* transcript type on response to first-line TKI with the patients expressing e14a2 transcripts having superior molecular responses to those harboring e13a2 transcripts; however, the impact on overall survival remains unclear [23, 24]. This theory has been extrapolated to those patients attempting TFR with one recent study suggesting that the e14a2 *BCR-ABL1* transcript, as expressed in the above case, favourably impacts on sustained TFR upon TKI discontinuation [25].

Table 1: Minimum criteria for tyrosine kinase inhibitor discontinuation outside of a clinical trial.

Criteria for TKI cessation	ESMO guidelines [18]	NCCN guidelines [19]
Consultation	CML speciality centre	CML speciality centre
Age	Not specified	≥18 years
Risk category or phase at diagnosis	Non-high Sokal score	Chronic phase
On TKI therapy	>5 years	>3 years
BCR-ABL1 transcript	e13a2, e14a2 or other transcript quantifiable over 4.5 log range	Evidence of quantifiable transcript
Molecular response achieved & duration	MR4.5 achieved/MR4.0 ≥ 2 years	MR4.0 ≥ 2 years
BCR-ABL1 test sensitivity/ turnaround	At least MR4.5/4 weeks	At least MR4.5/2 weeks
Monitoring frequency	Monthly for 6 months/6 weekly for next 6 months/3 monthly thereafter	Monthly for one year/6 weekly for second year/3 monthly thereafter
TKI resumption	Not specified	Within 4 weeks of loss of MMR with monthly monitoring

TKI: tyrosine kinase inhibitor; ESMO: European Society for Medical Oncology; NCCN: National Comprehensive Cancer Network; CML: chronic myeloid leukemia; MR: molecular response; MMR: major molecular response.

The initial molecular response to TKI in this case was slow and would be considered as a warning under current European LeukemiaNet guidelines, yet this did not prevent the patient achieving a subsequent TFR [26]. It is known that early molecular response and female sex strongly predict stable undetectable *BCR-ABL1* transcripts (the criteria for TKI discontinuation) [27, 28] but whether this actually translates to maintaining TFR upon cessation is not yet apparent. Most TKI discontinuation trials intuitively conclude that both the depth and duration of molecular response are key indicators of successful TFR [5] although a sustained MR4 prior to TKI cessation was not apparent in this case. While rare instances of TFR have been recently described in CML patients in only MMR [29], TFR trials to date have required deep molecular responses of a minimum of MR4 for entry. For those patients not achieving MR4, the possibility exists of clinical trials that facilitate switching to an alternative TKI in order to improve and sustain the molecular response before TFR. It is in patients with significant long-term side effects that such an approach may be beneficial.

Many factors contribute to the decision to attempt TFR in patients who are eligible and include risk of relapse, side effects, financial considerations, polypharmacy, and willingness to change something that is already working [30]. In an analysis of real-world experience of unplanned TKI discontinuation, patient request was one of the most frequent reasons for stopping with information on TFR clinical trials increasingly available through multiple media sources [31]. Acknowledging patient preference, TKI discontinuation should always follow a full assessment and consultation with patient-initiated discontinuation firmly discouraged.

Given the expected increased prevalence of CML in the forthcoming years driven by both population aging and a relative survival improvement, TFR is likely to become an increasingly sought long-term option and goal [32]. From a clinical practice perspective, an up-to-date survey of oncologists and hematologists regarding TKI therapy discontinuation practice including molecular monitoring, adequate response for discontinuation, and relapse and symptoms following discontinuation suggested discontinuation was often attempted under suboptimal conditions underscoring the requirement for clinician education [33]. Given the heterogeneity of inclusion criteria in previous TFR studies, further clinical trials, including biological investigations, are warranted to establish the optimal preconditions for achieving TFR [5]. Adherence to existing guidelines is recommended though these are likely to evolve with refinement and harmonization of TKI discontinuation trials.

References

[1] J. F. Apperley, “CML and tyrosine kinase inhibition: the hope becomes reality,” *The Lancet Haematology*, vol. 2, no. 5, pp. e176–e177, 2015.

[2] F. Efficace, M. Baccarani, M. Breccia et al., “Health-related quality of life in chronic myeloid leukemia patients receiving long-term therapy with imatinib compared with the general population,” *Blood*, vol. 118, no. 7, pp. 4554–4560, 2011.

[3] F.-X. Mahon, D. Réa, J. Guilhot et al., “Discontinuation of imatinib in patients with chronic myeloid leukaemia who have maintained complete molecular remission for at least 2 years: the prospective, multicentre Stop Imatinib (STIM) trial,” *The Lancet Oncology*, vol. 11, no. 11, pp. 1029–1035, 2010.

[4] P. Laneuville, “When to stop tyrosine kinase inhibitors for the treatment of chronic myeloid leukemia,” *Current Treatment Options in Oncology*, vol. 19, no. 3, p. 15, 2018.

[5] K. K. Chen, T. F. Du, P. S. Xiong, G. H. Fan, and W. Yang, “Discontinuation of tyrosine kinase inhibitors in chronic myeloid leukemia with losing major molecular response as a definition for molecular relapse: a systematic review and meta-analysis,” *Frontiers in Oncology*, vol. 9, p. 372, 2019.

[6] J. C. Hernández-Boluda, A. Pereira, I. Pastor-Gálan et al., “Feasibility of treatment discontinuation in chronic myeloid leukemia in clinical practice: results from a nationwide series of 236 patients,” *Blood Cancer Journal*, vol. 8, no. 10, p. 91, 2018.

[7] N. Cerveira, B. Loreiro, S. Bizarro et al., "Discontinuation of tyrosine kinase inhibitors in CML patients in a real-world clinical practice at a single institution," *BMC Cancer*, vol. 18, no. 1, p. 1245, 2018.

[8] K. Chamoun, H. Kantarjian, R. Atallah et al., "Tyrosine kinase inhibitor discontinuation in patients with chronic myeloid leukemia: a single-institution experience," *Journal of Hematology & Oncology*, vol. 12, no. 1, p. 1, 2019.

[9] D. Rea and F. X. Mahon, "How I manage relapse of chronic myeloid leukaemia after stopping tyrosine kinase inhibitor therapy," *British Journal of Haematology*, vol. 180, no. 1, pp. 34–32, 2018.

[10] M. Ilander, U. Olsson-Strömberg, H. Schlums et al., "Increased proportion of mature NK cells is associated with successful imatinib discontinuation in chronic myeloid leukemia," *Leukemia*, vol. 31, no. 5, pp. 1108–1116, 2017.

[11] E. Cayssials, F. Jacomet, N. Piccirilli et al., "Sustained treatment-free remission in chronic myeloid leukaemia is associated with an increased frequency of innate CD8(+) T-cells," *British Journal of Haematology*, vol. 186, no. 1, pp. 54–59, 2019.

[12] V. Kota and E. Atallah, "Musculoskeletal pain in patients with chronic myeloid leukemia after tyrosine kinase inhibitor therapy cessation," *Clinical Lymphoma Myeloma and Leukemia*, vol. 19, no. 8, pp. 480–487, 2019.

[13] A. Hochhaus, S. Saussele, G. Rosti et al., "Corrections to "Chronic myeloid leukaemia: ESMO Clinical Practice Guidelines for diagnosis, treatment and follow-up"," *Annals of Oncology*, vol. 29, no. 4, p. iv261, 2018.

[14] J. P. Radich, M. Deininger, C. N. Abboud et al., "Chronic myeloid leukemia, version 1.2019, NCCN clinical practice guidelines in oncology," *Journal of the National Comprehensive Cancer Network*, vol. 16, no. 9, pp. 1108–1135, 2018.

[15] S. Soverini, R. Bassan, and T. Lion, "Treatment and monitoring of Philadelphia chromosome-positive leukemia patients: recent advances and remaining challenges," *Journal of Hematology & Oncology*, vol. 12, no. 1, p. 39, 2019.

[16] J. Cortes, D. Rea, and J. H. Lipton, "Treatment-free remission with first- and second-generation tyrosine kinase inhibitors," *American Journal of Hematology*, vol. 94, no. 3, pp. 346–357, 2019.

[17] D. Marin, A. Bazeos, F.-X. Mahon et al., "Adherence is the critical factor for achieving molecular responses in patients with chronic myeloid leukemia who achieve complete cytogenetic responses on imatinib," *Journal of Clinical Oncology*, vol. 28, no. 14, pp. 2381–2388, 2010.

[18] M. E. O'Dwyer, R. Swords, A. Nagler et al., "Nilotinib 300 mg BID as frontline treatment of CML: prospective analysis of the Xpert BCR-ABL Monitor system and significance of 3-month molecular response," *Leukemia Research*, vol. 38, no. 3, pp. 310–315, 2014.

[19] L. Foroni, G. Wilson, G. Gerrard et al., "Guidelines for the measurement of BCR-ABL1 transcripts in chronic myeloid leukaemia," *British Journal of Haematology*, vol. 153, no. 2, pp. 179–190, 2011.

[20] N. C. P. Cross, H. E. White, D. Colomer et al., "Laboratory recommendations for scoring deep molecular responses following treatment for chronic myeloid leukemia," *Leukemia*, vol. 29, no. 5, pp. 999–1003, 2015.

[21] D. M. Ross, T. Masszi, M. T. Gómez Casares et al., "Durable treatment-free remission in patients with chronic myeloid leukemia in chronic phase following frontline nilotinib: 96-week update of the ENESTfreedom study," *Journal of Cancer Research and Clinical Oncology*, vol. 144, no. 5, pp. 945–954, 2018.

[22] R. E. Clark, F. Polydoros, J. F. Apperley et al., "De-escalation of tyrosine kinase inhibitor therapy before complete treatment discontinuation in patients with chronic myeloid leukaemia (DESTINY): a non-randomised, phase 2 trial," *The Lancet Haematology*, vol. 6, no. 7, pp. e375–e383, 2019.

[23] P. Jain, H. Kantarjian, K. P. Patel et al., "Impact of BCR-ABL transcript type on outcome in patients with chronic-phase CML treated with tyrosine kinase inhibitors," *Blood*, vol. 127, no. 10, pp. 1269–1275, 2016.

[24] M. Pfirrmann, D. Evtimova, S. Saussele et al., "No influence of BCR-ABL1 transcript types e13a2 and e14a2 on long-term survival: results in 1494 patients with chronic myeloid leukemia treated with imatinib," *Journal of Cancer Research and Clinical Oncology*, vol. 143, no. 5, pp. 843–850, 2017.

[25] M. D'Adda, M. Farina, F. Schlepped F et al., "The e13a2 BCR-ABL transcript negatively affects sustained deep molecular response and the achievement of treatment-free remission in patients with chronic myeloid leukemia who receive tyrosine kinase inhibitors," *Cancer*, vol. 125, no. 10, pp. 1674–1682, 2019.

[26] M. Baccarani, M. W. Deininger, G. Rosti et al., "European LeukemiaNet recommendations for the management of chronic myeloid leukemia: 2013," *Blood*, vol. 122, no. 6, pp. 872–884, 2013.

[27] S. Branford, D. T. Yeung, D. M. Ross et al., "Early molecular response and female sex strongly predict stable undetectable BCR-ABL1, the criteria for imatinib discontinuation in patients with CML," *Blood*, vol. 121, no. 19, pp. 3818–3824, 2013.

[28] H.-X. Lin, J. Sjaarda, J. Dyck et al., "Gender and BCR-ABL transcript type are correlated with molecular response to imatinib treatment in patients with chronic myeloid leukemia," *European Journal of Haematology*, vol. 96, no. 4, pp. 360–366, 2016.

[29] M. Dragani, G. Rege-Cambrin, D. Ferrero et al., "Beyond the comfort zone of deep molecular response: discontinuation in major molecular response chronic myeloid leukemia," *Leukemia & Lymphoma*, vol. 60, no. 13, pp. 3330–3332, 2019.

[30] K. E. Flynn, J. M. Myers, A. D'Souza, C. A. Schiffer, J. E. Thompson, and E. Atallah, "Exploring patient decision making regarding discontinuation of tyrosine kinase inhibitors for chronic myeloid leukemia," *The Oncologist*, vol. 24, no. 9, pp. 1253–1258, 2019.

[31] M. Iino, T. Yamamoto, and Y. Sakamoto, "Outcomes of unplanned tyrosine kinase inhibitor discontinuation in patients with chronic myeloid leukemia: retrospective analysis of real-world experience in a single institution," *Hematology*, vol. 24, no. 1, pp. 355–361, 2019.

[32] M. Delord, S. Foulon, J.-M. Cayuela, P. Rousselot, and J. Bonastre, "The rising prevalence of chronic myeloid leukemia in France," *Leukemia Research*, vol. 69, pp. 94–99, 2018.

[33] E. K. Ritchie, D. Latremouille-Viau, A. Guerin et al., "Tyrosine kinase inhibitor therapy treatment and discontinuation in patients with chronic myeloid leukemia in chronic phase in the United States: a clinical practice perspective," *Leukemia & Lymphoma*, vol. 60, no. 6, pp. 1476–1484, 2019.

42

Pituitary Gland and Neurological Involvement in a Case of Hemophagocytic Syndrome Revealing an Intravascular Large B-Cell Lymphoma

Sylvain Raoul Simeni Njonnou,[1,2,3] Bruno Couturier,[2,3] Yannick Gombeir,[2,3] Sylvain Verbanck,[2,3] France Devuyst,[3] Georges El Hachem,[2] Ivan Theate,[4] Anne-Laure Trepant,[5] Virginie De Wilde,[6] and Frédéric-Alain Vandergheynst[2]

[1]*Department of Internal Medicine and Specialties, Faculty of Medicine and Biomedical Sciences, University of Yaounde I, Yaoundé, Cameroon*
[2]*Department of Internal Medicine, Hôpital Erasme, Université Libre de Bruxelles, Brussels, Belgium*
[3]*Department of Endocrinology, Hôpital Erasme, Université Libre de Bruxelles, Brussels, Belgium*
[4]*Institute of Pathology and Genetics, Gosselies, Charleroi, Belgium*
[5]*Department of Pathology, Hôpital Erasme, Université Libre de Bruxelles, Brussels, Belgium*
[6]*Department of Hematology, Hôpital Erasme, Université Libre de Bruxelles, Brussels, Belgium*

Correspondence should be addressed to Sylvain Raoul Simeni Njonnou; raoulsims@yahoo.fr

Academic Editor: Kiyotaka Kawauchi

Intravascular large B-cell lymphoma is a rare entity characterized by the proliferation of neoplastic lymphocytes in the lumen of small blood vessels and high mortality. Diagnosis of intravascular lymphoma is often delayed or established postmortem. Here, we report the case of a 48-year-old woman presenting hemophagocytic syndrome, with pituitary gland and neurological involvement. Diagnosis of intravascular large B-cell lymphoma was made on perisplenic vessels, while liver and bone marrow biopsy was noncontributive. This case demonstrates the importance of thorough histopathologic investigations in the setting of high suspicion.

1. Introduction

Intravascular large B-cell lymphoma (IVLBCL) is defined as a rare subtype of diffuse extranodal large B-cell lymphoma [1]. It is characterized by proliferation of neoplastic cells in the lumen of small blood vessels in several organs including the skin, central nervous system, and endocrine system [2–4]. The reason of this peculiar localization is not known. Given the fact that IVLBCL does not produce a mass or lymphadenopathy, the diagnosis is often nonevoked or is particularly difficult to confirm. Another pitfall lies in the variety of clinical presentation, which includes fever of unknown origin.

Hemophagocytic syndrome (HPS) is a severe disease, caused by phagocytosis of hematopoietic cells by activated macrophages not controlled by the usual immune system regulation. It is classified into primary (familial) or secondary forms (associated with infections or malignancies or systemic diseases or immunodeficiencies). Identification and treatment of the underlying etiology of secondary HPS is critical for treatment and prognosis [5].

Here, we present a case of IVLBCL in an immunosuppressed patient (treated by methotrexate and etanercept for seronegative rheumatoid arthritis) who was referred to the emergency department for fever and bicytopenia.

2. Case Presentation

A 48-year-old woman was referred to the emergency department with a one-week history of fever and cytopenia

(Hb 8.7 g/dL, normal range 11.8–15.5; platelet count 77×10^9/L, normal range 155–346). Clinical examination found a huge splenomegaly, confirmed by abdominal CT scan but no arthritis. 18F-fluorodeoxyglucose positron emission tomography/computed tomography (^{18}FDG PET-CT) showed an enlarged hypermetabolic spleen and perisplenic and hilar hepatic hypermetabolic lymph nodes with hypermetabolism around the cervix (Figure 1). Biological investigations revealed mild anemia (Hb 8.4 g/dL), severe thrombopenia (platelet count 40×10^9/L), elevated CRP (200 mg/L, normal range <10), acute liver cytolysis (GPT 57 U/L, normal range <34), hyperferritinemia (ferritin 4724 μg/L, normal range 30–350), increased LDH (4482 U/L, normal range <214), increased soluble CD25 or soluble IL-2 receptor (>30000 pg/mL, normal range 632–4883), and biological intravascular disseminated coagulation (PT<50%, normal range >70% and fibrinogen 77 mg/dL, normal range 160–400). H-score, according to those results, was 99.6% [6, 7]. All this pattern was suggestive of HPS [8, 9]. Bone marrow aspiration and biopsy initially did not confirm and were not contributive for the etiology of HPS. All the infectious serologies including HTLV 1 and 2, HHV 6 and 8, parvovirus B19, *Toxoplasma*, and *Borrelia* were negative. EBV PCR and CMV PCR were negative. Evolution was marked by apparition of jaundice, worsening of liver function (total and conjugated bilirubin, alkaline phosphatase, gamma glutamyl transferase, and glutamic oxaloacetic transaminase were 4–6 times above normal range), and unexplained lactic acidemia (lactacte 8.9 mmol/L, normal range <2 mmol/l) without any clinical manifestation. Liver biopsy was performed, finding cholestasis without any inflammation probably due to toxic etiology. Etoposide (2 courses: first 300 mg and then 200 mg eight days later) and dexamethasone were given with good evolution. The patient was discharged on reduced doses of prednisone, with prednisone 8 mg/day planned to be gradually tapered.

She was readmitted 3 weeks after discharge and 1 week after discontinuation of prednisone, for nausea and vomiting in the setting of inflammatory syndrome (CRP 117 mg/L). Clinical examination was unremarkable. New biological investigations were suggestive of HPS (sCD25 at 15000 pg/mL and ferritin at 1740 μg/L) with evidence of hemophagocytosis at bone marrow aspirates, with acute renal failure and hypopituitarism (Figure 2), clearly concerning gonadotropic axis and thyrotropic axis. Gonadotropic hormone levels were as follows: estradiol <25 ng/L, progesterone <0.2 mcg/L (corresponding to menopause values), LH 2.5 IU/L (normal range: 7.7–58.5), and FSH 7 IU/L (normal range: 25.8–134.8). FSH and LH levels were inappropriate regarding progesterone and estradiol levels, although the patient was not taking oral contraceptives. Regarding thyrotropic axis, TSH was 0.1 mU/L (normal range: 0.3–4.2); free T4, 0.5 ng/dL (normal range 0.9–1.7); and free T3, 1.8 pmol/L (normal range 3.1–6.8). Growth hormone was 0.68 mcg/L (normal range 0.06–6.88), and IGF-1 dosage was performed. Corticotropic axis seemed to be normal: cortisol was 350 nmol/L in the morning (normal range 166–507) and ACTH was 11.4 ng/L (normal range 7.2–63.3). Finally, there was no diabetes insipidus. Brain MRI presented an enlarged pituitary gland and pituitary stalk with nonspecific lesions (Figure 3). A new ^{18}FDG PET-CT showed a reduction of size and hypermetabolism of the spleen but no pituitary hypermetabolism. Levothyroxine and hydrocortisone substitution were started, the latter considered given the concern of an increased steroid need due to pyrexia and the diagnostic splenectomy rapidly planned. A rapid onset of paraparesis with urinary and fecal incontinence led us to perform a new brain MRI. It showed a hypersignaling (T2/flair) medial medullary lesion associated with cortico-subcortical prerolandic homogeneous lesion (Figure 4). Analysis of CSF showed an inflammatory liquid with increased protein (0.80 g/L normal < 0.40) but normal cell count (2 cells/mL).

Given the result of histological examination, the patient has been treated by two courses of R-CHOEP with a three-week interval (rituximab 375 mg/m^2; cyclophosphamide 750 mg/m^2; doxorubicin 50 mg/m^2; vincristine 1.4 mg/m^2; etoposide 100 mg/m^2 on day 1, 2, and 3; and methylprednisolone 80 mg/day), together with weekly intrathecal infusion of methotrexate 15 mg, cytarabine 40 mg, and methylprednisolone 40 mg. Under this treatment, a marked decrease in the size of the pituitary gland and pituitary stalk was noted. Nevertheless, two months after beginning this treatment, the patient died from several infections in the context of persistent medullary toxicity. No autopsy was performed.

3. Pathological Findings

Histological examination revealed the following:

At the spleen level: extramedullary hematopoiesis (with megakaryocytes, erythroblasts, and neutrophils). There was no intravascular infiltration by IVLBCL in the splenic tissue (Figure 5).

At the periganglionic tissue level around the spleen: large atypical cells and hyperchromatic nucleolus, present inside the lumen of small vessels. These morphologic features were consistent with IVLBCL features. On immunostaining, tumor cells were histologically positive for CD20, PAX5, and MUM1 (Figure 6). EBV research was negative by "EBER (Epstein–Barr virus-encoded small RNA) in situ hybridization."

4. Discussion

We describe a case of IVLBCL with neurologic symptoms and hypopituitarism occurring in a patient treated for seronegative rheumatoid arthritis. At the beginning, we considered the hypothesis of adult-onset Still's disease (AOSD) to explain both the HPS and the seronegative rheumatoid arthritis. But the lack of fever and elevated inflammatory parameters at the onset of arthritis a few years ago were not consistent with this hypothesis.

IVLBCL is a rare disease. It has been mainly described in the setting of case reports or short case series [4, 10, 11]. Its

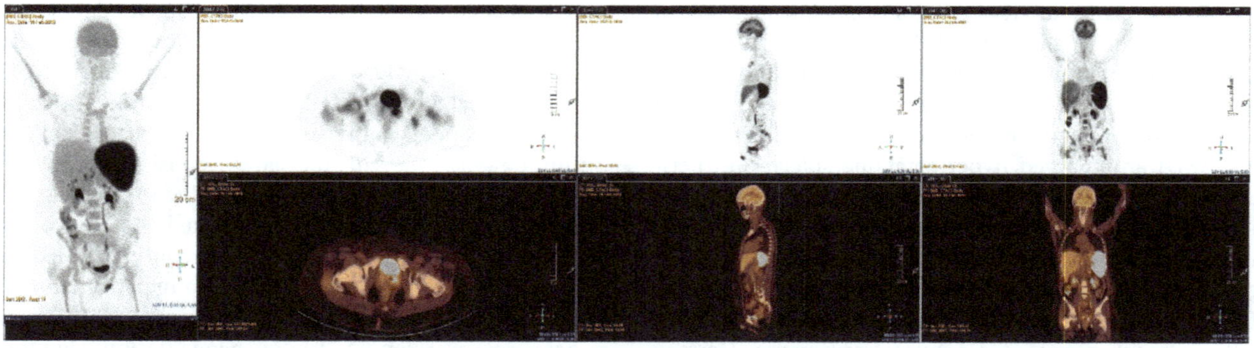

FIGURE 1: PET-CT hypermetabolic splenomegaly, perihepatic hypermetabolic lymph nodes, and cervical hypermetabolism.

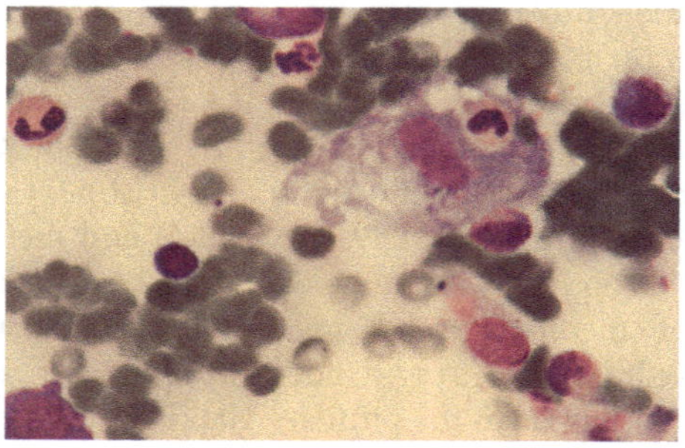

FIGURE 2: Hemophagocytosis at bone marrow aspiration.

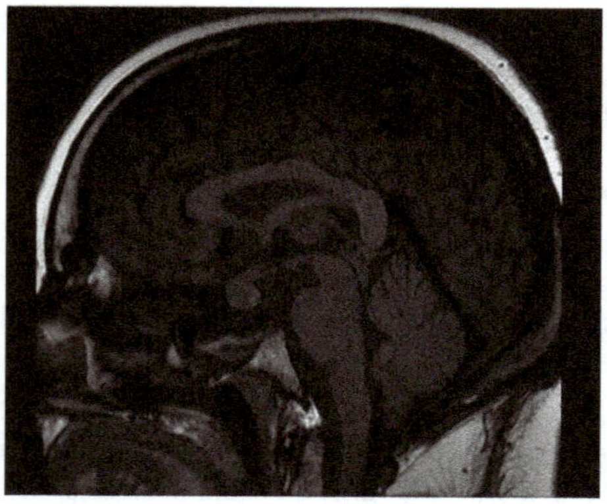

FIGURE 3: Brain MRI showing enlargement of the pituitary gland and pituitary stalk without evidence of adenoma.

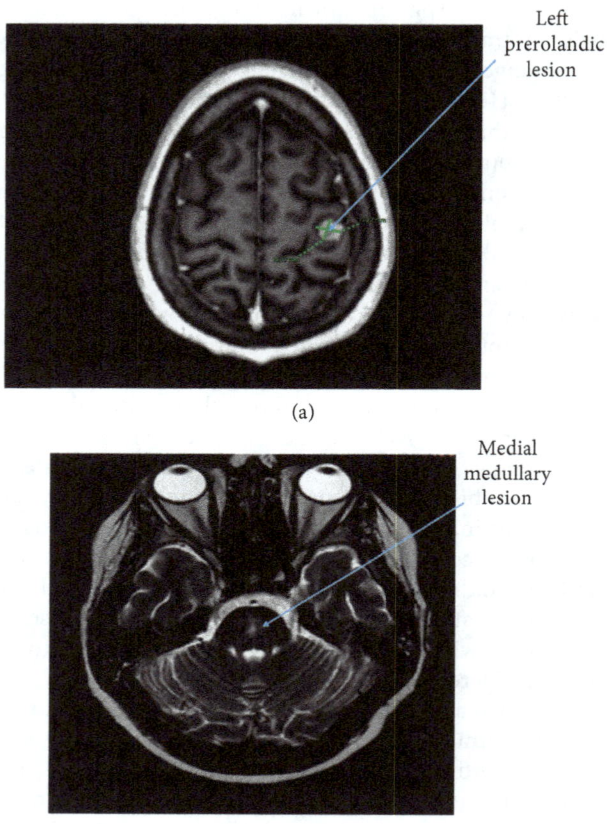

FIGURE 4: Brain MRI showing left prerolandic lesion and medial medullary hypersignal. (a) Prerolandic lesion with homogeneous corticosubcortical ring enhancement. (b) Medial medullary hypersignal in T2 and flair.

association with HPS has been reported several times [2, 12, 13]. Neurological involvement, mainly the central nervous system (CNS), represents 52% of the presentations. CNS is the main affected site. Cognitive impairment (61%), motor impairment (22%), and seizures (13.4%) are the most frequent CNS signs [14]. CNS localization of IVLBCL on the one hand and HPS on the other hand are confounding [3, 5]. It is difficult to affirm that the neurologic impairment in this patient is directly related to IVLBCL rather than HPS without any histological examination. However, given the rather good control of HPS for 3 months (on the basis of blood count), the neurological impairment is more likely related to the lymphoma than HPS. The treatment given for HPS—consisting in two courses of etoposide and steroids (first high-dose dexamethasone and then methylprednisolone)—had probably an impact on the clinical course of IVLBCL.

Pituitary gland involvement due to IVLBCL is exceptionally diagnosed on the basis of clinical and biological findings and rather evidenced postmortem [4, 15–18]. It could be isolated or associated in some cases with involvement of other endocrine glands (adrenal gland and ovaries) [4, 10, 18, 19]. The reason of the preferential tropism of clonal lymphocytes for the endocrine gland is not known. A transsphenoidal biopsy of the pituitary gland is not routinely performed because of the obvious risk of inducing or increasing panhypopituitarism. However, it is not established that pituitary involvement has an impact on

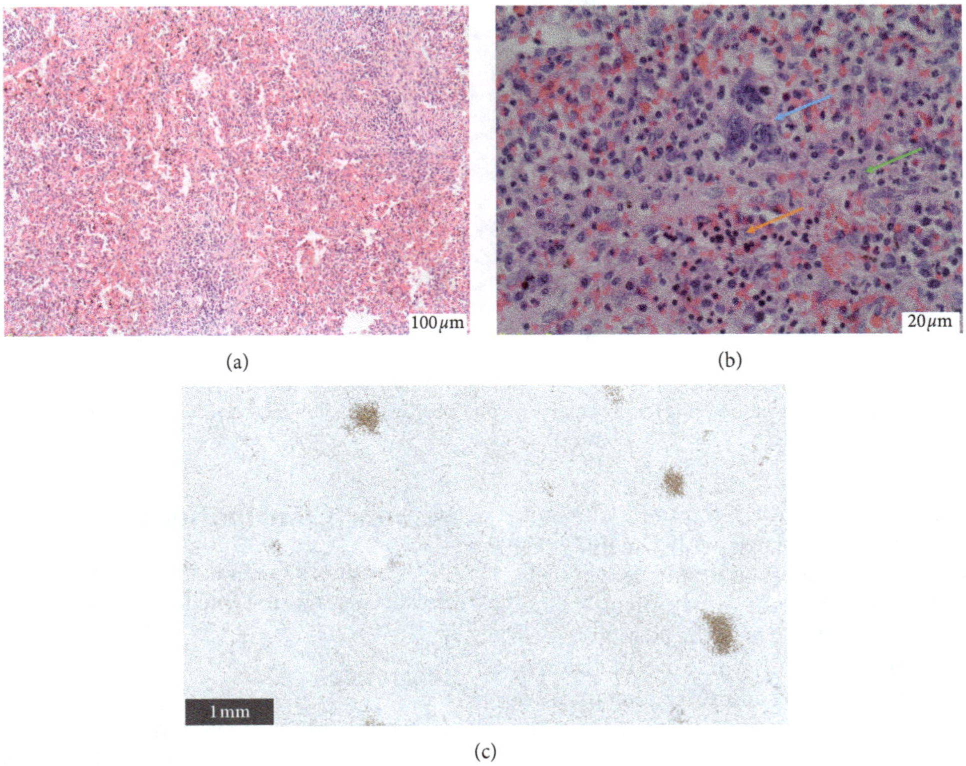

FIGURE 5: Histopathology of a splenectomy piece. (a) Extramedullary hematopoiesis (H&E, 10x). (b) Extramedullary hematopoiesis (H&E, 40x) with megakaryocytes (blue arrow), erythroblasts (orange arrow), and neutrophils (green arrow). (c) CD20 immunostaining showing no spleen infiltration (scale on image).

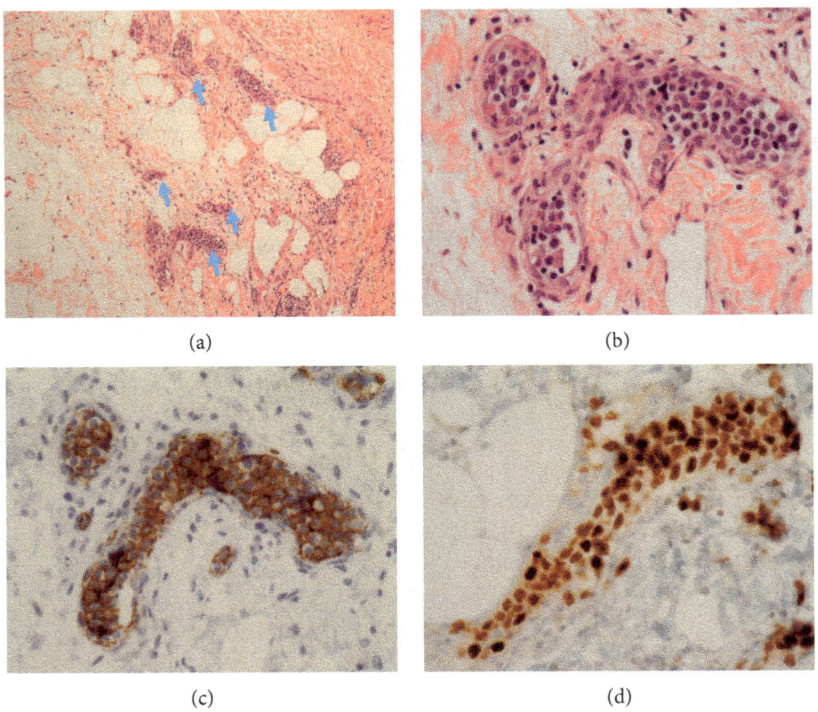

FIGURE 6: Continued.

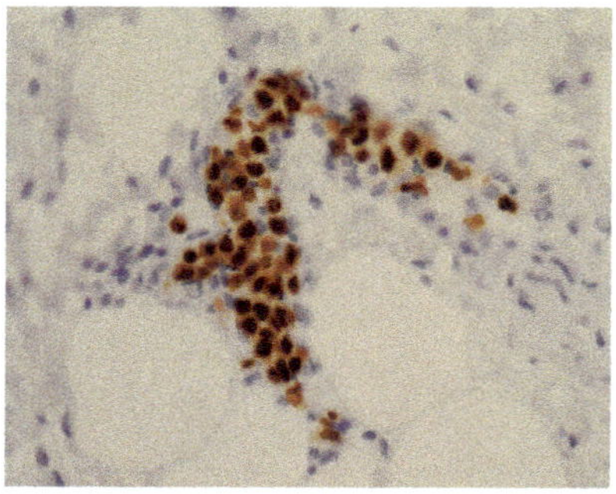

(e)

FIGURE 6: Histopathology of perisplenic tissues. (a) Tumoral intravascular infiltration (arrows) (H&E, 10x). (b) Large hyperchromatic cell inside small vessels around splenic lymph nodes (H&E, 40x). (c) Strong positive CD20 B-cell surface expression. (d) Positive expression of MUM1. (e) Positive expression of PAX5.

the prognosis of patient [14]. Findings of pituitary imaging in case of hypopituitarism associated with IVLBCL vary from suprasellar mass, sellar mass, partially empty sella, or normal [20]. Despite the absence of pathological findings, the marked reduction in the size of the pituitary gland and pituitary stalk with treatment would be in favor of IVLBCL-related disease. Cases of complete resolution of pituitary involvement under treatment have been described [18–20].

However, pituitary gland involvement related to HPS, although exceptional, has been described in some case reports. The usual manifestation is diabetes insipidus, which is lacking in this case [21].

The most effective treatment of IVLBCL involving the CNS is a combination of R-CHOP and intrathecal methotrexate, which could even be administered in prophylaxis of CNS involvement [22]. Etoposide has been administered in relapse protocol in some patients, but in this case, the choice was driven by the association with HPS [23]. Overall survival of patients with CNS involvement of IVLBCL, treated (with classical treatment) or not, is very poor (<1 year), but complete remission has been reported in some cases [14, 18, 19]. Autologous hematopoietic stem cell transplantation is reported to be successful in almost all cases [24].

5. Conclusion

The particularity of our patient is the association of endocrine and neurologic involvement in the context of HPS. This case supports the recommendation of a thorough etiological workup in an adult HPS patient.

Disclosure

This work has been presented as a poster at the 23rd Annual Congress of the Belgian Society of Internal Medicine, 14-15 December 2018, Dolce La Hulpe, La Hulpe, Belgium.

Authors' Contributions

All the authors made a major contribution to the patient's clinical care and the intellectual content of this manuscript.

References

[1] M. Ponzoni, A. J. M. Ferreri, E. Campo et al., "Definition, diagnosis, and management of intravascular large B-cell lymphoma: proposals and perspectives from an international consensus meeting," *Journal of Clinical Oncology*, vol. 25, no. 21, pp. 3168–3173, 2007.

[2] S. Nakamura, T. Murase, and T. Kinoshita, "Intravascular large B-cell lymphoma: the heterogeneous clinical manifestations of its classical and hemophagocytosis-related forms," *Haematologica*, vol. 92, no. 4, pp. 434–436, 2007.

[3] M. Fischer, S. Iglseder, A. Grams et al., "Intravascular large B-cell lymphoma mimicking central nervous system vasculitis," *Human Pathology: Case Reports*, vol. 8, pp. 3–8, 2017.

[4] A. Sakakibara, Y. Inagaki, E. Imaoka et al., "Autopsy case report of intravascular large B-cell lymphoma with neoplastic PD-L1 expression," *Journal of Clinical and Experimental Hematopathology*, vol. 58, no. 1, pp. 32–35, 2018.

[5] M. George, "Hemophagocytic lymphohistiocytosis: review of etiologies and management," *Journal of Blood Medicine*, vol. 5, pp. 69–86, 2014.

[6] L. Fardet, L. Galicier, O. Lambotte et al., "Development and validation of the HScore, a score for the diagnosis of reactive hemophagocytic syndrome," *Arthritis & Rheumatology*, vol. 66, no. 9, pp. 2613–2620, 2014.

[7] F. Debaugnies, B. Mahadeb, A. Ferster et al., "Performances of the H-score for diagnosis of hemophagocytic lymphohistiocytosis in adult and pediatric patients," *American Journal of Clinical Pathology*, vol. 145, no. 6, pp. 862–870, 2016.

[8] J.-I. Henter, A. Horne, M. Aricó et al., "HLH-2004: diagnostic and therapeutic guidelines for hemophagocytic lymphohistiocytosis," *Pediatric Blood & Cancer*, vol. 48, no. 2, pp. 124–131, 2007.

[9] M. Ramos-Casals, P. Brito-Zerón, A. López-Guillermo, M. A. Khamashta, and X. Bosch, "Adult haemophagocytic syndrome," *The Lancet*, vol. 383, no. 9927, pp. 1503–1516, 2014.

[10] K. Matsue, N. Asada, M. Takeuchi et al., "A clinicopathological study of 13 cases of intravascular lymphoma: experience in a single institution over a 9-yr period," *European Journal of Haematology*, vol. 80, no. 3, pp. 236–244, 2008.

[11] K. Poropatich, D. Dittmann, Y.-H. Chen, K. Raparia, K. Wolniak, and J. Gao, "A small case series of intravascular large B-cell lymphoma with unexpected findings: subset of cases with concomitant extravascular central nervous system (CNS) involvement mimicking primary CNS lymphoma," *Journal of Pathology and Translational Medicine*, vol. 51, no. 3, pp. 284–291, 2017.
[12] T. Murase, S. Nakamura, K. Kawauchi et al., "An Asian variant of intravascular large B-cell lymphoma: clinical, pathological and cytogenetic approaches to diffuse large B-cell lymphoma associated with haemophagocytic syndrome," *British Journal of Haematology*, vol. 111, no. 3, pp. 826–834, 2000.
[13] K.-M. Fung, J. H. Chakrabarty, W. F. Kern, H. Magharyous, B. C. Gehrs, and S. Li, "Intravascular large B-cell lymphoma with hemophagocytic syndrome (Asian variant) in a Caucasian patient," *International Journal of Clinical and Experimental Pathology*, vol. 5, no. 5, pp. 448–454, 2012.
[14] E. Fonkem, S. Dayawansa, E. Stroberg et al., "Neurological presentations of intravascular lymphoma (IVL): meta-analysis of 654 patients," *BMC Neurology*, vol. 16, no. 1, pp. 1–7, 2016.
[15] M. Svajdler, I. Lazúrová, P. Bohus, and M. Pal'ko, "Intravascular variant of diffuse large B-cell lymphoma with combined endocrine involvement," *Wiener Klinische Wochenschrift*, vol. 118, no. 13-14, pp. 422–425, 2006.
[16] S. Pekic, S. Milicevic, N. Colovic, M. Colovic, and V. Popovic, "Intravascular large B-cell lymphoma as a cause of hypopituitarism: gradual and late reversal of hypopituitarism after long-term remission of lymphoma with immunochemotherapy," *Endocrine*, vol. 34, no. 1–3, pp. 11–16, 2008.
[17] Y. Nakashima, M. Shiratsuchi, I. Abe et al., "Pituitary and adrenal involvement in diffuse large B-cell lymphoma, with recovery of their function after chemotherapy," *BMC Endocrine Disorders*, vol. 13, no. 1, pp. 1–7, 2013.
[18] S. Hussain, S. Hallam, L. Beltran et al., "Intravascular large B-cell lymphoma presenting as a pituitary mass with bilateral adrenal enlargement and haemophagocytic lymphohistiocytosis," *British Journal of Haematology*, vol. 181, no. 6, pp. 851-852, 2018.
[19] D. A. Pattison, M. S. Hofman, A. Bazargan, P. Colman, and R. J. Hicks, "Intense focal pituitary FDG uptake due to intravascular large B-cell lymphoma in pyrexia of unknown origin," *American Journal of Hematology*, vol. 91, no. 11, pp. 1167-1168, 2016.
[20] Y. Sawada, S. Ishii, Y. Koga et al., "Reversible hypopituitarism associated with intravascular large B-cell lymphoma: case report of successful immunochemotherapy," *The Tohoku Journal of Experimental Medicine*, vol. 238, no. 3, pp. 197–203, 2016.
[21] U. Pajvani, M. Lipton, and M. Grajower, "Diabetes insipidus associated with hemophagocytic lymphohistiocytosis: first case report," *Endocrine Practice*, vol. 17, no. 5, pp. e118–e122, 2011.
[22] D. Nizamutdinov, N. P. Patel, J. H. Huang, and E. Fonkem, "Intravascular lymphoma in the CNS: options for treatment," *Current Treatment Options in Neurology*, vol. 19, no. 10, pp. 1-8, 2017.
[23] V. Brunet, S. Marouan, J.-P. Routy et al., "Retrospective study of intravascular large B-cell lymphoma cases diagnosed in Quebec," *Medicine*, vol. 96, no. 5, article e5985, 2017.
[24] J. Meissner, H. Finel, S. Dietrich et al., "Autologous hematopoietic stem cell transplantation for intravascular large B-cell lymphoma: the european society for blood and marrow transplantation experience," *Bone Marrow Transplantation*, vol. 52, no. 4, pp. 650–652, 2017.

The Use of Etoposide, Ara-Cytarabine and Melphalan (EAM) Conditioning Chemotherapy in Autologous Stem Cell Transplantation (ASCT) for a Patient with Relapsed Hodgkin's Lymphoma

Eko A. Pangarsa,[1] **Ridho M. Naibaho**,[2,3] **Vina Yunarvika**,[1] **Budi Setiawan**,[1] **Damai Santosa**,[1] **and Catharina Suharti**[1]

[1]*Subdivion of Hematology and Medical Oncology, Medical Faculty of Diponegoro University, Dr. Kariadi General Hospital, Semarang, Indonesia*
[2]*Trainee in Hematology and Medical Oncology, Medical Faculty of Diponegoro University, Dr. Kariadi General Hospital, Semarang, Indonesia*
[3]*Department of Internal Medicine, Parikesit Hospital, Mulawarman School of Medicine, Samarinda, East Kalimantan, Indonesia*

Correspondence should be addressed to Eko A. Pangarsa; ekopangarsa90@gmail.com

Academic Editor: Kostas Konstantopoulos

Up to 20–40% of patients with Hodgkin's lymphoma will eventually relapse after treatment, among which early relapse confers a poor outcome. With salvage chemotherapy followed by autologous stem cell transplantation (ASCT), the long-term remission rate is 30%. We report our experience of using a modified-BEAM conditioning regimen without BCNU consisting of etoposide, cytarabine, and melphalan (EAM) in a patient with relapsed Hodgkin's lymphoma. Before transplantation, the patient achieved second complete remission (CR2) using brentuximab vedotin and ESHAP (BR-ESHAP) chemotherapy. The ASCT went well without significant complications. This case demonstrated the considerable efficacy of EAM protocol as a conditioning regimen in terms of sufficient ablative capabilities, and the patient showed a successful hematopoietic engraftment. Although durability of the disease-free survival needs further observation, it had nearly 18 months of complete remission and the patient was in good performance status at the time of writing this manuscript.

1. Background

BEAM (carmustine (BCNU), etoposide, Ara-cytarabine, and melphalan) is considered as the standard conditioning regimen for autologous stem cell transplantation (ASCT) in malignant lymphoma [1, 2]. Unexpectedly, since 2010, the oncological community faced the issue of shortage of some essential chemotherapy drugs, among which was BCNU, one of the central components of the BEAM protocol. Physicians were, thus, forced to change their standard for those regimens in which a component was no longer available: two common solutions were to replace the missing drug with a substitutive agent or even to skip the unavailable drug, trusting that the modified regimen would yield a noninferior result in terms of efficacy and better toxicity profile [3].

BCNU shortage was also reported in Indonesia. So far, we have always been hindered to perform hematopoietic stem cell transplants by the unavailability of this particular drug in the national formularies [4]. We then employed a BEAM-like myeloablative protocol without the letter "B" consisting of etoposide, Ara-cytarabine, and melphalan (EAM) for a preparative ASCT regimen [5], of which one of the cases will be reported here in a patient with Hodgkin's lymphoma.

2. Case Presentation

We report a young female patient with bone marrow "only" Hodgkin's lymphoma relapsed within 12 months after frontline ABVD chemotherapy; initial staging was unfavourable, Ann-Arbor II-B with International Prognostic Score (IPS) = 3. A previous pathological report (March 2017) from cervical lymphadenopathy revealed a mixed cellularity classical Hodgkin's lymphoma. Immunohistochemistry showed expression of CD15+, CD30+, CD3+, and high Ki67. The interim evaluation after treatment assessed by an 18-FDG PET scan is shown in Figure 1 and revealed a first complete remission (CR1) upon completion of 6 cycles of ABVD.

At relapse, she was staged as Ann-Arbor IV-B-E by PET/CT scan (Deauville score 5) and showed bone marrow involvement "only." As salvage therapy, we treated her with ICE protocol showing partial remission (Interim PET/CT resulted in Deauville score 4) and then we switched to anti-CD30 brentuximab vedotin in combination with ESHAP (BR-ESHAP regimen) for the second salvage. After 2 BR-ESHAP courses, examination by PET/CT demonstrated a negative metabolic activity of the bone marrow (Deauville score 2), see Figure 2.

She agreed to proceed to ASCT with her second complete remission (CR2) status. Peripheral blood stem cell (PBSC) harvest was performed in October 2019 by obtaining a CD34+ of 2.31×10^6 per kg of body weight. Our original uncontrolled rate freezing protocol with only 5% dimethyl sulfoxide (DMSO) by using the Planer 560–16 equipment (Planer products Ltd., UK) was used for stem cell cryopreservation, and the transplant was performed in December 2019. The cryopreserved stem cell was planned to be reinfused to the patient after EAM conditioning at least after 24 hours of free-chemo day. The EAM protocol consisted of intravenous etoposide ($200\,mg/m^2$ q24 hours) and Ara-cytarabine ($200\,mg/m^2$ q12 hours) administered for 4 consecutive days (days −6 to −3) followed by melphalan $140\,mg/m^2$ given as a single dose at day −2. The protocol and drug sequence administration are illustrated in Figure 3.

We summarized the transplant course day-by-day until hematopoietic engraftment, as shown in Figure 4. Following EAM chemotherapy and stem cell infusion, the ablative phase of transplant can be observed at day +2. The absolute neutrophil count (ANC) began to decline to $<500/\mu L$ from day +4, while platelet count kept going down to $<20{,}000/\mu L$ and reached its lowest point from day +5. During transplantation, the patient is treated in a positive pressure isolation room and all supportive measures were adopted per local, including the administration of granulocyte colony-stimulating factor (G-CSF) and infectious disease prophylaxis regimen. The posttransplantation period was uneventful though multiple packed red cells and platelet units were required to maintain hemoglobin concentration around 8–10 g/dL and platelet count above $10{,}000/\mu L$ during this critical phase. No other significant nonhematological toxicities except nausea (grade 2), mucositis (grade 2), and diarrhea (grade 1) were reported. Neutrophil engraftment occurred at day +15, and stable platelet count above $20{,}000/\mu L$ was noted from day +20. With a follow-up of 18 months, the patient is in good health with complete and durable hematopoietic resolution with brentuximab vedotin was continued as the consolidation treatment after ASCT.

3. Discussion

Hodgkin's lymphoma accounts for approximately 10% of newly diagnosed malignant lymphoma [6]. Up to 20–40% of these patients will eventually relapse after treatment, among which early relapse confers a poor outcome [1, 7]. For patients who exhibited chemosensitivity, salvage treatment and then high-dose (conditioning) chemotherapy followed by ASCT is the current standard treatment [1, 2, 6]. We followed the methods of Wu et al. [8] utilizing brentuximab vedotin therapy to achieve clinical remission. Related to the conditioning regimen, the two randomized controlled phase III clinical studies with BEAM, mini-BEAM, Dexa-BEAM, or high-dose BEAM found that compared with conventional chemotherapy, salvage high-dose chemotherapy combined with ASCT can significantly increase the disease-free survival (DFS) of relapsed/refractory Hodgkin's lymphoma patients [9, 10].

There are several other commonly used regimens as conditioning chemotherapy for malignant lymphoma, namely, high-dose ICE (h-ICE; ifosfamide, carboplatin, and etoposide) [11], CMV (cyclophosphamide, melphalan, and etoposide) [12], CLV (cytarabine, lomustine and etoposide) [13], CBV (cyclophosphamide, BCNU, and etoposide), combination regimens including total body irradiation (TBI) [7, 12], rituximab or iodine-131-tositumomab combined with BEAM [14], and so forth. However, head-to-head comparisons of different conditioning regimens in relapsed/refractory lymphoma patients before ASCT are sparse.

Generally speaking, the BEAM regimen is currently recognized as the best conditioning regimen for Hodgkin's lymphoma [15, 16]. The overall survival (OS) rate of the BEAM pretreatment regimen for Hodgkin's lymphoma patients is the highest with a 3-year progression-free survival (PFS) of 62% and a 3-year OS of 79% [17]. The BEAM regimen has also been compared to three-drug regimen such as CEB (carboplatin, etoposide, and bleomycin) or CLV (cytarabine, lomustine, and etoposide) regimen with better OS in favor of BEAM [13, 18].

Many countries have also experienced temporary shortage of BCNU; the question is that could we simply omit the BCNU. A number of retrospective studies have tried to address the issue. Unfortunately, EAM conditioning in 12 Hodgkin's lymphoma and 11 non-Hodgkin's lymphoma patients by Loke et al. [19] gave disappointing results (mOS 29 months compared to 77 months for the matched BEAM group). A more recent study by Bekadja et al. [20] demonstrated comparable results in efficacy and toxicity with EAM, but the Ara-C total dose was $8\,gr/m^2$. Other groups studied the replacement of BCNU in the BEAM regimen by

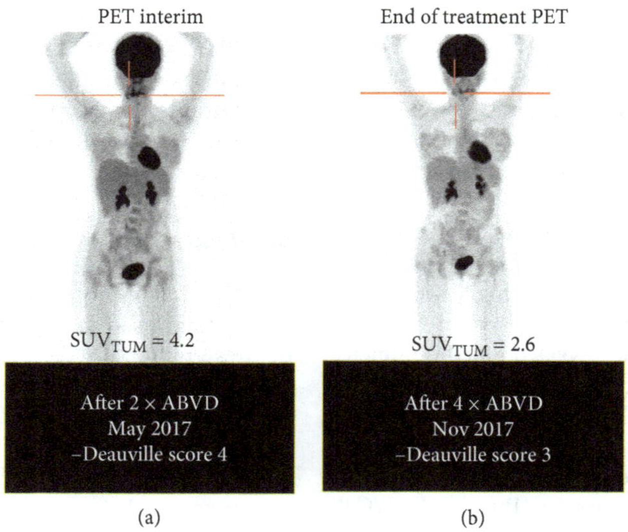

FIGURE 1: Clinical course of the patient after front-line treatment showing (a) PET-interim partial remission after induction ABVD chemotherapy; (b) PET/CT after completion of 6 cycles reveals complete remission and clinical improvement.

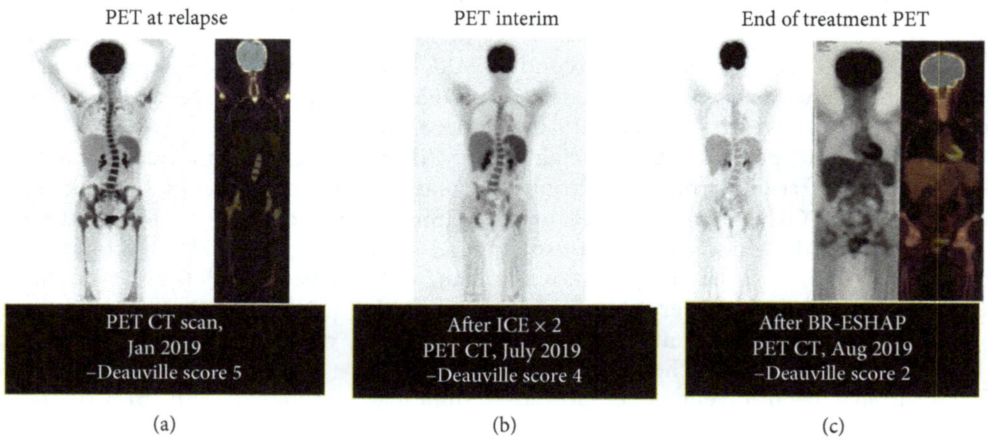

FIGURE 2: Clinical course of the patient at relapse. (a) First early relapse showing bone marrow progression (Ann-Arbor IVB-E); (b) partial remission after 2 cycles of the first ICE salvage treatment, with faint uptake over the bone marrow; and (c) complete remission after 2 cycles of second salvage using the brentuximab vedotin-ESHAP protocol.

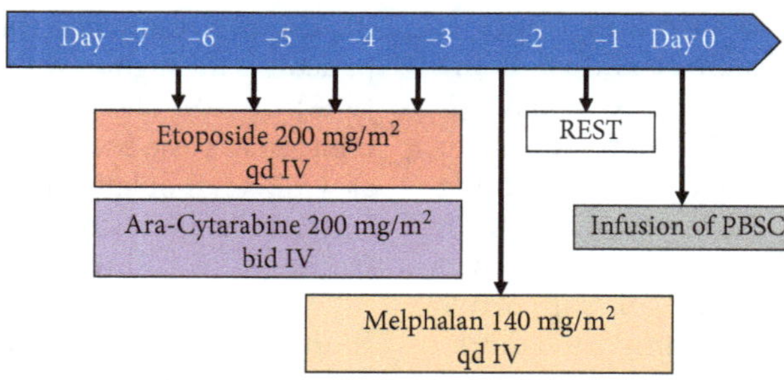

FIGURE 3: EAM protocol scheme at glance. Preharvested autologous stem cells were infused after 1 full day rest without chemotherapy (day zero). BMT, bone marrow transplantation; PBSC, peripheral blood stem cell.

lomustine or thiotepa and stated that although the BEAM group showed a lower rate of transplant-related mortality at day 100, the difference did not reach statistical significance and the 3 regimens had similar results in terms of toxicity and efficacy [21].

This case describes our attempt at modifying the conditioning regimen for relapsed Hodgkin's lymphoma. In the absence of the BCNU component of the BEAM (BCNU, etoposide, cytarabine, and melphalan) [15, 22] or BEAC (BCNU, etoposide, Ara-cytarabine, and cyclophosphamide)

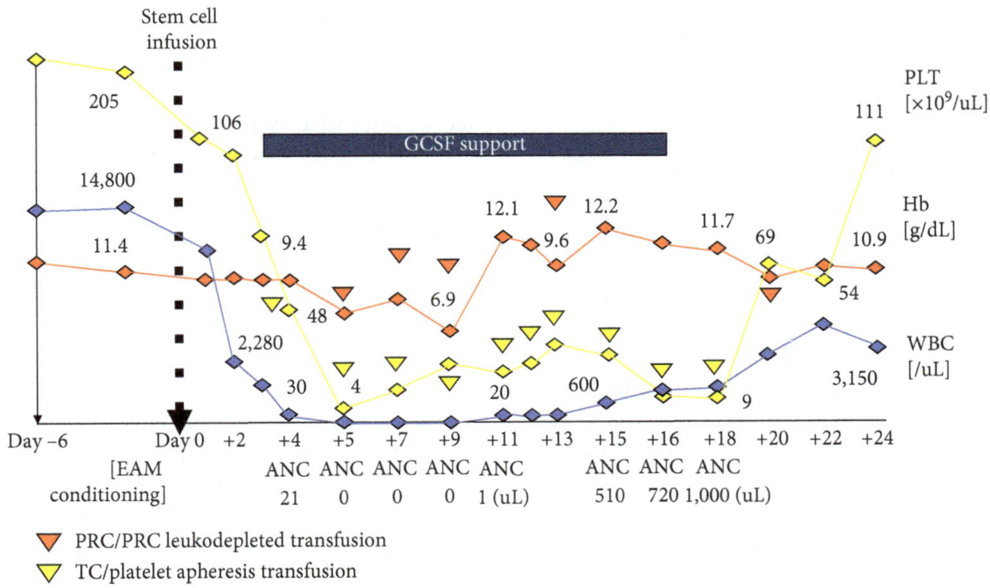

Figure 4: Day-to-day transplant evaluation from conditioning chemotherapy until engraftment. ANC, absolute neutrophil count; Hb, hemoglobin concentration; Plt, platelet count; PRC, packed red cells; and WBC, white blood cell count.

[14], the second most important consideration was drug availability while still maintaining effectiveness. The regimen should facilitate a successful transplant, create enough space for preharvested stem cell to regrowth, repopulate, and restore hematopoietic reconstitution or engraftment.

There are several adverse prognostic factors identified on patients with relapsed Hodgkin's lymphoma, among which others are short duration of CR after initial treatment [6]. The five-year-survival rates for early-relapse patients in the German Hodgkin Study Group (GHSG) cohort were below 50% [23]. In this patient, short remission duration (<12 months) was also reported along with presence of B symptoms, extranodal disease, and stage III/IV as predictors for another relapse post-ASCT [24]. A possible explanation for the favorable result of ASCT in the AETHERA study might be due to exclusion of poor-risked patients with refractory disease, good performance status, young age, sufficient stem cell harvest, and no life-threatening toxicity on salvage treatment. According to these clinical pre-ASCT risk factors, we planned to continue brentuximab vedotin up to a total of 16 cycles for better 5-year PFS based on the AETHERA study [25].

In this case report, we ablated the BCNU from the original BEAM regimen without altering either the dosage or drug sequence of the rest component, identical to Loke et al.'s protocol [19]. The details of our protocol can be found elsewhere [5]. Engraftment can be observed in day +15 and day +20 for neutrophils and platelets, respectively. Overall, the EAM scheme was well tolerated. As expected, nausea, mucositis, and diarrhea were the most prominent non-hematologic toxicity and fortunately manageable. These complications occur in frequent occasion with high-intensity regimens [13–23]. Considering the effectiveness of this three-drug regimen in longer-term outcome for PFS or even OS cannot be simply answered from this single case description. But, as depicted in Figure 4, the patient tolerated the expected ablative phase following the EAM regimen, and the cryopreserved stem cells successfully reconstituted hematopoietic engraftment without significant complications. We should admit that the utilization of brentuximab vedotin as the maintenance agent has made a significant survival advantage after ASCT as she is still in good condition until today.

4. Conclusions

We report a case of early-relapsed Hodgkin's lymphoma that underwent ASCT following CR2. The main message of this report is that the EAM protocol has the potential to be successful and effectively used in countries with limited access to BCNU. EAM was sufficient in terms of ablative capability to produce space for autograft to restore the hematopoiesis following ASCT.[4]In the meantime, ASCT has not been widely carried out in Indonesia for several reasons; thus, this publication is needed at least to hand in a simpler and feasible conditioning protocol. Further noninferiority trial and prospective study could be specifically designed to provide both a more powerful evidence and survival outcome on the use of EAM in broader clinical practice.

Abbreviations

ABVD:	Adriamycin, bleomycin, vinblastin, and dacarbazine
ANC:	Absolute neutrophil count
ASCT:	Autologous stem cell transplantation
BCNU:	Bis-chloroethyl nitrosurea
BEAC:	BCNU (carmustine, etoposide, cytarabine, and cyclophosphamide)
BEAM:	BCNU (carmustine, etoposide, cytarabine, and melphalan)

CEB: Cyclophosphamide, etoposide, and BCNU (carmustine)
CBV: Cyclophosphamide, BCNU (carmustine), and etoposide
CLV: Cyclophosphamide, lomustine, and etoposide
CMV: Cyclophosphamide, melphalan, and etoposide
CR: Complete remission
DFS: Disease-free survival
DMSO: Dimethyl sulfoxide
EAM: Etoposide, Ara-cytarabine, and melphalan
G-CSF: Granulocyte colony-stimulating factor
GHSG: German Hodgkin study group
ICE: Ifosfamide, carboplatin, and etoposide
IPS: International Prognostic Score
ESHAP: Etoposide, methylprednisolone, cytarabine, and cisplatin
PBSC: Peripheral blood stem cell
18-FDG PET: Positron emission tomography 18-fluorodeoxyglucose positron emission tomography scan
PFS: Progression-free survival
TBI: Total body irradiation
OS: Overall survival.

Consent

The manuscript has been sufficiently anonymized, and no identifiable information has been included in the manuscript. Moreover, informed consent was obtained from the patient and her legal guardians.

Disclosure

Preliminary data of this case have been previously presented in the 2020 Lymphoma, Leukemia, and Myeloma Congress, October 21–24, 2020, in the abstract form.

Authors' Contributions

EAP was responsible for clinical management of the patient and drafting the paper. RMN who is currently working as trainee in hematology and medical oncology has participated in the patient's management, performing literature research, and drafting the first manuscript. VY has kindly assisted RMN and provided significant input in the creation of the first draft of the manuscript. BS, DS, and CS have supervised the work, edited the content, and provided their expertise. All authors approved the final version of the manuscript submitted for publication.

Acknowledgments

The authors would like to thank all the Dr. Kariadi Transplant Unit personnel who were involved in patient care and Stem Cell Laboratory staff. Special acknowledgements belong to the patient and her family for accepting and consenting to the publication of this manuscript. Publication fee was granted by the Indonesian Society of Hematology and Medical Oncology of Semarang Chapter.

References

[1] M. Caballero, V. Rubio, J. Rifon et al., "BEAM chemotherapy followed by autologous stem cell support in lymphoma patients: analysis of efficacy, toxicity and prognostic factors," *Bone Marrow Transplantation*, vol. 20, no. 6, pp. 451–458, 1997.

[2] J. W. Sweetenham, "High dose chemotherapy and stem cell transplantation in Hodgkin's disease," in *High Dose Chemotherapy: Principles and Practice*, P. Lorigan and E. Vanderberghe, Eds., Martin Dunitz Ltd., London, UK, 2002.

[3] M. L. Gatesman and T. J. Smith, "The shortage of essential chemotherapy drugs in the United States," *New England Journal of Medicine*, vol. 365, no. 18, pp. 1653–1655, 2011.

[4] H. Hariman, "Thehematopoieticstemcelltransplantation inIndonesia: an unsolved dilemma," *Bone Marrow Transplantation*, vol. 42, no. Suppl. 1, pp. S85–S88, 2008.

[5] D. Santosa, E. A. Pangarsa, B. Setiawan et al., "Establishing the hematopoietic stem cell transplantation(HSCT)inadevelopingcountry;thejourneyofHSCT in Semarang, Indonesia," *Bone Marrow Transplantation*, vol. 56, no. Suppl. 1, pp. 1–4, 2020.

[6] A. Sureda and C. Martines, "Classical Hodgkin's lymphoma," in *The EBMT Handbook: Hematopoietic Stem Cell Transplantation and Cellular Therapies*, E. Carrera, C. Dufour, M. Mohty, and N. Kroger, Eds., Springer, Gewerbestrasse, Switzerland, 2019.

[7] A. Sureda, M. Constans, A. Iriondo et al., "Prognostic factors affecting long-term outcome after stem-cell transplantation in Hodgkin's lymphoma autografted after a first relapse," *Annals of Oncology*, vol. 16, no. 4, pp. 625–633, 2005.

[8] H. B. Wu, S. A. Yeh, and H. Y. Chen, "Brentuximab vedotin treatment for primary refractory Hodgkin lymphoma," *Case Reports in Hematology*, vol. 2013, Article ID 351292, 2013.

[9] D. C. Linch, D. Winfield, A. H. Goldstone et al., "Dose intensification with autologous bone-marrow transplantation in relapsed and resistant Hodgkin's disease: results of a BNLI randomised trial," *The Lancet*, vol. 341, no. 8852, pp. 1051–1054, 1993.

[10] N. Schmitz, B. Pfistner, M. Sextro et al., "Aggressive conventional chemotherapy compared with high-dose chemotherapy with autologous haemopoietic stem-cell transplantation for relapsed chemosensitive Hodgkin's disease: a randomised trial," *The Lancet*, vol. 359, no. 9323, pp. 2065–2071, 2002.

[11] K. K. Fields, G. J. Elfenbein, H. M. Lazarus et al., "Maximum-tolerated doses of ifosfamide, carboplatin, and etoposide given over 6 days followed by autologous stem-cell rescue: toxicity profile," *Journal of Clinical Oncology*, vol. 13, no. 2, pp. 323–332, 1995.

[12] P. J. Stiff, S. Dahlberg, S. J. Forman et al., "Autologous bone marrow transplantation for patients with relapsed or refractorydiffuse aggressive non-Hodgkin's lymphoma: value of augmented preparative regimens--a Southwest Oncology Group trial," *Journal of Clinical Oncology*, vol. 16, no. 1, pp. 48–55, 1998.

[13] A. Colita, A. Colita, H. Bumbea et al., "LEAM vs. BEAM vs. CLV conditioning regimen for autologous stem cell transplantation in malignant lymphomas. Retrospective comparison of toxicity and efficacy on 222 patients in the first 100 days after transplant, on behalf of the Romanian Society of Bone Marrow Transplantation," *Frontiers in Oncology*, vol. 9, no. 892, pp. 1–10, 2019.

[14] J. M. Vose, S. Carter, L. J. Burns et al., "Phase III randomized study of rituximab/carmustine, etoposide, cytarabine, and melphalan (BEAM) compared with iodine-131 tositumomab/BEAM with autologous hematopoietic cell transplantation for relapsed diffuse large B-cell lymphoma: results from the BMT CTN 0401 trial," *Journal of Clinical Oncology*, vol. 31, no. 13, pp. 1662–1668, 2013.

[15] J.-C. Jo, B. W. Kang, G. Jang et al., "BEAC or BEAM high-dose chemotherapy followed by autologous stem cell transplantation in non-Hodgkin's lymphoma patients: comparative analysis of efficacy and toxicity," *Annals of Hematology*, vol. 87, no. 1, pp. 43–48, 2008.

[16] E. Jantunen, T. Kuittinen, and T. Nousiainen, "BEAC or BEAM for high-dose therapyin patients with non-Hodgkin's lymphoma? A single centre analysis on toxicity and efficacy," *Leukemia and Lymphoma*, vol. 44, no. 7, pp. 1151–1158, 2003.

[17] Y.-B. Chen, A. A. Lane, B. R. Logan et al., "Impact of conditioning regimen on outcomes for patients with lymphoma undergoing high-dose therapy with autologous hematopoietic cell transplantation," *Biology of Blood and Marrow Transplantation*, vol. 21, no. 6, pp. 1046–1053, 2015.

[18] E. H. Wang, Y. A. Chen, S. Corrigan et al., "High-dose CEB vs BEAM with autologous stem cell transplant in lymphoma," *Bone Marrow Transplantation*, vol. 34, no. 7, pp. 581–587, 2004.

[19] J. Loke, J. Ward, P. Mahendra, S. Chaganti, and R. Malladi, "Outcomes of EAM conditioned autologous haematopoietic SCT for lymphoma: a matched pair retrospective single-centre study analysis," *Bone Marrow Transplantation*, vol. 48, no. 11, pp. 1486-1487, 2013.

[20] M. A. Bekadja, S. Talhi, K. Amani et al., "Outcomes of modified-eam conditioned autologous non-cryopreserved hematopoietic hematopoietic sct for lymphoma. A retrospective single-centre study," *Bone Marrow Transplantation*, vol. 53, no. 12, pp. 1596–1598, 2018.

[21] G. C. Seval, D. G. Sahin, E. A. Soydan et al., "Comparing conditioning remigens for autologous stem cell transplantation in lymphoma patients," *Clinical Lymphoma, Myeloma & Leukemia*, vol. 18, no. Suppl. 1, p. S306, 2018.

[22] F. Abdel-Rahman, A. Hussein, M. Aljamily, A. Al-Zaben, N. Hussein, and A. Addasi, "High-dose therapy and autologous hematopoietic progenitor cells transplantation for recurrent or refractory Hodgkin's lymphoma: analysis of King Hussein Cancer Center results and prognostic variables," *ISRN Oncology*, vol. 12, no. 3, Article ID 249124, 2012.

[23] A. Josting, U. Rueffer, J. Franklin, M. Sieber, V. Diehl, and A. Engert, "Prognostic factors and treatment outcome in primary progressive Hodgkin lymphoma: a report from the German Hodgkin Lymphoma Study Group," *Blood*, vol. 96, no. 4, pp. 1280–1286, 2000.

[24] E. Van Den Neste, O. Cassasnovas, M. Andre et al., "Classical Hodgkin's lymphoma: the Lymphoma Study Association (LYSA) guidelines for relapsed and refractory adult patients eligible for transplant," *Haematologica*, vol. 98, no. 8, pp. 1–12, 2013.

[25] C. H. Moskowitz, J. Walewski, A. Nademanee et al., "Five-year PFS from the AETHERA trial of brentuximab vedotin for Hodgkin lymphoma at high risk of progression or relapse," *Blood*, vol. 132, no. 25, pp. 2639–2642, 2018.

44

Primary Cutaneous Anaplastic Large Cell Lymphoma of the Oral Cavity Successfully Treated with Brentuximab Vedotin

Federico Meconi, Roberto Secchi, Raffaele Palmieri, Sara Vaccarini, Vito Mario Rapisarda, Laura Giannì, Fabiana Esposito, Ida Provenzano, Daniela Nasso, Livio Pupo, and Maria Cantonetti

Department of Biomedicine and Prevention, Haematology Division, University of Tor Vergata, Viale Oxford 81, Rome, Italy

Correspondence should be addressed to Federico Meconi; federico.meconi89@gmail.com

Academic Editor: Sergio Storti

Primary cutaneous anaplastic large cell lymphoma is a CD-30 positive lymphoproliferative disorder with good prognosis, usually treated with radiation therapy and surgery. Head, neck, and extremities are the most frequently involved sites. In this paper, we describe an unusual case of oral localization, recurring after skin-involving radiotherapy, successfully treated with sixteen cycles of brentuximab vedotin. This could be a more effective approach with a less detrimental toll for treating these rare disorders.

1. Introduction

Primary cutaneous CD-30 positive lymphoproliferative disorders are a rare and heterogeneous group of primary skin tumors, accounting for about 30% of all cases of primary cutaneous T-cell lymphomas (PCTCL) [1]. The group comprises primary cutaneous anaplastic large cell lymphoma (PCALCL), lymphomatoid papulosis (LyP), and borderline cases.

PCALCL is most commonly found in adults (median age at diagnosis is 60 years old), occurring more often in men than women (3 : 1). Macroscopically, PCALCL usually presents itself with red to violaceous lesions, rapidly growing and frequently ulcerative. Head, neck, and extremities are the most frequently involved sites, both for solitary lesions or for multiple grouped nodules. Systemic symptoms, such as fever, fatigue, and mucosal involvement, are rare in PCALCL. However, in at least 10% of cases, neoplastic CD30+ cells can be found in locoregional lymph nodes. Its course is generally indolent (dissemination is uncommon); spontaneous regression occurs in about 40% of cases, even though partial remission is documented more frequently than complete ones [2–4].

The first line treatment currently accepted is radiation therapy or surgical removal, whenever possible. In case of multifocal lesions, methotrexate is accepted followed by low-dose maintenance [1]. However, brentuximab vedotin (BV) was recently included in the National Comprehensive Cancer Network Guidelines as a first line treatment. Recurrences are common in both the same or in different cutaneous sites. PCALCL carries a favorable prognosis with a 5-year survival rate over 90% [5].

Histopathologically and microscopically, PCALCL exhibits a high expression rate of CD30+ antigen (CD30 positivity is required for diagnosis in at least 75% of atypical cells), positivity for CD4+ antigen and does not present ALK positivity [6]. In this article, we describe a rare case of PCALCL of the hard palate that was successfully treated with BV.

2. Case Report

In November 2016, a 40-year-old Caucasian male came to our attention for a nodular, erythematous, nonulcerated, well-defined, and indurated lesion localized in his right forearm.

A skin punch biopsy of the lesion was performed, showing an inflammatory multinodular infiltration of lymphohistiocytic cells in both deep and superficial dermis, including many large, atypical, anaplastic cells with frequent mitosis, characterized by the following immunohistochemistry: CD45+, CD2+, CD3+/–, CD7+/–, CD20–, CD30+, and ALK–. To rule out systemic anaplastic large cell lymphoma, we performed a bone marrow biopsy (negative for malignant cells) and a CT/PET scan that revealed a significant and singular uptake of ^{18}F-FDG in the right forearm region (matching precisely the tumor localization). As we made diagnosis of PCALCL, the patient began radiation therapy (dose of 3600 cGy), achieving complete response.

A new nodular erythematous lesion of 1 cm appeared in March 2017 in the right inguinal region and was unsuccessfully treated with topical steroids. One month later, when it expanded up to 3 cm, a new CT/PET scan was performed and revealed the lesion as the only pathological uptake in the right inguinal region. The patient underwent another radiation therapy of 3600 cGy, obtaining complete response again.

In May 2017, two more nodular lesions appeared in the patient's oral cavity, in the left hard palate (Figure 1). A punch biopsy showed histopathological and immunohistochemical findings consistent with PCALCL. As the lesions did not show spontaneous regression in one month of clinical observation and the patient was experiencing oral discomfort in eating and chewing, it was decided to proceed with treatment.

To avoid radiation therapy and its side effects and taking into account the short time to relapse that the patient experienced with previous radiation therapy in different sites, it was decided to start systemic immunochemotherapy with brentuximab vedotin (BV) 1.8 mg/Kg every 21 days. Interesting later reviews about reduction in doses and numbers of cycles of BV have been published recently [7], showing these protocols could be as effective as the standard therapy. After only two cycles of BV, the patient showed complete regression of nodular lesions with reappearance of normal mucosa of the oral cavity (Figure 2). The final CT/PET scan evaluation was negative for any disease localization.

Since the patient did not present any neuropathy and experienced early relapse after initial remission obtained with radiotherapy, we continued treatment with BV for sixteen cycles [8] with no reduction in dose. All sixteen cycles were performed since we could not find any data showing that the reduction of cycles could lead to the same disease-free survival, trying to ensure our patient the longest possible complete remission.

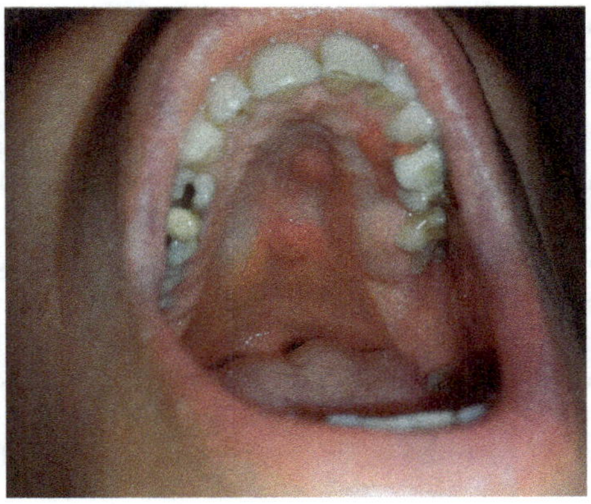

Figure 1: Oral cavity before therapy with BV.

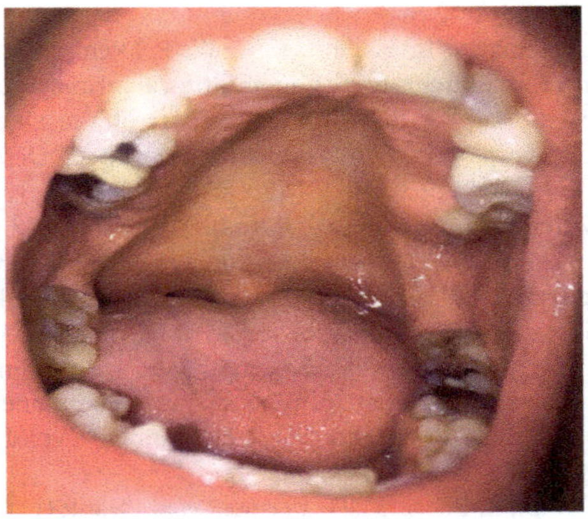

Figure 2: Oral cavity after the 2nd cycle of BV.

3. Conclusions

To the best of our knowledge, this is the first documented case of PCALCL present only in the hard palate, while other few cases of similar processes involving mucosal sites of the head and neck have been previously reported with one case of systemic anaplastic large cell lymphoma involving the hard palate [9].

We demonstrated that oral PCALCL could be successfully treated with systemic immune-chemotherapy with brentuximab vedotin, an anti-CD30 antibody conjugated to monomethyl auristatin E and an effective antimicrotubule agent that was previously approved for Hodgkin lymphoma, ALK-positive anaplastic large cell lymphoma [10], and other cutaneous lymphoproliferative disorders, such as mycosis fungoides.

Using immune-chemotherapy instead of radiation therapy can prevent several side effects, such as mucositis, candidosis, dysgeusia, radiation caries, osteoradionecrosis, soft tissue necrosis, progressive periodontal attachment loss, trismus, and xerostomia, which are all well documented while treating mucosal lesions with radiations [11].

Brentuximab's most common side effect is peripheral sensitive neuropathy that can lead to dose reduction or even drug withdrawal. However, our patient did not experience such neuropathy and could complete therapy within the sixteen cycles at full dose.

Due to the rarity of this group of cutaneous lymphoproliferative disorders (even rarer if we consider those found in the oral cavity), it is still a challenge to make a trial comparing radiation therapy with immune-chemotherapy using BV. From this case, we can infer that although BV is not side-effect free, it offers a safe choice to treat primary cutaneous CD-30 positive lymphoproliferative disorders no longer responding to radiation therapy and standard chemotherapy or cases where the anatomic site involved does not allow RT or must be avoided due to its side effects.

References

[1] R. C. Melchers, R. Willemze, M. W. Bekkenk et al., "Evaluation of treatment results in multifocal primary cutaneous anaplastic large cell lymphoma: report of the Dutch Cutaneous Lymphoma Group," *British Journal of Dermatology*, vol. 179, no. 3, pp. 724–731, 2018.

[2] R. Willemze, L. Cerroni, W. Kempf et al., "The 2018 update of the WHO-EORTC classification for primary cutaneous lymphomas," *Blood*, vol. 133, no. 16, pp. 1703–1714, 2019.

[3] D. Gilson, S. J. Whittaker, F. J. Child et al., "British Association of Dermatologists and U.K. Cutaneous Lymphoma Group guidelines for the management of primary cutaneous lymphomas 2018," *British Journal of Dermatology*, vol. 180, no. 3, pp. 496–526, 2019.

[4] W. Kempf, K. Pfaltz, M. H. Vermeer et al., "EORTC, ISCL, and USCLC consensus recommendations for the treatment of primary cutaneous CD30-positive lymphoproliferative disorders: lymphomatoid papulosis and primary cutaneous anaplastic large-cell lymphoma," *Blood*, vol. 118, no. 15, pp. 4024–4035, 2011.

[5] M. W. Bekkenk, F. A. Geelen, P. C. van Voorst Vader et al., "Primary and secondary cutaneous CD30(+) lymphoproliferative disorders: a report from the Dutch Cutaneous Lymphoma Group on the long-term follow-up data of 219 patients and guidelines for diagnosis and treatment," *Blood*, vol. 95, no. 12, pp. 3653–3661, 2000.

[6] R. Willemze, E. S. Jaffe, G. Burg et al., "WHO-EORTC classification for cutaneous lymphomas," *Blood*, vol. 105, no. 10, pp. 3768–3785, 2005.

[7] R. Stranzenbach, E. Dippel, M. Schlaak, and R. Stadler, "Brentuximab vedotin in CD30+ cutaneous lymphoma: how do we treat, how shall we treat? A review of the literature," *British Journal of Dermatology*, vol. 177, no. 6, pp. 1503–1509, 2017.

[8] R. Dummer, Y. H. Kim, S. M. Horwitz et al., "Brentuximab vedotin or physician's choice in CD30-positive cutaneous T-cell lymphoma (ALCANZA): an international, open-label, randomised, phase 3, multicentre trial," *The Lancet*, vol. 390, no. 10094, pp. 555–566, 2017.

[9] A. P. Sciallis, M. E. Law, D. J. Inwards et al., "Mucosal CD30-positive T-cell lymphoproliferations of the head and neck show a clinicopathologic spectrum similar to cutaneous CD30-positive T-cell lymphoproliferative disorders," *Modern Pathology*, vol. 25, no. 7, pp. 983–992, 2012.

[10] P. L. Zinzani, S. Sasse, J. Radford, O. Shonukan, and V. Bonthapally, "Experience of brentuximab vedotin in relapsed/refractory Hodgkin lymphoma and relapsed/refractory systemic anaplastic large-cell lymphoma in the named patient program: review of the literature," *Critical Reviews in Oncology/Hematology*, vol. 95, no. 3, pp. 359–369, 2015.

[11] E. de Souza Tolentino, B. S. Centurion, L. H. C. Ferreira, A. P. de Souza, J. H. Damante, and I. R. F. Rubira-Bullen, "Oral adverse effects of head and neck radiotherapy: literature review and suggestion of a clinical oral care guideline for irradiated patients," *Journal of Applied Oral Science*, vol. 19, no. 5, pp. 448–454, 2011.

45

Mimicking Myelodysplastic Syndrome: Importance of Differential Diagnosis

Thomas Luo,[1] Joanna Zurko,[1] John Astle,[2] and Nirav N. Shah[1]

[1]*BMT & Cellular Therapy Program, Division of Hematology & Oncology, Medical College of Wisconsin, Milwaukee, WI, USA*
[2]*Department of Pathology, Medical College of Wisconsin, Milwaukee, WI, USA*

Correspondence should be addressed to Nirav N. Shah; nishah@mcw.edu

Academic Editor: Kostas Konstantopoulos

Copper deficiency is a rare nutritional deficiency with hematological manifestations that mimic those found in myelodysplastic syndrome, a hematological malignancy incurable without allogeneic hematopoietic stem cell transplantation. Bone marrow biopsy findings and peripheral blood counts are oftentimes insufficient to differentiate the two conditions. Moreover, the symptoms of copper deficiency can arise years after the surgery, making diagnosis a challenge. In patients with new-onset pancytopenia, copper deficiency must be considered on the differential, especially in the setting of known risk factors such as bariatric surgery, zinc supplementation, and celiac disease. Herein, we present a case of a 61-year-old female with a remote history of gastric bypass being evaluated for MDS in the context of progressive pancytopenia and new-onset paresthesias. The patient was found to have low serum copper and ceruloplasmin. Copper supplementation largely resolved the hematological abnormalities, but the limb paresthesias remain. This case highlights the need to identify copper deficiency early and distinguish it from MDS in order to prevent permanent neurological deficits and catastrophic response should the patient undergo hematopoietic stem cell transplantation.

1. Introduction

Myelodysplastic syndrome (MDS) is a hematological malignancy that presents with pancytopenia, ineffective hematopoiesis, and cytogenetic abnormalities; the condition is considered incurable without an allogeneic stem cell transplant (allo-HCT) [1]. The diagnosis is made through bone marrow biopsy evaluation and requires appropriate exclusion of other causes of cytopenias, e.g., nutritional deficiencies, drug toxicities, infection, and autoimmune disease [2]. Several conditions can mimic MDS with potentially catastrophic consequences should the patient proceed towards allo-HCT [3]. In this report, we describe a case of copper deficiency initially diagnosed as MDS to emphasize the need to rule out nutritional deficiency in the workup of patients with suspected MDS. IRB submission was deferred per institutional policy for case series including less than 3 patients.

2. Case Report

A 61-year-old female with a history of alcoholism, vitamin B12 deficiency, and remote gastric bypass was referred to hematology with a two-month history of shortness of breath and cytopenias. She admitted to consuming 2–4 alcoholic drinks weekly and had just recently resumed B12 supplementation. Complete blood count revealed a severe macrocytic anemia (6.6 g/dL), MCV (108 fl), and neutropenia (ANC 520/μL). She had an elevated vitamin B12 level reflective of recent intramuscular supplementation (Table 1). Bone marrow biopsy was performed and revealed a hypercellular marrow for age (75%) and dyserythropoiesis but without cytogenetic and dysplastic changes characteristic of MDS. However, early MDS could not be ruled out. Despite two months of B12 supplementation, her anemia and leukopenia did not improve, and she required further transfusion. Direct Coombs testing, lactate

TABLE 1: Laboratory values.

	Initial presentation	+2 months	+4 months allo-HCT consult	1 month postcopper replacement
WBC, K/μL	**1.3**	**1.4**	**0.8**	4.3
ANC, K/μL	**0.7**	**0.4**	**0.29**	3.3
MCV	**108**	96	97	93
Hgb, g/dL	**6.6**	**7.1**	**7.3**	**11.6**
PLT, K/μL	222	191	**144**	157
Vit B12 (211–911)	>2000	—	507	—
Copper (80–155)	—	—	**<10**	107
Ceruloplasmin (17–54)	—	—	**<3**	—

WBC, white blood cell; ANC, absolute neutrophil count; MCV, mean corpuscular volume; Hgb, hemoglobin; PLT, platelet; Vit, vitamin. Bolded values are abnormal.

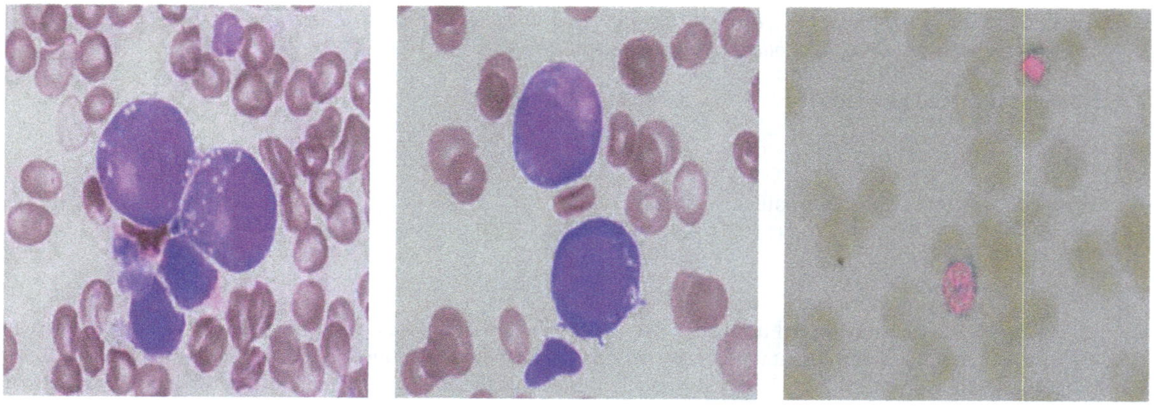

(a) (b) (c)

FIGURE 1: (a-b) Wright Giemsa-stained bone marrow aspirate smear slide (l000x magnification) showing neutrophil precursors (a) and an erythroid precursor (b) bottom with cytoplasmic vacuoles. (c) Prussian blue-stained bone marrow aspirate smear slide (l000x magnification) showing ring sideroblasts.

dehydrogenase, reticulocyte count, haptoglobin, and methylmalonic acid testing revealed no significant abnormalities. Daily prednisone (40 mg) was started as empiric treatment for potential occult autoimmune condition with no efficacy. The patient's anemia continued to worsen (5.7 g/dL) requiring further transfusion with progressive neutropenia. Additionally, she developed bilateral foot paresthesias, which were felt to be due to Raynaud's phenomena. A repeat bone marrow biopsy now revealed a hypocellular bone marrow (20–30%) with erythroid hyperplasia and dyserythropoiesis. A presumptive diagnosis of MDS (R-IPSS 3) was made, and the patient was referred for allo-HCT evaluation.

At time of consultation, the patient reported taking a daily zinc supplement for several years for a previously diagnosed deficiency. The combined history of gastric bypass and high zinc intake raised suspicion for copper deficiency, and additional labs were drawn. Both serum ceruloplasmin (<3 mg/dL) and copper (10 μg/dL) were below the lower limits of diagnostic testing, and serum zinc (151 μg/dL) was elevated. Hematopathology review of the second bone marrow biopsy showed vacuolated precursors and ring sideroblasts commonly seen in copper deficiency (Figure 1). Accordingly, the patient was started on IV cupric chloride (2 g) daily for 5 days and then once weekly for four weeks. At one-month follow-up, the patient's anemia improved and leukopenia resolved (Table 1). Although her energy level improved, her paresthesia remained.

3. Discussion

Copper deficiency is a rare nutritional condition that results in reversible hematologic findings—anemia and neutropenia—and often irreversible neurologic manifestations—optic neuropathy, paresthesia, and spasticity [4]. The most common etiologies of copper deficiency in the United States are gastric bypass surgery, excessive zinc intake, and celiac disease [4, 5]. Since the majority of copper is absorbed in the stomach and duodenum, gastric bypass surgery significantly increases risk of copper deficiency [4, 6]. The utility of prophylactic oral copper supplementation or serum copper monitoring in bariatric surgery patients is well established [6, 7]. Zinc primarily upregulates expression of metallothionein in enterocytes, which binds copper to a greater extent than zinc, thereby sequestering copper within the intestinal tract [4, 8].

While our patient had risk factors for development of copper deficiency, her age and clinical presentation were suggestive of MDS [9]. The early signs of insufficiency of hematopoiesis seen in copper deficiency—cytopenias and dysplastic changes—mimic those seen in clonal expansion driven diseases such as MDS—a condition encountered more frequently [10, 11]. Although not pathognomonic for copper deficiency, intracytoplasmic vacuoles in precursor cells and ring sideroblasts are subtle findings often observed on bone marrow biopsy as found in this patient; cytogenetic changes are not found in copper deficiency [10, 12]. Although the mechanism of copper deficiency anemia is unclear, copper is a vital coenzyme in the function of hephaestin—responsible for the oxidation of dietary iron—and ceruloplasmin—responsible for the transfer of iron from macrophages/monocytes to plasma [4, 13].

4. Conclusion

In this report, we highlight the clinical progression of occult copper deficiency. Although our patient's copper deficiency was initially misdiagnosed, prompt treatment with IV cupric chloride ameliorated the hematological and constitutional symptoms of low copper. Since delayed treatment of copper deficiency can result in permanent neurological impairment, clinicians should promptly rule out copper deficiency in patients being evaluated for MDS, especially if presenting with neurological symptoms [4, 14]. The steady rise of bariatric surgeries performed to curb the obesity epidemic will likely increase the prevalence of nutritional deficiencies, including copper deficiency [15]. Most importantly, early diagnosis can alleviate symptoms and spare patients' toxicities associated with chemotherapeutic agents or allo-HCT.

Disclosure

This study was performed as part of employment or enrollment at the Medical College of Wisconsin.

References

[1] M. Cazzola, "Myelodysplastic syndromes," *New England Journal of Medicine*, vol. 383, no. 14, pp. 1358–1374, 2020.

[2] G. Montalban-Bravo and G. Garcia-Manero, "Myelodysplastic syndromes: 2018 update on diagnosis, risk-stratification and management," *American Journal of Hematology*, vol. 93, no. 1, pp. 129–147, 2018.

[3] D. P. Steensma, "Dysplasia has A differential diagnosis: distinguishing genuine myelodysplastic syndromes (MDS) from mimics, imitators, copycats and impostors," *Curr Hematol Malig Rep*, vol. 7, no. 4, pp. 310–320, 2012.

[4] Z. W. Myint, T. H. Oo, K. Z. Thein, A. M. Tun, and H. Saeed, "Copper deficiency anemia: review article," *Annals of Hematology*, vol. 97, no. 9, pp. 1527–1534, 2018.

[5] M. Altarelli, N. Ben-Hamouda, A. Schneider, and M. M. Berger, "Copper deficiency: causes, manifestations, and treatment," *Nutrition in Clinical Practice*, vol. 34, no. 4, pp. 504–513, 2019.

[6] P. Kumar, N. Hamza, and B. Madhok, "Copper deficiency after gastric bypass for morbid obesity: a systematic review," *Obesity Surgery*, vol. 26, no. 6, pp. 1335–1342, 2016.

[7] V. Tatineni, J. Y. An, M. R. Leffew, and S. A. Mahesh, "Anemia from A to zinc: hypocupremia in the setting of gastric bypass and zinc excess," *Clinical Case Reports*, vol. 8, no. 4, pp. 745–750, 2020.

[8] H. N. Hoffman, R. L. Phyliky, and C. R. Fleming, "Zinc-induced copper deficiency," *Gastroenterology*, vol. 94, no. 2, pp. 508–512, 1988.

[9] X. Ma, "Epidemiology of myelodysplastic syndromes," *The American Journal of Medicine*, vol. 125, no. 7, pp. S2–S5, 2012.

[10] G. D'Angelo, "Copper deficiency mimicking myelodysplastic syndrome," *Blood Research*, vol. 51, no. 4, pp. 217–219, 2016.

[11] R. P. Hasserjian, "Myelodysplastic syndrome updated," *Pathobiology*, vol. 86, no. 1, pp. 7–13, 2019.

[12] V. Visconte, R. V. Tiu, and H. J. Rogers, "Pathogenesis of myelodysplastic syndromes: an overview of molecular and non-molecular aspects of the disease," *Blood Research*, vol. 49, no. 4, pp. 216–227, 2014.

[13] G. J. Anderson, D. M. Frazer, A. T. McKie, and C. D. Vulpe, "The ceruloplasmin homolog hephaestin and the control of intestinal iron absorption," *Blood Cells Molecules and Diseases*, vol. 29, no. 3, pp. 367–375, 2002.

[14] K. Juhasz-Pocsine, S. A. Rudnicki, R. L. Archer, and S. I. Harik, "Neurologic complications of gastric bypass surgery for morbid obesity," *Neurology*, vol. 68, no. 21, pp. 1843–1850, 2007.

[15] W. J. English, E. J. DeMaria, and M. M. Hutter, "American Society for Metabolic and Bariatric Surgery 2018 estimate of metabolic and bariatric procedures performed in the United States," *Surgery for Obesity and Related Diseases*, vol. 16, no. 4, pp. 457–463, 2020.

Durable Leukemic Remission and Autologous Marrow Recovery with Random Chromosomal Abnormalities after Allogeneic Hematopoietic Stem Cell Transplantation for Chronic Lymphocytic Leukemia

Hidekazu Nishikii,[1] Naoki Kurita,[1] Atsushi Shinagawa,[2] Tatsuhiro Sakamoto,[1] Manabu Kusakabe,[1] Yasuhisa Yokoyama,[1] Takayasu Kato,[1] Mamiko Sakata-Yanagimoto,[1] Naoshi Obara,[1] Yuichi Hasegawa,[1] Naoya Nakamura,[3] and Shigeru Chiba[1]

[1]*Department of Hematology, Faculty of Medicine, University of Tsukuba, Tsukuba, Japan*
[2]*Department of Hemato-Oncology, Hitachi General Hospital, Hitachi, Japan*
[3]*Department of Pathology, Tokai University, Tokyo, Japan*

Correspondence should be addressed to Shigeru Chiba; schiba-t@md.tsukuba.ac.jp

Academic Editor: Yusuke Shiozawa

A 38-year-old woman with aggressive clinical course of chronic lymphocytic leukemia (CLL) was treated with 8 courses of R-CHOP. Clinical remission was achieved, while B-cell clonality remained. Allogeneic hematopoietic stem cell transplantation was performed with reduced intensity conditioning (fludarabine and 2-Gy total body irradiation). However, autologous hematopoietic recovery occurred within a month after the transplant. Nevertheless, B-cell clonality became undetectable at 14 days after transplant, which has been kept so for over 10 years with clinical remission. Cytogenetic analyses were repeatedly performed and demonstrated nonclonal chromosomal aberrations, although the patient did not develop any secondary malignancies. One possible explanation for the clinical course is a very short-term allogeneic immune reaction helping eradication of residual CLL cells.

1. Introduction

Chronic lymphocytic leukemia (CLL) is a clonal B-cell neoplasm, which is generally slowly progressive but difficult to be cured even with current chemoimmunotherapy. Allogeneic hematopoietic stem cell transplantation (allo-HSCT) is a possible therapeutic choice for disease cure, although the indication of allo-HSCT for CLL is limited because of the advances of treatment options with lower morbidity. Here, we report a case of durable molecular remission of CLL with autologous marrow recovery after allo-HSCT. The patient demonstrated the recovery of recipient-derived hematopoietic system within one month after allo-HSCT but did not show any signs of CLL relapse even 10 years after allo-HSCT. This is a report of a rare case implying that a cure of CLL could be achieved possibly by a very short-term allogeneic immune reaction. Repeated cytogenetic studies after autologous recovery are accompanied with a detailed description of random chromosomal abnormalities.

2. Case Presentation

A 38-year-old woman with systemic lymphadenopathy and fever was admitted to a local hospital. Performance status was 2 according to the Eastern Cooperative Oncology Group criteria [1]. White blood cell count (WBC) was 21×10^9/L, with 91% of nucleated cells being small and mature lymphocytes. Mild anemia (hemoglobin, 10.8 g/dl) and moderate thrombocytopenia (platelet number, 46×10^9/L) were also observed (Table 1). Flow cytometric analysis revealed that the increased lymphocytes were positive for CD5, CD19, CD20, CD23, and IgGλ (Figure 1(a)). *IgH/cyclinD1* translocation was negative in fluorescence in situ hybridization analysis. Cytogenetic analysis of bone marrow cells demonstrated the normal karyotype. She also demonstrated elevated levels of aspartate transaminase (156 IU/l; normal 13–30 U/l), alanine transaminase (139 IU/l; normal, 7–23 U/l), lactate dehydrogenase (595 IU/l; normal, 124–232 U/l), and total bilirubin (1.8 g/dl; normal, 0.4–1.5 mg/dl). Soluble interleukin-2 receptor was also markedly elevated (10,400 U/ml; normal, 190–650 U/ml; Table 1 and Figure 2). Contrast computed tomography revealed multiple lymphadenopathy, hepatosplenomegaly, bilateral pleural effusion, and massive ascites. Bone marrow biopsy demonstrated a remarkable infiltration of small mature lymphocytes (57% of the total bone marrow cells). Immunophenotype of the major population was the same as that of peripheral blood lymphocytes. A small number of relatively large, blastic lymphocytes were diffusely observed in the bone marrow. Polymerase chain reaction (PCR) analysis demonstrated a single complementarity determining region (CDR-III) signal, indicating clonal B-cell proliferation. Taken together, she was diagnosed to have CLL (Rai stage IV and Binet stage C).

Because of her aggressive disease presentation and suspect of Richter syndrome, R-CHOP therapy (rituximab 375 mg/m^2, cyclophosphamide 750 mg/m^2, daunorubicin 50 mg/m^2 for one day, and prednisolone 100 mg/body for 5 days) was chosen as an initial therapy. After the treatment, her lymphadenopathy, hepatosplenomegaly, pleural effusion, and ascites were improved and 8 courses of R-CHOP were given. Morphologic CLL cells disappeared in peripheral blood. However, flow cytometric analysis revealed that 0.17% of the total bone marrow cells were leukemic cells and that the same single CDR-III signal as the one detected at the diagnosis was confirmed by PCR. These observations suggested the presence of minimum residual diseases (MRD), even after additional three courses of rituximab monotherapy.

Because of young age, suspect of Richter syndrome, and remaining MRD, the patient was referred to the University of Tsukuba Hospital 21 months after the diagnosis for allo-HSCT. The graft was bone marrow from an unrelated female donor with one-allele mismatched HLA. Nonmyeloablative conditioning regimen was chosen containing fludarabine 30 mg/m^2 for 3 days and 2-Gy total body irradiation. Tacrolimus and short-term methotrexate were used for graft-versus-host disease (GVHD) prophylaxis (Figure 2). On day 14, neutrophil engraftment was achieved, and the MRD judged by PCR for CDR-III became undetectable with the bone marrow cells. Donor-cell chimerism in the bone marrow was 70.4%, when evaluated by short tandem repeat-(STR-) PCR analysis. However, a progressive neutropenia was observed from day 20, when peripheral blood cells showed decreased donor chimerism down to 14.2%. On day 24, STR-PCR of bone marrow cells revealed 100% recipient type, suggesting rejection of the donor graft. Favorably, however, the multilineage cytopenia was gradually improved, and single CDR-III signal was never detected after the transplant. On day 62, WBC was 34×10^9/L with 42.7% neutrophils and 41.8% lymphocytes. Hemoglobin was 10.2 g/dl, and the platelet number was 146×10^9/L. These observations suggested that autologous bone marrow recover with remission of CLL. No apparent acute GVHD was observed. Leukemic cells were never detected in the bone

Table 1: Laboratory findings at the initial diagnosis.

Peripheral blood	
WBC	**21 × 109/l**
Seg	**3%**
Band	**1%**
Lymph	**70%**
A-lym	**21%**
Mono	**2%**
Eos	0%
Baso	1%
RBC	**308 × 104/μl**
Hb	**10.8 g/dl**
Plt	**46 × 109/l**
Coagulation	
PT	12.1 sec
APTT	27.1 sec
Fib	241 mg/dl
AT	86%
FDP	5.1 μg/ml
Blood chemistry	
TP	**6.0 g/dl**
Alb	3.8 g/dl
AST	**156 U/l**
ALT	**139 U/l**
LDH	**595 IU/l**
GGT	**319 U/l**
ALP	**2022 U/l**
ChE	**163 U/l**
T-bil	**1.8 mg/dl**
D-bil	**1.1 mg/dl**
AMY	58 U/l
CK	29 U/l
BUN	16 mg/dl
Cre	0.7 mg/dl
Na	142 mEq/l
K	4.0 mEq/l
Ca	9.1 mg/dl
CRP	**1.19 mg/dl**
β2MG	**5.41 mg/l**
Ferritin	102.5 ng·ml
sIL-2R	**10400 U/ml**
Immunology	
IgG	615 mg/dl
IgA	**50 mg/dl**
IgM	**17 mg/dl**
C3	**124 mg/dl**
C4	36 mg/dl
CH50	**51.5 U/ml**

Bold means the abnormal laboratory value.

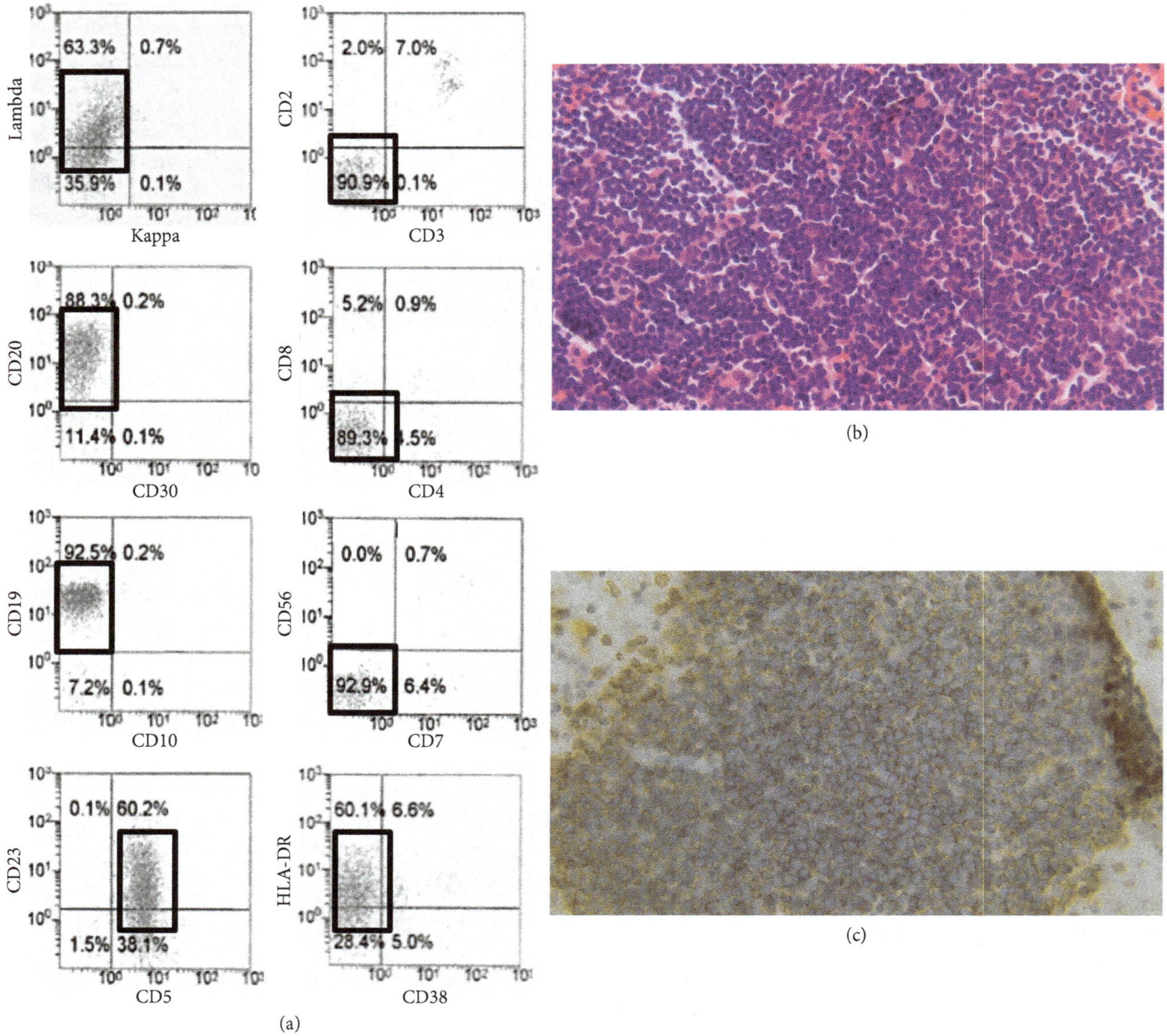

FIGURE 1: (a). Flow cytometric analysis of peripheral blood at diagnosis. □ means leukemic cell gate. Leukemic cells are positive in IgGλ, CD20, CD19, CD23, CD5, and HLA-DR. (b) Hematoxylin and eosin staining of leukemic cells in the bone marrow clot (× 400). (c) Immunostaining of CD20 (× 400).

marrow or peripheral blood in flow cytometry even 10 years after the transplant. There were no chronic GVHD-like symptoms or signs. Cytogenetic studies were repeated 15 times over 10 years for the screening purpose to detect emergence of clonal cells. In total, 299 metaphase cells were analyzed, and abnormalities were found in 50 cells (16.7%, Table 2). Abnormalities in 7q22 were found in four cells at 3 independent studies performed at 53 through 61 months after the transplant. However, the 7q22 abnormalities were detected only temporarily and were never found thereafter until 136 months after the transplant. All the other abnormalities were seen only one time. All this agrees with the concept of random chromosomal abnormalities (RCA) seen in automarrow recovery after receiving high-dose ionizing radiation exposure [2]. Despite the careful follow-up, the patient has been evaluated not to develop any clonal disorders such as myelodysplastic syndromes (MDS). Her blood cell counts and lymphocytes number were within the normal range at the last visit (140 months after the transplant), and there was no dysplastic changes in peripheral blood and bone marrow cells.

3. Discussion

CLL, the most common mature B-cell neoplasm in Caucasians, is generally prevalent in elderly people, although it is also present in younger adults. In the current therapeutic strategy for CLL [3–5], the indication of allo-HSCT is very limited. In the report from Fred Hutchinson Cancer Research Center, allo-HSCT with fludarabine plus low-dose total body irradiation regimen improved overall survival (OS; 5-year OS, 50%) and progression-free survival (PFS; 5-year PFS, 39%) in CLL patients [6]. However, the other literatures reported that the risk of graft rejection in

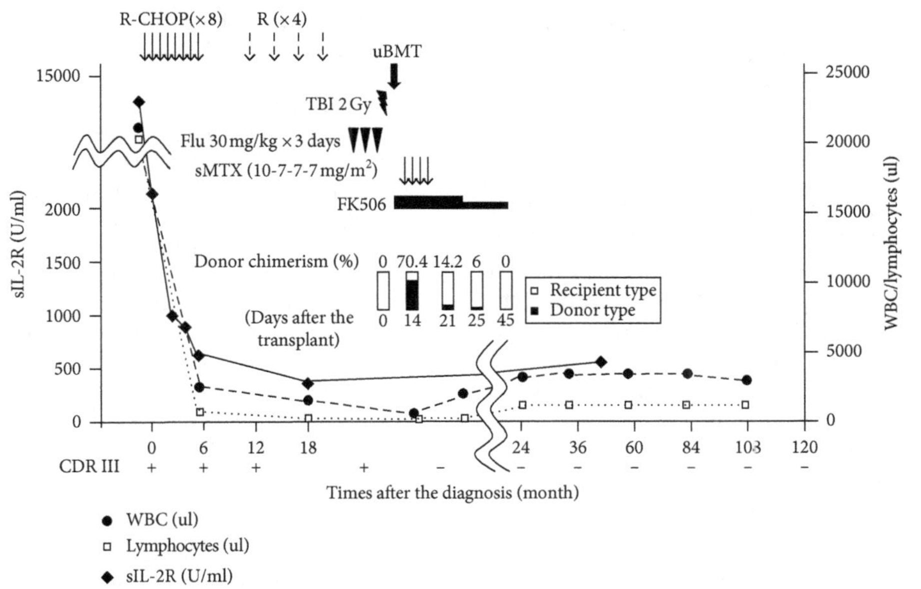

FIGURE 2: Clinical course. Absolute number or white blood cells (WBC, ●), lymphocytes (□), and soluble IL2-receptor (sIL-2R, ◆) were shown in graph. R-CHOP, rituximab, cyclophosphamide, doxorubicin, vincristine, and prednisolone; Flu, fludarabine; TBI, total body irradiation; uBMT, unrelated bone marrow transplantation; sMTX, short-term methotrexate; CDR III, complementarity determining region III.

TABLE 2: Random chromosomal abnormalities after autologous hematopoietic recovery.

Days after the transplant (month)	Karyotype (number of cells)	Number of abnormal karyotypes	Number of the metaphase
At diagnosis	46,XX[20]	(0)	(20)
45 (1)	46,XX,t(8;11)(p23;p21)[1] / 46,XX,t(8;22)(p21;p13)[1] / 46,XX[18]	2	20
172 (24)	46,XX,t(2;3)(p23;q29)[1] / 46,XX[19]	1	20
886 (29)	46,XX,add(1)(p11),add(2)(p11.2),−8,add(12)(q13),+mar1[3] / 46,XX [17]	3	20
1257 (41)	46,XX,t(3;3)(p11;p25)[2] / 46,X,t(X;8)(p22.3;q13)[1] / 46,XX,t(11;15)(q23;q15)[1] / 46,XX[15]	4	19
1623 (53)	46,XX,del(7)(q?)[3]* / 46,XX,t(12;15)(q24.1;q22)[1] / 46,XX,add(4)(q12),add(6)(p21),der(6) t(4;6)(q12;q21)[1] / 46,XX[15]	5	20
1819 (59)	46,XX,add(7)(q22)[1]*/46,XX,t(1;3)(p36.3;p21)[1] / 46,X,?t(X;16)(q22;q24),t(1;13)(p35.3;q14) [1] / 46,XX,t(13;20)(q14;q13.1)[1] / 46,X,?inv(X)(p11.2q21),t(5;16)(q31;p13.3)[1] / 46,XX[15]	5	20
1861 (61)	46,XX,add(7)(q22)[2]*/ 46,XX,del(7)(q22),add(19)(q13.3)[1]*/ 46,XX[17]	3	20
2022 (66)	46,XX,t(5;11)(q13;q21)[1] / 46,XX,t(5;13)(q13;q21)[1] / 46,XX,t(5;9)(q22;q34)[1] / 46XX,t(1; 15;13;13)(q32;q15;p12;q12),?t(4;11)(p16;q23)[1] / 46, XX[16]	4	20
2169 (71)	46,XX,t(3;3)(p25; q21)[1]/46,XX,t(7;11)(p13;q22)[1] / 46,XX,t(9;16)(q22;q24)[1] / 46,XX,t(16; 21)(q12-13;q22)[1] / 46,XX[16]	4	20
2358 (77)	46,XX,t(4;5)(q35;q11.2)[2] / 46,XX,t(3;6)(q24;p25)[1] / 46,XX, add(10)(p13),−15,+mar[1] / 46,XX[16]	4	20
2547 (83)	46,XX,t(2;16)(q13;q24)[1] / 46,XX, t(2;4)(q37;q31)[1] / 46,XX,add(1)(p13),? add(3)(p25),der(22)t(1;22)(p22;q11.2)[1] / 46,XX[17]	3	20
2792 (91)	46,XX,der(1)inv(1)(p13;q21)t(1;5)(p13;q11.2),der(5)t(1;5)(p13;q11.2)[1] / 46,XX[19]	3	20
3184 (104)	46,XX,−4,add(5)(p15),−10,der(11)(q23),−12,−13,+4mar[1] / 46,XX,t(16;22)(q24;q11.2)[1] / 46,XX[18]	2	20
3821 (125)	45,XX,−2,t(3;9)(p25;q22)[1] / 46,XX,inv(11)(p15;q13)[1]/46, XX t(1;5)(p32;q13)[1] / 46,XX,−4,−5,−8,−10,−22,+5mar[1] / 47,XX,+5[1] / 46,XX[15]	5	20
4211 (138)	44,XX,t(1;6)(q12;q21),−4,−13[1] / 46,XX,inv(10)(q11.2q24)[1] / 46,XX[18]	2	20
	Total number of analyzed cells after the transplant	50	299

*Potential clone. The results of chromosomal analysis of bone marrow cells at several time points after allo-HSCT are shown above.

nonmyeloablative allo-HSCT for CLL was relatively high (12–25% with T-cell depleted grafts and 5–6% with unmanipulated grafts) [7]. High incidences of infectious complication are also concerned in allo-HSCT for CLL. Moreover, the recent advances of chemoimmunotherapy with lower morbidity decrease the indication of allo-HSCT for CLL. Therefore, allo-HSCT is currently considered only for the relapsing patients with *TP53* mutations and/or del

(17p), or patients who are refractory to repeated chemo-immunotherapies [4]. Transformation into more aggressive lymphoma, called as Richter syndrome, also could be considered for the indication of allo-HSCT [8].

In the current case, non-myeloablative allo-HSCT was performed after achieving first hematological remission of CLL based on the aggressive clinical presentation at diagnosis with the suspect of Richter syndrome and the persistence of MRD. Later, Richter syndrome was thought to be inaccurate because the frequencies of blastic lymphocytes at the diagnosis did not fulfill the criteria, and thus, arguments may remain regarding the clinical decision for allo-HSCT. Such patient would be treated with the other treatment options if current chemoimmunotherapies would be applicable. Anyhow, autologous bone marrow recovery resulted. No donor-type hematopoiesis was detectable at the level with STR-PCR, and there was no apparent GVHD. Autologous marrow recovery after allo-HSCT is sometimes observed in patients with chronic myelogenous leukemia, in the majority of those who eventually demonstrate the disease relapse [9, 10]. However, the long-term consequence after the post-allo-HSCT autologous marrow recovery in CLL is unclear. Given that we were not able to find any report describing a long-term outcome after autologous marrow recovery in CLL, the clinical course of the current case is considered to be extremely rare. There is no good evidence-based scenario that explains the mechanism how CLL cells were eradicated and have been controlled for a long time. One possibility may be that a very short-term allogeneic immune reaction soon after the transplantation has helped eradicate residual CLL cells. In any case, low tumor burden and non-myeloablative regimen with very weak cytotoxicity may have caused the recovery of patient's own hematopoietic system and durable remission of disease.

We also showed the results of repeated cytogenetic analyses, demonstrating RCA over 10 years after autologous marrow recovery (Table 2). RCA represents nonclonal chromosomal aberrations and are caused by external factors such as radiation, chemical, or others [11, 12], among which experiences of high-dose ionizing radiation are the most abundant [13, 14]. In the literature regarding cord blood transplant for a lethally irradiated nuclear accident victim [15], clonal and nonclonal chromosomal aberrations within 100 days after the transplant were documented. Given the fact that irradiation exposure is associated with an increased risk for MDS development even 40–60 years after the exposure [2], and careful follow-up is mandatory.

References

[1] M. M. Oken, R. H. Creech, D. C. Tormey et al., "Toxicity and response criteria of the eastern cooperative Oncology Group," *American Journal of Clinical Oncology*, vol. 5, no. 6, pp. 649–656, 1982.

[2] M. Iwanaga, W.-L. Hsu, M. Soda et al., "Risk of myelodysplastic syndromes in people exposed to ionizing radiation: a retrospective cohort study of nagasaki atomic bomb survivors," *Journal of Clinical Oncology*, vol. 29, no. 4, pp. 428–434, 2011.

[3] N. Jain and S. O'Brien, "Targeted therapies for CLL: practical issues with the changing treatment paradigm," *Blood Reviews*, vol. 30, no. 3, pp. 233–244, 2016.

[4] M. Hallek, "Chronic lymphocytic leukemia: 2015 Update on diagnosis, risk stratification, and treatment," *American Journal of Hematology*, vol. 90, no. 5, pp. 446–460, 2015.

[5] W. G. Wierda, A. D. Zelenetz, L. I. Gordon et al., "NCCN guidelines insights: chronic lymphocytic leukemia/small lymphocytic lymphoma, version 1.2017," *Journal of the National Comprehensive Cancer Network*, vol. 15, no. 3, pp. 293–311, 2017.

[6] M. L. Sorror, B. E. Storer, B. M. Sandmaier et al., "Five-year follow-up of patients with advanced chronic lymphocytic leukemia treated with allogeneic hematopoietic cell transplantation after nonmyeloablative conditioning," *Journal of Clinical Oncology*, vol. 26, no. 30, pp. 4912–4920, 2008.

[7] J. Delgado, D. W. Milligan, and P. Dreger, "Allogeneic hematopoietic cell transplantation for chronic lymphocytic leukemia: ready for prime time?," *Blood*, vol. 114, no. 13, pp. 2581–2588, 2009.

[8] J. El-Asmar and M. A. Kharfan-Dabaja, "Hematopoietic cell transplantation for richter syndrome," *Biology of Blood and Marrow Transplantation*, vol. 22, no. 11, pp. 1938–1944, 2016.

[9] C. Brunstein, B. Hirsch, J. Miller et al., "Non-leukemic autologous reconstitution after allogeneic bone marrow transplantation for Ph-positive chronic myelogenous leukemia: extended remission preceding eventual relapse," *Bone Marrow Transplantation*, vol. 26, no. 11, pp. 1173–1177, 2000.

[10] S. Maury, K. Belhadj, I. Chami, M. Kuentz, C. Cordonnier, and D. Bories, "Autologous reconstitution combined with durable leukemic remission after allogeneic BMT for CML: absence of persistence of a donor-derived T cell effector population," *Bone Marrow Transplantation*, vol. 28, no. 7, pp. 717–720, 2001.

[11] Z. Chen, R. Morgan, J. F. Stone, and A. A. Sandberg, "FISH: a useful technique in the verification of clonality of random chromosome abnormalities," *Cancer Genetics and Cytogenetics*, vol. 66, no. 1, pp. 73-74, 1993.

[12] T. S. McConnell, M. H. Duncan, and K. Foucar, "Do random (non-clonal) chromosome abnormalities in bone marrow predict a clone to come?," *Cancer Genetics and Cytogenetics*, vol. 53, no. 2, pp. 257–263, 1991.

[13] S. Chiba, A. Saito, S. Ogawa et al., "Transplantation for accidental acute high-dose total body neutron- and γ-radiation exposure," *Bone Marrow Transplantation*, vol. 29, no. 11, pp. 935–939, 2002.

[14] M. Horai, S. Satoh, M. Matsuo et al., "Chromosomal analysis of myelodysplastic syndromes among atomic bomb survivors in Nagasaki," *British Journal of Haematology*, vol. 180, no. 3, pp. 381–390, 2017.

[15] H. Nagayama, K. Misawa, H. Tanaka et al., "Transient hematopoietic stem cell rescue using umbilical cord blood for a lethally irradiated nuclear accident victim," *Bone Marrow Transplantation*, vol. 29, no. 3, pp. 197–204, 2002.

47

Salvage Therapy in Early Relapse of T-Lymphoblastic Leukemia/Lymphoma using Daratumumab/Nelarabine Combination: Two Consecutive Cases

Ingolf Molle, Irma Petruskevicius, Peter Kamper, and Francesco d'Amore

Department of Haematology, University Hospital of Aarhus, Aarhus, Denmark

Correspondence should be addressed to Ingolf Molle; ingolf.moelle@rm.dk

Academic Editor: Chihaya Imai

Treatment of early relapses of T lymphoblastic leukemia/lymphoma is often unsuccessful. We tested an experimental regimen containing daratumumab and nelarabine in two young patients with early relapses of T lymphoblastic lymphoma and T-ALL, respectively. Both patients achieved a deep complete remission. Combining daratumumab with chemotherapy may have a role in relapsing T lymphoblastic leukemia/lymphoma.

1. Introduction

Relapsing T lymphoblastic lymphoma/leukemia has a poor prognosis with up to 10% survivors after 2 years [1, 2]. In early relapses, the prognosis is extremely poor [1].

In relapsing young patients, possible remission induction treatments include traditional high-dose chemotherapy, such as FLAG-IDA or combination chemotherapy based on high-risk ALL protocols. Nelarabine, the prodrug of the deoxyguanosine analogue 9-beta-d-arabinofuranosylguanine used alone or more recently in combination chemotherapy, is another option [3].

Results are far from satisfying with roughly one-third of patients achieving a new remission [1, 2]. Second remissions are often short-lived, and subsequent relapses hamper stem cell transplant (SCT) in many patients.

T lymphoblasts usually express high levels of CD38 on the cell surface [4]. The human IgG1k monoclonal anti-CD38 antibody daratumumab has proven very potent in multiple myeloma, and a few observations have suggested a possible future role in T lymphoblastic leukemia/lymphoma [5–9].

We tested an experimental regimen based on daratumumab/nelarabine combination in two early relapses of T lymphoblastic leukemia/lymphoma. Both cases strongly expressed CD38 on the majority of the cancer cells, but a fraction of blasts was CD38 negative. A combination of daratumumab and nelarabine was therefore chosen.

2. Case 1

A 38-year-old male with no medical history presented with T lymphoblastic lymphoma with a large mediastinal bulk tumor but no bone marrow or CNS involvement. Though not registered in the NOPHO database (no bone marrow involvement), he was treated with NOPHO2008 high-risk induction (dexamethasone, daunorubicin, and vincristine) and achieved a complete structural and metabolic response after 30 days. He received consolidation chemotherapy per protocol (NOPHO.org), but unfortunately he had an early relapse during high-risk maintenance after 1 year of intense poly-chemotherapy. Bone marrow (73% infiltration), mediastinum, and pleurae were affected.

The prognosis was considered very poor. Treatment had already encompassed FLAG-IDA during the course, and nelarabine monotherapy was initially considered treatment of choice. Led by a brisk CD38 expression on 96% of the cancer cells in the bone marrow, we combined daratumumab, nelarabine, pegylated asparaginase, and dexamethasone as described in Table 1.

Table 1: Overview of salvage therapy with daratumumab/nelarabine combination.

	Case 1	Case 2
Daratumumab	16 mg/kg i.v., d1 weekly for 13 weeks (till start of conditioning)	16 mg/kg i.v., d1 weekly for 8 weeks and thereafter every 2 weeks till relapse (total 17 infusions)
Nelarabine	1500 mg/m2, d1, 3, 5 every 3 weeks, 4 courses	1500 mg/m2, d1, 3, 5 every 3 weeks, 2 courses
Dexamethasone	40 mg, d1–4 every 3 weeks, 4 courses	40 mg, d1–4 every two weeks, 2 courses
PEG-asparaginase	1000 mg/m2 i.m., d1 every 3 weeks, 4 courses	not used
PEG-filgrastim	6 mg s.c., d7 every 3 weeks, 4 courses	6 mg s.c., d7 every 3 weeks, 2 courses
Effect on relapse of T-lymphoblast disease	CR : bone marrow after 3 weeks CR : PET/CT scan after 6 weeks	Partial remission after 3 weeks CR, neg. PCR after 6 weeks CR, neg. PCR and FC after 9 weeks Second relapse d196
Side effects, first 3 weeks	Bone marrow impairment, need for transfusions	Fatigue, sore muscles first few days Thrombocytopenia
Side effects, subsequent weeks	Grade I-II sensory polyneuropathy (hands, feet) Bone marrow impairment Uncomplicated neutropenic fever Weakness	Grade III GVHD (liver, intestine) Bacteremia x 2 Bone marrow impairment Grade I sensory polyneuropathy (hands)
Side effects, after conditioning	Grade III-IV neurological impairment (see text)	No re-SCT

Treatment was well tolerated initially, and clinically the patient improved considerably within a few days. A complete remission with a negative bone marrow test after 3 weeks and a negative PET/CT scan after 6 weeks was seen. At this point, Grade I sensory poly-neuropathic symptoms in the hands were reported by the patient (CTCAE v5.0).

SCT was scheduled, and treatment was continued as described in Table 1 for 13 weeks. After nine weeks, the patient had an uncomplicated episode of neutropenic fever.

General weakness interfering with daily life and Grade II sensory polyneuropathy in hands and feet were seen until conditioning consisting of involved-field radiotherapy (mediastinum, 18 Gy in total), TBI (12 Gy in total) (testes 4 Gy), and cyclophosphamide (120 mg/kg).

During conditioning, over a few days, the patient developed a progressive severe neurological disability with a combination of spinal and peripheral ataxia, sensory loss, and pareses of upper and lower extremities. Sphincter functions were impaired. The symptoms were progressive till 3 weeks after SCT and then became stable for months. Some improvement has taken place later, but the patient remains considerably disabled—most neurological symptoms are still Grade III. He is alive with no signs of relapse 3½ years after transplantation. A moderate chronic GvHD is still treated with immunosuppressive drugs.

The neurological impairment was characterized by neurologists after MR scan showing medullopathy, as well as clinical and neurophysiological examinations. It was presumably caused by a combination of nelarabine and radiotherapy as reported earlier [10, 11]. A possible complicating role of daratumumab cannot be excluded but is not considered likely, given the well-known neurotoxic potential of nelarabine.

3. Case 2

A 25-year-old female with no medical history presented with T-ALL with 80% bone marrow involvement but no CNS affection. She was treated as per NOPHO2008 protocol. Due to a poor bone marrow response on day 15, she was referred to the high-risk arm aiming for a myeloablative SCT. She received 5 high-risk blocks but remained MRD positive. At SCT, her MRD was 1.7%, but the procedure was carried out, since we lacked an obvious better alternative. Conditioning regimen was etoposide 1800 mg/m^2 and TBI 12.5 Gy. No GvHD was seen in the course.

After 3 months, she had a bone marrow relapse (35% infiltration on flowcytometry, and 71% of cancer cells were strongly positive for CD38) without CNS infiltration.

As a consequence of the neurotoxicity seen in Case 1, we modified the combination regimen and treated with weekly daratumumab, only two three-day courses of nelarabine, and less dexamethasone as shown in Table 1.

The regimen was well tolerated. After 6 weeks, she had a complete remission, and for the first time in the entire treatment period, a negative MRD (flow cytometry and TCR gene rearrangement PCR) was seen after 9 weeks.

Daratumumab was continued as monotherapy weekly for 8 courses and then every two weeks. After a few weeks, she developed Grade III acute GvHD affecting liver and intestine. Daratumumab was stopped for 2 weeks while GvHD was diagnosed but was then started again. High-dose prednisolone and ciclosporine were administered without response. Four courses of infliximab 10 mg/kg weekly was added, and steroid was tapered. She had two episodes of septicaemia with *Aeromonas* and *Bacteroides*. Furthermore, a fungal infection was suspected and treated with posaconazole. The bone marrow function was weak, but neutrophils responded well to filgrastim, and gradually her condition improved.

We initially aimed for a second SCT, but due to the severe GvHD and her general condition after this complication, we went for long-term daratumumab treatment instead. Unfortunately, the leukemia relapsed 196 days after starting salvage therapy. MRD was 0.047% in multicolour flowcytometry and similar in PCR. At this second relapse, she was physically quite well, and ciclosporine was tapered without recurrence of GvHD. She did not want further medical treatment at this point but received homeopathic therapy abroad.

Ten weeks later, she was admitted with a clinical superior vena cava syndrome. A CT scan revealed large mediastinal lymphomas, pleural effusion, and lymphoma masses in mammary glands, around the large vessels, and within the posterior thoracic wall. She was treated with dexamethasone, nelarabine, and palliative radiotherapy (12 Gy in total). A short relief was seen, but ultimately, she died 5 months after positive MRD was identified.

4. Discussion

The two cases suggest a possible role for daratumumab/nelarabine combination in treatment of relapsing T lymphoblastic leukemia/lymphoma as a path to SCT in Case 1. Re-transplant had to be abandoned in Case 2 due to GvHD and the patient's general condition. Nevertheless, the duration of her second remission was long enough for a re-transplant, had it been possible. The usual short duration of CR2, hampering SCT, is a major challenge in these patients, and therefore we consider the apparent effect of combining daratumumab and nelarabine meaningful. In Case 2, however, a possible graft-versus-leukemia effect may have had a role in maintaining the CR2 for several months.

The treatment was effective as re-induction and initially well tolerated even in these heavily treated patients. Neurological side effects seen in Case 1 were most likely caused by an additive effect of nelarabine, total burden of other chemotherapy, and radiotherapy. For this reason, Case 2 only had two courses of nelarabine, and she only had a Grade I sensory polyneuropathy.

There were no indications of interactions between the two drugs, but this topic still needs attention.

A few case reports have suggested that daratumumab monotherapy may be effective as re-induction and palliative therapy in T lymphoblastic leukemia/lymphoma [5–7]. Use of daratumumab/nelarabine combination is addressed in two publications, but in the 4 cases described, the drugs were separated in time, as daratumumab was administered 3 weeks after de-bulking chemotherapy. The results were promising [8, 9]. One case had failed monotherapy with daratumumab just prior to chemotherapy with a large amount of leukemia in the bone marrow, but the drug seemed effective in diminishing MRD afterwards [8].

Conclusively, the role of daratumumab, alone or in combination, in relapsing T lymphoblastic leukemia/lymphoma is not clear at present. A prospective phase 2 trial of daratumumab monotherapy in relapsing ALL has enrolled 47 patients so far and will hopefully bring important new knowledge on monotherapy with daratumumab (ClinicalTrial.gov (NCT03384654)). Combining daratumumab with nelarabine or other chemotherapy may also be an emerging therapeutic option in relapsing T lymphoblastic leukemia/lymphoma, and results so far merit further tests.

References

[1] A. Oriol, S. Vives, J. M. Hernandez-Rivas et al., "Outcome after relapse of acute lymphoblastic leukemia in adult patients included in four consecutive risk-adapted trials by the PETHEMA Study Group," *Haematologica*, vol. 95, no. 4, pp. 589–596, 2010.

[2] D. I. Marks, E. M. Paietta, A. V. Moorman et al., "T-cell acute lymphoblastic leukemia in adults: clinical features, immunophenotype, cytogenetics, and outcome from the large randomized prospective trial (UKALL XII/ECOG 2993)," *Blood*, vol. 114, no. 25, pp. 5136–5145, 2009.

[3] C. M. McMahon and S. M. Luger, "Relapsed T cell ALL: current approaches and new directions," *Current Hematologic Malignancy Reports*, vol. 14, no. 2, pp. 83–93, 2019.

[4] K. L. Bride, T. L. Vincent, S.-Y. Im et al., "Preclinical efficacy of daratumumab in T-cell acute lymphoblastic leukemia," *Blood*, vol. 131, no. 9, pp. 995–999, 2018.

[5] s Mirgh, R. Ahmed, N. Agrawal et al., "Will Daratumumab be the next game changer in early thymic precursor-acute lymphoblastic leukaemia?" *British Journal of Haematology*, vol. 187, pp. e33–e34, 2019.

[6] A. Bonda, S. Punatar, A. Gokarn et al., "Daratumumab at the frontiers of post-transplant refractory T-acute lymphoblastic leukemia-a worthwhile strategy?" *Bone Marrow Transplantation*, vol. 53, no. 11, pp. 1487–1489, 2018.

[7] Y. Ofran, S. Ringelstein-Harlev, I. Slouzkey et al., "Daratumumab for eradication of minimal residual disease in high-risk advanced relapse of t-cell/cd19/cd22-negative acute lymphoblastic leukemia," *Leukemia*, vol. 34, pp. 293–295, 2020.

[8] J. Fulcher, P. Berardi, G. Christou, P. J. A. Villeneuve, C. Bredeson, and M. Sabloff, "Nelarabine-containing regimen followed by daratumumab as an effective salvage therapy and bridge to allogeneic hematopoietic stem cell transplantation for primary refractory early T-cell precursor lymphoblastic leukemia," *Leukemia and Lymphoma*, vol. 62, no. 9, pp. 2295–2297, 2021.

[9] Y. Ofran, C. Ganzel, S. Harlev et al., "Daratumumab in combination with vincristine or nelarabine as effective salvage therapy for patients with acute lymphoblastic leukemia at high risk for relapse," *Blood*, vol. 132, no. suppl 1, p. 5206, 2018.

[10] M. C. Tisi, G. Ausoni, M. G. Vita et al., "Clinical reversible myelopathy in T-cell lymphoblastic lymphoma treated with nelarabine and radiotherapy: report of a case and review of literature of an increasing complication," *Mediterranean Journal of Hematology and Infectious Diseases*, vol. 7, 2015.

[11] M. Kawakami, K. Taniguchi, S. Yoshihara et al., "Irreversible neurological defects in the lower extremities after haploidentical stem cell transplantation: possible association with nelarabine," *American Journal of Hematology*, vol. 88, no. 10, pp. 853–857, 2013.

Unusual B-Lymphoid Blastic Crisis as Initial Presentation of Chronic Myeloid Leukemia Imposes Diagnostic Challenges

Nouran Momen,[1] Bora Baysal,[2] Sheila Jani Sait,[2] Joseph Tario,[2] and You-Wen Qian[2]

[1]*Clinical & Chemical Pathology Department, Cairo University, Giza, Egypt*
[2]*Department of Pathology, Roswell Park Cancer Institute, 665 Elm Street, Buffalo, NY 14203, USA*

Correspondence should be addressed to You-Wen Qian; you-wen.qian@roswellpark.org

Academic Editor: Massimo Breccia

Chronic myeloid leukemia (CML) is a clonal hematopoietic stem cell disorder, characterized by reciprocal translocation *t*(9,22) (q34; q11), leading to increased myeloid proliferation. Most cases are diagnosed in the chronic phase (CP). However, a minority of cases can be present in the blastic phase (BP). In most patients with CML-BP, the blasts have a myeloid phenotype, however, in 20–30% of cases, the blasts have a lymphoid phenotype, mostly a B-cell phenotype. It is challenging to differentiate CML B-lymphoblastic phase (CML-BLP) from Ph + primary B-acute lymphoblastic leukemia (B-ALL) especially when the CML-BLP is the initial presentation of the disease, which is uncommon. We report here an unusual case of CML-BLP as an initial presentation of the disease without typical CML morphological findings. This case demonstrates diagnostic challenges and emphasizes the importance of an integrated approach using morphology, multiparametric flow cytometry, cytogenetic studies, and molecular studies to render an accurate diagnosis.

1. Introduction

Chronic myeloid leukemia (CML) is a myeloproliferative disorder characterized by the presence of the Philadelphia (Ph) chromosome generated by the reciprocal translocation *t*(9,22) (q34; q11), leading to the proliferation of granulocytes and their precursors. Around 50% of newly diagnosed CML patients are asymptomatic and are usually diagnosed when a white blood cell (WBC) count is found to be elevated during a routine medical examination [1]. Detection of BCR-ABL1 fusion is required for the diagnosis of CML. Meanwhile, Ph chromosome/BCR-ABL1 fusion is also the most common recurrent cytogenetic abnormality in B-lymphoblastic leukemia (B-ALL) in adults, representing around 25–30% of adult B-ALL cases [2]. Different fusion proteins are produced from different BCR-ABL1 fusion transcripts depending on the breakpoints within the breakpoint cluster region (BCR). The most common fusion proteins are p210 and p190, in which the breakpoints are located within the major BCR (M-BCR) and minor BCR (m-BCR), respectively. In CML, almost all cases are associated with the p210, and p190 is rarely detected, whereas in Ph + B-ALL, almost all cases are associated with p190, and p210 is detected in a minority of adult cases [3].

The natural progression of the disease usually follows a triphasic course; a chronic phase (CP), an accelerated phase (AP), and a blastic phase (BP). Most CML cases are diagnosed in the CP. Patients in AP have a blast count of 10–19% in the blood or bone marrow, and BP is characterized by more than 20% blasts in the blood or bone marrow. In most patients with CML-BP, the blasts show a myeloid phenotype, however, in 20–30% of cases the blasts show a lymphoid phenotype, usually B-lymphoblasts [4]. The BP can be the initial presentation of the disease in approximately 15% of adults and 5% of children, with blasts expressing a lymphoid phenotype in 20 to 30% of these cases [5], with rare *T* or mixed phenotypes [6]. In those cases, with AP or BP as the initial presentation with no prior history of CML, the presence of basophilia, myeloid hyperplasia, and

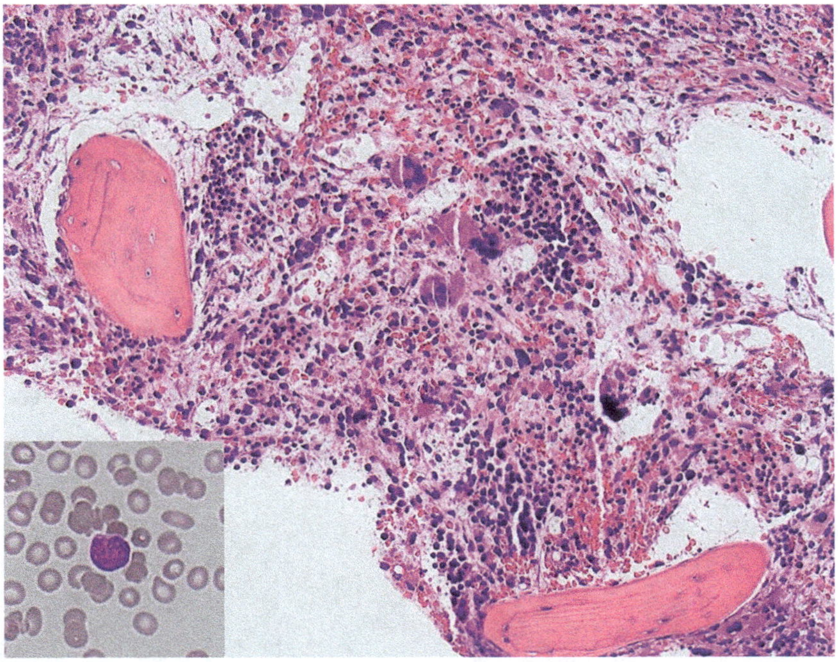

FIGURE 1: Hematoxylin and Eosin (H & E) stained bone marrow biopsy section showing hypercellular marrow with myeloid hypoplasia, erythroid hyperplasia, and increased atypical megakaryocytes (x200). An enclosed picture shows the morphology of the immature cells on a Wright-Giemsa-stained bone marrow aspirate smear (x400).

micromegakaryocytes ("dwarf" megakaryocytes) may be suspicious of underlying CML [4].

Here, we describe a case which had none of the above findings and yet was diagnosed as a case of CML-BLP to discuss the challenges we faced to reach a final diagnosis.

2. Case Presentation

We report a 69-year-old female with a history of atrial fibrillation and hyperlipidemia, presenting with a 1-month history of shortness of breath with an acute worsening of the condition. When she came to the emergency room (ER), she was hemodynamically stable and her oxygen saturation was 95% on room air. No organomegaly on the physical exam. Her complete blood count (CBC) showed pancytopenia with a white blood cell (WBC) of 1100/μL, a hemoglobin (Hg) level of 4.5 g/dL, and a platelet count of 107,000/μL. The differential count was within the normal ranges and no abnormal cells were seen on the blood smear. Her INR was 1.85 and her prothrombin time (PT) was 20.8 seconds. A bone marrow aspirate and biopsy (BMAB1) revealed about 6% immature cells on examination of the aspirate smears, while the biopsy examination showed a hypercellular bone marrow (80% cellularity) with a population of atypical immature B-cells (about 20–25%) together with myeloid hypoplasia, erythroid hyperplasia, atypical megakaryocytes, and marrow fibrosis (MF-2) as shown in Figure 1. These cells showed positive expression of CD34, TdT, CD20, PAX-5, and c-MYC by immunohistochemistry as seen in Figure 2.

Immunophenotyping by flow cytometry was performed on the bone marrow aspirate sample. A low-sensitivity leukemia panel was initially performed where a population of immature B-cells was identified. Although a hematogone population phenotype was considered in the differential, the moderate intensity of CD38 and homogenous expression of CD10 were concerning. A high-sensitivity COG B-precursor leukemia minimal residual disease (MRD) panel was subsequently performed, where 281,400 events were collected. B cells were measured at 10.7% of total cells and exhibited a spectrum of maturation. However, a subset of B cells expressed an atypical phenotype with heterogenous expression of CD45, CD34, and CD20 together with positive expression of CD19, CD10, CD38, CD9, CD24, bright expression of CD58, and dim expression of CD22. This population showed negative expression of CD13 and CD33. This immature population represented around 1.9% of total cells and was suspicious of a B-lymphoblastic leukemia/lymphoma (Figure 3).

Karyotyping performed on the bone marrow aspirate sample revealed a female karyotype with *t*(9,22) detected in 3/20 cells as illustrated in Figure 4.

Fluorescence in situ hybridization (FISH) studies were positive for BCR/ABL1 fusion seen in 24/200 cells examined. Among the BCR/ABL1 fusion positive cells, some have morphologic features of blasts, while cells with features of band neutrophils are also noted (Figure 5). and was negative for immunoglobulin heavy chain (IGH) gene rearrangements.

A subsequent bone marrow aspirate and biopsy (BMAB2) performed a few days later showed similar morphologic and immunophenotypic findings to those seen in BMAB1. Karyotyping detected *t*(9; 22) in 3/20 cells. PCR for BCR/ABL performed on the bone marrow aspirate sample was positive for BCR-ABL1 e13a2 (b2a2, p210)

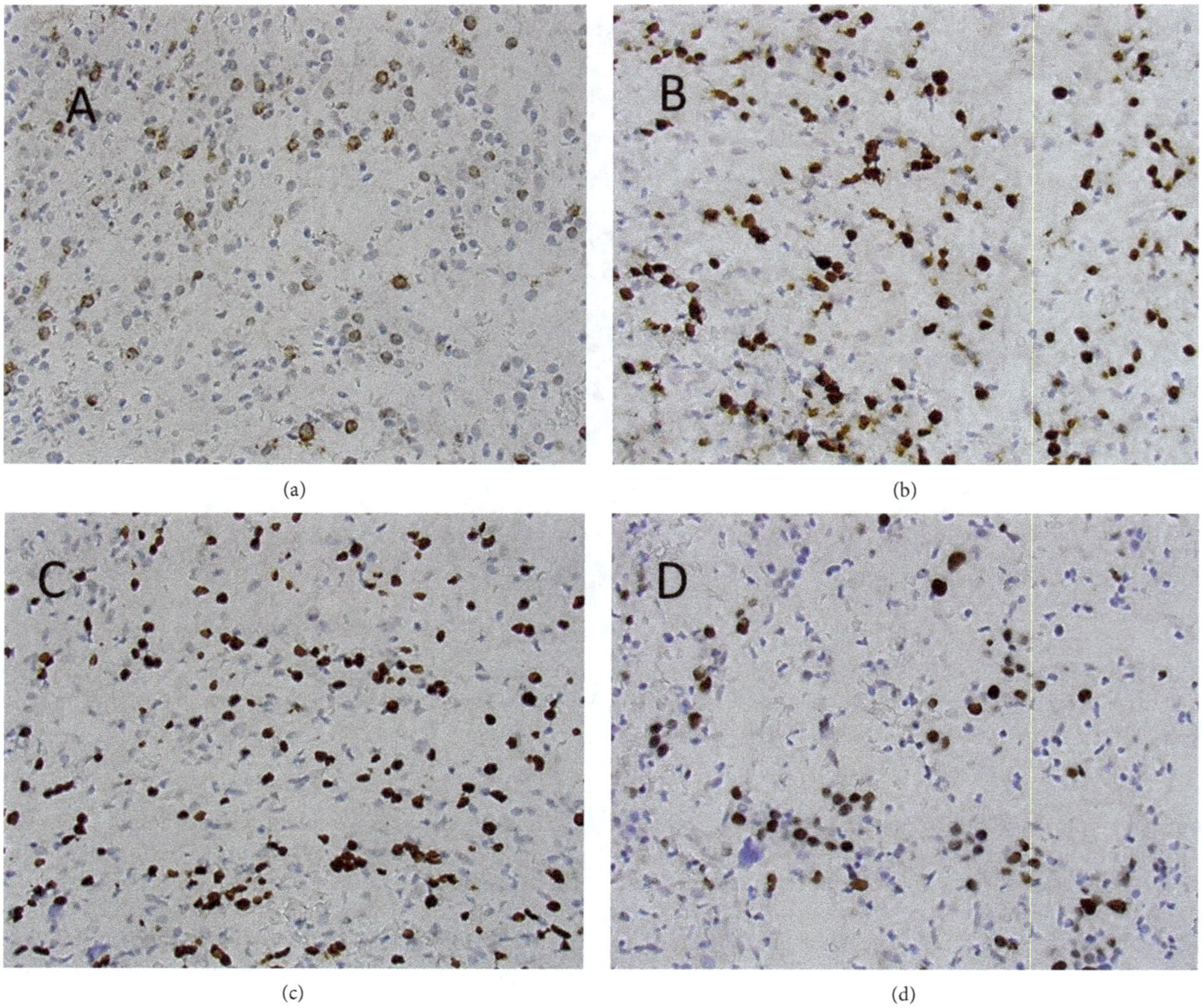

Figure 2: Immunohistochemistry-stained bone marrow biopsy sections showing: A-Positive CD34 staining in immature cells, B- Positive TdT staining in immature cells, C- Positive PAX-5 staining in immature cells, and D- Positive c-MYC staining in immature cells (x200).

fusion transcript, detected at an International Scale (IS) of more than 55%. A bone marrow aspirate and biopsy performed after 2 weeks (BMAB3) also showed similar findings to those noted in BMAB2.

A PET/CT skull-base to mild-thigh was done after BMAB3 that showed an intense hypermetabolic left axillary lymph node (LN) measuring 1.5 × 1 cm, while the spleen was normal in size with no metabolic signature of a tumor. A needle biopsy was taken from the left axillary LN and revealed a non-necrotizing granuloma with no evidence of lymphoid infiltrate (Figure 6). FISH studies done on the LN touch imprints were positive for BCR/ABL1 fusion in 22/200 cells.

Two months later, the patient came for a follow-up. Examination of the blood smear showed mildly left-shifted neutrophilia with 2% blasts. Bone marrow aspirate and biopsy (BMAB4) at this time revealed a hypercellular marrow (70%) with myeloid hyperplasia, 5% blasts, reduced erythroid precursors, and mild fibrosis (MF-1). Immunostains on the BM biopsy for CD34, TdT, and PAX-5 were positive in around 5% of immature B-cells. Immunophenotyping on the bone marrow aspirate revealed an abnormal population comprising 2.4% of total cells with positive expression of CD45 (dim), CD19, HLADR, CD7 (dim), CD13, CD34, CD38, CD10 (subset), CD33 (heterogenous), CD15 (dim subset), CD123 (dim), CD71 (heterogenous), CD117 (dim subset), TdT, cCD22 (dim) and cCD79a (heterogenous). This population is consistent with abnormal B-lymphoblasts with aberrant myeloid antigen expression. Karyotyping detected *t*(9; 22) in 11/20 cells. In addition, deletion 7 was detected in 8/20 cells. FISH studies were positive for BCR/ABL1 fusion in 162/200 cells and deletion 7 was detected in 52/200 cells analyzed. The emergence of deletion 7 by karyotyping and FISH as a new cytogenetic abnormality, along with the abnormal population detected morphologically and phenotypically, was highly suggestive of a case of CML in an accelerated phase.

Therapy was initiated with daily Dasatinib. Follow-up CBC around two months later showed normocytic normochromic anemia and leukopenia. Bone marrow examination (BMAB5) revealed a mildly hypercellular bone marrow for age (50%) with progressive trilineage

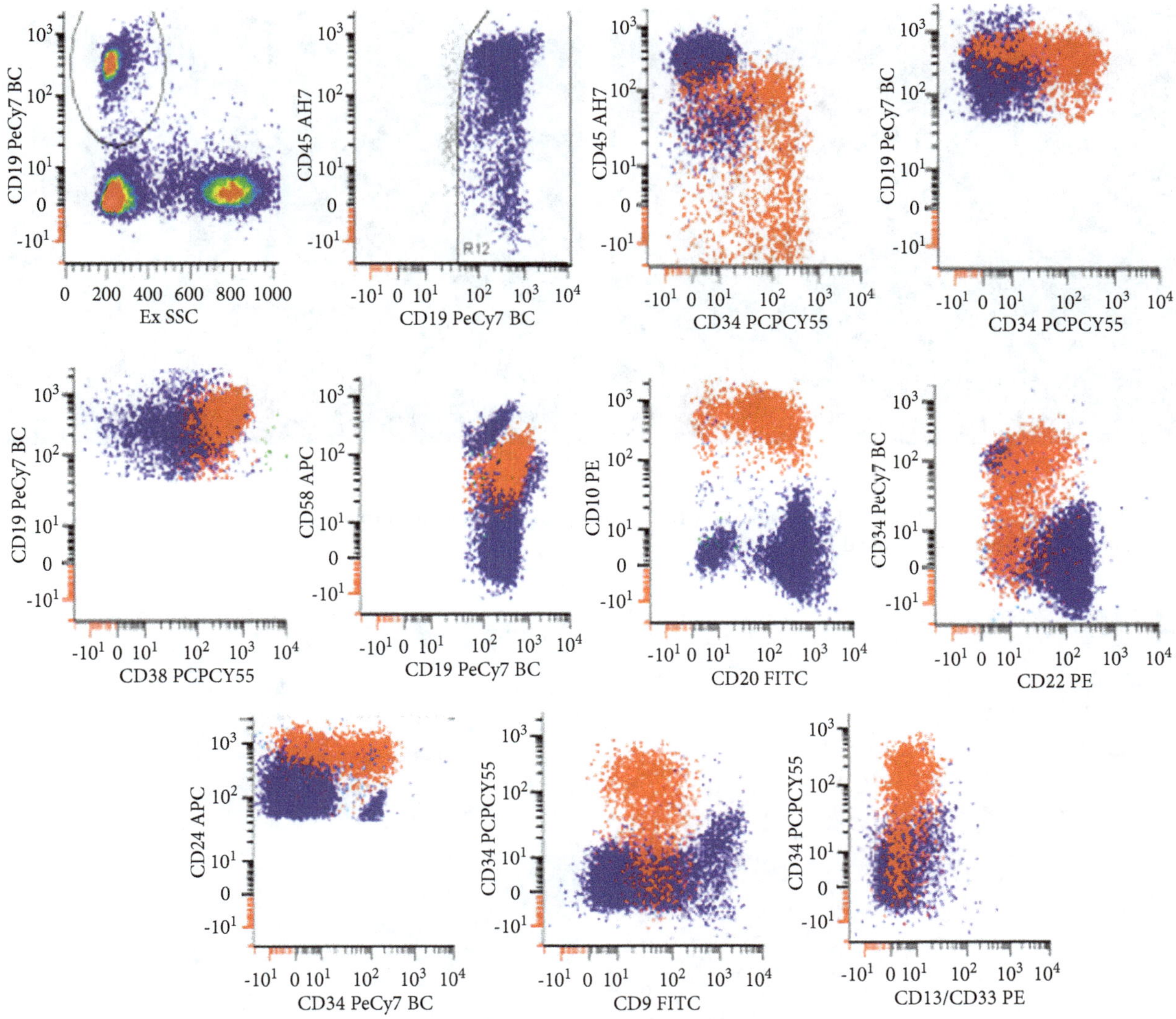

FIGURE 3: Flow cytometric immunophenotyping of the immature population in the bone marrow. The blasts express CD45 (heterogenous), CD19, CD34 (heterogeneous), CD38 (moderate), CD58 (bright), CD20, CD10, CD22 (dim), CD24 (heterogenous), CD9 (dim) and are negative for CD13 and CD33. B-lymphoblasts are red, mature B cells are blue.

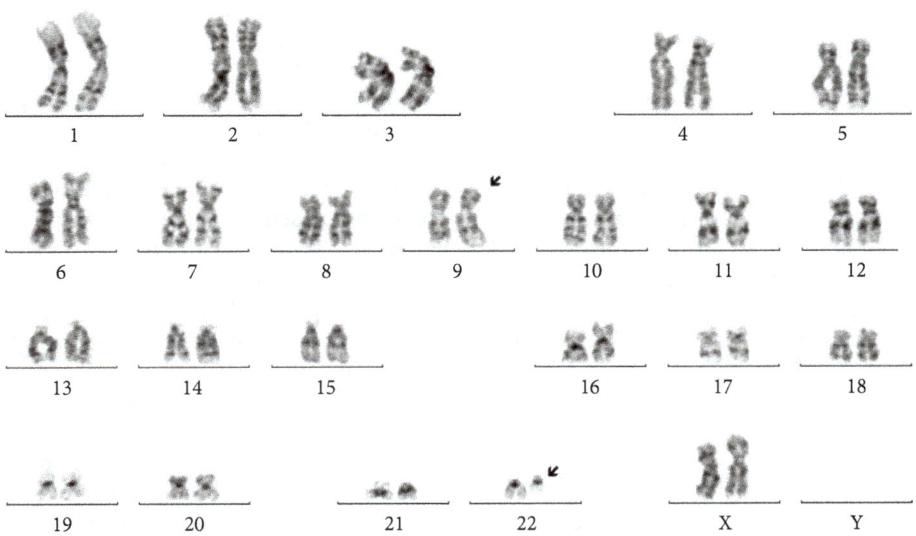

FIGURE 4: Conventional karyotyping shows positive $t(9, 22)$.

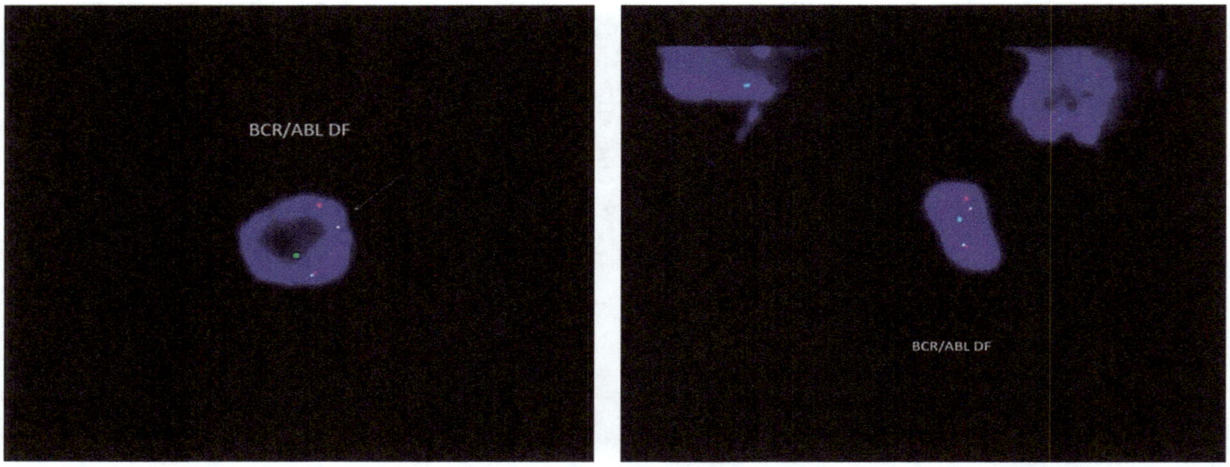

(a) (b)

FIGURE 5: FISH showing positive BCR/ABL1 translocation. (a) Fusion signal in a cell with morphologic feature of blast. (b) Fusion signal in a cell with morphologic features of a band neutrophil.

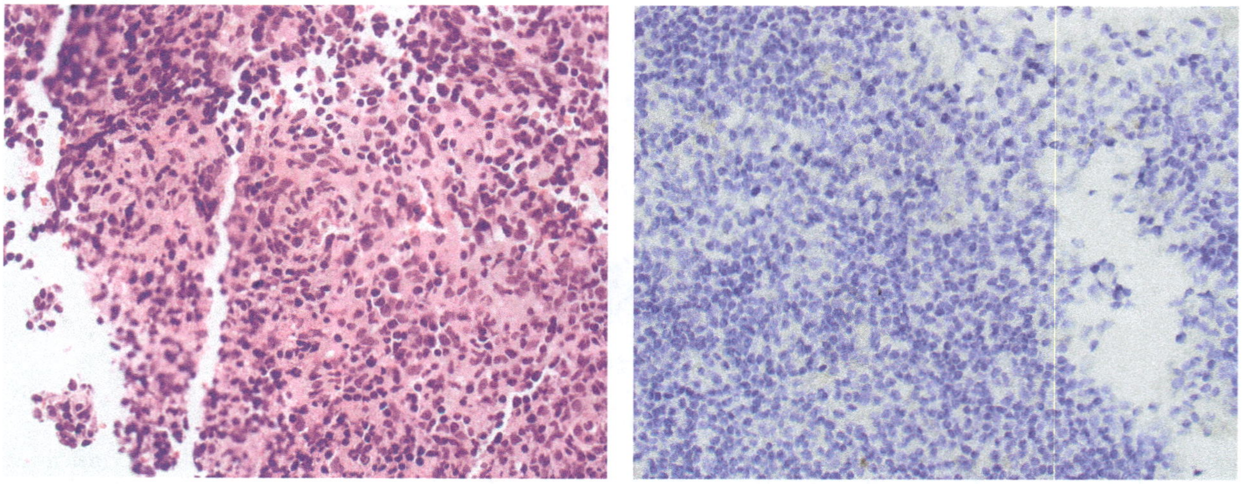

(a) (b)

FIGURE 6: (a) H&E stained LN needle biopsy section showing a non-necrotizing granuloma with no evidence of lymphoid infiltrate (x200). (b) Immunohistochemically stained lymph node needle biopsy section showing negative staining for TdT (x200).

hematopoiesis and 1% blasts. A flow cytometric evaluation using the COG MRD panel, where 542,700 events were collected, showed no evidence of relapsed/residual disease. B cells represented around 2% of total cells and exhibited a spectrum of differentiation. FISH studies were positive for BCR/ABL1 fusion in 5/200 cells and for deletion 7 in 3/200 cells analyzed. PCR analysis revealed an evident reduction in BCR-ABL1 e13a2 (b2a2, p210) fusion transcript (detected at an IS of 1.25). The patient has been clinically stable for about 6 months on therapy and has been evaluated for transplant. All five bone marrow findings are summarized in Table 1.

3. Discussion

3.1. Differentiation between CML-BLP and de Novo B-ALL. Although CML remains an indolent illness in the majority of patients, the blastic phase still represents a serious and often life-threatening complication requiring aggressive measures to control the disease. Differentiation between Ph + B-ALL and CML-LBP is very important since it has a significant impact on the patient's management and outcome. CML patients presenting with BP often have a much worse prognosis. Patients with Ph + B-ALL are usually treated with frontline regimens for B-ALL and tyrosine kinase inhibitors (TKI). Patients with CML-LBP are usually treated with TKI combined with intensive chemotherapy followed by allo-SCT in qualified patients [7].

Our patient was diagnosed with a CML-BLP rather than Ph + B-ALL for several reasons. First, the p210 BCR-ABL1 fusion was detected instead of the p190 BCR-ABL1. A diagnosis of CML-BLP should always be considered when the transcripts are p210 [5]. Fusion gene p190 can be detected in less than 1% of CML cases and is often associated with monocytosis in CML-CP [7]. In B-ALL, Ph chromosome/

Table 1: The bone marrow aspirate and biopsy findings during the disease course.

Bone marrow	Date	Morphology on aspirate	IHC on biopsy	Flow cytometry	Karyotyping	FISH	Molecular by PCR
BMAB1	6-3-21	6% immature cells on aspirate	20–25% immature B-cells on biopsy	1.9% B-lymphoblasts by COG MRD	$t(9:22)$ in 1/20 cells	BCR/ ABL124/200 cells	Not done
BMAB2	6-7-21	10% blasts	About 10% blasts	No COG MRD	$t(9:22)$ in 3/20 cells	Not done	Positive for p210, IS of more than 55%.
BMAB3	6-24-21	2% blasts	2%	0.2% B-lymphoblasts by COG MRD	$t(9:22)$ in 9/20 cells	BCR/ABL1 22/200 cells	Not done
BMAB4	8-16-21	5% blasts	5% B-lymphoblasts	2% B-lymphoblasts by COG MRD	46, XX, $t(9; 22)$ [4/10] 45, XX, -7, $t(9; 22)$ [6/10]	BCR/ABL1 162/200 cells	Not done
BMAB5	10-14-21	1% blasts	1% blasts	Negative COG MRD	46, XX [15]	BCR/ABL1 5/200 cells	Positive for p21, IS of 1.25%.

BCR-ABL1 fusion is the most common recurrent cytogenetic abnormality in adults. In adults with B-ALL, p190 is detected in around 60–70% of cases, and p210 is detected in around 30–40% of cases [8]. Second, the discordance between the percentage of blasts and the size of the Ph + clone is supportive of a diagnosis of CML-BLP. In CML-BLP, BCR/ABL1 is detected in both lymphoblasts and myeloid cells since the myeloid cells are part of the proliferative process. Therefore, the Ph + clone count is often higher than the blast count. Whereas in de novo Ph + B-ALL, BCR/ABL1 is restricted to the lymphoblasts thus the Ph + clone size is often close to blast count. In our case, all four bone marrow evaluations showed a higher Ph + clone count compared to the blast count in the corresponding bone marrow aspirate morphological evaluations. For example, BMAB4 had 5% blasts yet karyotyping detected $t(9; 22)$ in 11/20 cells (55%), and the FISH studies were positive for BCR/ABL1 fusion in 162/200 cells analyzed (81%). Moreover, the $t(9,22)$ was detected in the LN biopsy using FISH in the absence of immature cell infiltrate. Even further, BCR/ABL1 fusion is also seen in cells with band form nuclear features. Third, the patient had atypical megakaryocytic morphology and marrow fibrosis in BMAB1 and neutrophilia with left-shift in BMAB4, which are suggestive of an underlying myeloid neoplasm. CML-BP tends to have high WBC, neutrophilia, and immature myeloid cells in the blood [5]. Although the diagnosis of CML-AP was made on BMAB4, retrospectively, the increased B-lymphoblasts to 20–25% in BMAB1 represents a CML-BLP. The blast count varied between 2% and 25% in the four bone marrow samples examined over a period of two months. This case demonstrated that the B-lymphoblast count in CML AP or BLP may not be stable or even decrease without therapy. NCCN guideline version 3.2022 [9] also states that an increase in lymphoblasts is concerning and should be considered as a sign of an impending transformation to frank BP.

In our case, the bone marrow initially showed myeloid hypoplasia and erythroid hyperplasia. It is difficult to explain these findings in a CML case. The megakaryocytic series did not show the typical "dwarf" morphology expected to be seen in cases of CML. According to the 2018 WHO classification, megakaryocytes in CML may be normal or slightly decreased in number, but 40–50% of the cases exhibit moderate to marked megakaryocytic proliferation. In the chronic phase, megakaryocytes are usually smaller than normal, have hyposegmented nuclei, and are referred to as "dwarf" megakaryocytes but they are not true micromegakaryocytes, such as those seen in cases of the myelodysplastic syndrome [4].

3.2. *Differentiation between B-Lymphoblasts and Hematogones.*

The other diagnostic challenge is to differentiate B lymphoblasts from hematogones (HGs). HGs may exhibit morphological characteristics indistinguishable from lymphoblasts. They may constitute 5% to more than 50% of the bone marrow differential count. It is especially difficult to distinguish minimal B-lymphoblastic involvement in bone marrow from HGs. It has been shown that B-lymphoblasts usually show overexpression of CD123, CD58, CD10, CD22, CD34, and underexpression of CD38, CD81, and CD45 compared to HGs. They may also show aberrant expression of other lineage markers. CD58 and CD81 are two important markers that can be used to improve the distinction between HGs and precursor B lymphoblasts. It was recommended that CD58 and CD81 should be included in flow cytometry panels done at the time of diagnosis, thus allowing reliable and rapid MRD monitoring, especially for patients with no aberrant markers on their lymphoblasts [10]. Another useful marker is CD38. It is brightly expressed on HGs throughout all stages of maturation until it is downregulated in mature B cells. Approximately 75% of B-ALL cases express CD38, with a dimmer intensity than that expressed on HGs. The applicability of the underexpression of CD38 in B-ALL as a discriminating marker has been demonstrated in various studies examining its utility in MRD testing [11].

Interestingly, in a study by Vrotsos et al., they reported detecting a small (less than 0.5%) abnormal B-lymphoblast population in cases of chronic phase CML in a significant minority of diagnostic bone marrow samples. After follow-up of patients, it was concluded that this finding does not inevitably herald progression to a B-lymphoblastic blast phase [12].

In our case, the initial low-sensitivity leukemia panel showed decreased CD38 intensity and homogenous CD10 expression, which was concerning. The subsequent COG MRD study detected a population of B-lymphoblasts with a bright expression of CD58 and a positive expression of CD9. Interestingly, the B-lymphoblastic population showed an antigenic shift after two months with aberrant expression of the myeloid antigen CD13. Our case also emphasizes the importance of CD38 intensity in differentiating B-lymphoblasts from HGs, especially when MRD evaluation is not available. CML-BLP with expression of antigens from more than 1 lineage is common and additionally expression of 1 or more myeloid-related antigens is frequently seen [4]. Nevertheless, the flow cytometry immunophenotypic profile was lacking the typical features of Ph + B-lymphoblasts where bright CD10 together with aberrant expression of CD13 and CD33 and loss of CD45 were frequently seen. CD117 and CD15 were positively expressed on the lymphoblasts in our case, which is not typical for cases of Ph + B-ALL.

3.3. C-MYC Expression on CML-BLP. In our case, the immature B cells showed positive expression of c-MYC by immunohistochemistry on BMAB1. Deregulated MYC is found in about half of human tumors, being more prevalent in hematological neoplasms. Approximately 2%–5% of cases of ALL show MYC rearrangements. A number of B-ALL cases, while not having MYC gene abnormalities, show high MYC expression [13]. It was also found that BCR-ABL upregulates MYC expression, which cooperates with BCR–ABL in the transformation from the chronic phase to the blastic phase in CML cases. Consistently, imatinib and other BCR–ABL inhibitors provoke downregulation of MYC [14]. It was found that MYC mRNA levels were elevated in cases of CML-BP and in CML-CP compared to healthy bone marrow samples and that high MYC expression levels correlate with poorer response to imatinib and progression to the blastic crisis [15]. While c-MYC may not help in differentiating between CML-BLP and Ph + B-ALL, it would be interesting to follow-up with the patient and assess MYC expression in the bone marrow.

3.4. Cytogenetic Changes in CML-BLP. At diagnosis, approximately 5% to 10% of cases of CML will show chromosomal abnormalities in addition to *t*(9; 22); however, additional chromosomal anomalies (ACAs) are identified in around 50% to 80% of CML-AP as the disease progresses. ACAs are also commonly acquired during the course of CML treatment. In fact, the acquisition of specific additional chromosomal abnormalities can be used as a criterion for advancement from CML-CP to CML-AP. The chromosomal changes that define a transformation to CML-AP include a second Philadelphia chromosome, isochromosome 17q, trisomy 8, trisomy 19, abnormalities of 3q 26.2, or a complex karyotype [16]. Some studies have shown that B-ALL with BCR-ABL1 is associated with a greater number of additional chromosomal changes when compared with CML in BLP [17]. Additionally, gains in chromosome 9 are associated with B-ALL with BCR-ABL1, whereas deletions in chromosome 9p are more commonly seen in CML in BLP. This chromosomal abnormality is postulated to play an important role in CML-BLP because 9p is home to genes important in B-cell differentiation (PAX5 and CDKN1A). Lymphoid BP has also been associated with deletion of p16/CDKN2A and numerical gains and breakpoints involving chromosomes 1q and 7p. However, neither of these changes can be used to definitively distinguish between CML-BLP and B-ALL [18].

Our patient developed Del 7 around two months after the first presentation. It was reported that monosomy 7 in CML is rare, with only a few reported cases [19]. It was also reported that in adult ALL cases, the presence of monosomy 7, as a sole secondary abnormality, was associated with a poor prognosis and shorter survival [20]. However, the emergence of del (7) in our case does not seem to correlate with disease progression. The role of del (7) in CML disease progression may need further observation.

Detecting cytogenetic abnormalities plays an important role in the diagnosis of hematologic malignancies. It is worthy to point out that in rare instances, some of these abnormalities may be constitutional and are not necessarily linked to the neoplastic process, leading to a diagnostic dilemma. For instance, very few cases have been reported to have a constitutional balanced *t*(9; 22) (q34; q11.2) cytogenetically mimicking the acquired *t*(9; 22) (q34; q11.2), characteristic of CML. These findings prove the necessity of a detailed investigation of such cases together with correlation with all clinical findings to avoid an erroneous diagnosis of myeloid malignancies in the presence of rare constitutional cytogenetic abnormalities [21].

4. Conclusion

CML presenting with a B-lymphoblastic crisis as an initial presentation is very uncommon, and it may present without typical CML morphology. It is important to differentiate such cases from primary Ph + B-ALL due to the impact it has on the patient's management and prognosis. PCR testing, together with cytogenetic studies and multiparametric flow cytometry, serves as tools that help in reaching an accurate diagnosis. However, the importance of morphological evaluation and applying a comprehensive immunohistochemistry panel cannot be undermined. The prognosis of patients with CML-BP is poor and, without proper treatment, patients usually die. However, with TKI therapy, survival has markedly improved.

Authors' Contributions

The manuscript has been read and approved by the authors. No one has denied being an author. The authors agreed on the order that our names appeared in the manuscript. The authors respect that the corresponding author is the sole contact for the editorial process.

References

[1] P. Jain, H. M. Kantarjian, A. Ghorab et al., "Prognostic factors and survival outcomes in patients with chronic myeloid leukemia in blast phase in the tyrosine kinase inhibitor era: cohort study of 477 patients," *Cancer*, vol. 123, no. 22, pp. 4391–4402, 2017.

[2] M. J. Borowitz, J. K. C. Chan, J. R. Downing, M. M. Le Beau, and D. A. Arber, "B-lymphoblastic leukemia/lymphoma with recurrent genetic abnormalities," *WHO Classification of Tumours of Haematopoietic and Lymphoid Tissues*, International Agency for Research on Cancer (IARC), Lyon, France, 4th edition, 2017.

[3] J. Score, M. J. Calasanz, O. Ottman et al., "Analysis of genomic breakpoints in p190 and p210 BCR-ABL indicate distinct mechanisms of formation," *Leukemia*, vol. 24, no. 10, pp. 1742–1750, 2010.

[4] J. W. Vardiman, J. V. Melo, M. Baccarabu, J. P. Radich, and H. M. Kvasnicka, "Chronic myeloid leukemia, BCR-ABL1-positive," *WHO Classification of Tumours of Haematopoietic and Lymphoid Tissues*, International Agency for Research on Cancer (IARC), Lyon, France, 2017.

[5] Z. Chen, S. Hu, S. A. Wang et al., "Chronic myeloid leukemia presenting in lymphoblastic crisis, a differential diagnosis with Philadelphia-positive B-lymphoblastic leukemia," *Leukemia & Lymphoma*, vol. 61, no. 12, pp. 2831–2838, 2020.

[6] X. Qing, X. Qing, P. Ji, S. W. French, and H. Mason, "Mixed phenotype (T/B/myeloid) extramedullary blast crisis as an initial presentation of chronic myelogenous leukemia," *Experimental Ana Molecular Pathology*, vol. 104, no. 2, pp. 130–133, 2018.

[7] J. V. Melo, H. Myint, D. A. Galton, and J. M. Goldman, "P190 BCR-ABL chronic myeloid leukaemia: the missing link with chronic myelomonocytic leukaemia?" *Leukemia*, vol. 8, no. 1, pp. 208–211, 1994.

[8] G. P. Cimino and L. Elia, "The role of BCR-ABL isoforms in the presentation and outcome of patients with philadelphia-positive acute lymphoblastic leukemia," *Haematologica*, vol. 91, no. 3, pp. 377–380, 2006.

[9] National Comprehensive Cancer Network, *NCCN Clinical Practice Guidelines in Oncology, Chronic Myeloid Leukemia*, NCCN.Org, Jen kintown, PA, USA, 2022.

[10] C. Nagant, D. Casula, A. Janssens, V. T. P. Nguyen, and B. Cantinieaux, "Easy discrimination of hematogones from lymphoblasts in B-cell progenitor acute lymphoblastic leukemia patients using CD81/CD58 expression ratio," *International Journal of Laboratory Hematology*, vol. 40, no. 6, pp. 734–739, 2018.

[11] M. D. Don, W. Lim, A. Lo et al., "Improved recognition of hematogones from precursor B-lymphoblastic leukemia by a single tube flow cytometric analysis," *American Journal of Clinical Pathology*, vol. 153, no. 6, pp. 790–798, 2020.

[12] E. Vrotsos, M. Gorgan, and J. A. DiGiuseppe, "Detection of small abnormal B-Lymphoblast populations at diagnosis of chronic myelogenous leukemia, BCR–ABL1+: incidence, phenotypic features, and clinical implications," *Cytometry B Clinical Cytometry*, vol. 92, no. 4, pp. 275–278, 2017.

[13] D. Da Costa, A. Agathanggelou, T. Perry et al., "BET inhibition as a single or combined therapeutic approach in primary paediatric B-precursor acute lymphoblastic leukaemia," *Blood Cancer Journal*, vol. 3, p. e126, 2013.

[14] M. G. Cortiguera, A. Batlle-López, M. Albajar, M. D. Delgado, and J. León, "MYC as therapeutic target in leukemia and lymphoma," *Blood and Lymphatic Cancer*, vol. 5, pp. 75–91, 2015.

[15] M. Albajar, M. T. Gómez-Casares, J. Llorca et al., "MYC in chronic myeloid leukemia: induction of aberrant DNA synthesis and association with poor response to imatinib," *Molecular Cancer Research*, vol. 9, pp. 564–576, 2011.

[16] Z. Chen, J. E. Cortes, J. L. Jorgensen et al., "Differential impact of additional chromosomal abnormalities in myeloid vs. lymphoid blast phase of chronic myelogenous leukemia in the era of tyrosine kinase inhibitor therapy," *Leukemia*, vol. 30, pp. 1606–1609, 2016.

[17] E. Balducci, M. Loosveld, I. Rahal et al., "Interphase FISH for BCR-ABL1 rearrangement on neutrophils: a decisive tool to discriminate a lymphoid blast crisis of chronic myeloid leukemia from a de novo BCR-ABL1 positive acute lymphoblastic leukemia," *Hematological Oncology*, vol. 36, pp. 344–348, 2018.

[18] A. D. Ware, L. Wake, P. Brown, J. A. Webster, B. D. Smith, and A. S. Duffield, "B-lymphoid blast phase of chronic myeloid leukemia: a case report and review of the literature," *AJSP: Reviews & Reports*, vol. 24, no. 5, pp. 191–195, 2019.

[19] A. Alswied, A. Rehman, L. W. Lai, J. Duran, M. Sardar, and M. A. Proytcheva, "Rare monosomy 7 and deletion 7p at diagnosis of chronic myeloid leukemia in accelerated phase," *Cancer Genetics*, vol. 252, pp. 111–114, 2021.

[20] M. Wetzler, R. K. Dodge, K. Mrozek et al., "Additional cytogenetic abnormalities in adults with philadelphia chromosome positive acute lymphoblastic leukaemia: a study of the cancer and leukaemia group B," *British Journal of Haematology*, vol. 124, pp. 275–288, 2004.

[21] D. R. Czuchlewski, H. Farzanmehr, S. Robinett, S. Haines, and K. K. Reichard, "t(9;22) (q34;q11.2) is a recurrent constitutional non-Robertsonian translocation and a rare cytogenetic mimic of chronic myeloid leukemia," *Cancer Genetics*, vol. 204, pp. 572–576, 2011.

Nivolumab Effective for Gastric and Lung Cancers but Not for Multiple Myeloma in a Multiple Primary Cancer Patient

Tsukasa Yasuda,[1] **Junji Hiraga**,[2] **Michihiko Narita**,[3] **Yoshimasa Tanikawa**,[4] **and Tomoyuki Tsuzuki**[1]

[1]*Department of Gastroenterology, Toyota Kosei Hospital, Toyota, Japan*
[2]*Department of Hematology, Toyota Kosei Hospital, Toyota, Japan*
[3]*Department of Pathology, Toyota Kosei Hospital, Toyota, Japan*
[4]*Department of Respiratory Medicine, Toyota Kosei Hospital, Toyota, Japan*

Correspondence should be addressed to Tsukasa Yasuda; tksysd70142@gmail.com

Academic Editor: Håkon Reikvam

The case of a 76-year-old man with multiple primary cancers that were treated with nivolumab is presented. Six years earlier, he was diagnosed with multiple myeloma (MM) and was treated with several chemotherapies. He was also diagnosed with gastric cancer with liver metastasis and primary lung cancer by upper gastrointestinal endoscopy and computed tomography (CT). Nivolumab treatment was given as third-line therapy, and it was effective for gastric and lung cancers. But MM worsened, and the patient died. There is no standard treatment for multiple primary cancers, and the development of effective treatments for multiple primary cancers is important.

1. Introduction

Multiple myeloma (MM) is a hematological malignancy for which survival has been prolonged through the development of new agents such as proteasome inhibitors, immunomodulators, and antibody drugs [1–3]. The median survival of patients with MM has increased from 3 to 8 years in the last 15 years. However, second primary cancers have created problems with the long-term survival of patients with MM [4]. It has been reported that the risk of developing solid tumors remains unchanged, but the risk of developing hematological malignancies is significantly higher, especially in patients treated with immunomodulators such as lenalidomide [5–7]. In addition, the prognosis of patients with second primary cancers has been reported to be worse than that of patients without them [8, 9].

Nivolumab is classified as a checkpoint inhibitor that is a monoclonal antibody drug against programmed cell death-1 (PD-1). The indications for PD-1 antibody drugs have been expanded to various cancers, and it has become available from the second line for unresectable advanced or recurrent gastric cancer and the first line for unresectable advanced or recurrent non-small cell lung cancer [10, 11]. In contrast, unfortunately, pembrolizumab, a similar PD-1 antibody, was found not effective for MM in combination with lenalidomide [12], so the PD-1 antibody drugs are not approved for MM in the United States and Japan.

A rare case, in which a patient who had been treated with new agents for MM developed multiple primary cancers (gastric cancer and lung cancer) and was treated with nivolumab, which was effective for gastric and lung cancers, but not for MM, is presented.

2. Case Report

A 76-year-old man noticed melena and had a medical examination. He was found to have renal dysfunction 6 years earlier, and further evaluations showed serum albumin, 2.2 g/dL; urinary protein, 4+; urinary Bence Jones protein-(BJP-) λ-type M protein positivity; decreased serum IgG,

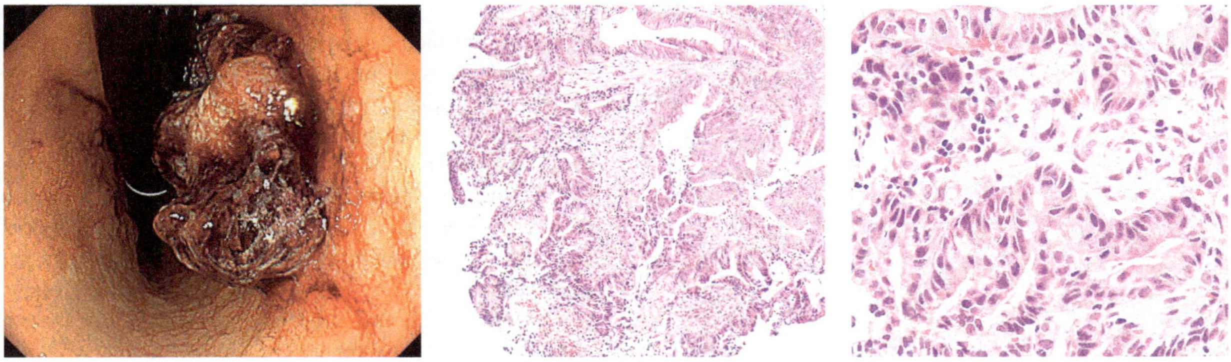

(a) (b) (c)

FIGURE 1: (a) Upper gastrointestinal endoscopy findings. A type 1 tumor with a diameter of 30 mm is found on the posterior wall of the gastric body. The tumor is easily bleeding. (b) Histopathologic findings of the biopsy specimens of gastric cancer. Findings of well-differentiated adenocarcinoma. Hematoxylin and eosin staining, ×100. (c) Hematoxylin and eosin staining, ×400.

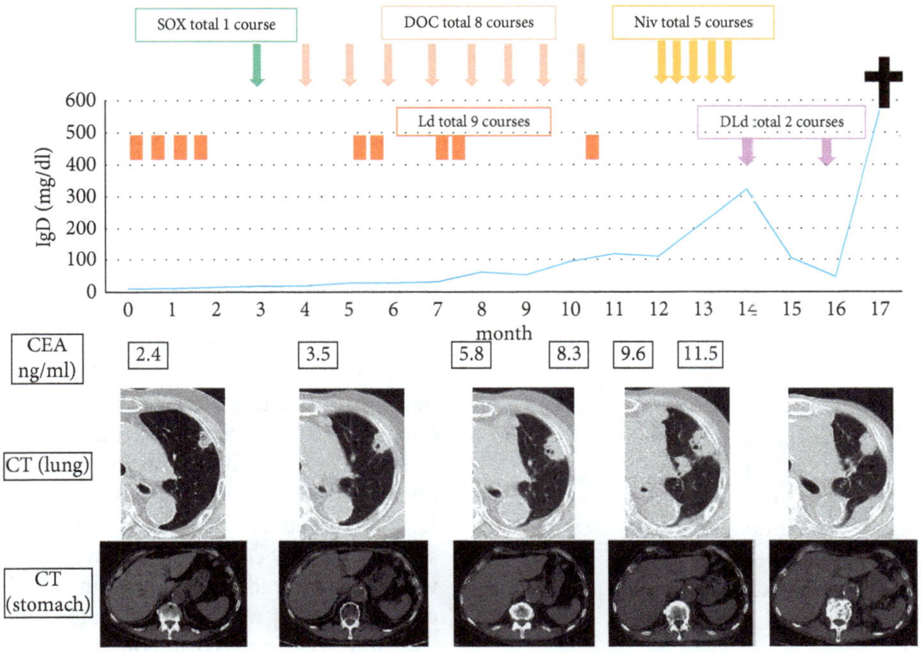

FIGURE 2: Clinical courses of the patient after gastric and lung cancers are diagnosed. The solid line indicates serum IgD level. Computed tomography (CT) shows the lung nodules and stomach. At the time of appearance, a pulmonary nodule with a diameter of 20 mm is found in the upper lobe of the left lung. The tumor grew over time, and a new intrapulmonary lesion appears after DOC treatment, but after nivolumab treatment, the new lesion almost disappeared and the primary lesion reduced. The gastric cancer could not be identified by CT at the start of treatment and had not changed since then. But 16 months after, gastric cancer increased. SOX: tegafur, gimeracil, oteracil potassium (TS-1), and oxaliplatin; DOC: docetaxel; Niv: nivolumab; Ld: lenalidomide and dexamethasone; DLd: daratumumab, lenalidomide, and dexamethasone, CEA: carcinoembryonic antigen.

IgA, and IgM levels; and an increased serum IgD (516 mg/dL) level. In addition, bone marrow aspiration showed clonal proliferation of plasma cells, so he was diagnosed with MM (IgD-λ type, BJP-λ type, International Staging System III). He was treated with 7 courses of bortezomib dexamethasone (BD) therapy, but due to recurrence, his therapy was changed to lenalidomide dexamethasone (Ld), and he was undergoing his 36th course. On upper gastrointestinal endoscopy, a type 1 tumor with a diameter of 30 mm was seen at the posterior wall of the corpus of the stomach, and the histopathological diagnosis of the tumor was tubular adenocarcinoma (Figures 1(a)–1(c)). And, the HER2 status of gastric cancer was negative, and MSI status of that was not examined. In addition, computed tomography (CT) showed liver metastasis of gastric cancer, so the gastric cancer was diagnosed as clinical stage IV (T3N2M1). Furthermore, CT showed a pulmonary nodule with a diameter of 20 mm in the upper lobe of the left lung, and the diagnosis of the nodule was primary lung cancer clinical stage IA2 (T1bN0M0) based on the imaging findings (Figure 2). Transbronchial lung biopsy could not be performed because the lesion of the lung cancer

Table 1: Laboratory data at the time of diagnosis of gastric cancer and lung cancer.

		Units	Reference range
		Hematology	
WBC	7,300	μL	4,000–9,000
Neut	52	%	38.0–71.9
Eos	2.0	%	0.2–6.8
Ba	0.0	%	0.0–1.0
Mono	8.0	%	2.3–7.7
Lymph	38	%	26.0–46.6
RBC	329	$\times 10^4/\mu L$	410–560
Hb	11.1	g/dL	13.5–17.5
Ht	33.5	%	40.0–53.0
MCV	89.6	fL	80.0–100.0
Platelets	20.1	$\times 10^4/\mu L$	14.0–40.0
		Biochemistry	
TP	5.3	g/dL	6.7–8.3
Alb	3.6	g/dL	4.0–5.0
T-bil	0.4	mg/dL	0.3–1.2
AST	16	U/L	13–33
ALT	27	U/L	6–30
LDH	243	U/L	119–229
γ-GTP	106	U/L	10–47
BUN	14.9	mg/dL	8.0–22.0
Cre	0.86	mg/dL	0.60–1.10
Na	142	mmol/L	138–146
K	3.7	mmol/L	3.6–4.9
Cl	110	mmol/L	99–109
Ca	8.9	mg/dL	8.7–10.3
P	3.1	mg/dL	2.5–4.7
IgG	453	mg/dL	870–1700
IgA	33	mg/dL	110–410
IgM	21	mg/dL	35–220
IgD	10.5	mg/dL	<9.0
		Tumor markers	
CEA	2.4	ng/mL	<5.0
CYFRA	1.4	ng/mL	<3.5
Pro-GRP	66.6	pg/mL	<81.0
		Urinalysis	
Protein	0.22	g/gCr	<0.15
RBC	(—)		
WBC	(—)		

WBC: white blood cells; Neut: neutrophils; Eos: eosinophils; Ba: basophils; Mono: monocytes; Lymph: lymphocytes; RBC: red blood cells; Hb: hemoglobin; Ht: hematocrit; MCV: mean corpuscular volume; TP: total protein; Alb: albumin; T-Bil: total bilirubin; AST: aspartate aminotransferase; ALT: alanine aminotransferase; LDH: lactate dehydrogenase; γ-GTP: gamma-glutamyl transpeptidase; BUN: blood urea nitrogen; Cre: creatinine; Na: sodium; K: potassium; Cl: chloride; Ca: calcium; P: phosphorus; IgG: immunoglobulin G; IgA: immunoglobulin A; IgM: immunoglobulin M; IgD: immunoglobulin D; CEA: carcinoembryonic antigen; CYFRA: cytokeratin-19; Pro-GRP: progastrin releasing peptide.

was a very difficult place for the examination, and the gastric cancer had advanced and a poor prognosis. So, immediate chemotherapy was needed. In conclusion, this patient was diagnosed as having primary gastric cancer and lung cancer that developed during the treatment of MM. The laboratory data at the time of diagnosis are shown in Table 1.

For this case of multiple primary cancers, the treatment plan was considered by the cancer board of our institute, and the treatment of the gastric cancer, which had the worst prognosis, was prioritized. First, one course of tegafur, gimeracil, oteracil potassium (TS-1), and oxaliplatin (SOX) was administered, but it was discontinued due to gastrointestinal symptoms and changed to docetaxel (DOC). He had a history of unstable angina and paroxysmal atrial fibrillation and had been treated for percutaneous coronary intervention two years ago. To avoid the onset of thrombosis, he was treated with monotherapy of docetaxel for second line. Since the serum IgD level also tended to increase gradually during the previous treatment, the treatment plan was re-examined, and the treatment for MM was resumed after the administration of a second course of DOC. Then, DOC and Ld treatment were administered alternately. However, due to progression of the lung cancer, the treatment was changed from DOC to nivolumab the following year. After the start of nivolumab, the lung cancer showed partial response, and the gastric cancer showed stable disease, but the MM gradually worsened. Although the serum IgD level decreased due to the addition of daratumumab, lenalidomide, and dexamethasone (DLd), the patient was unable to continue chemotherapy because of loss of appetite, which was thought to be an exacerbation of gastric cancer. The serum IgD level and carcinoembryonic antigen (CEA) level were increased. The patient died 17 months after the multiple primary cancers were diagnosed (Figure 2).

3. Discussion

A rare case, in which nivolumab treatment was administered for primary gastric cancer and primary lung cancer that developed during treatment for MM, and the gastric cancer and lung cancer responded, but the MM did not, was reported. Patients with second primary cancers that develop after treatment for MM have been reported to have a 2- to 6-fold increased risk of death compared to those without second primary cancers [8, 9]. In particular, patients treated with lenalidomide have a high incidence of secondary carcinogenesis, which is estimated to be 5–8% [5–7]. In addition, older age is also considered to be a significant risk factor for the development of second primary cancers [13]. According to a Swedish report, 1,547 of 26,627 patients with MM developed second primary cancers, but the rate of gastrointestinal cancers was low (364 patients, 1.4%) and that of respiratory cancers was also low (68 patients, 0.25%). A study of 2,732 patients with MM treated with lenalidomide found no gastric cancers, 5 (0.18%) lung cancers, and only 3 multiple primary solid cancer cases [13]. It is considered that cases such as the present one in which gastric cancer and lung cancer developed as second primary cancers are extremely rare. The present patient was an elderly patient who had been receiving long-term lenalidomide and dexamethasone treatments with relapse of MM after proteasome inhibitor treatment. Because the risk of death from MM is much higher than the risk of death from second primary cancers, lenalidomide treatment should be given aggressively for MM, but it is necessary to always keep in mind the onset of second primary cancers, especially in elderly patients receiving long-term lenalidomide treatment.

Nivolumab is classified as a checkpoint inhibitor that is a monoclonal antibody drug against PD-1. This drug can be used in first-line, second-line, and third-line treatments for unresectable gastric cancer and lung cancer [10, 11]. In the present case, there was no pathological proof of lung cancer, but the pulmonary nodule was likely to be primary lung cancer based on the CT findings. Gastric cancer and lung cancer were evaluated as stable disease and partial remission, respectively, based on clinical and imaging findings. However, nivolumab was not effective for MM, so daratumumab was also used, but it was also ineffective, and the patient died. Pembrolizumab, a PD-1 antibody similar to nivolumab, also failed to show efficacy against MM [12], which led to the discontinuation of clinical trials with nivolumab. Therefore, PD-1 antibody drugs are not indicated for MM. PD-1 antibody drugs have been reported to be effective for MM in some cases [14], but not in the present case. Other therapeutic approaches may be needed for MM, but in the present case, treatment for MM alone was associated with a high risk of exacerbation of other multiple cancers, so further approaches may have been difficult.

With the development of treatment for MM, the diagnosis and treatment of multiple primary cancers become very important issues. The present case was treated with nivolumab, but it was ineffective for MM. With the accumulation of more such multiple primary cancers cases, more effective treatments might be developed.

References

[1] S. K. Kumar, S. V. Rajkumar, A. Dispenzieri et al., "Improved survival in multiple myeloma and the impact of novel therapies," *Blood*, vol. 111, no. 5, pp. 2516–2520, 2008.

[2] I. Turesson, R. Velez, S. Y. Kristinsson, and O. Landgren, "Patterns of improved survival in patients with multiple myeloma in the twenty-first century: a population-based study," *Journal of Clinical Oncology*, vol. 28, no. 5, pp. 830–834, 2010.

[3] S. K. Kumar, A. Dispenzieri, M. Q. Lacy et al., "Continued improvement in survival in multiple myeloma: changes in early mortality and outcomes in older patients," *Leukemia*, vol. 28, pp. 1122–1128, 2014.

[4] O. Landgren, A. Thomas, and S. Mailankody, "Myeloma and second primary cancers," *New England Journal of Medicine*, vol. 365, no. 23, pp. 2241-2242, 2011.

[5] M. Attal, V. Lauwers-Cances, G. Marit et al., "Lenalidomide maintenance after stem-cell transplantation for multiple myeloma," *New England Journal of Medicine*, vol. 366, no. 19, pp. 1782–1791, 2012.

[6] P. L. McCarthy, S. A. Holstein, M. T. Petrucci et al., "Lenalidomide maintenance after autologous stem-cell transplantation in newly diagnosed multiple myeloma: a meta-analysis," *Journal of Clinical Oncology*, vol. 35, no. 29, pp. 3279–3289, 2017.

[7] T. Chen, M. Fallah, M. Fallah et al., "Risk of second primary cancers in multiple myeloma survivors in German and Swedish cancer registries," *Scientific Reports*, vol. 6, no. 1, Article ID 22084, 2016.

[8] L. J. Costa, K. N. Godby, S. Chhabra, R. F. Cornell, P. Hari, and S. Bhatia, "Second primary malignancy after multiple myeloma-population trends and cause-specific mortality," *British Journal of Haematology*, vol. 182, no. 4, pp. 513–520, 2018.

[9] G. Jonsdottir, S. H. Lund, M. Björkholm et al., "Survival in multiple myeloma patients who develop second malignancies: a population-based cohort study," *Haematologica*, vol. 101, no. 4, pp. e145–e148, 2016.

[10] E. C. Smyth, M. Nilsson, H. I. Grabsch, N. C. van Grieken, and F. Lordick, "Gastric cancer," *The Lancet*, vol. 396, no. 10251, pp. 635–648, 2020.

[11] L. Xia, Y. Liu, and Y. Wang, "PD-1/PD-L1 blockade therapy in advanced non-small-cell lung cancer: current status and future directions," *The Oncologist*, vol. 24, no. 1, pp. S31–S41, 2019.

[12] S. Z. Usmani, F. Schjesvold, A. Oriol et al., "Pembrolizumab plus lenalidomide and dexamethasone for patients with treatment-naïve multiple myeloma (KEYNOTE-185): a randomized, open-label, phase 3 trial," *Lancet Haematology*, vol. 6, pp. e448–e458, 2019.

[13] J. R. Jones, D. A. Cairns, D. A. Cairns et al., "Second malignancies in the context of lenalidomide treatment: an analysis of 2732 myeloma patients enrolled to the myeloma XI trial," *Blood Cancer Journal*, vol. 6, no. 12, p. e506, 2016.

[14] M. J. Pianko, S. A. Funt, D. B. Page et al., "Efficacy and toxicity of therapy immediately after treatment with nivolumab in relapsed multiple myeloma," *Leukemia & Lymphoma*, vol. 59, no. 1, pp. 221–224, 2018.

50

Recurrent Nasal-Type Extranodal Natural Killer/T-Cell Lymphoma with Meningeal Involvement

Sylvester Homsy[1] **Ralph Kamel**[1] **Mark Raden,**[2] **and Yevgeniy Skaradinskiy**[3]

[1]*Department of Internal Medicine, Staten Island University Hospital-Northwell Health, Staten Island, New York, NY, USA*
[2]*Department of Radiology, Staten Island University Hospital-Northwell Health, Staten Island, New York, NY, USA*
[3]*Division of Hematology/Oncology, Staten Island University Hospital-Northwell Health, Staten Island, New York, NY, USA*

Correspondence should be addressed to Sylvester Homsy; sylvester.homsy@gmail.com

Academic Editor: Kostas Konstantopoulos

Extranodal natural killer/T-cell lymphoma nasal type (NNKTL) is a type of non-Hodgkin's lymphoma that has been associated with Epstein–Barr virus (EBV). It has an aggressive behavior, known for predilection to metastasize to different organs. Central nervous system (CNS) spread from a primary location has been reported. Different modalities of treatment such as chemotherapy and radiation therapy have been employed in the management of this disease. Severe toxicities of currently available treatment have made clinicians seek more targeted therapies using molecular profiling. We present a 44-year-old Hispanic patient who was diagnosed with an early-stage NNKTL and treated with the modified SMILE regimen for 6 cycles. His EBV DNA PCR turned undetectable and remained so throughout the treatment. He sustained complete right vision loss due to right optic nerve invasion by the tumor, leading to prophylactic intravitreal methotrexate to the contralateral eye. The patient achieved good response with minimal residual disease. He was supposed to start radiation as a sequential therapy. However, the acute development of severe headache and confusion lead to a complete workup showing leptomeningeal spread. He eventually succumbed to the disease.

1. Introduction

Extranodal natural killer/T-cell lymphoma nasal type (NNKTL) occurs primarily in the nasal cavity or paranasal sinuses. It is characterized by ulceration and necrosis of the nasal cavity and midline facial tissues [1]. It is commonly observed in Asia and South America where it accounts for up to 10% of all non-Hodgkin lymphoma. In the United States, it only accounts for 3.3% of all T-cell lymphomas [2]. It is known to have an aggressive course which is often fatal due to rapid local progression and distant metastases mainly to the lymph nodes, lungs, liver, and the gastrointestinal tract [3].Central nervous system (CNS) involvement is rare and has only been reported in 7% of a Japanese cohort at presentation [4]. Herein, we report a case of an otherwise healthy male who was successfully treated for a primary NNKTL in his nasal cavity. He subsequently developed meningeal recurrence that was fatal.

2. Case Report

A 44-year-old Hispanic male from Mexico presented to the emergency department for progressive nasal congestion, rhinorrhea, ear fullness, facial swelling, and sore throat that has been ongoing for 2 months. He also noted gradual vision loss of his right eye and intermittent bloody discharge from both the nostrils. Bedsides, rhinoscopy showed swelling of the right nare and nasal turbinates along with small blood clots without active bleeding. A maxillofacial computed tomography (CT) scan showed phlegmonous change about the right lamina papyracea with an erosive change. Also shown was destruction and soft-tissue swelling that extends along the medial border of the right orbit (Figure 1). Biopsy of the right nasal vestibule was diagnostic for extranodal NK/T-cell lymphoma nasal type. The atypical cells were positive for CD2, CD3, CD4, CD56, CD43, and Bcl-2 and negative for CD5, CD7, CD8, CD10, CD20, CD30, and BCL-6. In situ

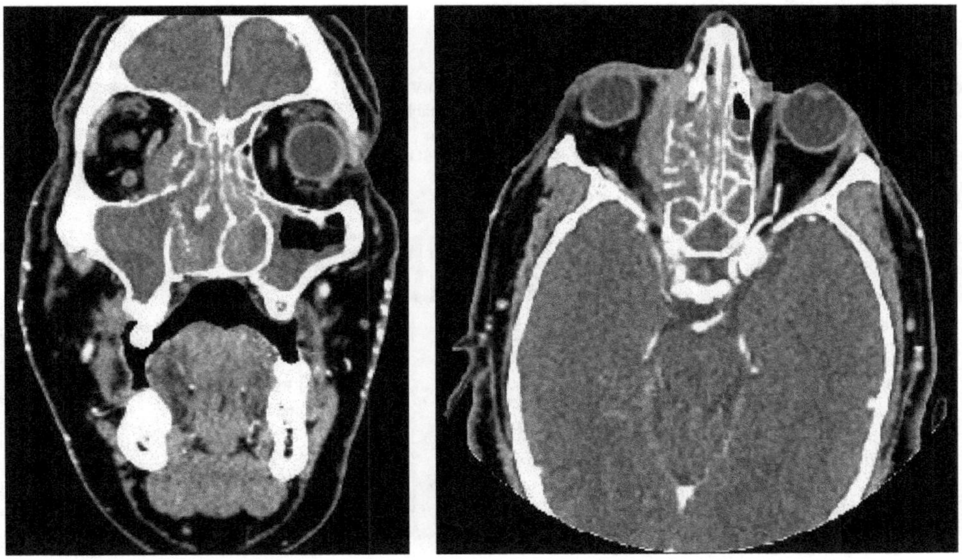

(a) (b)

Figure 1: CT maxillofacial with IV contrast showing opacified ethmoid sinuses with bone destruction of the right lamina papyracea with soft-tissue extension into the right orbit. (a) Coronal view; (b) axial view.

hybridization was positive for the Epstein–Barr encoding region (EBER). Bone marrow biopsy showed a normocellular bone marrow with trilineage hematopoiesis. Additional imaging with magnetic resonance imaging (MRI) of the head showed a vague enhancement over the frontal convexities. EBV DNA PCR in the blood was 4.90 log10 IU/mL (equivalent to 79,792 IU/mL). He was started on a modified SMILE (m-SMILE) regimen consistent of methotrexate 2 g/m^2 given on day 1, etoposide 100 mg/m^2, ifosfamide 1500 mg/m^2, dexamethasone 40 mg/d given on days 2 to 4, and pegasparagase 2000 U/m^2 given on day 8 of a 28-day cycle (Figure 2). He developed acute right-sided complete vision loss; magnetic resonance imaging of the orbits showed increased enhancement of the optic nerve sheath with a complex edema suspicious for optic nerve invasion. The case was discussed at an ENT oncology and other multidisciplinary oncology conferences; the decision was made to proceed with the same chemotherapy regimen. The patient then received prophylactic intravitreal methotrexate of the left eye. He completed his second cycle of m-SMILE, and a follow-up positron emission tomography-computed tomography (PET/CT) scan showed good response (Figure 3(a)). Methotrexate dose had to be reduced 50% on the third cycle of m-SMILE due to kidney injury. He subsequently received 4 more cycles of m-SMILE with 25% dose reduction of chemotherapeutic agents due to prolonged cytopenia from previous cycles. His EBV DNA PCR turned undetectable after the first cycle and remained so after the final (6th) cycle. A restaging PET/CT scan showed good response with faint residual disease in the paranasal sinuses and sinonasal cavity (Figure 3(b)). One month after he completed his last cycle, he developed new-onset severe headache, confusion, and shortness of breath. He was admitted to the emergency department where a CT scan of the head showed diffuse cerebral and cerebella edema. MRI of the brain with intravenous contrast revealed multiple focal cortical and subcortical signal abnormalities, with extensive gyral swelling involving the frontal, anterior parietal, and bilateral temporal lobe. Subtle enhancement in the sulci of the high frontoparietal region, particularly at the central sulcus, was noted (Figures 4 and 5). Cerebrospinal fluid examination was positive for CD 56+ cells and aberrant atypical lymphocytes. EBV DNA PCR was 14,800 IU/mL. His course was later complicated by respiratory failure and cerebellar tonsillar herniation; he subsequently succumbed after 19 days of hospitalization.

3. Discussion

NNKTL is an EBV-associated malignancy, and it was first reported in 1990 by Harabuchi et al. when EBV DNA PCR was found on the biopsies of nasal T-cell lymphoma of a series of patients diagnosed with this disease [5]. That led to the use of this simple blood test as a marker for tumor progression and surveillance for recurrences [6]. This disease was initially described as "lethal midline granuloma" in the USA because of its destructive property to the nose and face, with progression to a necrotic granuloma [7]. Later on, it has been shown that the neoplasm contains at least 2 lineages of cells: gamma delta T cell and NK cell. This has led to a change in its nomenclature [8]. Initially, diagnosis was made by finding angioinvasion and angiodestruction along with necrosis and apoptosis. However, with the advent of immunophenotyping, a more precise way to diagnose the

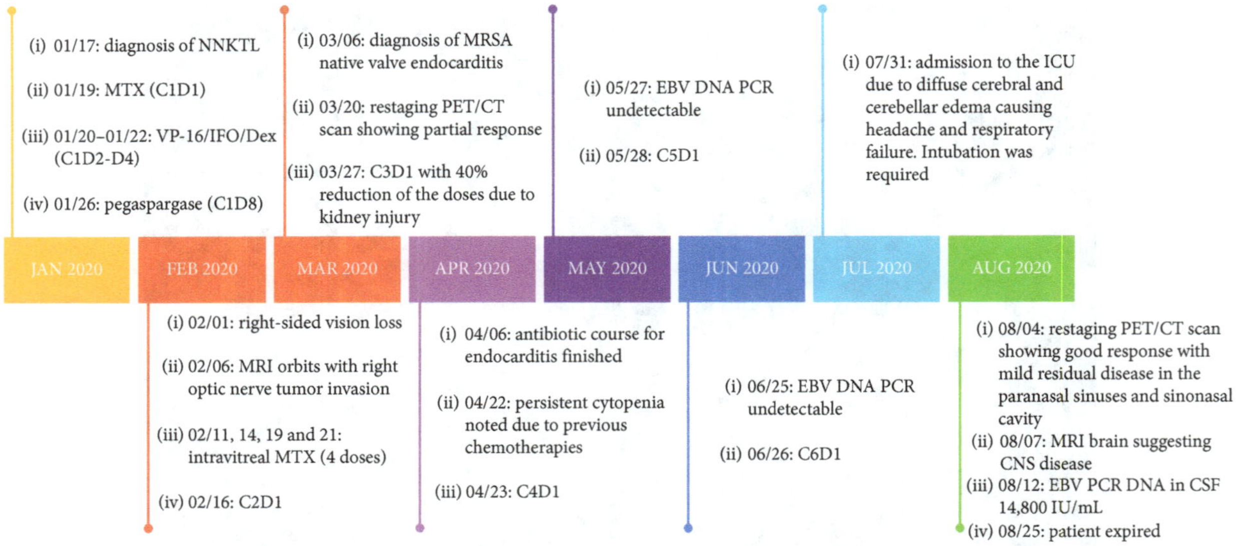

Figure 2: Timeline highlighting diagnosis, treatment schedule, disease course, and findings.

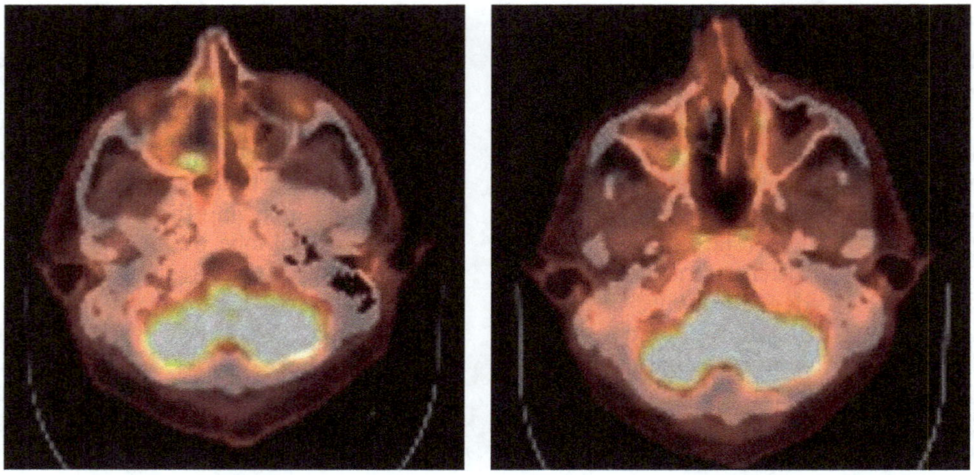

(a) (b)

Figure 3: PET/CT scan highlighting the maxillofacial structures. (a) After 2 cycles of mSMILE, a single 1.1 cm focus of increased FDG uptake was seen along the right sinonasal cavity, SUV max 9.3. (b) Restaging PET/CT scan after 6 cycles of mSMILE showing mild residual uptake in the right maxillary sinus, SUV max 4.2.

lymphoma had been since employed [9]. This tumor usually expresses CD2 and CD56 and lacks CD3 (but expresses cytoplasmic CD3ε). It is usually EBV positive [10].

One of the most common presentations is nasal obstruction followed by bloody rhinorrhea. B symptoms, including prolonged fevers and weight loss, can also be present in up to 50% of the cases [3, 11]. Ocular involvement represents mainly uveitis/vitritis; orbital infiltration has been reported in the literature as complication of NNKTL [12].CNS involvement has been reported as being a primary involvement as well as a progression or invasion from an existing primary tumor, which is mainly in the nasopharynx. In both instances, the prognosis is dismal and the overall survival drops from 20 months to 7 months [13]. Treatment of NNKTL depends on the stage of the disease at diagnosis. It usually involves chemotherapy, radiation, and bone marrow transplantation [14]. In this case, the patient had limited-stage disease (IE).This case was presented in the tumor board and ENT oncology sessions. The review of the questionable slight enhancement on the initial staging MRI of the head was deemed not significant and unlikely representing CNS disease. The plan was sequential therapy with chemotherapy (modified SMILE regimen) followed by radiation therapy, the so called "sandwich" approach. The decision was to proceed with regular-dose methotrexate ($2\,g/m^2$). The higher dose of $3\,g/m^2$ has a better CNS penetration [15]. Radiation was supposed to be given at a total dose of 50 Gy to the involved paranasal sinuses via intensity-modulated radiation therapy (IMRT) over 5 to 6 weeks. Compliance to clinical appointments as well as chemotherapy induced adverse events such as prolonged neutropenia and

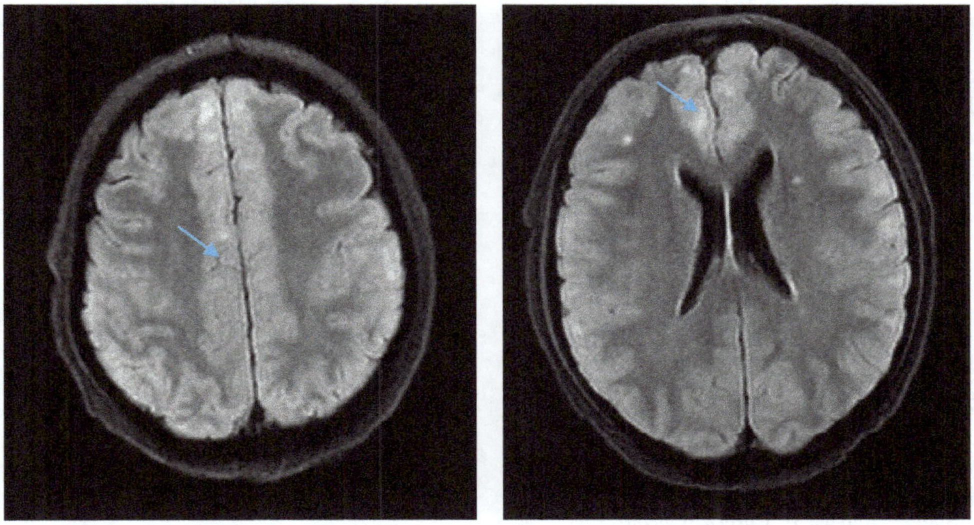

(a) (b)

FIGURE 4: MRI brain with IV contrast showing several scattered bilateral foci of increased T2/FLAIR signal in the bifrontal regions. Also noted, as shown by the blue arrows, was a diffuse swelling of the gyri involving bilateral frontal and anterior parietal lobes.

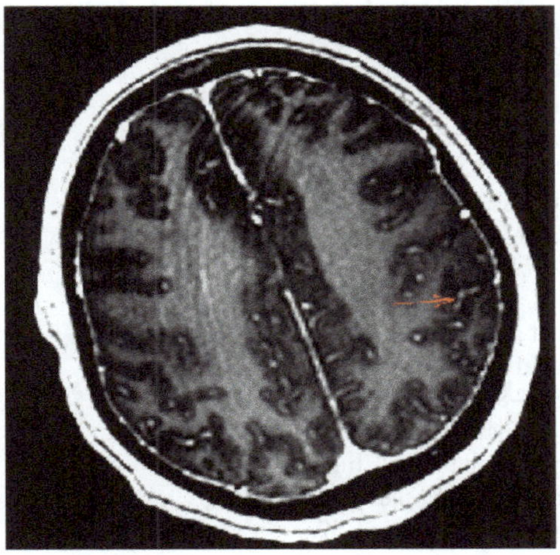

FIGURE 5: MRI brain with IV contrast suggesting sulcal enhancement of the gyrus representing underlying leptomeningeal disease.

fatigue delayed the process. A restaging PET/CT scan performed after the 6th cycle did not show any evidence of disease. The last hospital admission was shortly after the restaging PET scan was performed. It was until the patient was readmitted for headache and confusion that the MRI head was performed and showed evidence of leptomeningeal spread, which was late in the course. To note, that patient had complete right vision loss due to right optic nerve invasion by the tumor and received prophylactic intravitreal methotrexate in the left eye. To date, there is no consensus regarding treating ocular involvement as a CNS involvement with high-dose methotrexate, intrathecal methotrexate, or brain radiation.

4. Conclusions

NNKTL is an aggressive type of lymphoma that can spread to the CNS even when diagnosed at an earlier stage. A high index of suspicion is required when faced with a new onset of neurological symptoms where a more aggressive approach such as intravitreal injection of methotrexate and higher doses of its intravenous administration should be used. Although intensive chemotherapy and radiation therapy have provided good outcomes when it comes to survival, their toxicities remain the major limiting factor in the course of treatment; dose and schedule modifications should be proposed without affecting its benefits.

Additional Points

Sylvester Homsy is the author guarantor.

Authors' Contributions

Homsy S and Kamel R participated in writing and editing the manuscript. Raden M participated in editing the images and critically revising the manuscript. Skaradinskiy Y critically revised the article and approved the final version of the manuscript.

References

[1] Y. Harabuchi, M. Takahara, K. Kishibe, S. Moriai, T. Nagato, and H. Ishii, "Nasal natural killer (NK)/T-cell lymphoma: clinical, histological, virological, and genetic features," *International Journal of Clinical Oncology*, vol. 14, no. 3, pp. 181–190, 2009.

[2] S. V. Adams, P. A. Newcomb, and A. R. Shustov, "Racial patterns of peripheral T-cell lymphoma incidence and survival in the United States," *Journal of Clinical Oncology*, vol. 34, no. 9, pp. 963–971, 2016.

[3] Y. Harabuchi, S. Imai, J. Wakashima et al., "Nasal T-cell lymphoma causally associated with Epstein-Barr virus: clinicopathologic, phenotypic, and genotypic studies," *Cancer: Interdisciplinary International Journal of the American Cancer Society*, vol. 77, no. 10, pp. 2137–2149, 1996.

[4] K. Oshimi, K. Kawa, S. Nakamura et al., "NK-cell neoplasms in Japan," *Hematology*, vol. 10, no. 3, pp. 237–245, 2005.

[5] Y. Harabuchi, N. Yamanaka, A. Kataura, S. Imai, T. Kinoshita, and T. Osato, "Epstein-Barr virus in nasal T-cell lymphomas in patients with lethal midline granuloma," *Lancet*, vol. 335, no. 8682, pp. 128–130, 1990.

[6] H. Ishii, T. Ogino, C. Berger et al., "Clinical usefulness of serum EBV DNA levels of BamHI W and LMP1 for Nasal NK/T-cell lymphoma," *Journal of Medical Virology*, vol. 79, no. 5, pp. 562–572, 2007.

[7] Y. Harabuchi, A. Kataura, K. Kobayashi et al., "Lethal midline granuloma (peripheral T-cell lymphoma) after lymphomatoid papulosis," *Cancer*, vol. 70, no. 4, pp. 835–839, 1992.

[8] H. Nagata, A. Konno, N. Kimura et al., "Characterization of novel natural killer (NK)-cell and gamma delta T-cell lines established from primary lesions of nasal T/NK-cell lymphomas associated with the Epstein-Barr virus," *Blood*, vol. 97, no. 3, pp. 708–713, 2001.

[9] J. P. Greer, M. C. Kinney, and T. P. Loughran, "T cell and NK cell lymphoproliferative disorders," *Hematology (ASH Education Program)*, vol. 2001, no. 1, pp. 259–281, 2001.

[10] E. S. Jaffe, J. K. Chan, I. J. Su et al., "Report of the workshop on nasal and related extranodal angiocentric T/natural killer cell lymphomas. Definitions, differential diagnosis, and epidemiology," *American Journal of Surgical Pathology*, vol. 20, no. 1, pp. 103–111, 1996.

[11] X. Wu, P. Li, J. Zhao et al., "A clinical study of 115 patients with extranodal natural killer/T-cell lymphoma, nasal type," *Clinical Oncology*, vol. 20, no. 8, pp. 619–625, 2008.

[12] C. Hon, A. K. Kwok, T. W. Shek, J. C. Chim, and W. Y. Au, "Vision-threatening complications of nasal T/NK lymphoma," *American Journal of Ophthalmology*, vol. 134, no. 3, pp. 406–410, 2002.

[13] A. Kommalapati, S. H. Tella, A. K. Ganti, and J. O Armitage, "Natural killer/T-cell neoplasms: analysis of incidence, patient characteristics, and survival outcomes in the United States," *Clinical Lymphoma Myeloma and Leukemia*, vol. 18, no. 7, pp. 475–479, 2018.

[14] P. B. Allen and M. Jo Lechowicz., "Management of NK/T-cell lymphoma, nasal type," *Journal of Oncology Practice*, vol. 15, no. 10, pp. 513–520, 2019.

[15] M. Reni, A. J. Ferreri, N. Guha-Thakurta et al., "Clinical relevance of consolidation radiotherapy and other main therapeutic issues in primary central nervous system lymphomas treated with upfront high-dose methotrexate," *International Journal of Radiation Oncology*Biology*Physics*, vol. 51, no. 2, pp. 419–425, 2001.

Permissions

All chapters in this book were first published by Hindawi Publishing Corporation; hereby published with permission under the Creative Commons Attribution License or equivalent. Every chapter published in this book has been scrutinized by our experts. Their significance has been extensively debated. The topics covered herein carry significant findings which will fuel the growth of the discipline. They may even be implemented as practical applications or may be referred to as a beginning point for another development.

The contributors of this book come from diverse backgrounds, making this book a truly international effort. This book will bring forth new frontiers with its revolutionizing research information and detailed analysis of the nascent developments around the world.

We would like to thank all the contributing authors for lending their expertise to make the book truly unique. They have played a crucial role in the development of this book. Without their invaluable contributions this book wouldn't have been possible. They have made vital efforts to compile up to date information on the varied aspects of this subject to make this book a valuable addition to the collection of many professionals and students.

This book was conceptualized with the vision of imparting up-to-date information and advanced data in this field. To ensure the same, a matchless editorial board was set up. Every individual on the board went through rigorous rounds of assessment to prove their worth. After which they invested a large part of their time researching and compiling the most relevant data for our readers.

The editorial board has been involved in producing this book since its inception. They have spent rigorous hours researching and exploring the diverse topics which have resulted in the successful publishing of this book. They have passed on their knowledge of decades through this book. To expedite this challenging task, the publisher supported the team at every step. A small team of assistant editors was also appointed to further simplify the editing procedure and attain best results for the readers.

Apart from the editorial board, the designing team has also invested a significant amount of their time in understanding the subject and creating the most relevant covers. They scrutinized every image to scout for the most suitable representation of the subject and create an appropriate cover for the book.

The publishing team has been an ardent support to the editorial, designing and production team. Their endless efforts to recruit the best for this project, has resulted in the accomplishment of this book. They are a veteran in the field of academics and their pool of knowledge is as vast as their experience in printing. Their expertise and guidance has proved useful at every step. Their uncompromising quality standards have made this book an exceptional effort. Their encouragement from time to time has been an inspiration for everyone.

The publisher and the editorial board hope that this book will prove to be a valuable piece of knowledge for researchers, students, practitioners and scholars across the globe.

List of Contributors

Kartik Anand
Houston Methodist Cancer Center, Weill Cornell Medicine, Houston, TX, USA

Sai Ravi Pingali
Houston Methodist Cancer Center, Weill Cornell Medicine, Houston, TX, USA
Houston Methodist Cancer Center, 6445 Main St Floor 24, Houston, TX 77030, USA

Barry Trachtenberg
Division of Cardiology, DeBakey Heart & Vascular Institute, Houston Methodist Hospital, Houston, TX, USA

Swaminathan Padmanabhan Iyer
Houston Methodist Cancer Center, Weill Cornell Medicine, Houston, TX, USA
Department of Lymphoma/Myeloma, UT MD Anderson Cancer Center, Houston, TX, USA

Bruna Cristine Duarte Rodrigues, Pedro José Galvão Freire, Beatriz Pinto e Siqueira Campos and Pedro Alves da Cruz Gouveia
Internal Medicine Service, Federal University of Pernambuco, Recife, PE, Brazil

Juliana Oliveira Vieira
Hematology Service, Federal University of Pernambuco, Recife, PE, Brazil

Ethan A. Burns and Saro Kasparian
Houston Methodist Hospital, Department of Medicine, 6550 Fannin St, Ste 1101, Houston, TX 77030, USA

Cesar Gentille
Houston Methodist Cancer Center, 6445 Main St Floor 24, Houston, TX 77030, USA

Nii Boi-Doku Pepra-Ameyaw
Department of Haematology, Korle Bu Teaching Hospital, Accra, Ghana

William Kwasi Ghunney
Ghana Institute of Clinical Genetics, Korle Bu, Accra, Ghana

Eugene Baafi Ampofo
National Cardiothoracic Centre, Korle Bu Teaching Hospital, Accra, Ghana

Edeghonghon Olayemi
Department of Haematology, University of Ghana Medical School, Accra, Ghana

Nan Chen, Mike Perez and Martha Mims
Baylor College of Medicine, 1 Baylor Plaza, Houston, TX 77030, USA

Rajesh Essrani
General Internal Medicine, Lehigh Valley Health Network, Allentown, PA, USA

Matthew J. Sullivan and Hiral Shah
Department of Gastroenterology, Lehigh Valley Health Network, Allentown, PA, USA

Michael Youssef and Reid C. Gallant
Faculty of Medicine, University of Toronto, Toronto, Canada

Tyler W. Stratton
Schulich School of Medicine & Dentistry, Western University, London, ON, Canada

Christine Young
Department of Pharmacy, Trillium Health Partners, Mississauga, Ontario, Canada

Daniel Y. Li
Department of Laboratory Medicine and Pathobiology, University of Toronto, Toronto, Canada

Siavash Piran
Department of Medicine, Division of Hematology, University of Toronto, Toronto, Canada

Matthew Lee
UCSF Fresno, Department of Internal Medicine, Fresno, CA, USA

Beth A. Martin
Stanford University, Division of Hematology, Stanford, CA, USA

Haifaa Abdulhaq
University of California San Francisco-Fresno (UCSF Fresno), Fresno, California, USA
UCSF Fresno, Division of Hematology and Oncology, Fresno, CA, USA

Prasun Pudasainee and Bimatshu Pyakuryal
Department of Internal Medicine, Nepal Medical College, Kathmandu, Nepal

Yogesh Subedi
Department of Internal Medicine, Institute of Medicine, Kathmandu, Nepal

Jenisha Upadhyay and Subarna Adhikari
Mountain Medicine Society of Nepal, Kathmandu, Nepal

Teng Fong Ng, Benedict Carnley and Michael F. Leahy
Royal Perth Hospital, Perth, WA, Australia
Path West Laboratory Medicine, Perth, WA, Australia

Celia Green and Dominic Spagnolo
Path West Laboratory Medicine, Perth, WA, Australia

Stephen E. Langabeer, Lisa Lee Tokar, Laura Kearney and Cathal O'Brien
Cancer Molecular Diagnostics, St. James's Hospital, Dublin D08 W9RT, Ireland

Kowshika Thavarajah and John McManus
Department of Medicine for the Elderly, University Hospital Limerick, Limerick V94 F858, Ireland

Aisling Barrett and Hilary O'Leary
Department of Haematology, University Hospital Limerick, Limerick V94 F858, Ireland

Ronak H. Mistry
Department of Internal Medicine, Pennsylvania Hospital of the University of Pennsylvania, 800 Spruce Street, Philadelphia, PA 19107, USA

Elizabeth O. Hexner and James K. Mangan
Abramson Cancer Center, Perelman Center for Advanced Medicine, University of Pennsylvania, 34th Street and Civic Center Boulevard, 12th Floor South Pavilion, Philadelphia, PA 19104, USA

David Alejandro Vargas Gutiérrez and Priscila Joseline Pérez Vinueza
Department of Rheumatology, Instituto Nacional de Rehabilitación Luis Guillermo Ibarra Ibarra, CDMX, Mexico

Karina Ivonne Arias Callejas
Department of Rheumatology, Instituto Nacional de Cardiología Ignacio Chávez, CDMX, Mexico

Edwin Pavel Palacios Ruiz and Ingrid Salinas Zaldívar
Department of Internal Medicine, Hospital General de México: "Dr. Eduardo Liceaga", CDMX, Mexico

Juan Diego Muñoz Vega
Department of Hematology, Hospital General Mexico: "Dr. Eduardo Liceaga", CDMX, Mexico

Ana Karen G. Mejía Geraldo
Department of Pathological Anatomy, Hospital General Mexico: "Dr. Eduardo Liceaga", CDMX, Mexico

Heather Klocke and Craig O'Brien
Veterans Affairs Puget Sound Health Care System, Seattle, WA, USA

Zhao Ming Dong
Veterans Affairs Puget Sound Health Care System, Seattle, WA, USA
Department of Pathology, University of Washington Medicine, Seattle, WA, USA

Nicholas Burwick and Robert E. Richard
Veterans Affairs Puget Sound Health Care System, Seattle, WA, USA
Division of Hematology, University of Washington Medicine, Seattle, WA, USA

Daniel Y. Wu, Thomas R. Chauncey and Solomon A. Graf
Veterans Affairs Puget Sound Health Care System, Seattle, WA, USA
Division of Medical Oncology, University of Washington Medicine, Seattle, WA, USA
Clinical Research Division, Fred Hutch Cancer Research Center, Seattle, WA, USA

Habib Moshref Razavi
Division of Hematopathology, Department of Pathology and Laboratory Medicine, University of British Columbia, Vancouver, British Columbia, Canada
Fraser Health Authority, Royal Columbian Hospital, Department of Laboratory Medicine, New Westminster, British Columbia, Canada

Reza Alaghehbandan
Fraser Health Authority, Royal Columbian Hospital, Department of Laboratory Medicine, New Westminster, British Columbia, Canada
Division of Anatomical Pathology, Department of Pathology and Laboratory Medicine, University of British Columbia, Vancouver, British Columbia, Canada

Mounir Ababou, Hicham El Maaroufi, Adnane Hammani, Selim Jennane, El Mehdi Mahtat and Kamal Doghmi
Department of Clinical Hematology, Military Hospital Mohammed V, Mohammed V University, Rabat, Morocco

Mohammed Mikdame
Faculty of Medicine and Pharmacy of Rabat, Mohammed V University, Rabat, Morocco

Steve Biko Otieno
The University of Tennessee Health Science Center, Department of Hematology/Oncology, 19 S. Manassas, Memphis, TN 38103, USA
The Veterans Affairs Medical Center, 1030 Jefferson Ave, Memphis, TN 38104, USA
The West Cancer and Research Institute, 7945 Wolf River Blvd, Germantown, TN 38138, USA

Alva Weir
The University of Tennessee Health Science Center, Department of Hematology/Oncology, 19 S. Manassas, Memphis, TN 38103, USA
The Veterans Affairs Medical Center, 1030 Jefferson Ave, Memphis, TN 38104, USA

Syed Nasir and Robert Johnson
The University of Tennessee Health Science Center, Department of Hematology/Oncology, 19 S. Manassas, Memphis, TN 38103, USA
The West Cancer and Research Institute, 7945 Wolf River Blvd, Germantown, TN 38138, USA

Jinichi Mori
Department of Hematology, Jyoban Hospital, Tokiwa Foundation, Fukushima, Japan

Kumi Oshima
Department of Hematology, Jyoban Hospital, Tokiwa Foundation, Fukushima, Japan
Patient Safety Division, QI Center, St. Luke's International Hospital, Tokyo, Japan

Satoshi Kimura and Takayuki Ikezoe
Department of Hematology, Fukushima Medical University, Fukushima, Japan

Salimah Valliani, Mir Ali, Omar Mahmoo and Sanjay Hinduja
University of California San Francisco-Fresno (UCSF Fresno), Fresno, California, USA

Calvin K. Chen
Community Regional Medical Center (CRMC), Fresno, California, USA

Lloyd Damon
University of California San Francisco (UCSF), San Francisco, California, USA

S. A. Touré, M. Seck, A B. Diallo, E. H. D. Niang, M. Keita, M. F. Dabo, B. F. Faye and S. Diop
Hematology Department, Cheikh Anta Diop University, Dakar, Senegal

Meilen Chang Muñoz
Department of Internal Medicine, University of California Davis, School of Medicine, Sacramento, CA, USA

Jennifer A. Murphy
Department of Pharmacy Services, University of California Davis Medical Center, Sacramento, CA, USA
University of California Davis Comprehensive Cancer Center, Sacramento, CA, USA

Johannes E. Wolff
AbbVie Inc., North Chicago, IL, USA

Brian A. Jonas
Department of Internal Medicine, University of California Davis, School of Medicine, Sacramento, CA, USA
University of California Davis Comprehensive Cancer Center, Sacramento, CA, USA

Stephanie Wolanin, Mark J. Pettenati, Michael W. Beaty, Giovanni Insuasti-Beltran and Stacey S. O'Neill
Wake Forest Baptist Medical Center, Department of Pathology, Winston-Salem, NC, USA

Robert K. McCall
Molecular Pathology Laboratory Network, Maryville, TN, USA

Bayard L. Powell
Wake Forest Baptist Comprehensive Cancer Center, Section on Hematology and Oncology, Winston-Salem, NC, USA

Feryal Ibrahim
Department of Laboratory Medicine and Pathology, National Center for Cancer Care and Research, Hamad Medical Corporation, Doha, Qatar

Dina Soliman
Department of Laboratory Medicine and Pathology, National Center for Cancer Care and Research, Hamad Medical Corporation, Doha, Qatar
Weill Cornell Medicine, Doha, Qatar
Department of Clinical Pathology, National Cancer Institute, Cairo University, Cairo, Egypt

Sherin Sallam
Weill Cornell Medicine, Doha, Qatar

Deena Mudawi
Department of Hematology and Medical Oncology, National Center for Cancer Care and Research, Hamad Medical Corporation, Doha, Qatar

Susanna Akiki
Department of Laboratory Medicine and Pathology, National Center for Cancer Care and Research, Hamad Medical Corporation, Doha, Qatar
Weill Cornell Medicine, Doha, Qatar

Parikshit Padhi
Memorial Medical Cancer Center, 2530 S Telshor Blvd, Las Cruces, NM 88011, USA

Radwa El-Behery
Integrated Oncology, 5005 S 40th St, Phoenix, AZ 85040, USA

Constantine N. Logothetis
Department of Internal Medicine, University of South Florida Morsani College of Medicine, 17 Davis Blvd, Suite 308, Tampa,FL 33606, USA

Charles Pizanis
Division of Hospital Medicine Department of Internal Medicine, University of New Mexico School of Medicine, University of New Mexico, MSC10 5550, Albuquerque, NM 87131, USA

Brenda Mai, Michaelangelo Friscia, Pamela Younes, Jaiyeola Thomas-Ogunniyi and Lei Chen
Department of Pathology and Laboratory Medicine, McGovern Medical School at the University of Texas Health Science Center,6431 Fannin Street, Houston, TX, USA

Jiankun Tong and Jean Luo
Department of Pathology, New York Presbyterian Queens, 56-45 Main Street, Flushing, NY 11355, USA

Pierre F. Saldinger
Department of Surgery, New York Presbyterian Queens, 56-45 Main Street, Flushing, NY 11355, USA
Weill Cornell Medical College, 525 East 68th Street, New York, NY 10065, USA

William H. Rodgers
Department of Pathology, New York Presbyterian Queens, 56-45 Main Street, Flushing, NY 11355, USA
Weill Cornell Medical College, 525 East 68th Street, New York, NY 10065, USA

Jorge Labrador, Gerardo J. Hermida, Rodolfo Alvarez, Victor Anso, Pilar de Vicente, Mercedes Goñi and Tomas Jose Gonzalez-Lopez
Department of Hematology, University Hospital of Burgos, Burgos, Spain

Cláudia L. Pedrosa, Patrícia Seabra, Luísa Regadas, Cláudia Casais and Jorge Coutinho
Department of Clinical Hematology, Centro Hospitalar Universitário Do Porto, Porto, Portugal

Patrícia Rosinha and Cláudia Rosado
Department of Internal Medicine, Centro Hospitalar Do Baixo Vouga, Aveiro, Portugal

Gisela Ferreira
Department of Clinical Hematology, Centro Hospitalar Do Baixo Vouga, Aveiro, Portugal

Norisato Hashimoto, Tomoki Ueda and Kenji Yokoyama
Department of Hematology/Oncology, Tokai University Hachioji Hospital, 1838 Ishikawa-machi, Hachioji 1920032, Japan

Shinichiro Hiraiwa and Takuma Tajiri
Department of Pathology, Tokai University Hachioji Hospital, 1838 Ishikawa-machi, Hachioji 1920032, Japan

Naoya Nakamura
Department of Pathology, Tokai University, School of Medicine, 143 Shimokasuya, Isehara 2591193, Japan
Department of Pathology, Tokai University, Tokyo, Japan

Ranathunga
Professorial Medical Unit, Colombo South Teaching Hospital, Colombo, Sri Lanka

N. R. Muthumala and H. W. C. K. Kulathilake
Department of Haematology, Faculty of Medicine, University of Sri Jayewardenepura, Colombo, Sri Lanka

S. Weerasinghe
Cancer Institute, Maharagama, Colombo, Sri Lanka

N. L. A. Shyamali
Department of Medicine, Faculty of Medicine, University of Sri Jayewardenepura, Colombo, Sri Lanka

Marcus A. Healey
Edward Via College of Osteopathic Medicine, Blacksburg, VA, USA

Daniel J. Allendorf
Alabama Oncology, Alabaster, AL, USA

Uma Borate
School of Medicine, Oregon Health & Science University, Portland, OR, USA

Ankit Madan
SOVAH Cancer Center, Danville, VA, USA

L. Ballotta, S. M. Trisolini, A. P. Iori, U. La Rocca, A. Micozzi, G. Gentile, A. Guarini, R. Foà and S. Capria
Hematology, Department of Translational and Precision Medicine, Sapienza University of Rome, Rome, Italy

T. De Giacomo
Department of Cardiovascular and Thoracic Surgery "Paride Stefanini", Sapienza University, Policlinico Umberto I, Rome, Italy

Rūta Čepulytė and Andrius Žučenka
Vilnius University Hospital Santaros Klinikos, Center of Hematology, Oncology and Transfusion Medicine, Santariškių 2, Vilnius 08661, Lithuania

Valdas Pečeliūnas
Vilnius University Hospital Santaros Klinikos, Center of Hematology, Oncology and Transfusion Medicine, Santariškių 2, Vilnius 08661, Lithuania
Vilnius University Faculty of Medicine, Institute of Clinical Medicine, Clinic of Internal Diseases, Family Medicine and Oncology, Santariškių 2, Vilnius 08661, Lithuania

Stephanie L. Pritzl, Daniel R. Matson, Mark B. Juckett and David J. Ciske
University of Wisconsin School of Medicine and Public Health, Madison, Wisconsin, USA

Yukiko Komeno and Tomiko Ryu
Department of Hematology, Japan Community Healthcare Organization (JCHO) Tokyo Yamate Medical Center, Hyakunin-cho, Shinjuku, Tokyo 169-0073, Japan

Minako Akiyama
Department of Nephrology, JCHO Tokyo Yamate Medical Center, Hyakunin-cho, Shinjuku, Tokyo 169-0073, Japan

Yasumi Okochi and Hitoshi Tokuda
Department of Respiratory Medicine, JCHO Tokyo Yamate Medical Center, Hyakunin-cho, Shinjuku, Tokyo 169-0073, Japan

Keiko Abe and Kuniko Iihara
Department of Pathology, JCHO Tokyo Yamate Medical Center, Hyakunin-cho, Shinjuku, Tokyo 169-0073, Japan

Clara Bertuzzi, Elena Sabattini, Francesco Bacci and Claudio Agostinelli
Hematopathology Unit, Sant'Orsola University Hospital, Bologna, Italy

Gian Gaetano Ferri
ENT and Audiology Unit, Department of Experimental, Diagnostic and Specialty Medicine, Sant' Orsola Hospital, University of Bologna, Bologna, Italy

Waqas Jehangir and Elvira Umyarova
University of Vermont Medical Center, Hematology and Medical Oncology, 89 Beaumont Ave., Burlington,VT 05405-0068, USA

Alexander Karabachev
University of Vermont College of Medicine, Larner College of Medicine. 89 Beaumont Ave., Burlington, VT 05405-0068, USA

Taimoor Jahangir
University Hospitals of Leicester NHS Trust, Groby Rd., Leicester LE3 9QP, UK

Guillaume Beziat, Suzanne Tavitian, Christian Recher and Françoise Huguet
Service d'Hématologie Clinique, Institut Universitaire du Cancer Oncopole, Toulouse, France

Muriel Picard
Réanimation et Soins Intensifs, Institut Universitaire du Cancer Oncopole, Toulouse, France

Stanislas Faguer
Secteur de Réanimation de l'Unité de Transplantation d'Organes, CHU Rangueil, Toulouse, France

Eleni Thodou
Department of Pathology, Medical School, University of essaly, Viopolis, 41500 Larisa, Greece

Maria Befani
Hematology, Private Practice, 61 Koumoundourou Str., 38221 Volos, Greece

George Triantafyllidis
Radiology, Private Practice, 29 Glavani Str., 38221 Volos, Greece

Theodosia Choreftaki
Department of Pathology, "G. Genimmatas", Athens General Hospital, 154 Mesogeion Ave., 11527 Athens, Greece

George Kanellis
Department of Hematopathology, "Evangelismos", General Hospital, 45 Ypsilantou Str., 10676 Athens, Greece

Nikolaos Giannakoulas
Department of Hematology, Medical School, University of Thessly, Viopolis, 41500 Larisa, Greece

Rehman Faryal and Sorcha Ní Loingsigh
Department of Haematology, University Hospital Galway, Galway H91 YR71, Ireland

Michael O'Dwyer
Department of Haematology, University Hospital Galway, Galway H91 YR71, Ireland
National University of Ireland, Galway H91 TK33, Ireland

Sylvain Raoul Simeni Njonnou
Department of Internal Medicine and Specialties, Faculty of Medicine and Biomedical Sciences, University of Yaounde I, Yaoundé, Cameroon
Department of Internal Medicine, Hôpital Erasme, Université Libre de Bruxelles, Brussels, Belgium
Department of Endocrinology, Hôpital Erasme, Université Libre de Bruxelles, Brussels, Belgium

Bruno Couturier, Yannick Gombeir and Sylvain Verbanck
Department of Internal Medicine, Hôpital Erasme, Université Libre de Bruxelles, Brussels, Belgium
Department of Endocrinology, Hôpital Erasme, Université Libre de Bruxelles, Brussels, Belgium

France Devuyst
Department of Endocrinology, Hôpital Erasme, Université Libre de Bruxelles, Brussels, Belgium

Anne-Laure Trepant
Department of Pathology, Hôpital Erasme, Université Libre de Bruxelles, Brussels, Belgium

Virginie De Wilde
Department of Hematology, H^oôpital Erasme, Université Libre de Bruxelles, Brussels, Belgium

Ivan Theate
Institute of Pathology and Genetics, Gosselies, Charleroi, Belgium

Georges El Hachem and Frédéric-Alain Vandergheynst
Department of Internal Medicine, Hôpital Erasme, Université Libre de Bruxelles, Brussels, Belgium

Eko A. Pangarsa, Vina Yunarvika, Budi Setiawan, Damai Santosa and Catharina Suharti
Subdivion of Hematology and Medical Oncology, Medical Faculty of Diponegoro University, Dr. Kariadi General Hospital,Semarang, Indonesia

Ridho M. Naibaho
Trainee in Hematology and Medical Oncology, Medical Faculty of Diponegoro University, Dr. Kariadi General Hospital,Semarang, Indonesia
Department of Internal Medicine, Parikesit Hospital, Mulawarman School of Medicine, Samarinda, East Kalimantan, Indonesia

Federico Meconi, Roberto Secchi, Raffaele Palmieri, Sara Vaccarini, Vito Mario Rapisarda, Laura Giannì, Fabiana Esposito, Ida Provenzano, Daniela Nasso, Livio Pupo and Maria Cantonetti
Department of Biomedicine and Prevention, Haematology Division, University of Tor Vergata, Viale Oxford 81, Rome, Italy

Thomas Luo, Joanna Zurko and Nirav N. Shah
BMT & Cellular Therapy Program, Division of Hematology & Oncology, Medical College of Wisconsin, Milwaukee, WI, USA

John Astle
Department of Pathology, Medical College of Wisconsin, Milwaukee, WI, USA

Hidekazu Nishikii, Naoki Kurita, Tatsuhiro Sakamoto, Manabu Kusakabe, Yasuhisa Yokoyama, Takayasu Kato, Mamiko Sakata-Yanagimoto, Naoshi Obara, Yuichi Hasegawa and Shigeru Chiba
Department of Hematology, Faculty of Medicine, University of Tsukuba, Tsukuba, Japan

Atsushi Shinagawa
Department of Hemato-Oncology, Hitachi General Hospital, Hitachi, Japan

Ingolf Molle, Irma Petruskevicius, Peter Kamper and Francesco d'Amore
Department of Haematology, University Hospital of Aarhus, Aarhus, Denmark

Nouran Momen
Clinical & Chemical Pathology Department, Cairo University, Giza, Egypt

Bora Baysal, Sheila Jani Sait, Joseph Tario and You-Wen Qian
Department of Pathology, Roswell Park Cancer Institute, 665 Elm Street, Bu alo, NY 14203, USA

Tsukasa Yasuda and Tomoyuki Tsuzuki
Department of Gastroenterology, Toyota Kosei Hospital, Toyota, Japan

Junji Hiraga
Department of Hematology, Toyota Kosei Hospital, Toyota, Japan

Michihiko Narita
Department of Pathology, Toyota Kosei Hospital, Toyota, Japan

Yoshimasa Tanikawa
Department of Respiratory Medicine, Toyota Kosei Hospital, Toyota, Japan

Sylvester Homsy and Ralph Kamel
Department of Internal Medicine, Staten Island University Hospital-Northwell Health, Staten Island, New York, NY, USA

Mark Raden
Department of Radiology, Staten Island University Hospital-Northwell Health, Staten Island, New York, NY, USA

Yevgeniy Skaradinskiy
Division of Hematology/Oncology, Staten Island University Hospital-Northwell Health, Staten Island, New York, NY, USA

Index

M

N

P

R

S

T

V